Intelligent User Interfaces: Adaptation and Personalization Systems and Technologies

Constantinos Mourlas
National & Kapodistrian University of Athens, Greece

Panagiotis Germanakos
National & Kapodistrian University of Athens, Greece

Information Science REFERENCE

INFORMATION SCIENCE REFERENCE

Hershey · New York

Director of Editorial Content:	Kristin Klinger
Managing Development Editor:	Kristin M. Roth
Assistant Development Editor:	Deborah Yahnke
Editorial Assistant:	Rebecca Beistline
Senior Managing Editor:	Jennifer Neidig
Managing Editor:	Jamie Snavely
Assistant Managing Editor:	Carole Coulson
Typesetter:	Michael Brehm
Cover Design:	Lisa Tosheff
Printed at:	Yurchak Printing Inc.

Published in the United States of America by
Information Science Reference (an imprint of IGI Global)
701 E. Chocolate Avenue, Suite 200
Hershey PA 17033
Tel: 717-533-8845
Fax: 717-533-8661
E-mail: cust@igi-global.com
Web site: http://www.igi-global.com

and in the United Kingdom by
Information Science Reference (an imprint of IGI Global)
3 Henrietta Street
Covent Garden
London WC2E 8LU
Tel: 44 20 7240 0856
Fax: 44 20 7379 0609
Web site: http://www.eurospanbookstore.com

Library of Congress Cataloging-in-Publication Data

Intelligent user interfaces : adaptation and personalization systems and technologies / Constantinos Mourlas and Panagiotis Germanakos, editors.
p. cm.
Includes bibliographical references and index.
Summary: "This book identifies solutions and suggestions for the design and development of adaptive applications and systems that provides more usable and qualitative content and services adjusted to the needs and requirements of the various users"--Provided by publisher.
ISBN 978-1-60566-032-5 (hardcover) -- ISBN 978-1-60566-033-2 (ebook)
1. Human-computer interaction. 2. Artificial intelligence. 3. Adaptive computing systems. I. Mourlas, Constantinos. II. Germanakos, Panagiotis.
QA76.9.H85I5833 2008
004.01'9--dc22

2008010314

British Cataloguing in Publication Data
A Cataloguing in Publication record for this book is available from the British Library.

Editorial Advisory Board

Table of Contents

Section II
Adaptive Content and Services

Section III
Adaptive Processing and Communication

Section V
Security, Privacy, and Personalization

Detailed Table of Contents

User profiles serves as the main component of most Web personalization systems. With the use of various techniques that are based on given user preferences, navigation behaviour and the Web-based content returns the requested personalized result. Main scope of this chapter is to present the various techniques employed by such systems with regards to user profiles extraction and introduce a comprehensive user profile, which includes User Perceptual Preference Characteristics. It further analyzes the main intrinsic users' characteristics like visual, cognitive, and emotional processing parameters incorporated as well as the "traditional" user profile characteristics that together tend to give the most optimized, adapted and personalized outcome. It finally presents a Web adaptation and personalization system that implements the proposed comprehensive user profile as well as evaluation results that further support their importance and impact in the information space.

Navigation, search, and recommendation each have their own set of challenges when it comes to facilitating fast and efficient information access. This chapter considers a number of these challenges and describes how they can be addressed by using techniques that allow information services to respond more intelligently to the needs and preferences of individuals and groups of users. Each challenge is being addressed in the form of a case study focusing on one particular mode of information access (navigation, search, and recommendation) and an application scenario (mobile portals, Web search, and e-commerce), to describe how user profiling, personalization, and adaptive interface design can be combined to produce a more efficient and effective information service.

Web-based instruction is prevalent in educational settings, with many issues that still need to be investigated. One of them is the significance of human factors, and how they influence learners' performance and perception in Web-based instruction. In this vein, the study presented in this chapter investigates this issue in a Web-based instructional program, which was applied to teach students how to use HyperText Markup Language (HTML) in a United Kingdom (UK) university.

Innovative personalization services are required to extend the traditional user profiling techniques with semantic-based information. Using semantic-based information provides additional clues as to the reasons the user may or may not be interested in certain objects. The primary goal of this chapter is to present a comprehensive overview of the state-of-the art techniques and methodologies which integrate personalization technologies with semantic knowledge, exploring the challenges that such research areas pose to today's information society.

The diversity of service access contexts, which is inevitable in the era of pervasive, "anywhere" computing, and the co-existence of different technologies caused by the evolutionary character of the transition to next generation systems, will lead to the heterogeneity of the networks and systems that support end-user application provision. The current mobile communications paradigm was not built to support this evolution, and therefore this chapter supports that intelligent mechanisms should exist for identifying the context and the particular high-level requirements of an application and mapping them to appropriate reconfiguration operations on the underlying hardware and software infrastructure. To this end, context management, knowledge building and the respective decision making process are key factors for the service personalisation and system adaptation in future mobile communications. A need for middleware platforms, that will abstract this management load and complexity and enable an end-user seamless service experience, emerges.

Information users are different in nature—they manifest heterogeneous information seeking behaviours, needs and expectations. Yet, most information retrieval services purport a one size fits all model whereby the same information is disseminated to a wide range of information users despite the individualistic nature of each user's needs, goals, interests, preferences, intellectual levels and information consumption capacity. This leads to a sub-optimal model because information users,who are intrinsically distinct, are not only compelled to experience a generic outcome but are further required to manually adjust and adapt the recommended information artifacts according to their immediate needs or preferences in order to achieve the desired results. Therefore, this chapter argues that there is both a case and the need to design information services that take into account the individuality of information users, and in turn aim to personalize the information seeking experiences and outcomes for users.

Citizens possess, amongst others, different access possibilities, skills, expectations and motivation, during their navigation to an e-government portal while searching for a public e-service or during the actual service provision. This variety in citizens' skills, expectations and in problems they face has as consequence that each citizen has different perceptions concerning the quality of public e-services. It is apparent, therefore, that a "one fits all" e-government services' assessment is not efficient, since their evaluation should be organized in a way to serve every citizen individually. This chapter supports that for the realization of such a customized and adaptive evaluation of e-government services, an intelligent, semantic-based platform is needed which allows each citizen to put emphasis in quality dimensions related with the problems he/she faces, depending on his/her skills and expectations. It further presents a semantically adaptive interface for measuring portal quality in e-Government.

The solution to the WWW cognitive overload, and more specifically to e-Government services, it seems that is the issue of personalization. On these grounds, this chapter introduces the design and implementation of Web information systems supporting personalized access to multi-version resources in an e-Government scenario. Personalization is supported by means of Semantic Web techniques and relies on an ontology-based profiling of users. Resources that considers are collections of norm documents in XML format but can also be generic Web pages and portals or e-Government transactional services. It further introduces a reference infrastructure, describes the organization and presents performance figures of a prototype system the authors have been developed.

The presented work introduces new techniques for supporting the adaptation and personalization issues in the design and development of Intelligent User Interfaces, mainly by adapting services to user preferences and device characteristics of the user. The user characteristics, the data collection particularities and the system capabilities are matched with the visualization method properties in a context-based adaptive visualization environment to be used in the Historical Archive of the University of Athens, in order to support information seeking tasks.

The integration of semantic knowledge is the primary challenge for the next generation of personalization systems and the automatic collection of data. This chapter provides an overview of approaches for incorporating semantic knowledge into Web usage mining and the personalization processes. It discusses

Limitation of the human memory is a well-known issue that anybody has experienced. Some of these can be addressed by exploiting one of the strengths of computers: the ability to store huge amounts of information for an unlimited time without loss of precision. And actually, state-of-the-art mobile devices in general provide features for creating reminders, linking notes to time and dates, and for managing time. However, these techniques require the user to capture this data manually, and thus the quality of such memories greatly depends on her cognition and carefulness. Thus, this chapter provides a discussion of various challenges related to building and exploiting such augmented personal memories in everyday's life. It concentrates on a number of crucial aspects: the importance of abstraction processes for building this memory and the design of a user interface for supporting interaction between user and memory. It further illustrates authors' approach with examples of processing and exploiting information about the user's location in the shopping assistant SPECTER.

Learner models, understood as digital representations of learners, have been at the core of intelligent tutoring systems from their original inception. Learner models facilitate the knowledge about the learner necessary for achieving any personalisation through adaptation, while most intelligent tutoring systems have been designed to support the learning modelling process. Learner modelling is a necessary process to achieve the adaptability, personalisation and efficacy of intelligent tutoring systems. This chapter provides an analysis of the migration of open learner modelling technology to common e-learning settings, the implications for modern e-learning systems in terms of adaptations to support the open learner modelling process, and the expected functionality of a new generation of intelligent learning environments. This analysis is grounded on the authors' recent experience on an e-learning environment called LeActiveMath, aimed at developing a web-based learning environment for Mathematics in the state of the art.

sirable principles in the context of privacy protection, it discusses privacy concerns and how different privacy principles address them, and further describes the techniques that have been used in the main types of privacy-enhancing personalization solutions, and how they relate to the major privacy concerns and privacy principles, with the necessary analysis findings.

Foreword

Access to online information is now a pervasive part of many of our lives, whether at work or at play. Indeed, the Internet has become such an important influence that it hardly seems possible to remember a time before the World-Wide Web, even though the first browsers only arrived on the scene less than 15 years ago. Today, billions of users access the Internet on a daily basis, with the leading search engines handling tens of billions of queries per month, and the volume of online information continues to grow at near exponential rates.

Unfortunately, for many, finding the right information quickly and easily continues to be a challenge and the *one-size-fits-all* nature of most information services does little to acknowledge the distinctive information needs that we all invariably have. In this context the idea that information services can adapt to the needs and preferences of individuals, or groups of users, has attracted considerable attention and so-called *personalized* user interfaces represent an important step forward in the development of online services that are capable of proactively responding to the needs of the individual.

The prospect of personalized information services and interfaces, which can intelligently adapt to our changing circumstances and contexts, has the potential to dramatically change the way that we interact with a wide range of online services. Already, a number of organizations have made great strides when it comes to offering their customers more personalized online experiences. For example, Amazon's now famous recommendation engine drives significant additional sales by promoting products that are relevant to individual customers, given their past purchases. Set-top-boxes such as Tivo have changed the way that people watch television, by recommending and proactively recording TV shows based on their learned viewing preferences. And, more recently, mobile telephone operators such as Vodafone and O_2 provide their subscribers with access to mobile portals that automatically adapt their structure, so that relevant content and services are promoted to individual subscribers, based on their access patterns. These are just a few of the examples of large-scale personalization deployments within the different consumer markets. In each case the benefits of personalized and adaptive information services have been enjoyed by consumers (through more efficient access to relevant information) and operating companies, through increased sales or growth in user activity.

What is especially exciting about this book is that it brings together, in a single volume, a diverse collection of research on a variety of topics that drives developments in the area of personalized and intelligent user interfaces. These chapters have been written by leading researchers and cover a wide range of applications areas, from e-government to e-commerce, as well as providing a comprehensive account of the component technologies that underpin intelligent user interface technology. Indeed the reader will also benefit from an understanding of the various human factors associated with adaptivity and personalization, from user perceptions of adaptive systems to the privacy and security issues that are associated with user profiling and personalization.

This book is accessible to a wide range of individuals and should be read by academics, students, and professionals with an interest in the design and development of intelligent user interfaces and the applications of personalization technology. For the reader it provides a comprehensive account of the core challenges facing the development of the next generation of personalized and adaptive information services. And whether researcher or practitioner, the reader will come away with an appreciation and understanding of the major strands of work that make up this exciting area of research.

Barry Smyth
University College Dublin
Ireland

Preface

The explosive growth in size and use of the World Wide Web as a communication medium has been enthusiastically adopted by the mass market. The new developments in ICT along with the growth of mobile and wireless communication allowed service providers to meet these challenges developing new ways of interactions through a variety of channels enabling users to become accustomed to new means of service consumption in an "anytime, anywhere and anyhow" manner. However, the nature of most information structures is static and complicated, and users often lose sight of the goal of their inquiry, look for stimulating rather than informative material, or even use the navigational features unwisely. Hence, a number of researchers and practitioners studied adaptivity and personalization to address the comprehension and orientation difficulties presented in such systems; to alleviate navigational difficulties and satisfy the heterogeneous needs of the users, allowing at the same time Web applications of this nature to survive.

During the last years there has been huge effort from researchers to identify the peculiarities of each user group, analyze and design methodologies and systems that could alter the given raw content, and deliver them up-to-date personalized information as such, or with regards to products or services. Nonetheless, to date, there has not been a concrete definition of personalization. So far, the many adaptive hypermedia and Web personalization solutions offering personalisation features seem to meet an abstract common goal: to provide users with what they want or need without expecting from them to ask for it explicitly. There is a necessity therefore for further consideration and analysis of parameters and contexts such as users' intellectuality, mental capabilities, socio-psychological factors, emotional states and attention grabbing strategies to be extensively investigated. All these characteristics could affect the apt collection of users' customization requirements and along with the 'traditional' user characteristics (i.e. name, age, education, experience, interests, etc.), to constitute a comprehensive user profile that serves as the ground element of most of these systems offering in return the best adaptive environments to their preferences and demands.

Besides the content and services, which figure as the main personalization substance, also processes and communication need to become adaptive. New systems need to adapt their execution at run time according to new system requirements and requests that arrive from a dynamic and complex runtime environment where other processes coexist and share the same resources. The network resources and protocols should adapt their transmission according to the communication needs and characteristics of the connection of the individual user. The mobility of the user, the variation of bandwidth during communication, the loose connections and the network congestion are some of the main factors that network adaptation should be taken into account.

CHALLENGES

The field of adaptive systems and networks has received great attention from the research community in the last years with the explosion of new applications and services which have to be executed in a dynamic and continuous changing environment. It further covers a wide spectrum of applications with similar behaviour and properties where the term adaptivity is met in three different variations:

Adaptivity of content and services; in this category the content and services have to be adapted according to user preferences and system constraints. Adaptive hypermedia, Web personalization and Intelligent User Interfaces are some of the main representatives of this category where content, navigation and appearance / aesthetics have adapt according to (i) the user profile and (ii) the device characteristics of the user (e.g. monitor resolution, bandwidth allocation, etc.) also referred as QoS constraints. Adaptive and personalized services share in this case the same basic goal; that is to provide users with the desirable or necessary content without requiring from them to ask for it explicitly. Thus, adaptivity of content and services is the provision to the individual of tailored products, Web-based content, multimedia-based services, information or information relating to products or services. The issue of adaptivity of content and services is a complex one with many aspects that need to be examined. Such issues include, amongst others: (i) what content to present to the user, (ii) how to show the content to the user, (iii) how to ensure the user's privacy, (iv) how to create a global personalization scheme, etc.

At the higher level, adaptivity of content and services is realized in one of two ways: (i) Services or Web sites that require users to register and provide explicitly information about their interests and needs, and (ii) Services or Web sites that automatically extract the user profile by tracking the behavioural navigation pattern of the users. At the lower level, adaptivity of systems and processing is required for the implementation of such applications and services.

Adaptivity of systems and processing; the current interest on systems and processing is focused on the ability of these systems to adapt their execution at run time according to changing system requirements and requests that arrive from the dynamic and complex runtime environment where other objects or processes are running concurrently and share the same computational as well as other resources. The emphasis here is not to the adaptive content but to the adaptive execution of the processes. The traditional systems although they perform well in static information spaces they appear inadequate for new and evolving environments like multimedia servers, streaming media presentations, ubiquitous computing, soft real-time systems, agent computing and Grid computing. Recent research has given interesting results in the above areas where new operating systems and programming environments have been implemented supporting high levels of adaptivity without sacrificing the predictability and the correctness of the system during execution.

Adaptivity of networks and communication; current interest in network technology is focused on the development of new distributed applications like distributed multi-media information systems, media streaming, desktop conferencing and video-on-demand services. Each such application needs adaptive behaviour and Quality of Service (QoS) guarantees, otherwise users may not accept them since these applications are expected to be judged against the quality of traditional services (e.g. radio, television, telephone services). Some of these issues become even more complicated once viewed from a mobile user's perspective, when wireless communication media and mobile device constraints are involved and the demand for adaptive communication "anytime, anywhere and anyhow" is presupposed. The emphasis here is on the communication and transportation of information along with the ability of the network resources and protocols to adapt their transmission according to the communication needs and the characteristics of the connection of the individual user and the others. The mobility of the user, the variation of bandwidth during communication, loose connections and the network congestion are some of the main factors that adaptation should take into account.

Henceforth, the main focus of this book is to concentrate on the various aspects of adaptivity in one place. The book provides a very broad view of adaptive systems and networks with main focus on adaptivity. It attempts to present all the research results produced in the area of adaptive systems and networks covering a wide spectrum of applications, systems and networks starting from the higher level applications and personalization issues and then presenting the lower level issues of adaptive operating systems and processing and the adaptivity of networks and communication.

ORGANIZATION OF THE BOOK

This book is composed of five sections, with a total of seventeen chapters, each of which is described briefly below:

Section I: Theoretical Aspects of Adaptive and Personalized User Interfaces

Chapter I realizes the importance of the various techniques implemented by most Web personalization systems nowadays to extract the user profiles. User profiles serve as the main component of such systems. With the use of various techniques that are based on given user preferences, the navigation behaviour and the Web-based content they return the requested personalized result. Main scope of this chapter is to present the various techniques employed by such systems with regards to user profiles extraction and introduce a comprehensive user profile, which includes User Perceptual Preference Characteristics. It further analyzes the main intrinsic users' characteristics like visual, cognitive, and emotional processing parameters incorporated as well as the "traditional" user profile characteristics that together tend to give the most optimized, adapted and personalized outcome. Finally, it presents a Web adaptation and personalization system that implements the proposed comprehensive user profile as well as evaluation results that further support their importance and impact of cognitive and emotional factors in the information space.

Chapter II considers a number of challenges with regards information access, such as navigation, search and recommendation. It describes how they can be addressed by using techniques that allow information services to respond more intelligently to the needs and preferences of individuals and groups of users. Each challenge is being addressed in the form of a case study focusing on one particular mode of information access (navigation, search, and recommendation) and an application scenario (mobile portals, Web search, and e-commerce), to describe how user profiling, personalization, and adaptive interface design can be combined to produce a more efficient and effective information service.

Chapter III underlines the significance of human factors and how they influence learners' performance and perception in Web-based instruction. In this vein, the study presented in this chapter, investigates this issue in a Web-based instructional program that was designed to teach students how to use HyperText Markup Language (HTML) in a United Kingdom (UK) university.

Chapter IV identifies the importance that innovative personalization services are required to extend the traditional user profiling techniques with semantic-based information. The use of semantic-based information provides additional clues as to the reasons the user may or may not be interested in certain objects. The primary goal of this chapter is to present a comprehensive overview of the state-of-the art techniques and methodologies which integrate personalization technologies with semantic knowledge, exploring the challenges that such research areas pose to today's information society.

Section II: Adaptive Content and Services

Chapter V realizes that the current mobile communications paradigm has not been built to support the co-existence of different technologies caused by the evolutionary character of the transition to next generation systems, leading eventually to the heterogeneity of the networks and systems. Therefore, it argues that intelligent mechanisms should exist for identifying the context and the particular high-level requirements of an application and mapping them to appropriate reconfiguration operations on the underlying hardware and software infrastructure. To this end, context management, knowledge building and the respective decision making process are key factors for the service personalisation and system adaptation of future mobile communications. A need for middleware platforms, that will abstract this management load and complexity and enable an end-user seamless service experience, emerges.

Chapter VI underlines that most information retrieval services purport a *one size fits all* model whereby the same information is disseminated to a wide range of information users despite the individualistic nature of each user's needs, goals, interests, preferences, intellectual levels and information consumption capacity. This leads to a sub-optimal model because information users, who are intrinsically distinct, are not only compelled to experience a generic outcome but are further required to manually adjust and adapt the recommended information artifacts according to their immediate needs or preferences in order to achieve the desired results. Therefore, this chapter argues that there is both a case and a need to design information services that take into account the individuality of information users, and in turn aim to personalize the information seeking experiences and outcomes for users.

Chapter VII supports that the variety in citizens' skills and expectations along with the problems they face has as consequence that each citizen has different perceptions concerning the quality of public e-services. It is apparent, therefore, that a "one fits all" e-government services' assessment is not efficient, since their evaluation should be organized in a way to serve every citizen individually. Consequently, it further suggests that for the realization of such a customized and adaptive evaluation of e-government services, an intelligent, semantic-based platform is needed which allows each citizen to put emphasis in quality dimensions related with the problems he/she faces, depending on his/her skills and expectations. This part further presents a semantically adaptive interface for measuring portal quality in e-Government.

Chapter VIII discusses the solution to the WWW cognitive overload, and more specifically to e-Government services, is most probably an issue of personalization. On this ground, it introduces the design and implementation of Web information systems supporting personalized access to multi-version resources in an e-Government scenario. Personalization is supported by means of Semantic Web techniques and relies on an ontology-based profiling of users. It further introduces a reference infrastructure, describes the organization and presents performance figures of a prototype system the authors have been developed.

Chapter XI introduces new techniques for supporting the adaptation and personalization issues in the design and development of Intelligent User Interfaces, mainly by adapting services based on user preferences and user device characteristics. The user characteristics, the data collection particularities and the system capabilities are matched with the visualization method properties, in a context-based adaptive visualization environment to be used in the Historical Archive of the University of Athens, in order to support information seeking tasks.

Section III: Adaptive Processing and Communication

Chapter X argues that the integration of semantic knowledge is the primary challenge for the next generation of personalization systems and the automatic collection of data. Therefore, it provides an overview of approaches for incorporating semantic knowledge into Web usage mining and the personalization processes. It discusses the issues and requirements for successful integration of semantic knowledge using different sources, such as the content and the structure of Web sites for personalization. It further presents a general framework for fully integrating domain ontologies with Web usage.

Chapter XI investigates the development of adaptive software focusing on a design strategy for the implementation of parallel media servers with an adaptable behavior. This strategy makes the timing properties and the quality of presentation of a set of media streams predictable. The proposed adaptive scheduling approach exploits the performance of parallel environments and seems a promising method that brings the advantages of parallel computation in media servers. It further presents an efficient placement strategy for data frames as well as an adaptability strategy that allows appropriate frames to be dropped without sacrificing the ability to present multimedia applications predictably in time.

Section IV: Innovative Applications with Adaptive Behavior

Chapter XII supports that information transfer constitutes, in most cases, an important side of multimedia applications. Nonetheless, a dimension that is often overlooked in such cases, particularly in respect of quality considerations is the one of cognitive style, especially since it affects the ways through which people organize and perceive information. Accordingly, in this chapter, it is explored the impact of cognitive style on a user's perception of quality for dynamic multimedia content. In particular, it focuses on two dimensions of cognitive style: the Verbalizer / Imager and Field Dependent / Field Independent, because the first refers to information representation, while the latter relates to information organization.

Chapter XIII discusses about the limitation of the human memory, a well-acknowledged experience by everyone. In terms of computers, however there is the ability to store huge amounts of information for an unlimited time without loss of precision, and there are state-of-the-art mobile devices in general that provide features for creating reminders, linking notes to time and dates, and for managing time. However, these techniques require from the user to capture this data manually, and thus the quality of such memories greatly depends on his/her cognition and carefulness. This chapter provides a discussion on the various challenges related to building and exploiting augmented personal memories in everyday life. It concentrates on a number of crucial aspects: the importance of abstraction processes for building this memory and the design of a user interface for supporting interaction between user and memory. It further illustrates the authors' approach with examples of processing and exploiting information about the user's location in the shopping assistant SPECTER.

Chapter XIV discusses that learner models, understood as digital representations of learners, have been at the core of intelligent tutoring systems since from their original inception. Learner models facilitate the knowledge about the learner necessary for achieving any personalisation through adaptation, while most intelligent tutoring systems have been designed to support the learning modelling process. In this respect, this chapter provides an analysis of the migration of open learner modelling technology to common e-learning settings, the implications for modern e-learning systems in terms of adaptations to support the open learner modelling process, and the expected functionality of a new generation of intelligent learning environments. This analysis is supported by authors' recent experience on an e-learning environment called LeActiveMath, aimed at developing a web-based learning environment for Mathematics in the state of the art.

Chapter XV underlines the fact and discusses that even though humans need assistance in Web-based learning, most current IT systems appear as more or less complex tools. The more ambitious the problems in the application domain are, the more complex the tools are. This is one of the key obstacles to a wider acceptance of technology enhanced learning approaches. In e-learning, they need to "learn" about the learner and to build in accordance an internal model as a basis of adaptive system behavior. Steps toward assistance in e-learning are systematically illustrated by means of the authors' e-learning projects and systems eBuT and DaMiT. These steps are summarized in some process model proposed to the e-learning community.

Chapter XVI identifies that the process of training and learning in Web-based and ubiquitous environments brings a new sense of adaptation. With the development of more sophisticated environments, the need for them to take into account the user's traits, as well as the user's devices on which the training is executed, has become an important issue in the domain of building novel training and learning environments. This chapter introduces a system called eQ, to the realization of personalized adaptation, in terms of dealing with the stereotypes of e-learners, having in mind emotional intelligence concepts to help in adaptation to the e-learners real needs and known preferences.

Section V: Security, Privacy and Personalization

Chapter XVII supports that privacy and personalization are currently at odds, with the technical solutions for privacy protection to represent a special kind of so-called Privacy-Enhancing Technologies (PET). This chapter proposes an evaluation framework for PETs that considers the following dimensions: (a) What high-level principles the solution follows, (b) what privacy concerns the solution addresses, and (c) what basic privacy-enhancing techniques the solution employs. It describes and categorizes major privacy principles from privacy laws as well as other desirable principles in the context of privacy protection. It discusses privacy concerns and how different privacy principles address them. It further describes the techniques that have been used in the main types of privacy-enhancing personalization solutions, addressing how they relate to the major privacy concerns and privacy principles, with the necessary analysis findings.

IN SUMMARY

The contribution of this book may considered innovative and multi-fold since it brings together the three broad research areas of (a) adaptive content and services, (b) adaptive systems and processing and (c) adaptive communication and networks sharing the same goal of adaptation and personalization. It contains: (a) extensive investigations of the adaptation and personalization fields, based on researches and reviews; (b) further considerations and analysis of parameters and contexts identifying relationships between these two areas of research which effectively share the same goal: to adapt according to the specific user characteristics; (c) systems, technologies and methodologies assigned to a number of application areas trying to approach the topic from a more global perspective, including their advantages and disadvantages, efficiency, effectiveness, share-ability and interoperability as well as other vital attributes and capabilities that will help someone to finally distinguish the most prominent approach to the specific personalization problem; and finally it (d) offers solutions and suggestions for the design and development of adaptive applications and systems that could provide more usable and qualitative content and services adjusted to the needs and requirements of the various users and the execution environment.

This book is a useful tool for academics, teachers and researchers, professionals in the field of intelligent user interfaces and technology, and to people that belong to the broader field of the information communication technologies (ICT). The book covers a large number of topics in the area of adaptation and personalization of the content, processing and communication. It provides pragmatic references, analysis, new methodologies, and architectures that tend to approach the subject more comprehensively providing latest suggestions and solutions.

Constantinos Mourlas and Panagiotis Germanakos
Athens, 2008

Acknowledgment

We would like to truly thank and express our deepest gratitude to the people involved for the successful completion of this project. Without their tireless, continuous engagement and constant assistance, this book would likely not have realized.

We would like to thank all authors for their dedication, interest and excellent work. This book is successfully completed due to their timely responses to the strict deadlines imposed throughout the process as well as patience during the editing, corrections and communications.

Also, we would like to thank all reviewers for their constructive, comprehensive comments and objective suggestions. Their role has been instrumental in allowing this book to mature.

Furthermore, we would like to thank our colleagues from the Laboratory of New Technologies, Faculty of Communication & Media Studies – National & Kapodistrian University of Athens and the Department of Computer Science, University of Cyprus for their facilitation, availability, feedback and invaluable insights throughout the implementation of this book.

Finally, we would like to thank the publishing team at IGI Global for discussing this project and giving us their full support from the inception of this idea to the final publication. In particular, many thanks to Mehdi Khosrow-Pour, Kristin Roth, Deborah Yahnke and Rebecca Beistline for their invaluable assistance and guidance.

Most important, this book would be impossible to conclude without the support, patience, love and understanding of our families and beloved friends.

Constantinos Mourlas and Panagiotis Germanakos
Athens, Hellas
January, 2008

Section I

Theoretical Aspects of Adaptive and Personalized User Interfaces

Chapter I
An Assessment of Human Factors in Adaptive Hypermedia Environments

Nikos Tsianos
National & Kapodistrian University of Athens, Greece

Panagiotis Germanakos
National & Kapodistrian University of Athens, Greece

Zacharias Lekkas
National & Kapodistrian University of Athens, Greece

Constantinos Mourlas
National & Kapodistrian University of Athens, Greece

George Samaras
University of Cyprus, Cyprus

ABSTRACT

The plethora of information and services as well as the complicated nature of most Web structures intensify the navigational difficulties that arise when users navigate their way through this large information space. Personalized services that are highly sensitive to the immediate environment and the goals of the user can alleviate the orientation and presentation difficulties experienced by the relatively diverse user population. User profiles serves as the main component of most Web personalization systems. Main scope of this chapter is to present the various techniques employed by such systems with regards to user profiles extraction and introduce a comprehensive user profile, which includes User Perceptual Preference Characteristics. It further analyzes the main intrinsic users' characteristics like visual, cognitive, and emotional processing parameters incorporated as well as the "traditional" user profile characteristics that together tend to give the most optimized personalization outcome. It finally overviews a Web adaptation and personalization system and presents evaluation results that further support the importance of human factors in the information space.

INTRODUCTION

The unprecedented and constant expansion of the World Wide Web coupled with the obscure and multi-component nature of its structure, result in orientation difficulties, as users often lose sight of the goal of their inquiry, look for stimulating rather than informative material, or even use the navigational features unwisely. As the e-Services sector is rapidly evolving, the need for such Web structures that satisfy the heterogeneous needs of its users is becoming more and more evident.

To alleviate such navigational and presentation difficulties, researchers have put huge amounts of effort to identify the peculiarities of each user group and analyze and design methodologies and systems that could deliver up-to-date adaptive and personalized information, with regards to products or services. Since to date, there has not been a concrete definition of personalization. The many adaptive hypermedia and Web personalization solutions offering personalization features meet an abstract common goal: to provide users with what they want or need without expecting them to ask for it explicitly (Mulvenna et al., 2000). Further consideration and analysis of parameters and contexts such as users intellectuality, mental capabilities, socio-psychological factors, emotional states and attention grabbing strategies, that could affect the apt collection of users' customization requirements offering in return the best adaptive environments to their preferences and demands should be extensively investigated. All these characteristics, along with the "traditional" user characteristics that is, name, age, education, experience, etc., constitute a comprehensive user profile that serves as the ground element of most of these systems.

Some noteworthy, mostly commercial, applications in the area of Web personalization that collects information with various techniques from the users based on which they construct their user profile and further adapt the services content provided, are amongst others the Broadvision's One-To-One, a commercial tool for identification of on-line users; Microsoft's Firefly Passport (developed by the MIT Media Lab); the Macromedia's LikeMinds Preference Server, which identifies behaviours of on-line customers and it further predicts new purchases of a user; Apple's WebObjects, which adapts the content to user preferences, etc. Other, more research oriented systems, include ARCHIMIDES (Bogonicolos et al., 1999), which adapts the raw content based on the structure reorganization of a Web server. The structure is depicted as a semantic tree through of which there is a dynamic selection of the content nodes according to the users' preferences; Proteus (Anderson et.al., 2001), is a system that construct user models using artificial intelligence techniques and adapts the content of a Web site taking into consideration also wireless connections; WBI (Maglio & Barret, 2000; Barret et. al, 1997) and BASAR (Thomas & Fischer, 1997), use static agents for the personalization of the content while other systems employ mobile agents over mobile networks for this purpose, like mPERSONA (Panayiotou & Samaras, 2003). Significant implementations have also been developed in the area of adaptive hypermedia, with regards to the provision of adapted educational content to students using various adaptive hypermedia techniques. Such systems are amongst others, INSPIRE (Papanikolaou et al., 2003), ELM-ART (Weber & Specht, 1997), AHA! (De Bra & Calvi, 1998), Interbook (Brusilovsky et. al., 1998), and so on.

Although one-to-one Web-based content provision may be a functionality of the distant future, user segmentation is a very valuable step in the right direction. User segmentation means that the user population is subdivided, into more or less homogeneous, mutually exclusive subsets of users who share common user profile characteristics enabling the possibility of providing them a more personalized content. The subdivisions could be based on: Demographic characteristics (i.e. age, gender, urban or rural based, region); socio-economic characteristics (i.e. income, class, sector, channel access); psychographic characteristics (i.e. life style, values, sensitivity to new trends); individual physical and psychological characteristics (i.e. disabilities, attitude, loyalty). Moreover, the issue of personalization is a complex one with many aspects and viewpoints that need to be analyzed and resolved. Some of these issues become even more complicated once viewed from a moving user's perspective, in other words when constraints of mobile channels and devices are involved. Such issues include, but are not limited to: What content to present to the user, how to show the content to the user, how to ensure the user's privacy, how to create a global personalization scheme. As clearly viewed, user characteristics and needs, determining user segmentation and thus provision of the adjustable information delivery, differ according to the circumstances and they change over time (Panayiotou & Samaras, 2004). There are many approaches to address these issues of personalization but usually, each one is focused upon a specific area, i.e. whether this is profile creation, machine learning and pattern matching, data and Web mining or personalized navigation.

This chapter overviews adaptive hypermedia and Web personalization, investigating their relationship and presenting techniques used to monitor and extract user profiles which serves as their most essential and common element. Furthermore, it outlines the importance of user profiles and presents a comprehensive user profile that incorporates intrinsic user characteristics, such as user perceptual preferences (visual, cognitive and emotional processing parameters), on top of the "traditional" ones. Eventually, it introduces an adaptation and personalization architecture, AdaptiveWeb, emphasizing on the significance and peculiarities of the various user profiles aspects it employs, considered necessary for the provision of a most optimized personalization Web-based result. Based on this system, a further evaluation analysis is presented revealing the impact of human factors in the information space.

ADAPTIVE HYPERMEDIA OVERVIEW

Adaptivity is a particular functionality that alleviates navigational difficulties by distinguishing between interactions of different users within the information space (Eklund & Sinclair, 2000; Brusilovsky & Nejdl, 2004). Adaptive Hypermedia Systems employ adaptivity by manipulating the link structure or by altering the presentation of information, based on a basis of a dynamic understanding of the individual user, represented in an explicit user model (Eklund & Sinclair, 2000; De Bra et al., 1999; Brusilovsky, 2001; Brusilovsky, 1996a; Brusilovsky, 1996b). In the 1997 discussion forum on Adaptive Hypertext and Hypermedia, an agreed definition of adaptive hypermedia systems was reached after Brusilovsky (Eklund & Sinclair, 2000) as follows: "By Adaptive Hypermedia Systems we mean all hypertext and hypermedia systems which reflect some features of the user in the user model and apply this model to adapt various visible and functional aspects of the system to the user" (Eklund & Sinclair, 2000; Brusilovsky, 1996b).

A system can be classified as an Adaptive Hypermedia System if it is based on hypermedia, has an explicit user-model representing certain characteristics of the user, has a domain model which is a set of relationships between knowledge elements in the information space, and is capable of modifying some visible or functional part of the system based on the information maintained in the user-model (Eklund & Sinclair, 2000; Brusilovsky & Nejdl, 2004; Brusilovsky, 1996b).

In 1996, Brusilovsky identified four user characteristics to which an Adaptive Hypermedia System should adapt (Brusilovsky, 1996b; Brusilovsky, 2001). These were user's knowledge, goals, background and hypertext experience, and user's preferences. In 2001, further two sources of adaptation were added to this list, user's interests and individual traits, while a third source of different nature having to deal with the user's environment had also been identified.

Generally, Adaptive Hypermedia Systems can be useful in application areas where the hyperspace is reasonably large and the user population is relatively diverse in terms of the above user characteristics (Brusilovsky, 2001; Brusilovsky, 1996a; Brusilovsky and Nejdl, 2004; Brusilovsky, 1996b). A review by Brusilovsky has identified six specific application areas for adaptive hypermedia systems since 1996 (Brusilovsky, 2001). These are educational hypermedia, on-line information systems, information retrieval systems, institutional hypermedia and systems for managing personalized view in information spaces. Educational hypermedia and on-line information systems are the most popular, accounting for about two thirds of the research efforts in adaptive hypermedia.

Adaptation effects vary from one system to another. These effects are grouped into three major adaptation technologies - adaptive content selection (Brusilovsky & Nejdl, 2004), adaptive presentation (or content-level adaptation) and adaptive navigation support (or link-level adaptation) (Eklund & Sinclair, 2000; De Bra et al., 1999; Brusilovsky, 2001; Brusilovsky & Peylo, 2003; Brusilovsky, 1999; Brusilovsky, 1996a; Brusilovsky, 1996b; Brusilovsky & Nejdl, 2004; Brusilovsky, 2003; Bailey *et al.*, 2002; Brusilovsky & Pesin, 1998; Bulterman et al., 1999) and are summarized in Figure 1.

The first of these three technologies comes from the field of adaptive information retrieval (IR) and is associated with a search-based access to information. When the user searches for relevant information, the system can adaptively select and prioritize the most relevant items (Brusilovsky & Nejdl, 2004).

The idea of adaptive presentation is to adapt the content of a page to the characteristics of the user according to the user model (Eklund &

Figure 1. Adaptive hypermedia techniques

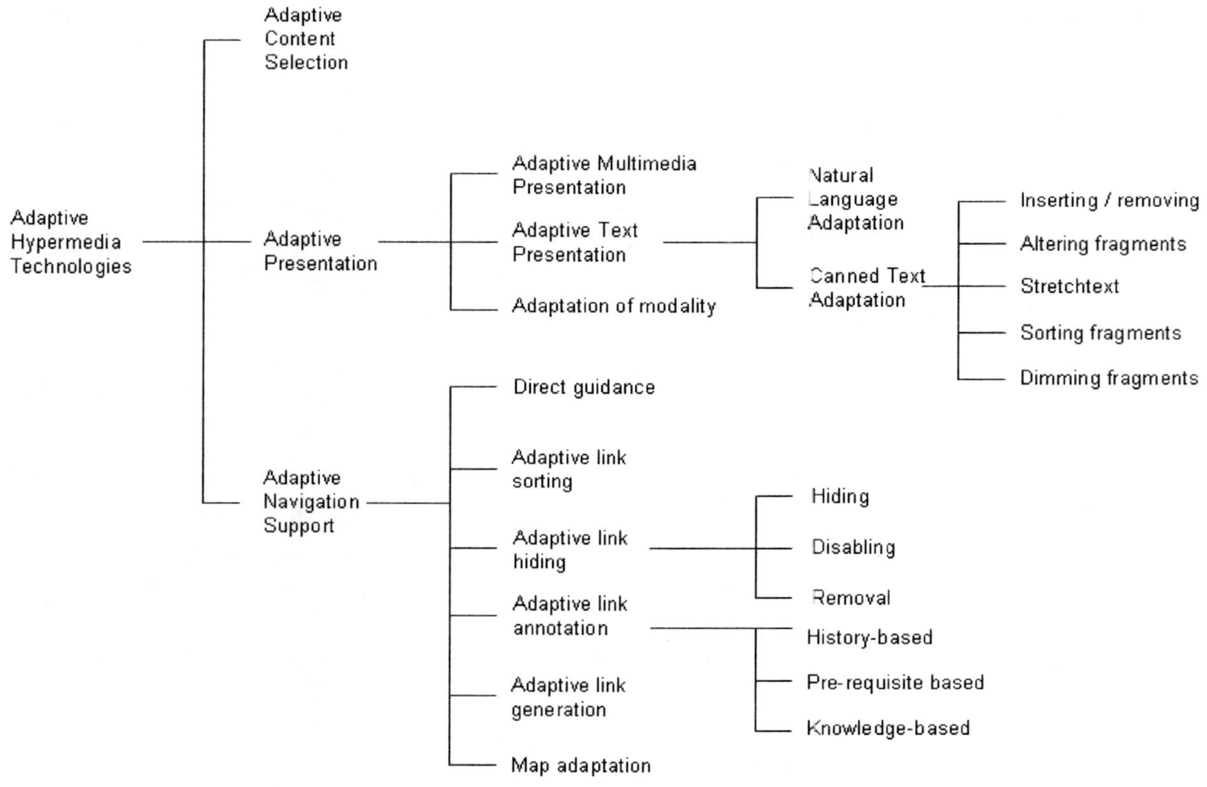

Sinclair, 2000; De Bra *et al.*, 1999; Brusilovsky, 2001; Brusilovsky & Pesin, 1998). With such techniques the content is individually generated or assembled from pieces for each user, to contain additional information, pre-requisite information or comparative explanations by conditionally showing, hiding, highlighting or dimming fragments on a page (De Bra *et al.*, 1999). The granularity may vary from word replacement to the substitution of pages to the application of different media. Adaptive presentation techniques have been classified into: (a) adaptive multimedia presentation, (b) adaptive text presentation, and (c) adaptation of modality (Brusilovsky & Nejdl, 2004; Brusilovsky & Pesin, 1998).

Adaptive navigation techniques have been classified according to the way they adapt the presentation of links, ranging from methods that restrict the user's interactions with the content to techniques that aid the user in their understanding of the information space, aiming provide either orientation or guidance (Eklund & Sinclair, 2000). Orientation informs the user about their place in the hyperspace while guidance is related to a user's goal. These techniques are: direct guidance (Eklund & Sinclair, 2000; Brusilovsky & Pesin, 1998); adaptive link sorting (Eklund & Sinclair, 2000; Brusilovsky & Pesin, 1998); adaptive link hiding (Eklund & Sinclair, 2000; Brusilovsky & Pesin, 1998); adaptive link annotation (Brusilovsky & Pesin, 1998); adaptive link generation (Brusilovsky, 2001; Brusilovsky & Nejdl, 2004); and map adaptation (Brusilovsky, 1996b).

WEB PERSONALIZATION OVERVIEW

Web personalization is the process of customizing the content and structure of a Web site to the specific needs of each user by taking advantage of the user's navigational behaviour. Being a multi-dimensional and complicated area a universal definition has not been agreed to date. Nevertheless, most of the definitions given to personalization (Cingil et al., 2000; Blom, 2000; Kim, 2002; Wang & Lin, 2002) agree that the steps of the Web personalization process include: (1) the collection of Web data, (2) the modelling and categorization of these data (pre-processing phase), (3) the analysis of the collected data, and the determination of the actions that should be performed. Moreover, many argue that emotional or mental needs, caused by external influences, should also be taken into account.

Personalization could be realized in one of two ways: (a) Web sites that require users to register and provide information about their interests, and (b) Web sites that only require the registration of users so that they can be identified (De Bra et al., 2004). The main motivation points for personalization can be divided into those that are primarily to facilitate the work and those that are primarily to accommodate social requirements. The former motivational subcategory contains the categories of enabling access to information content, accommodating work goals, and accommodating individual differences, while the latter eliciting an emotional response and expressing identity (Wang & Lin, 2002). Personalization levels have been classified into: Link Personalization, Content Personalization, Context Personalization, Authorized Personalization and Humanized Personalization.

Link personalization involves selecting the links that are more relevant to the user, changing the original navigation space by reducing or improving the relationships between nodes. E-commerce applications use link personalization to recommend items based on the clients' buying history or some categorization of clients based on ratings and opinions. Link personalization is widely used in Amazon.com to link the home page with recommendations, new releases, shopping groups, etc. (Rossi et al., 2001).

When *content* becomes personalized, user interface can present different information for different users providing substantive information in a node, other than link anchors. Most of the content personalization research is relative to text and hypertext personalization and can be further classified into two types: (a) Node structure customization (personalization), usually appears in those sites that filter the information that is relevant for the user, showing only sections and details in which the user may be interested. The user may explicitly indicate their preferences, or these may be inferred (semi-) automatically either from the user profile or navigation activity. For example, in my.yahoo.com or in www.mycnn.com users choose a set of "modules" and further personalize those modules by choosing a set of attributes of the module to be perceived. Some "automatic" customization may occur based on location information (e.g. by using the zip code of the user to select local to the user sport events). The outcome of these applications is that the user should be able to "build" their own page; and (b) Node content customization (personalization), occurs when different users perceive different values for the same node attribute; this kind of content personalization is finer grained than structure personalization. A good example can be found in online stores that give customers special discounts according to their buying history (in this case the attribute price of item is personalized) (Rossi et al., 2001).

Personalizing navigational *contexts* is critical when the same information (node) can be reached in different situations (Rossi et al., 2001). A navigational context is a set of nodes that usually share some property. For example in a Conference Paper Review Application, it is possible to access papers etc. Notice that one paper may appear in different sets and that different users may have different access restrictions according to their role in the Review application. Context personalization can also be adapted to the preferences of the learner and semantics of the learner's current environment. One sub-category of context personalization is terminal adaptivity. That is adapting information to the characteristics of a device. It is applied on the mobile devices to satisfy learner's demand for "learning as you go". Terminal Personalization occurs on a per session basis. Personalization can be achieved by applying many axes of adaptation effecting both the navigational structure and appearance of the learning experience. It involves the tailoring of a resource to the current environment of the learner (Lankhorst et al., 2002).

With *authorized* personalization, different users have different roles and therefore they might have different access authorizations. For example, in an academic application, instructors and students have different tasks to perform. Instructors want to access their class materials, such as upload, edit their class syllabus and give students' grades etc. On the other hand, students want to access the interface to find out their current GPA, their enrolment status, and their course work status etc.

Humanized personalization involves human computer interaction. If this dimension of the "emotional user interface" could be involved, it will be a huge step towards a concrete and universal definition of Web personalization. Unquestionably, this category of personalization still needs to be explored, with an extensive use of Artificial Intelligence technologies (Kaplan et al., 1999). Kaplan et al. (1999) made a first step towards exploring this area when they implemented an intelligent interactive telephone system (Telephone-Linked Care (TLC)) that provided information whether they were talking to a machine or to a person during TKC relationships with the TLC system (Hjelsvold et al., 2001).

Web Personalization Technologies

Some of the most common paradigms used for Web personalization and most broadly serving as methods to extract user profile are the following:

Content-Based Filtering

Systems that are implementing these kinds of techniques are solely based on individual users' preferences. The system tracks each user's behaviour and recommends items that are similar to items the user liked in the past. It is based on description analysis of the items rated by the user and correlations between the content of these items and user's preferences. It is an alternative paradigm that has been used mainly in the context of recommending items such as books, Web pages, news, etc. for which informative content descriptors exist (Pazzani, 2005; Basilico & Hofmann, 2004; Shardanand & Maes, 1995). This technique is primarily characterized by two weaknesses, content Limitations and over-Specialization. There are content limitations like IR methods that can only be applied to a few kinds of content, such as text and image, and the extent aspects can only capture certain aspects of the content. On the other hand content-based recommendation systems provide recommendations merely based on user profiles, therefore, users have no chance of exploring new items that are not similar to those items included in their profiles and thus leading to over-specialization. Consequently, some more drawbacks that have been identified in time are (Shahabi & Chen, 2003; Shardanand & Maes, 1995; Mobasher et al., 2002):

1. Search-based models build keyword, category, and author indexes offline, but fail to provide recommendations with interesting, targeted titles. They also scale poorly for customers with numerous purchases and ratings.
2. User input may be subjective and prone to bias.
3. Explicit (and non-binary) user ratings may not be available.
4. Profiles may be static and can become outdated quickly.
5. May miss other semantic relationships among objects.

At this point it would be noteworthy to mention a complementary technique of Content-based filtering, namely Social Information filtering. It essentially automates the process "word-of-mouth" recommendations: items are recommended to a user based upon values assigned by other people with similar taste. The system determines which users have similar taste via standard formulas for computing statistical correlations. Social Information filtering overcomes some of the limitations of content-based filtering. Items being filtered need not be amenable to parsing by a computer. Furthermore, the system may recommend items to the user which are very different (content-wise) from what the user has indicated liking before. Finally, recommendations are based on the quality of items, rather than more objective properties of the items themselves (Shardanand & Maes, 1995; Mobasher et al., 2002). Some of the most popular systems using content-based filtering are WebWatcher, and client-side agent Letizia (Lieberman, 1995).

Rule-Based Filtering

The users are asked to answer a set of questions. These questions are derived from a decision tree, so as the user proceeds to answer them. What he finally receives is a result (e.g. list of products) tailored to his/her needs. Content-based, rule-based, and collaborative filtering may also be used in combination, for deducing more accurate conclusions. Some of the rule-based filtering drawbacks are: User input may be subjective and prone to bias, explicit (and non-binary) user ratings may not be available, profiles may be static and can become outdated quickly, and for large systems it becomes burdensome to manage. Related interesting systems include Dell, Apple Computer, and Broadvision.

Collaborative Filtering

Systems invite users to rate the objects or divulge their preferences and interests and then return information that is predicted to be of interest to them. This is based on the assumption that users with similar behavior (e.g. users that are rating similar objects) have analogous interests. There are two general classes of collaborative filtering algorithms, memory-based methods and model-based methods (Wang & Lin, 2002; Eirinaki & Vazirgiannis, 2003, Pazzani, 2005; Basilico & Hofmann, 2004). Moreover, the goals in a collaborative filtering system are basically focused upon the reduction of computation time, the increase of the extent in which predictions can be computed in parallel, and the increase of prediction accuracy. Collaborative filtering can further refine the process of giving each individual personal recommendation compared to rule-based filtering. It overcomes the drawbacks of the content-based filtering because it typically does not use the actual content of the items for recommendation. It usually works based on assumptions. With this algorithm the similarity between the users is evaluated based on their ratings of products, and the recommendation is generated considering the items visited by nearest neighbors of the user. In its original form, the nearest-neighbor algorithm uses a two-dimensional user-item matrix to represent the user profiles. This original form suffers from three problems, scalability, sparsity, and synonymy (Shahabi & Chen, 2003; Papagelis et al., 2004). Some more highlighted drawbacks of collaborative filtering are focused upon: (a) Collaborative-filtering techniques are often based in matching in real-time the current user's profile against similar records obtained by the systems over time from other users. However, as noted in recent studies, it becomes hard to scale collaborative filtering techniques to a large number of items, while maintaining reasonable prediction performance and accuracy. Part of this is due to the increasing sparsity in the data as the number of items increase. One potential solution to this problem is to first cluster user records with similar characteristics, and focus the search for nearest neighbors only in the matching clusters. In the context of Web personalization this task involves clustering user transactions identified in the preprocessing stage; (b) traditional collaborative filtering does little or no offline computation, and its online computation scales with the number of customers and catalog items. The algorithm is impractical on large data sets, unless it uses dimensionality reduction, sampling, or partitioning–all of which reduce recommendation quality; (c) user input may be subjective and prone to bias; (d) explicit (and non-binary) user ratings may not be available; (e) profiles may be static and can become outdated quickly; (f) they are not able to recommend new items that have not already been rated by other users. An object will become available for recommendation only when many users have seen it and rated it, making it part of their profiles first ("latency problem"); (g) they are not satisfactory when dealing with a user that is not similar enough with any of the existing users (Mobasher et al., 2002; Mobasher et al., 2000; Vozalis et al., 2001). Some systems applied with this technique are Yahoo, Excite, Microsoft Network, Net Perceptions, Amazon.com, and CDNOW.

Web Usage Mining

The typical sub-categorization of the Web mining research field falls into the following three categories: Web-content mining, Web-structure mining, and Web usage mining. The prerequisite step to all of the techniques for providing users with recommendations is the identification of a set of user sessions from the raw usage data provided by the Web server. Web usage mining is the only category related to Web Personalization. This process relies on the application of statistical and data mining methods to the Web log data, resulting in a set of useful patterns that indicate users' navigational behavior. The data mining methods that are employed are: Association rule-mining, sequential pattern discovery, clustering, and classification. Given the site map structure and usage logs, a Web usage miner provides results regarding usage patterns, user behavior, session and user clusters, click stream information, and so on. Additional information about the individual users can be obtained by the user profiles (Deshpande & Karypis, 2004; Eirinaki & Vazirgiannis, 2003; Cingil et al., 2000). The overall process can be divided into two components. (a) The offline component is comprised of the pre-processing and data preparation tasks, including data cleaning, filtering, and transaction identification, resulting in a user transaction file, and (b) the data mining stage in which usage patterns are discovered via specific usage mining techniques such as association-rule mining, association-rule discovery and usage clustering (Mobasher et al., 2000). The increasing focus on Web-usage mining as the time passes derives from some key characteristics which are summarized as follows: (a) the profiles are dynamically obtained, from user patterns, and thus the system performance does not degrade over time as the profiles age; (b) using content similarly alone as a way to obtain aggregate profiles may result in missing important relationships among Web objects based on their usage. Thus, Web usage mining will reduce the need for obtaining subjective user ratings or registration-based personal preferences; (c) profiles are based on objective information (how users actually use the site); (d) there is no explicit user ratings or interaction with users (saves time and other complications); (e) it helps preserve user privacy, by making effective use of anonymous data; (f) the usage data captures relationships missed by content-based approaches; (g) it can help enhance the effectiveness of collaborative or content-based filtering techniques. Nevertheless, usage-based personalization can be problematic when little usage data is available pertaining to some objects or when the site content attributes of a site must be integrated into a Web mining framework and used by the recommendation engine in a uniform manner (Mobasher et al., 2002). Noteworthy applications are Alta-Vista, Lycos, WebSift, and SpeedTracer.

Demographic-Based Filtering

This specific technique could be roughly described as an approach that uses demographic information to identify the types of users that prefers a certain object and to identify one of the several pre-existing clusters to which a user belongs and to tailor recommendations based on information about others in this cluster (Pazzani, 2005; Basilico & Hofmann, 2004).

Agent Technologies

Agents are processes with the aim of performing tasks for their users, usually with autonomy, playing the role of personal assistants (Delicato et al. 2001; Panayiotou and Samaras, 2004). Agents usually solve common problems users experience on the Web such as personal history, shortcuts, page watching and traffic lights. Some of the agents' main characteristics could be distinguished according to their abilities used and according to the tasks they execute. The former include characteristics such as intelligence, autonomy, social capacity (inter-agent communication), and mobility; while the latter classify the agents into information filtering agents, information retrieval agents, recommendation agents, agents for electronic market, and agents for network management (Delicato et al. 2001). Pioneer personalization systems implemented with agents are: ARCHIMIDES, Proteus, WBI, BASAR, 1:1 Pro, Haystack, eRACE, mPersona, Fenix system, and SmartClient.

Cluster Models

These types of techniques are found mostly in the area of eCommerce and could be characterized as eCommerce recommendation algorithms. To find customers who are similar to the user, cluster models divide the customer base into many segments and treat the task as a classification problem. The algorithm's goal is to assign the user to the segment containing the most similar customers. It then uses the purchases and ratings of the customers in the segment to generate recommendations. The segments typically are created using a clustering or other unsupervised learning algorithm, although some applications use manually determined segments. Using a similarity metric, a clustering algorithm groups the most similar customers together to form clusters or segments. Because optimal clustering over large data sets is impractical, most applications use various forms of greedy cluster generation. These algorithms typically start with an initial set of segments, which often contain one randomly selected customer each. They then repeatedly match customers to the existing segments, usually with some provision for creating new or merging existing segments. For very large data sets–especially those with high dimensionality–sampling or dimensionality reduction is also necessary. Once the algorithm generates the segments, it computes the user's similarity to vectors that summarize each segment, chooses the segment with the strongest similarity and classifies the user accordingly. Some algorithms classify users into multiple segments and describe the strength of each relationship (Perkowitz & Etzioni, 2003). Cluster models have better online scalability and performance than collaborative filtering because they compare the user to a controlled number of segments rather than the entire customer base. The complex and expensive clustering computation is run offline. However, recommendation quality is relatively poor. To improve it, it is possible to increase the number of segments, but this makes the online user segment classification expensive. Typical examples of eCommerce systems are Amazon.com, Dell, and IBM.com.

SIMILARITIES AND DIFFERENCES

After having seen a brief overview of Adaptive Hypermedia and Web Personalization and their methodologies employed to deliver an adapted and optimized content to the user, it would be essential at this point to spot out their similarities and differences. Furthermore, to identify their convergence point which is their objective to develop techniques to adapt what is presented to the user based on the specific user needs identified in the extracted user profile.

Generally, Adaptive Hypermedia refers to the manipulation of the link or content structure of an application to achieve adaptation and makes use of an explicit user model (Eklund & Sinclair, 2000; De Bra et al., 1999; Brusilovsky, 2001; Brusilovsky, 1996a; Brusilovsky, 1996b). Adaptive Hypermedia is a relatively old and well established area of research counting three generations: The first "pre-Web" generation of adaptive hypermedia systems explored mainly adaptive presentation and adaptive navigation support and concentrated on modeling user knowledge and goals. The second "Web" generation extended the scope of adaptive hypermedia by exploring adaptive content selection and adaptive recommendation based on modeling user interests. The third "New Adaptive Web" generation moves adaptive hypermedia beyond traditional borders of desktop hypermedia systems embracing such modern Web trends as "mobile Web", "open Web", and "Semantic Web" (Brusilovsky, 2003). On the other hand, Web Personalization refers to the whole process of collecting, classifying and analyzing Web data, and determining based on these the actions that should be performed so that the user is presented with personalized information. As inferred from its name, Web Personalization refers to Web applications solely, and is a relatively new area of research. One could also argue that the areas of application of these two research areas are different, as Adaptive Hypermedia has found popular use in educational hypermedia and on-line information systems (Brusilovsky, 2001), where as Web Personalization has found popular use in eBusiness services delivery. From this, it could be inferred that Web Personalization has a more extended scope that Adaptive Hypermedia, exploring adaptive content selection and adaptive recommendation based on modeling user interests. Also, the reason for the need of such areas to be researched is the quite similar.

The most evident technical similarity is that they both make use of a user model to achieve their goal. However, the way they maintain the user profile is different; Adaptive Hypermedia requires a continuous interaction with the user, while Web Personalization employs algorithms that continuously follow the users' navigational behavior without any explicit interaction with the user. Technically, two of the adaptation / personalization techniques used are the same. These are adaptive-navigation support (of Adaptive Hypermedia and else referred to as link-level adaptation) and Link Personalization (of Web Personalization) and adaptive presentation (of Adaptive Hypermedia and else referred to as content-level adaptation) and Content Personalization (of Web Personalization). Last but not least, it is noteworthy to mention that they both make use of techniques from machine learning, information retrieval and filtering, databases, knowledge representation, data mining, text mining, statistics, and human-computer interaction (Mobasher et al., 2007).

THE USER PROFILE IMPERATIVE

User profile serves as the core element of most systems and especially the adaptive and personalization ones. This prompts us to have a better insight of the user profile itself and the dimensions incorporated.

The user population is not homogeneous, nor should be treated as such. To be able to deliver quality knowledge, systems should be tailored to the needs of individual users providing them personalized and adapted information based on their perceptions, reactions, and demands. Therefore, a serious analysis of user requirements has to be undertaken, documented and examined, taking into consideration their multi-application to the various delivery channels and devices. Some of the user requirements and arguments anticipated could be clearly distinguished into (CAP Gemini Ernst & Young, 2004): (a) General User Service Requirements (flexibility: anyhow, anytime, anywhere; accessibility; quality; and security), and (b) Requirements for a Friendly and Effective User Interaction (information acquisition; system controllability; navigation; versatility; errors handling; and personalization).

One of the key technical issues in developing personalization applications is the problem of how to construct accurate and comprehensive profiles of individual users and how these can be used to identify a user and describe the user behaviour, especially if they are moving (Adomavicious & Tuzhilin, 1999). According to Merriam- Webster dictionary the term profile means "a representation of something in outline". User profile can be thought of as being a set of data representing the significant features of the user. Its objective is the creation of an information base that contains the preferences, characteristics, and activities of the user. A user profile can be built from a set of keywords that describe the user preferred interest areas compared against information items.

User profile can either be static, when it contains information that rarely or never changes (e.g. demographic information), or dynamic, when the data change frequently. Such information is obtained either explicitly, using online registration forms and questionnaires resulting in static user profiles, or implicitly, by recording the navigational behaviour and / or the preferences of each user. In the case of implicit acquisition of user data, each user can either be regarded as a member of group and take up an aggregate user profile or be addressed individually and take up an individual user profile. The data used for constructing a user profile could be distinguished into: (a) the Data Model which could be classified into the demographic model (which describes who the user is), and the transactional model (which describes what the user does); and (b) the Profile Model which could be further classified into the factual profile (containing specific facts about the user derived from transactional data, including the demographic data, such as "the favorite beer of customer X is Beer A"), and the behavioral profile (modeling the behavior of the user using conjunctive rules, such as association or classification rules. The use of rules in profiles provides an intuitive, declarative and modular way to describe user behavior (Adomavicious & Tuzhilin, 1999)).

Still, could current user profiling techniques be considered complete incorporating only these dimensions? Do designers and developers of Web-based applications take into consideration the real users' preferences in order to provide them a really personalized Web-based content? Many times this is not the case. How can a user profile be considered complete, and the preferences derived optimized, if it does not contain parameters related to the user perceptual preference characteristics? We could define User Perceptual Preference Characteristics as all the critical factors that influence the visual, mental and emotional processes liable of manipulating the newly information received and building upon prior knowledge, that is different for each user or user group. These characteristics determine the visual attention, cognitive and emotional processing taking place throughout the whole process of accepting an object of perception (stimulus) until the comprehensive response to it (Germanakos et al., 2005).

In further support of the aforementioned concepts, one cannot disregard the fact that, besides the parameters that constitute the "traditional" user profile (composed of parameters like knowledge, goals, background, experience, preferences, activities, demographic information, socio-economic characteristics, device-channel characteristics etc.), each user carries his/her own perceptual and cognitive characteristics that have a significant effect on how information is perceived and processed. Information is encoded in the human brain by triggering electrical connections between neurons, and it is known that the number of synapses that any person activates each time is unique and dependant on many factors, including physiological differences (Graber, 2000). Since early work on the psychological field has shown that research on actual intelligence and learning ability is hampered by too many limitations, there have been a "number of efforts to identify several styles or abilities and dimensions of cognitive and perceptual processing" (McLoughlin, 1999), which have resulted in what is known as learning and cognitive styles. Learning and cognitive styles can be defined as relatively stable strategies, preferences and attitudes that determine an individual's typical modes of perceiving, remembering and solving problems, as well as the consistent ways in which an individual memorizes and retrieves information (Pithers, 2002). Each learning and cognitive style typology defines patterns of common characteristics and implications in order to overcome difficulties that usually occur throughout the procedure of information processing. Therefore, in any Web-based informational environment, the significance of the fore mentioned users' differences, both physiological and preferential, is distinct and should be taken into consideration when designing such adaptive environments.

It is true that nowadays, there are not researches that move towards the consideration of user profile incorporating optimized parameters taken from the research areas of visual attention processing and cognitive psychology in combination. Some serious attempts have been made though on approaching e-Learning systems providing adapted content to the students but most of them are lying to the analysis and design of methodologies that consider only the particular dimension of cognitive learning styles, including Field Independence vs. Field Dependence, Holistic-Analytic, Sensory Preference, Hemispheric Preferences, and Kolb's

Learning Style Model (Yuliang & Dean, 1999), applied to identified mental models, such as concept maps, semantic networks, frames, and schemata (Ayersman & Reed, 1998; Reed et al., 1996). In order to deal with the diversified students' preferences such systems are matching the instructional materials and teaching styles with the cognitive styles and consequently they are satisfying the whole spectrum of the students' cognitive learning styles by offering a personalized Web-based educational content.

CONSIDERING THE IMPORTANCE OF HUMAN FACTORS IN FURTHER COMPLETING THE USER PROFILE

Based on the abovementioned considerations we introduce the Comprehensive User Profile that combines the User Perceptual Preference Characteristics described above along with the "Traditional" User Profile Characteristics since they are affecting the way a user approaches an object of perception (Germanakos et al., 2007a).

The Comprehensive User Profile could be considered as the main raw content filtering module of an Adaptive Web-based Architecture. At this module all the requests are processed, being responsible for the custom tailoring of information to be delivered to the users, taking into consideration their habits and preferences, as well as, for mobile users mostly, their location ("location-based") and time ("time-based") of access (Panayiotou & Samaras, 2006). The whole processing varies from security, authentication, user segmentation, content identification, user perceptual characteristics (visual, cognitive and emotional processing parameters) and so forth. This module could accept requests from an 'Entry Point' module and after the necessary processing and further communication with a 'Semantic Web-based Content' module, to provide the requested adapted and personalized result. The Comprehensive User Profile is comprised of two main components:

The "Traditional" User Profile

It contains all the information related to the user, necessary for the Web Personalization processing. It is composed of two elements, the (a) User Characteristics (the so called "traditional" characteristics of a user: knowledge, goals, background, experience, preferences, activities, demographic information (age, gender), socio-economic information (income, class, sector etc.), and the (b) Device / Channel Characteristics (contains characteristics that referred to the device or channel the user is using and contains information like: Bandwidth, displays, text-writing, connectivity, size, power processing, interface and data entry, memory and storage capacity, latency (high / low), and battery lifetime. These characteristics are mostly referred to mobile users and are considered important for the formulation of a more integrated user profile, since it determines the technical aspects of it). Both elements are completing the user profile from the user's point of view.

The User Perceptual Preference Characteristics

This is the new component / dimension of the user profile defined above. It contains all the visual attention and cognitive psychology processes (cognitive and emotional processing parameters) that completes the user preferences and fulfills the user profile. User Perceptual Preference Characteristics could be described as a continuous mental processing starting with the perception of an object in the user's attentional visual field and going through a number of cognitive, learning and emotional processes giving the actual response to that stimulus, as depicted in Figure 2, below. As it can be observed, its primary parameters formulate a three-dimensional approach to the problem. The first dimension investigates the visual and cognitive processing of the user, the second his/her cognitive style, while the third captures his/her emotional processing during the interaction process with the information space (Germanakos et al., 2007a)

It is considered a vital component of the user profile since it identifies the aspects of the user that is very difficult to be revealed and measured but, however, might determine his/her exact preferences and lead to a more concrete, accurate and optimized user segmentation. As mentioned above, it is composed of three elements:

Cognitive Processing Speed Efficiency

The Actual Speed of Processing parameters could be primarily determined by (i) the visual processing, whereby special emphasis is given to the visual attention that is responsible for the tracking of the user's eye movements and in particular the scanning of his/her eye gaze on the information environment (Gulliver & Ghinea, 2004). It is composed of two serial phases: the pre-attentive and the limited-capacity stage. The pre-attentive stage of vision subconsciously defines objects from visual primitives, such as lines, curvature, orientation, color and motion and allows definition of objects in the visual field. When items pass from the pre-attentive stage to the limited-capacity stage, these items are considered as selected. Interpretation of eye movement data is based on the empirically validated assumption that when a person is performing a cognitive task, while watching a display, the location of his/her gaze corresponds to the symbol currently being processed in working memory and, moreover, that the eye naturally focuses on areas that are most likely to be informative; (ii) the control of processing (refers to the processes that identify and register goal-relevant information and block out dominant or appealing but actually irrelevant information); and (iii) the speed of processing (refers to the maximum speed at which a given mental

Figure 2. User perceptual preference characteristics: Three-dimensional approach

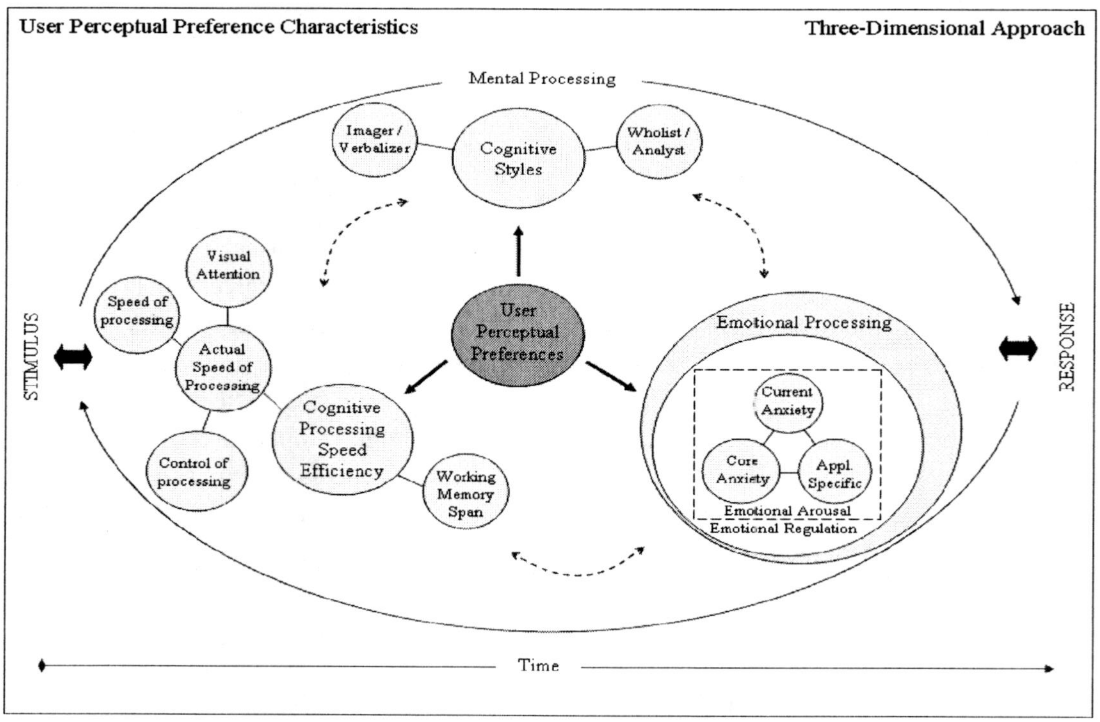

act may be efficiently executed). The Working Memory Span refers to the processes that enable a person to hold information in an active state while integrating it with other information until the current problem is solved. Many researches (Demetriou et al., 1993; Demetriou & Kazi, 2001) have identified that the speed of cognitive processing and control of processing it is directly related to the human's age, as well as to the continuous exercise and experience, with the former to be the primary indicator. Therefore, as it is depicted in Figure 3a, the processing development speed increases non-linearly in the age of 0–15 (1500 msec), it is further stabilized in the age of 15 - 55-60 (500 msec) and decreases from that age on (1500 msec). However, it should be stated that the actual cognitive processing speed efficiency is yielded from the difference (maximum value 0.8 msec) between the peak value of the speed of processing and the peak value of control of processing, as it is depicted in Figure 3b.

Cognitive Style

Since early work on the psychological field has shown that research on actual intelligence and learning ability is hampered by too many limitations, there have been a "number of efforts to identify several styles or abilities and dimensions of cognitive and perceptual processing" (McLoughlin, 1999), which have resulted in what is known as learning and cognitive styles. *Learning and cognitive styles* can be defined as relatively stable strategies, preferences and attitudes that determine an individual's typical modes of perceiving, remembering and solving problems, as well as the consistent ways in which an individual memorizes and retrieves information (Pithers, 2002). Each learning and cognitive style typology defines patterns of common characteristics and implications in order to overcome difficulties that usually occur throughout the procedure of information processing. Therefore, in any Web-based informational environment, the significance of

Figure 3a. Speed of processing

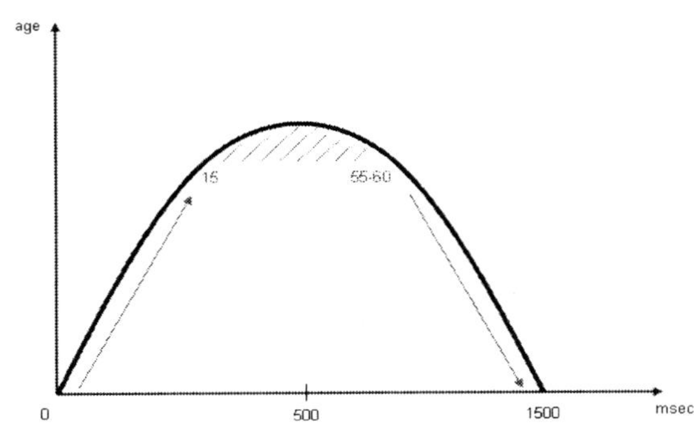

Figure 3b. Actual cognitive processing speed efficiency

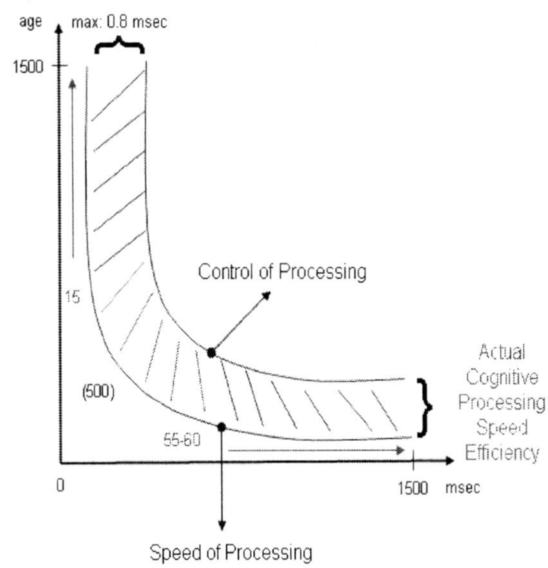

the fore mentioned users' differences, both physiological and preferential, is distinct and should be taken into consideration when designing such adaptive environments.

It is true that nowadays, there are not researches that move towards the consideration of user profile incorporating optimized parameters taken from the research areas of visual attention processing and cognitive psychology in combination. Some serious attempts have been made though on approaching e-Learning systems providing adapted content to the students but most of them are lying to the analysis and design of methodologies that consider only the particular dimension of cognitive learning styles, including Field Independence vs. Field Dependence, Holistic-Analytic, Sensory Preference, Hemispheric Preferences, and Kolb's Learning Style Model (Yuliang & Dean, 1999), applied to identified mental models, such as concept maps, semantic networks, frames, and schemata (Ayersman & Reed, 1998; Reed et al., 1996). In order to deal with the diversified students' preferences such systems are matching the instructional materials and teaching styles with the cognitive styles and consequently they are satisfying the whole spectrum of the students' cognitive learning styles by offering a personalized Web-based educational content.

They represent the particular set of strengths and preferences that an individual or group of people have in how they take in and process information. By taking into account these preferences and defining specific learning strategies, empirical research has shown that more effective learning can be achieved (Boyle et al., 2003), and that learning styles nevertheless correlate with performance in an e-Learning environment (Wang et al., 2006). A selection of the most appropriate and technologically feasible learning styles (those that can be projected on the processes of selection and presentation of Web-content and the tailoring of navigational tools) has been studied, such as Riding's Cognitive Style Analysis (Verbal-Imager and Wholistic-Analytical–Riding, 2001), Felder / Silverman Index of Learning Styles (4 scales: Active vs Reflective, Sensing vs Intuitive, visual vs Verbal and Global vs Sequential–Felder & Silverman, 1988), Witkin's Field-Dependent and Field-Independent (Witkin et al., 1977), and Kolb's Learning Styles (Converger, Diverger, Accommodator, and Assimilator), in order to identify how users transforms information into knowledge (constructing new cognitive frames).

The most prominent to be used seemed to be Riding's CSA since it can be mapped on the information space more precisely (the implications are consisted of distinct scales that respond to different aspects of the Web-space) and can be applied on most cognitive informational processing tasks (rather than strictly educational). The CSA implications are quite clear in terms of hypermedia design (visual/verbal content presentation and wholist/analyst pattern of navigation), and is probably one of the most inclusive theories, since it is actually derived from the common axis of a number of previous theories.

Learning style theories that define specific types of learners, as Kolb's Experiential Learning Theory, and Felder/Silverman's ILS (at least the active/reflective and sensing/intuitive scales) have far more complex implications, since they relate strongly with personality theories, and therefore cannot be adequately quantified and correlated easily with Web objects and structures.

The CSA main characteristics as well as their implication into the information space are summarized in Figure 4 (Sadler-Smith & Riding , 1999).

Emotional Processing

Research on modelling affect and on interfaces adaptation based on affective factors has matured considerably over the past several years, so that even designers of commercial products are now

Figure 4. Riding's cognitive learning styles characteristics and implications

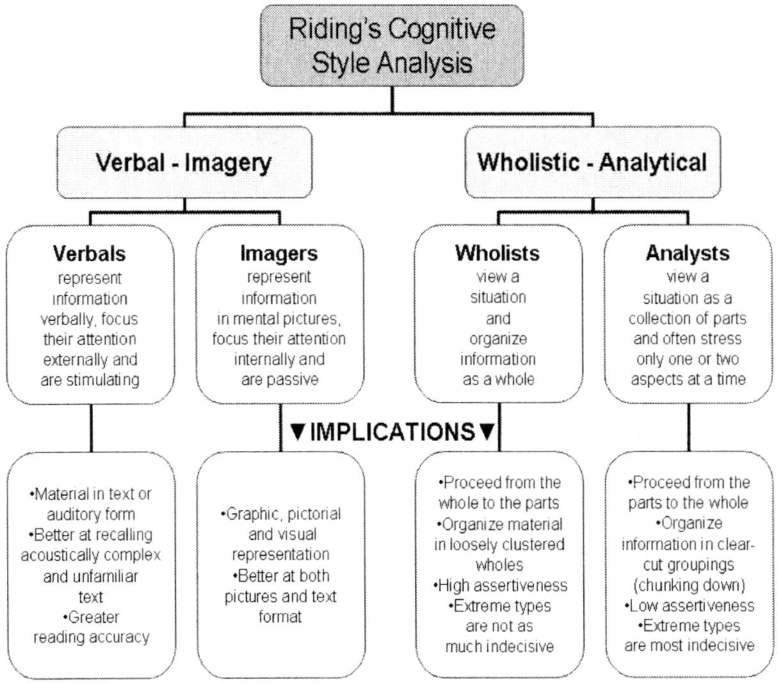

considering the inclusion of components that take affect into account. Emotions are considered to play a central role in guiding and regulating behaviour and decision making, by modulating numerous cognitive and physiological activities. By coordinating specific instances of cognitive processing and physiological functioning, emotions are one of the tools that allow agents to make adaptive inferences in the design of Web-based systems.

In our study, we are interested in the way that individuals process their emotions and how they interact with other elements of their information-processing system. Emotional processing is a pluralistic construct which is comprised of two mechanisms: emotional arousal, which is the capacity of a human being to sense and experience specific emotional situations, and emotion regulation, which is the way in which an individual perceives and controls his/her emotions. We focus on these two sub-processes because they are easily generalized, inclusive and provide some indirect measurement of general emotional mechanisms. These sub-processes manage a number of emotional factors like anxiety boredom effects, anger, feelings of self efficacy and user satisfaction etc. Among these, our current research concerning emotional arousal emphasizes on anxiety, which is probably the most indicative, while other emotional factors are to be examined within the context of a further study.

Anxiety is an unpleasant combination of emotions that includes fear, worry and uneasiness and is often accompanied by physical reactions such as high blood pressure, increased heart rate and other body signals like shortness of breath, nausea and increased sweating. The anxious person is not able to regulate his/her emotional state since he feels and expects danger all the time. The systems underlying anxiety are being studied and examined continuously and it has been found that their foundations lie in the more primitive regions of the brain. However, given the complexity of the human nature, anxiety is characterized as a difficult to be understood construct of emotions which is at a balance between nature and nurture and between higher perception and animal instinct.(Kim & Gorman, 1995).

Similar to Bandura's (1986) theory of self-efficacy, Barlow (2002) describes anxiety as a cognitive-affective process in which the individual has a sense of unpredictability, a feeling of uncertainty and a sense of lack of control over emotions, thoughts and events. This cognitive and affective situation is associated as well with physiological arousal and research has shown that an individual's perception is influenced in specific domains such as attentional span, memory, performance in specific tasks etc. In relation to performance, the findings are controversial. There is a number of studies that has shown no relationship between anxiety and performance, especially academic, although there is strong evidence that even if performance is not correlated with anxiety, they have indirect connection through a construct defined as cognitive effort. Although the final result is not altered, individuals with high anxiety level, in order to perform as required or fulfil the task assigned to them, need to try more, which means that they have to spend more of their cognitive resources. Performance is impaired in cases that the task is highly demanding and the individual needs to "mobilize" all his/her cognitive powers to respond. This way, the extra resources that would be probably needed because of high anxiety levels, would have been already occupied because of the demanding nature of the task itself. Another body of research supports that anxiety is strongly correlated to performance and academic achievement. High levels of anxiety impair concentration, attention, memory and finally performance itself. Low levels of anxiety mean lack of motivation, interest and goals.

Accordingly, in order to measure emotion regulation, we are using the cognominal construct of emotional regulation. An effort to construct a model that predicts the role of emotion, in general, is beyond the scope of our research, due to the complexity and the numerous confounding variables that would make such an attempt rather impossible. However, there is a considerable amount of references concerning the role of emotion and its implications on academic performance (or achievement), in terms of efficient learning (Kort & Reilly, 2002). Emotional Intelligence seems to be an adequate predictor of the aforementioned concepts, and is surely a grounded enough construct, already supported by academic literature. Additional concepts that were used are the concepts of self-efficacy, emotional experience and emotional expression.

On the basis of the research conducted by Goleman (1995), as well as Salovey & Mayer (1990), who have introduced the term, we are in the process of developing an EQ questionnaire that examines the 3 out of 5 scales that comprise the Emotional Intelligence construct (according to Goleman), since factors that deal with human to human interaction (like empathy) are not present in our Web- application - at least for the time being. As a result, our variation of the EQ construct, which we refer to as Emotional Control, consists of: (a) The Self- Awareness scale, (b) The Emotional Management scale, and (c) The Self- Motivation scale. While our sample is still growing, Crombach's alpha, which indicates scale reliability, is currently 0.714. Revisions on the questionnaire are expected to increase reliability.

Self-efficacy is defined as people's beliefs about their capabilities to produce and perform. Self-efficacy beliefs determine how people feel, think, motivate themselves and behave. Such beliefs produce these diverse effects through four major processes. They include cognitive, motivational, affective and selection processes. *Emotional experience* is the conceptualization of an emotion, the way in which the individual is dealing with it and how he perceives it. *Emotional expression* is the way in which the individual is reacting after an emotion triggers. It is his/her behaviour after an affective stimulus. It can be argued that emotional expression is the representation of an emotion.

Still, there is a question about the role of emotions, and their cognitive and / or neuro-physiologic intrinsic origins (Damasio, 1994). Emotions influence the cognitive processes of the individual, and therefore have certain effect in any educational setting. Again, bibliographic research has shown that anxiety is often correlated with academic performance (Cassady, 2004), as well with performance in computer mediated learning procedures (Smith & Caputi, 2005; Chang, 2005). Subsequently, different levels of anxiety have also a significant effect in cognitive functions. We believe that combining the level of anxiety of an individual with the moderating role of Emotional Control, it is possible to clarify, at some extent, how emotional responses of the individual hamper or promote learning procedures. Thus, by personalizing Web-based content, taking into account emotional processing, we can avoid stressful instances and take full advantage of his/her cognitive capacity at any time.

Anxiety is a complex term and in order to measure it accurately and validly (measure the kind of anxiety we are interested in), it has to be adapted to our research. For this reason we included in our model not only a general anxiety measure (Stait-Trait Anxiety Inventory (STAI) test (Spielberger, 1983)) but a situation-specific measure of anxiety as well (i.e. educational). Additionally, we are interested in measuring anxiety as a predisposition (trait-anxiety) and as a generated (state-anxiety) set of emotions as well. This way, we can see the differences between the individual's evaluation of anxiety and what actually happens during the task. Individuals with high trait anxiety, report heightened perceptions of negative outcomes across a range of possible contexts and scenarios (Lerner and Keltner, 2000), so they tend to be subjective and negative to their judgement.

Still, since we are interested also in his/her emotional state during the Web-based learning procedures, real- time monitoring of anxiety levels (Current Anxiety) would also provide us useful indications. This is done by a self-reporting instrument (e.g. by giving the user the possibility to define his/her anxiety level on a bar shown on the computer screen).

Since our research examines learning process and how to improve performance through a personalization system, the situation-specific measure of anxiety that we are interested in is test anxiety. Test anxiety has been defined as one element of general anxiety composed of cognitive processes that interferes with performance in academic or assessment situations (Spielberger & Vagg, 1995). It includes both cognitive and physiological activity (Spielberger, 1972). Its two components are worry and emotionality. Worry is the cognitive concern about performance and emotionality is somatic reactions to task demands and stress (Schwarzer, 1984). Test anxiety research has shown a relationship between anxiety and performance (Sapp, 1993).

A DATA–IMPLICATIONS CORRELATION DIAGRAM

For a better understanding of the three dimensions' implications and their relation with the information space a diagram that presents a high level correlation of these implications with selected tags of the information space (a code used in Web languages to define a format change or hypertext link) is depicted in Figure 5. These tags (images, text, information quantity, links–learner control, navigation support, additional navigation support, and aesthetics) have gone through an extensive optimization representing group of data affected after the mapping with the implications. The particular mapping is based on specific rules created, liable for the combination of these tags and the variation of their value in order to better filter the raw content and deliver the most personalized Web-based result to the user.

As it can be observed from the diagram below each dimension has primary (solid line) and secondary (dashed line) implications on the information space altering dynamically the weight of the tags. It has to be mentioned at this point that we consider that this Data–Implications Diagram can be applied on multiple research fields. Therefore, we include in the Cognitive Styles dimension Riding's Cognitive Style Analysis, which applies in a greater number of information distribution circumstances, since it deals rather with cognitive than learning style. Henceforth, for example, the number of images (few or many) to be displayed has a primary implication on imagers, while text (more concise or abstract) has a secondary implication. An analyst may affect primarily the links–learner control and navigation support tag, which in turn is secondary affected by high and medium emotional processing, while might secondary affect the number of images or kind of text to be displayed, consequently. Actual speed of processing parameters (visual attention, speed of processing, and control of processing) as well as working memory span are primarily affecting information quantity. Eventually, emotional processing is primarily affecting additional navigation support and aesthetics, as visual attention does, while secondary affects information quantity.

A practical example of the Data–Implications Correlation Diagram could be as follows, a user might be identified that is: Verbalizer (V)–Wholist (W) with regards to the Cognitive Style, has an Actual Cognitive Processing Speed Efficiency of 1000 msec, and a fair Working Memory Span (weighting 5/7), with regards to his/her Cogni-

Figure 5. Data–implications correlation diagram

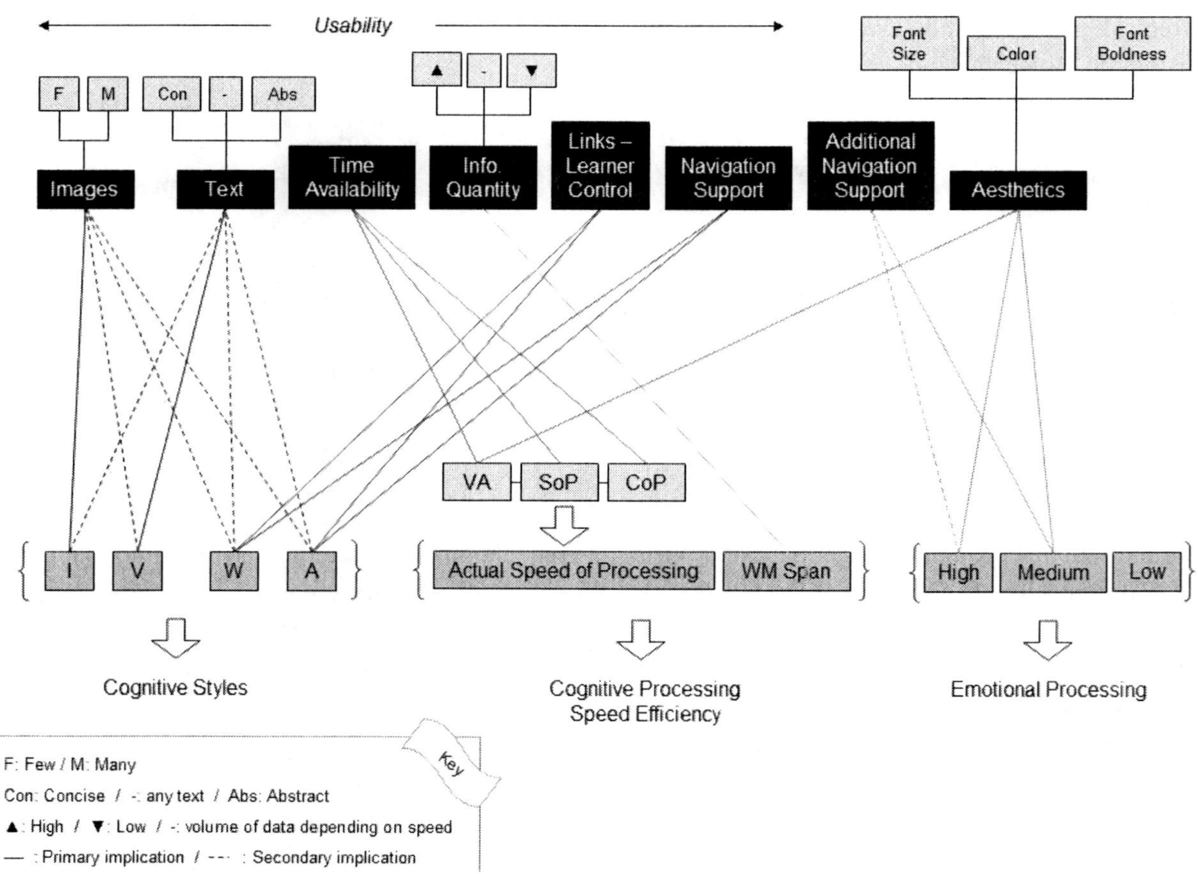

tive Processing Speed Efficiency, and (s)he has a High Emotional processing. The tags affected, according to the rules created and the Data–Implications Correlation Diagram, for this particular instance are the: Images (few images displayed), Text (any text could be delivered), Info Quantity (less info since his/her cognitive speed is moderate), Links–Learner Control (less learner control because (s)he is Wholist), Additional Navigation Support (significant because (s)he has high emotional processing), and high aesthetics (to give more structured and well defined information, with more colors, larger fonts, more bold text, since (s)he has high emotional processing). At this point it should be mentioned that in case of internal correlation conflicts primary implications take over secondary ones. Additionally, since emotional processing is the most dynamic parameter compared to the others, any changes occurring at any given time are directly affecting the yielded value of the adaptation and personalization rules and henceforth the format of the content delivered.

OVERVIEWING AN ADAPTIVE WEB ARCHITECTURE AND THE COMPREHENSIVE USER PROFILE CONSTRUCTION

In this section, an adaptive Web-based environment is overviewed trying to convey the essence and the peculiarities encapsulated above and further indicate the construction of a Comprehensive User Profile. The current system, AdaptiveWeb[1] (see Figure 6–Germanakos et al., 2007b), is a Web-based and mobile Web application. It is detached into four parts, interrelated components, each one representing a stand alone Web system briefly presented below. The technology used to build each Web system is ASP .Net.

Figure 6. AdaptiveWeb System Architecture

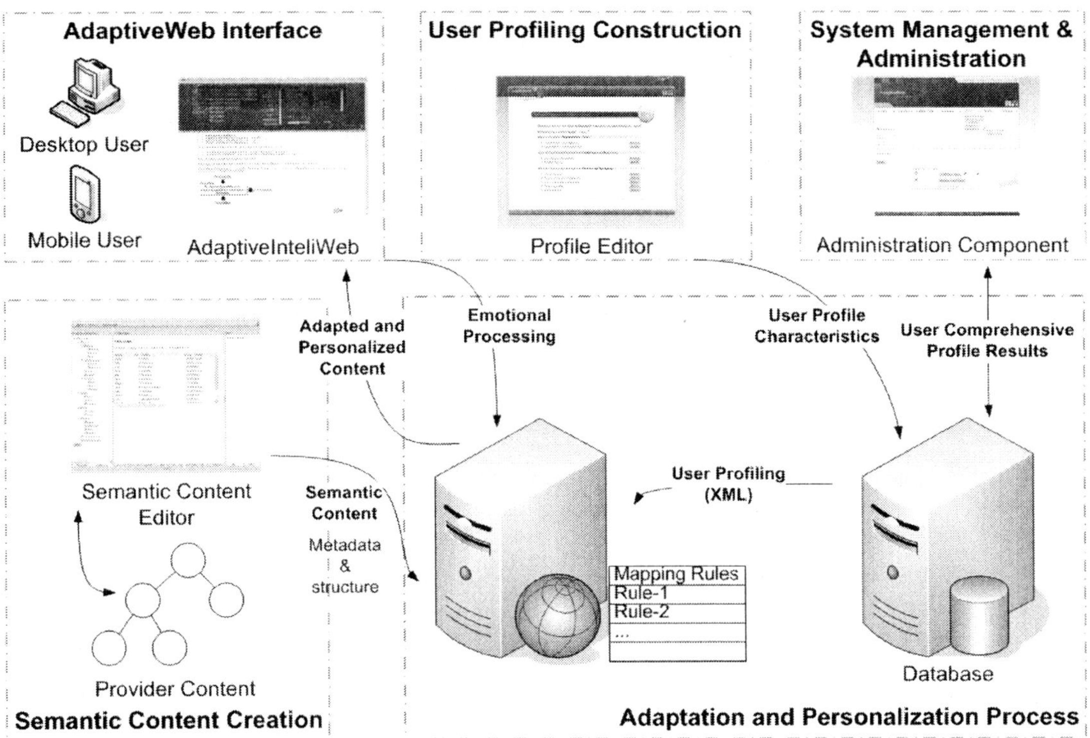

Figure 7. User profile construction

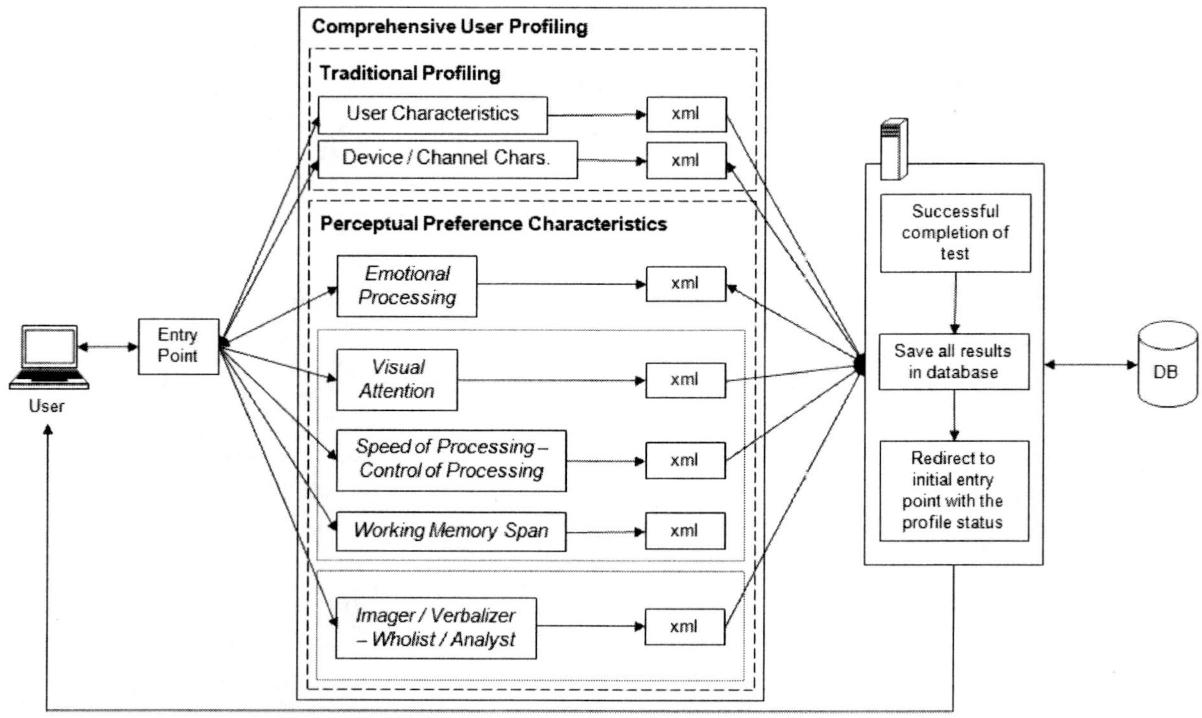

In order to get personalized and adapted content, a user has to create his/her comprehensive profile. Responsible for this part is the "User Profile Construction" component (see Figure 7). At this point the user has to give his/her "Traditional" and Device / Channel Characteristics and further complete a number of real-time tests as well as answer some questionnaires for identifying his/her Perceptual Preference Characteristics and consequently generating his/her cumulative profile. If a user has not completed all the tests available, the system will not be able to give him a Web-page reconstructed.

The second component is the system's "Semantic Content Editor", where the provider will build his/her Web site by defining the content as objects. The Web site structure has to be "well-formatted" and the objects have to be "well-defined" (based on given semantic tags) by the editor in order to give the best results to the end-user. The technology used for creating the personalized content is XML, which is a powerful and one of the most common markup languages nowadays, used for describing data and to focus on what data is. For a better insight, the Tree Structure of the Comprehensive User Profile, giving emphasis on the comprehensive user profile structure, is depicted in Figure 8. The author of the page uploads the content on the system's database, which will be mapped after with the system's "Mapping Rules". The system's "Mapping Rules" are functions that run on the AdaptiveWeb server and comprise the main body of the adaptation and personalization procedure of the provider's content, according to the user's comprehensive profile. In this section, all the system's components interact with each other in order to create and give personalized and adapted content to the end user.

The last component of the architecture is the "AdaptiveWeb Interface" which is a Web application used for displaying the raw or personalized and adapted content on the user's device. This can be a home desktop, laptop or a mobile device. Using this interface the user will navigate through

Figure 8. The tree structure of the comprehensive user profile XML document

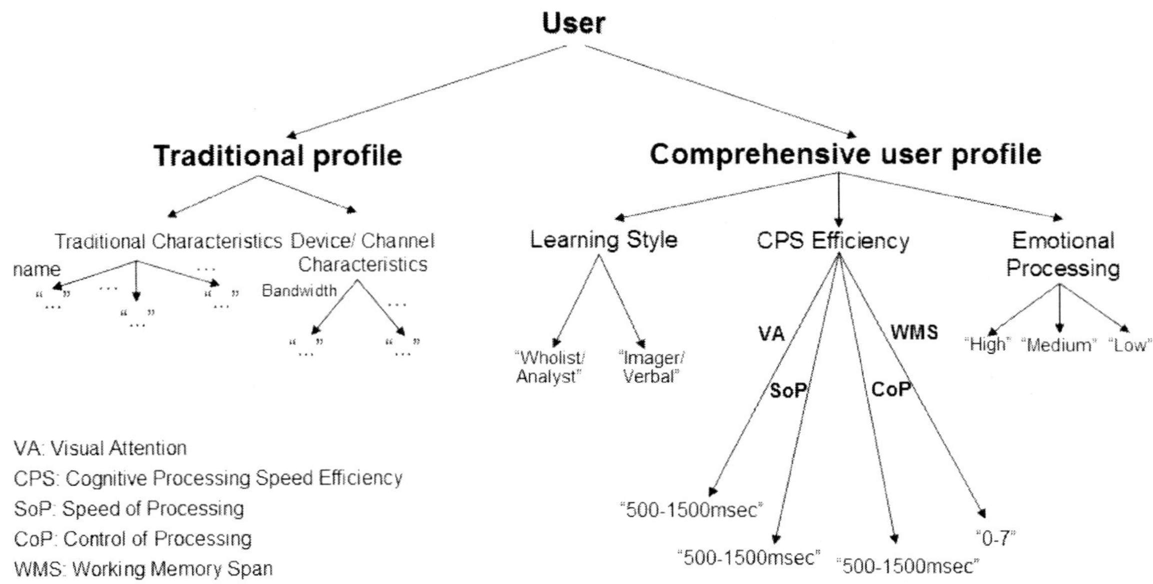

the provider's content. At the very beginning the interface will show the raw, not personalized content of the provider. When the user wants to personalize and adapt the content according to his/her comprehensive profile he / she will proceed by giving his username and password. The corresponding profile will be loaded onto the server and in proportion with his/her cumulative characteristics the content of the provider will be mapped with the "Mapping Rules". The content will be adapted according to the user's preferences. The new, adapted content will then be loaded onto the user's device. While navigating, the user will be able to change his/her emotional state through a dynamic slide bar on the system's toolbar. By changing his/her current emotional state, the server will be alerted and the content will be "shaped" and changed according to his/her emotional state.

EXPERIMENTAL EVALUATION

In order to manipulate the parameters of an adaptive system according to user characteristics, the research has to go through the stage of extracting quantified elements that represent deeper psychological cognitive and emotional abilities. These extracted elements cannot be directly used in a Web environment, but a numerical equivalent can define the parameters that are to be used in a personalization system.

The current experiment is consisted of two distinct phases: phase I was conducted at the University of Cyprus, while phase II was conducted at the University of Athens. The aim of the first experiment was to clarify whether matching (or mismatching) instructional style to users' cognitive style improves performance. The second experiment focused on the importance of matching instructional style to the remaining parameters of our model (working memory, cognitive processing efficiency, emotional processing).

All participants were students from the Universities of Cyprus and Athens; phase I was conducted with a sample of 138 students, whilst phase II with 82 individuals. 35% of the participants were male and 65% were female, and their age varied from 17 to 22 with a mean age of 19. The environment in which the procedure took place was an e-Learning course on algorithms. The course subject was chosen due to the fact that students of the departments where the experiment took place had absolutely no experience on computer science, and traditionally perform poorly. By controlling the factor of experience in that way, we divided our sample in two groups: almost half of the participants were provided with information matched to their Perceptual Preferences, while the other half were taught in a mismatched way. We expected that users in the matched condition, both in phase I and phase II, would outperform those in the mismatched condition.

In order to evaluate the effect of matched and mismatched conditions, participants took an online assessment test on the subject they were taught (algorithms). This exam was taken as soon as the e-Learning procedure ended, in order to control for long-term memory decay effects. The dependent variable that was used to assess the effect of adaptation to users' preferences was participants' score at the online exam.

At this point, it should be clarified that matching and mismatching instructional style is a process with different implications for each dimension of our model (see Table 1).

Questionnaires

In this specific e-Learning setting, Users' Perceptual Preferences were the sole parameters that comprised each user profile, since demographics and device characteristics were controlled for. In order to build each user profile according to our model, we used a number of questionnaires that address all theories involved.

- **Cognitive Style:** Riding's Cognitive Style Analysis, standardized in Greek and integrated in .NET platform
- **Cognitive Processing Efficiency:** Speed and accuracy task-based tests that assess control of processing, speed of processing, visual attention and visuospatial working memory. Originally developed in the E-prime platform, we integrated them into the .NET platform.
- **Core (general) Anxiety:** Spielberger's State-Trait Anxiety Inventory (STAI)–10 items (Only the trait scale was used) (Spielberger, 1983).

Table 1. Implications for matched/mismatched conditions

	Cognitive Style	Working Memory	**Cognitive Processing Speed Efficiency**	***Emotional Processing***
Matched Condition	Presentation and structure of information matches user's preference	Low Working Memory users are provided with segmented information	Each user has in his disposal the amount of time that fits his ability	*Users with moderate and high levels of anxiety receive aesthetic enhancement of the content and navigational help*
Mismatched Condition	*Presentation and structure of information does not coincide with user's preference*	*Low Working Memory users are provided with the whole information*	*Users' with low speed of processing have less time in their disposal (the same with "medium" users).*	*Users with moderate and high levels of anxiety receive no additional help or aesthetics*

- **Application Specific Anxiety:** Cassady's Cognitive Test Anxiety scale–27 items (Cassady & Johnson, 2002).
- **Current Anxiety:** Self-reported measures of state anxiety taken during the assessment phase of the experiment, in time slots of every 10 minutes–6 Time slots.
- **Emotion Regulation:** This questionnaire was developed by us; cronbach's α that indicates scale reliability reaches 0.718.

Results

As expected, in both experiments the matched condition group outperformed those of the mismatched group. Figure 9 displays the aggregated differences in performance (the dependent variable of exam score), in matched and mismatched conditions.

Table 2 shows the differences of means (one way ANOVA) and their statistical significance for the parameters of Cognitive Style, Cognitive Efficiency Speed, and Emotional Processing.

The relatively small sample that falls into each category and its distribution hamper statistical analysis of the working memory (WM) parameter. In any case, the difference between those with high WM and those with low WM, when both categories receive non-segmented (whole) content, approaches statistical significance: 57.06% for those with High WM, 47.37% for those with Low WM, Welch statistic= 3.988, p=0.054.

This demonstrates that WM has indeed some effect on an e-Learning environment. Moreover, if those with low WM receive segmented information, then the difference of means decreases and becomes non-significant (57.06% for High WM, 54.90% for those with Low WM, Welch statistic=0.165, p=0.687).

In the case of Emotional Processing, the results of experiments conducted within the actual learning environment, as we hypothesized, show that users with high or medium anxiety level, lacking the moderating role of emotion regulation, are in a greater need of enhancing the aesthetic aspects of our system and the provision of additional help, in order to perform as well as low anxiety users. Users with low anxiety levels focus more on usability aspects.

We can observe in Table 3 that all types of anxiety are positively correlated with each other and are negatively correlated with emotion regulation. These findings support our hypothesis and it can be argued that our theory concerning the relationship between anxiety and regulation has a logical meaning.

In Tables 4 and 5 we can see an even stronger relationship between emotion regulation and core and specific anxiety respectively. A statistically significant analysis of variance for each anxiety type shows that if we categorize the participants according to their emotional regulation ability, then the anxiety means vary significantly with the high regulation group scoring much higher than the low one.

Finally, in Table 6 we can see that the two conditions (matched aesthetics/mismatched aesthetics) are differentiating the sample significantly always in relation with performance. Participants in the matched category scored higher than the ones in the mismatched and additionally lower anxious (core or specific or both) scored higher than high anxious, always of course in relation to match/mismatch factor.

We also found that participants with low application specific anxiety perform better than participants with high specific anxiety in both matched and mismatched environments. Additionally, in categories that a certain amount of anxiety exists, match-mismatch factor is extremely important for user performance. Participants with matched environments scored highly while participants with mismatched environments had poor performance. Emotion regulation is negatively correlated with current anxiety. High emotion regulation means low current anxiety and low emotion regulation means high current anxiety. Finally, current anxiety is indicative of performance. High current

Figure 9. Aggregated differences in matched/mismatch condition

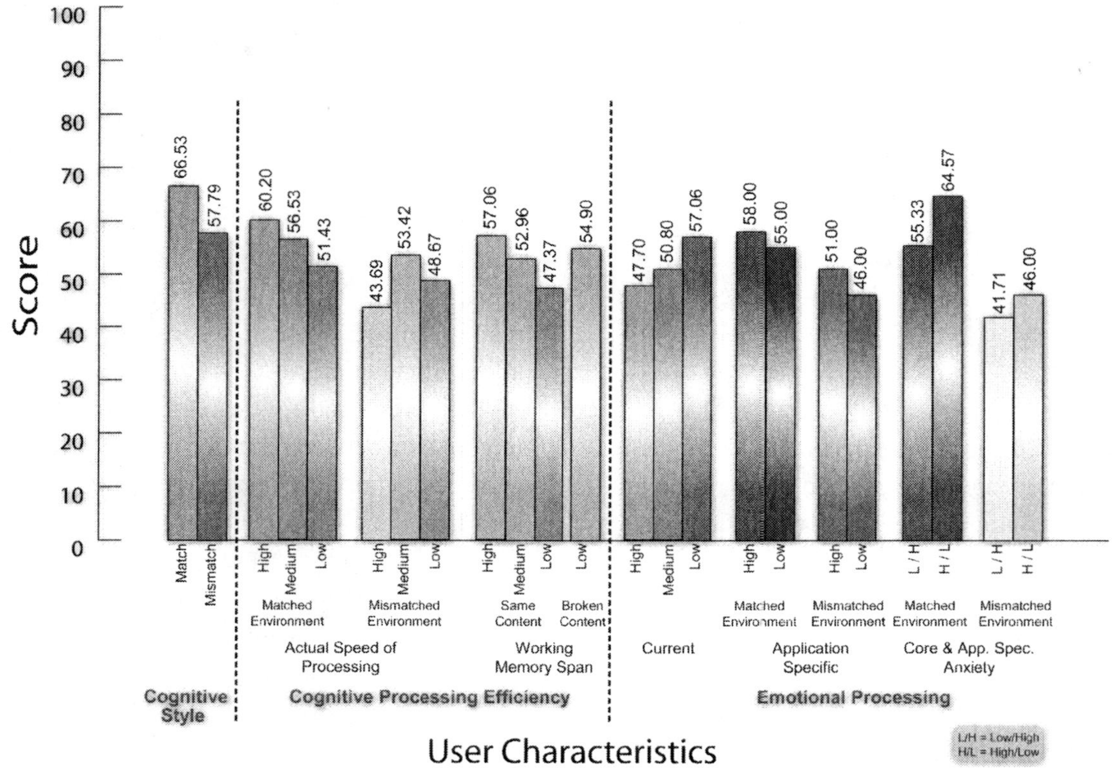

Table 2. Differences of means in the matched/mismatched condition for cognitive style and cognitive efficiency speed

	Match Score	Match n	Mismatch Score	Mismatch n	F	Sig.
Cognitive Style	66.53%	53	57.79%	61	6.330	0.013
Cognitive Processing Speed Efficiency	57.00%	41	48.93%	41	5.345	0.023

Table 3. Correlations of types of anxiety and emotion regulation

	Core Anxiety	**Application Specific Anxiety**	**Current Anxiety**	**Emotion Regulation**
Core Anxiety	1	.613(**)	.288(**)	-.569(**)
Application Specific Anxiety	.613(**)	1	.501(**)	-.471(**)
Current Anxiety	.288(**)	.501(**)	1	-.094
Emotion Regulation	-.569(**)	-.471(**)	-.094	1

** *Correlation is significant at the 0.01 level (2-tailed).*

Table 4. Analysis of variance between emotion regulation groups and core anxiety means

	Sum of Squares	df	Mean Square	F	Sig.
Between Groups	4.316	2	2.158	18.554	.000
Within Groups	10.700	92	.116		
Total	15.015	94			

Table 5. Analysis of variance between emotion regulation groups and specific anxiety means

	Sum of Squares	df	Mean Square	F	Sig.
Between Groups	8.345	2	4.173	15.226	.000
Within Groups	25.213	92	.274		
Total	33.558	94			

Table 6. Multifactorial ANOVA (factors-core anxiety, application specific anxiety and aesthetics)

Source	Type III Sum of Squares (a)	df	Mean Square	F	Sig.
MatchedAesthetics	1097.361	1	1097.361	4.238	.043
core_groups * specific_ groups * MatchedAesthetics	983.259	1	983.259	3.797	.055

Dependent Variable: Score %
(a) *R Squared = .102 (Adjusted R Squared = .017)*

anxiety means test scores below average while low current anxiety means high scores.

DISCUSSION AND CONCLUSION

Adaptive Hypermedia and Web personalization are two distinct well established areas of research both investigating methods and techniques to move conventional static systems beyond traditional borders to more intelligent, adaptive and personalized implementations. They share a common goal: to alleviate navigational difficulties and satisfy the heterogeneous needs of the user population by adapting according to user specific characteristics. In order to do that, the user profile construction is considered necessary.

The basic objective of this chapter was to make an extensive reference of a combination of concepts and techniques coming from different research areas, Adaptive Hypermedia and Web personalization, all of which focusing upon the user. It has been attempted to approach the theoretical considerations and technological parameters that can provide the most comprehensive user profile, under a common filtering element (User Perceptual Preference Characteristics), supporting the provision of the most apt and optimized user-centred Web-based result.

The proposed three-dimensional model (based on which the AdaptiveWeb system has been developed) seems to cover a wide area of human factors that are proven significant in computer mediated learning procedures, and may provide a basis for meaningful adaptation and personalization.

The current results of the evaluation, conducted in an e-Learning environment, show that it is possible to increase academic performance by taking into account cognitive and emotional parameters within the context of Web-based learning. Research in Adaptive Hypermedia often focuses on a single aspect of individual differences (such as cognitive style), resulting in limited effects on academic performance. However, the combination of multiple individual differences and emotional parameters in a comprehensive user model may promote effective learning, regardless of specific users' preferences and abilities, ensuring the success of e-Learning environments.

Also, the proposed model seems to cover a wide area of human factors that are proven significant in computer mediated learning procedures, and may provide a basis for meaningful personalization. Cognitive style is certainly of high importance, cognitive processing efficiency and Working Memory have an impact on the Web environment, and anxiety (as the main component of Emotional Processing) can be manipulated for optimization of performance. We believe that combining the level of anxiety of an individual with the moderating role of Emotion Regulation, it is possible to clarify, at some extent, how emotional responses of the individual hamper or promote learning procedures. Thus, by personalizing Web-based content, taking into account emotional processing, we can avoid stressful instances and take full advantage of his/her cognitive capacity at any time.

There are of course limitations in our approach, mainly due to the nature of the Web content that often limits radically differentiated adaptation, and the psychometric challenges of measuring a wide spectrum of human cognition and emotionality. The relationship between different dimensions of the model must be further investigated, and an experiment focused on the effect of working memory must be conducted.

There are of course limitations in our approach, mainly due to the nature of the Web content that often limits radically differentiated adaptation, and the psychometric challenges of measuring a wide spectrum of human cognition and emotionality. The relationship between different dimensions of the model must be further investigated, and an experiment focused on the effect of working memory must be conducted. Eventually, in order to further support the validity of the proposed model's effect, a number of experiments applied to Web information other than learning should be accomplished, identifying whether these parameters can be proven equally important in application areas such as news portals, e-Commerce, e-Services etc.

FUTURE RESEARCH DIRECTIONS

The initial evaluative results were really encouraging for the future of the current work since it has been identified that in many cases there is high positive correlation of matched conditions with performance, as well as between the dimensions of the various factors of the proposed model. This fact demonstrates the effectiveness of incorporating human factors in Web-based personalized environments. Synoptically, this holistic approach to information processing and learning in Web-based environments will lead to the formulation of adaptation rules, personalization techniques, designing principles, assessment methods, new practices, effective semantically enriched educational content, affective system responses and generally the enhancement of hypermedia with exceptionally important human cognitive and emotional factor.

Future and emerging trends include the further investigation of constraints and challenges arise from the implementation of such issues on mobile devices and channels; study on the structure of the metadata coming from the providers' side, aiming to construct a Web-based personalization architecture that will serve as an automatic filter adapting the received content based on a comprehensive user profile; the incorporation of physiological measurements of emotions and anxiety in such a model, with the use of biometrical sensors; as well as the use of an eye-tracker tool to clarify the role of Visual Attention in Web-based communication environments.

Our future work will embrace all the above-mentioned future research opportunities and directions aiming to develop a system that will provide a complete adaptation and personalization Web-based solution to the users satisfying their individual needs and preferences.

REFERENCES

Adomavicious, G., and Tuzhilin, A. (1999). User Profiling in Personalization Applications through Rule Discovery and Validation. *In Proceedings of the ACM Fifth International Conference on Data Mining and Knowledge Discovery (KDD'99)*, 377-381.

Anderson C. et.al. (2001). Personilizing Web Sites for Mobile Users. *In Proceedings of the 10th Conference on the World Wide Web*, 2001.

Ayersman, D., J. and Reed, W., M. (1998). Relationships among hypermedia-based mental models and hypermedia knowledge, *Journal of Research on Computing in Education*, 30 (3), pp.222-238.

Bailey C., Hall W., Millard D., & Weal M. (2002). Towards Open Adaptive Hypermedia. *In Proceedings of the Second International Conference on Adaptive Hypermedia and Adaptive Web Based Systems*, Malaga, Spain, LNCS 2347, Springer, pp. 36-46.

Bandura, A. (1986). Social foundations of thought and action: A social cognitive theory. Englewood Cliffs, NJ: Prentice-Hall.

Barret, R., Maglio, P. and Kellem, D. (1997). How to Personalize the Web. *In Proceedings CHI 97.*

Barlow, D. H. (2002). Anxiety and its disorders: The nature and treatment of anxiety and panic (2nd ed.). New York: The Guilford Press.

Basilico J., and Hofmann T. Unifying. (2004). Collaborative and content-based filtering. *In Proceedings of the 21st International Conference on Machine Learning*, Banff, Canada.

Blom J. Personalization–A Taxonomy, ACM 2000. ISBN:1-58113-248-4.

Bogonicolos N. et al. (1999). ARCHIMIDES : an intelligent agent for adaptive-personilized navigation within a WEB server, *In Proceedings of the 32nd Annual Hawaii Intl. Conf. On System Science, HICSS-32*, Vol 5.

Boyle, E. A., Duffy, T., Dunleavy, K. (2003). Learning styles and academic outcome: The validity and utility of Vermunt's Inventory of Learning Styles in a British higher education setting, *British Journal of Educational Psychology*, 73, 267–290.

Brusilovsky P. and Nejdl W. (2004). Adaptive Hypermedia and Adaptive Web, © 2004 CSC Press LLC.

Brusilovsky P. (2003).From Adaptive Hypermedia to the Adaptive Web, G.Szwillus, *J.Ziegler (Hrsg): Mensch & Computer 2003: Interaktion in Bewegung, Stuttgart: B. G. Teubner, 2003*, S. 21-24.

Brusilovsky P.,and Peylo C. (2003). Adaptive and Intelligent Web-based Educational Systems, *International Journal of Artificial Intelligence in Education* 13, 156-169.

Brusilovsky P. Adaptive Hypermedia. (2001). User Modeling and User-Adapted Interaction, 11: 87-110.

Brusilovsky, P., Eklund, J. and Schwarz, E. (1998). Web-based education for all: A tool for developing adaptive courseware. Computer Networks and ISDN Systems. Proceedings of the 7th International WWW Conference, 14-18 April, 30(1-7), 291-300.

Brusilovsky, P. and Pesin, L. (1998). Adaptive navigation support in educational hypermedia: An evaluation of the ISIS-Tutor, *Journal of Computing and Information Technology* 6 (1), 27-38.

Brusilovsky P. (1996). Adaptive Hypermedia: an attempt to analyse and generalize, *In P.*

Brusilovsky, P. Kommers, and Streitz (Eds.), Multimedia, Hypermedia, and Virtual Reality, Berlin: Springer-Verlag, 288-304.

Brusilovsky P. (1996b). Methods and techniques of adaptive hypermedia, *User Modeling and User Adapted Interaction*, 1996, v6, n 2-3, pp 87-129.

De Bra P., Brusilovsky P., and Houben G. (1999). Adaptive Hypermedia: From systems to framework, *ACM Computing Surveys* 31(4).

Bulterman D.C.A., Rutledge L., Hardman L., & Ossenbruggen J. (1999). Supporting adaptive and adaptable hypermedia presentantion semantics, *Database Semantics* 8 Submission.

CAP Gemini Ernst and Young. (2004). Online Availability of Public Services: How is Europe Progressing? European Commission DG Information Society.

Cassady, C.C. (2004). The influence of cognitive test anxiety across the learning–testing cycle, *Learning and Instruction 14,* 569–592.

Chaffee J., & Gauch S. (2000). Personal Ontologies for Web Navigation, *ACM 2000,* 1-58113-320-0/00/11.

Chang, S. E. (2005). Computer anxiety and perception of task complexity in learning programming-related skills, *Computers in Human Behavior 21,* 713–728.

Cingil I., Dogac A., and Azgin A. (2000). A broader approach to personalization, *Communications of the ACM*, Vol. 43, No. 8.

Damasio, A. R. (1994). Descartes' error: Emotion, reason, and the human brain. New York: Putnam Publishing Group.

De Bra, P. and Calvi, L. (1998). AHA ! An open Adaptive Hypermedia Architecture. *The New Review of Hypermedia and Multimedia*, 4, Taylor Graham Publishers, pp. 115-139.

Delicato F., Pirmez L., and Carmo L. (2001). Fenix–personalized information filtering system for WWW pages, Internet Research: Electronic Networking Applications and Policy, Vol. 11, No. 1, pp. 42-48.

Demetriou, A., Efklides, A. and Platsidou, M. (1993). The architecture and dynamics of developing mind: Experiential structuralism as a frame for unifying cognitive development theories. *Monographs of the Society for Research in Child Development*, 58 (Serial No. 234), 5-6.

Demetriou, A. and Kazi, S. (2001). Unity and modularity in the mind and the self: Studies on the relationships between self-awareness, personality, and intellectual development from childhood to adolescence. London: Routdledge.

Eklund J. and Sinclair K. (2000). An empirical appraisal of the effectiveness of adaptive interfaces of instructional systems. *Educational Technology and Society* 3 (4), ISSN 1436-4522.

Eirinaki M., & Vazirgiannis M. (2003). Web Mining for Web Personalization, *ACM Transactions on Internet Technology*, Vol. 3, No. 1, Pages 1-27.

Felder, R.M., and Silverman, L.K. (1988). Learning and Teaching Styles in Engineering Education, *Engineering Education* 78: 674-681.

Germanakos, P, Tsianos, N, Lekkas, Z, Mourlas, C, and Samaras, G. (2007a). Capturing Essential Intrinsic User Behaviour Values for the Design of Comprehensive Web-based Personalized Environments, *Computers in Human Behavior Journal*, Special Issue on Integration of Human Factors in Networked Computing, doi:10.1016/j.chb.2007.07.010.

Germanakos, P, Tsianos, N, Lekkas, Z, Mourlas, C, Belk, M, & Samaras, G. (2007b). An AdaptiveWeb System for Integrating Human Factors in Personalization of Web Content. *Demonstration in the Proceedings of the 11th International Conference on User Modeling (UM2007)*, Corfu, Greece, June 25-29.

Germanakos, P., Tsianos, N., Mourlas, C., and Samaras, G. (2005). New Fundamental Profiling Characteristics for Designing Adaptive Web-based Educational Systems, *In Proceeding of the IADIS International Conference on Cognition and Exploratory Learning in Digital Age (CELDA2005)*, Porto, December 14-16, pp. 10-17.

Goleman, D. (1995). Emotional Intelligence: why it can matter more than IQ, New York: Bantam Books.

Graber, D., A. (2000). Processing Politics. Chapter 2, The University of Chicago Press.

Gulliver, S., R., and Ghinea, G. (2004). Stars in their Eyes: What Eye-Tracking Reveals about Multimedia Perceptual Quality, *IEEE Transactions on Systems*, Man and Cybernetics, Part A, 34(4), 472-482.

Henke, H. (2001). Applying Kolb's Learning Style Inventory with Computer Based Training.

Sharp, J. E. (1998). Learning Styles and Technical Communication: Improving Communication and Teamwork Skills.

Hjelsvold R., Vdaygiri S., and Leaute Y. (2001). Web –based personalization and management of interactive video, ACM 1-58113-348-0/01/0005.

Hong H. and Kinshuk. (2004). Adaptation to Student Learning Styles in Web Based Educational Systems, *In L. Cantoni & C. McLoughlin, (Eds.) Proceedings of ED-MEDIA 2004–World Conference on Educational Multimedia, Hypermedia & Telecommunications* (June 21-26, 2004, Lugano, Switzerland).

Kaplan, B., Farzanfar, R. and Friedman R.H. (1999). Research and Ethical Issues Arising from Ethnographic Interviews of Patients' Reactions to an Intelligent Interactive Telephone Health Behavior Advisor System, *In: Ngwenyama, O., Introna, L.D., Myers, M.D. and DeGross, J.I. (Eds) New Information Technologies in Organizational Processes: Field Studies and Theoretical Reflections on the Future of Work*, Boston: Kluwer Academic Publishers, 67-77.

Karat M.C., Brodie C., Karat J., Vergo J., and Alpert S.R. (2003). Personalizing the user experience on ibm.com. *IBM Systems Journal*, Vol. 42, No. 4, 2003

Kim W. (2002). Personalization: Definition, Status, and Challenges Ahead, Published by ETH Zurich, Chair of Software Engineering JOT, ©2002, Vol. 1, No. 1.

Kolb, A.Y., and Kolb, D.A. (2005). The Kolb Learning Style Inventory–Version 3.1 2005 Technical Specifications, Experience Based Learning Systems, Inc.

Kort, B., and Reilly, R. (2002). Analytical Models of Emotions, Learning and Relationships: Towards an Affect-Sensitive Cognitive Machine. *Conference on Virtual Worlds and Simulation (VWSim 2002),* [on-line]: http://affect.media.mit.edu/projectpages/lc/vworlds.pdf.

Lankhorst M.M., Kranenburg, Salden A., and Peddemors A.J.H. (2002). Enabling Technology for Personalizing Mobile Services, *In Proceedings of the 35th Annual Hawaii International Conference on System Sciences* (HICSS-35'02).

Lerner, J. S., & Keltner, D. (2000). Beyond valence: Toward a model of emotion specific influences on judgment and choice. *Cognition and Emotion*, 14, 473–493.

Lieberman, H. (1995). Letizia: An Agent That Assists Web Browsing. *In 1995 International Joint Conference on Aritifical Intelligence*, Montreal, CA.

Liu Y. and Ginther, D. (1999). Cognitive Styles and Distant Education. *Online Journal of Distance Learning Administration*, Vo. 2(3)..

McLoughlin C. (1999). The implications of the research literature on learning styles for the design of instructional material. *Australian Journal of Educational Technology*, 15(3), p. 222-241.

Mulvenna, M. D., Anand S. S., and Buchner, A. G. (2002). Personalization on the net 23using Web mining. *Communications of the ACM*, 43, 8 (August), 123–125.

Maglio P., and Barret, R. (2000). Intermediaries Personalize Information Streams, Communications of the ACM, Vol. 43(8), pp. 96-101.

Mobasher B, Anand S.S., and Kobsa A. (2007). Intelligent Techniques for Web Personalization. *Proceedings of the 5th workshop ITWP 2007*, held in conjunction with the 22nd National Conference in Artificial Intelligence (AAAI2007).

Mobasher B., DaiH., Luo T.,Nakagawa M., and Wiltshire J. (2002). Discovery of aggregate usage profiles for Web personalization. *Data Mining and Knowledge Discovery*, Vol. 6 (1), pp. 61–82.

Panayiotou C., and Samaras G. (2006). Mobile User Personalization with Dynamic Profiles: Time and Activity. *On the Move to Meaningful Internet Systems 2006: OTM 2006 Workshops*, PerSys 2006, Montpellier, France, October 29 - November 3, 2006. Proceedings, Part II, pp. 1295-1304.

Panayiotou C., and Samaras G. (2004). mPersona: Personalized Portals for the Wireless User: An Agent Approach. *Journal of ACM/ Baltzer Mobile Networking and Applications* (MONET), special issue on "Mobile and Pervasive Commerce", (6), 663-677.

Pazzani J. M. (2005). A framework for collaborative, content-based and demographic filtering. *Artificial Intelligence Review*, December 1999, vol. 13, no. 5-6, pp. 393-408(16).

Papagelis M., Plexousakis D., Rousidis D., and Theoharopoulos E. (2004). Qualitative Analysis of User-based and Item-based Prediction Algorithms for Recommendation Systems, CIA 2004: 152-166.

Papanikolaou K.A., Grigoriadou M., Kornilakis H., and Magoulas G.D. (2003). Personalizing the Interaction in a Web-based Educational Hypermedia System: the case of INSPIRE. User-Modeling and User-Adapted Interaction, 13(3), 213-267.

Perkowitz M, and Etzioni O. (2003). Adaptive Websites, Towards Adaptive Web sites: Conceptual Framework and case study, [on-line]: http://www.cse.buffalo.edu/~sbraynov/ seninar2003/ presenttations/adaptive.pdf.

Pierrakos D., Paliouras G., Papatheodorou C., and Spyropoulos C.D. (2001). KOINOTITES: A Web Usage Mining Tool for Personalization, *Proceedings of the Panhellenic Conference on Human Computer Interaction*, Patra.

Pithers R. T. (2002). Cognitive Learning Style: A review of the field dependent- field independent approach. *Journal of Vocational Education and Training*, Vol. 54 (11), pp. 117-8.

Pu P., and Faltings B. (2002). Personalized Navigation of Heterogeneous Products Spaces using SmartClient, © 2002 ACM 1-58113-459-2/02/0001.

Reed W. M., Ayersman D. J. and Liu M. (1996). The effects of students' computer-based prior experiences and instructional exposures on the application of hypermedia-related mental models. *Journal of Educational Computing Research*, 14 (2), pp. 175-187.

Riding R. (2001). Cognitive Style Analysis–Research Administration, Published by Learning and Training Technology.

Rossi G., Schwade D., & Guimaraes M.R. (2001). Designing Personalized Web Applications, ACM 1-58113-348-0/01/0005.

Sadler-Smith E. & Riding R., (1999). Cognitive style and instructional preferences. Instructional Science Volume 27, Number 5, September 1999, 355-371.

Salovey, P., & Mayer, J. D. (1990). Emotional intelligence. *Imagination, Cognition and Personality*, 9, 185-211.

Sapp M. (1993). Test anxiety: Applied research, assessment, and treatment intervention. Lanham, MD: University Press of America.

Schwarzer R. (1984). Worry and emotionality as separate components in test anxiety. *International Review of Applied Psychology*, 33, 205-220.

Shahabi C. and Chen Y. (2003). Web Information Personalization: Challenges and Approaches, *In the 3nd International Workshop on Databases in Networked Information Systems* (DNIS 2003), Aizu-Wakamatsu, Japan.

Shardanand U. and Maes. (1995). Social information filtering: Algorithms for automating "Word of Mouth", *Proceedings of CHI'95 -- Human Factors in Computing Systems*, 210-217.

Smith B., Caputi P. (2005). Cognitive interference model of computer anxiety: Implications for computer-based assessment, *Computers in Human Behavior 21*, 713-728.

Spielberger C. D. (1983). Manual for the State-Trait Anxiety Inventory (STAI). PaloAlto, CA: Consulting Psychologists Press.Spielberger, C. D. (1972). Conceptual and methodological issues in anxiety research. *In C. D. Spielberger (Ed.), Anxiety. Current trends in theory and research (Vol. 2).* New York: Academic Press.

Spielberger C. D. (1972). Conceptual and methodological issues in anxiety research. *In C. D. Spielberger (Ed.), Anxiety. Current trends in theory and research (Vol. 2).* New York: Academic Press.

Spielberger C. D., andVagg P. R. (1995). Test anxiety: A transactional process model. *In C. D. Spielberger and P. R. Vagg (Eds.), Test anxiety: Theory, assessment, and treatment (pp. 3-14).* Washington, DC: Taylor & Francis.

Thomas C. and Fischer G. (1997). Using agents to personalize the Web, *In proceedings ACM IUI'97*, pp. 53-60, Florida Usa.

Vozalis E., Nicolaou A., and Margaritis K. G. (2001). Intelligent Techniques for Web Applications: Review and Educational Application, *presented at the Fifth Hellenic-European Conference on Computer Mathematics and its Applications* (HERCMA), Athens, Greece.

Wang J., and Lin J. (2002). Are personalization systems really personal?–Effects of conformity in reducing information overload, *Proceedings of the 36th Hawaii International Conference on Systems Sciences* (HICSS'03), 0-7695-1874-5/03, © 2002 IEEE.

Wang K. H., Wang T. H., Wang W. L., Huang S. C. (2006). Learning styles and formative assessment strategy: enhancing student achievement in Web-based learning. *Journal of Computer Assisted Learning*, 22, 207-217. (SSCI).

Weber G. & Specht M. (1997). User Modeling and Adaptive Navigation Support in WWW-Based Tutoring Systems. *In Proceedings of User Modeling '97*, pp. 289-300.

Witkin H., Moore C., Gooddenough D., Cox P. (1977). Field- dependent and field- independent cognitive styles and their educational implications. *Review of Educational Research* 47, pp 1-64.

Yuliang, L. and Dean, G. (1999). Cognitive Styles and Distance Education. *Online Journal of Distance Learning Administration*, Vol. 2 (3).

ADDITIONAL READING

Baddeley, A.D. (1997). Human Memory: Theory and Practice. Psychology Press.

Cassidy S. (2004). Learning Styles: An overview of theories, models, and measures. *In Educational Psychology*, Vol. 24 No 4, pp. 419-444.

Cooley R., Tan P.-N., and Srivastava, J. (1999). Websift: the Web site information filter system, *In Proceedings of the 1999 KDD Workshop on Web Mining*, San Diego, CA. Springer-Verlag

Desikan and Srivastava. (2005). Mining Temporally. Evolving Graphs, *In WebKDD 2005.*

Eysenck, M. W. & Keane, M. T. (2005), Cognitive Psychology. Psychology Press

Gardner, H. (1993). Frames of Mind: Theory of Multiple Intelligences, Fontana Press.

Jin and Zaiane. (2004). Using Distinctive Information Channels for a Mission-based Web Recommender System, *In WebKDD 2004.*

Lewis, M. & Haviland-Jones, J.M. (2004), The Handbook of Emotions. Guilford Press

Linden G., Smith B., and York, J. (2003). Amazon.com recommendations: item-to-item collaborative filtering, *IEEE Internet Computing*, Jan/Feb 2003, Volume: 7, Issue: 1,pp. 76- 80.

Mobasher B., Dai H., Luo T., Sun Y., and Zhu J. (2000). Combining web usage and content mining for more effective personalization, *In Proceedings of the International Conference on ECommerce and Web Technologies (ECWeb).*

Nasraoui O. and Pavuluri M. (2004). Complete this Puzzle: A Connectionist Approach to Accurate Web Recommendations based on a Committee of Predictors, *In Proceedings of WebKDD- 2004 workshop on Web Mining and Web Usage Analysis*, Seattle, WA, 2004.

Nasraoui O., and Petenes C. (2003). Combining Web Usage Mining and Fuzzy Inference for Website Personalization, *In Proceedings of WebKDD 2003–KDD Workshop on Web mining as a Premise to Effective and Intelligent Web Applications*, Washington DC, August 2003, p. 37.

Picard, R.W. (1997). Affective Computing, MIT Press, Cambridge.

Spielberger C. D. (1983). Manual for the State-Trait Anxiety Inventory (STAI). *Consulting Psychologists Press*, PaloAlto, CA.

Wu K., Yu P. S., and Ballman A. (1998). SpeedTracer: a Web usage mining and analysis tool. IBM Syst. J. 37, 1 (Jan. 1998), 89-105.

ENDNOTE

[1] http://www3.cs.ucy.ac.cy/adaptiveWeb

Chapter II
Case Studies in Adaptive Information Access: Navigation, Search, and Recommendation

Barry Smyth
University College Dublin, Ireland

ABSTRACT

Everyday hundreds of millions of users turn to the World-Wide Web as their primary source of information during their educational, business and personal lives. The Web is an essential source of business-critical information but has also changed our personal lives, influencing the way that we learn, play, shop and socialise. During the course of a typical day an increasing number of us will interact with a variety of information services on the Web as we hunt for the information that we need. Very often these services will offer a number of alternative modes of information access and associated interfaces— navigation, search, and recommendation being the most common — each designed to help the user to efficiently fulfilling their current information needs. Navigation, search, and recommendation each have their own set of challenges when it comes to facilitating fast and efficient information access. In this chapter we will consider a number of these challenges and describe how they can be addressed by using techniques that allow information services to respond more intelligently to the needs and preferences of individuals and groups of users. Each challenge will be addressed in the form of a case-study focusing on one particular mode of information access (navigation, search, and recommendation) and an application scenario (mobile portals, Web search, and e-commerce), to describe how user profiling, personalization, and adaptive interface design can be combined to produce a more efficient and effective information service.

INTRODUCTION

The Web is an essential source of business-critical information but has also had a significant impact on our personal lives, influencing the way that we learn, play, shop and socialise. During the course of a typical day an increasing number of us will interact with a variety of information services on the Web as we hunt for the information that we need. Very often these services will offer a number of alternative modes of information access and associated interfaces–navigation, search, and recommendation being the most common–each designed to help the user to efficiently fulfill their current information needs.

One familiar mode of information access sees users *navigating* or *browsing* through pages of content, following an appropriate sequence of links to locate the particular item of content that they are seeking. Indeed, for a long time navigation was the dominant form of information access, especially during the early years of the Web, when most users began their information quest at the home page of a major portal such as Yahoo or AOL; information access on the Mobile Internet is still largely dominated by navigation-based portal access (Church, Smyth, Cotter, & Bradley, 2007). Today however, with significant advances in search engine technologies, navigation has largely given way, at least on the traditional Web, to query-based *search,* which is now the primary form of information access for most Web users. In contrast to navigation, search-based information access aims to engage the user in a more targeted information access session, requesting their current information needs, up-front, in the form of a query, and using this to select and rank pages that are known to be relevant to this query.

Navigation and search are examples of *reactive* modes of information access, in that they both respond to explicit user input (link selection or search queries). The third mode of information access, *recommendation*, provides an more *proactive* information access strategy in which content is automatically suggested to a user in the form of a set of recommendations or suggestions. Recommendation interfaces are now a routine part of many information services, especially e-commerce services, where they are used to make product suggestions to users based on either their past purchase histories or on feedback as an effective mode of cross-selling and up-selling.

Navigation, search, and recommendation each have their own set of challenges when it comes to facilitating fast and efficient information access. In this chapter we will consider a number of these challenges and describe how they can be addressed by using techniques that allow information services to respond more intelligently to the needs and preferences of individuals and groups of users. Each challenge will be addressed in the form of a case-study focusing on one particular mode of information access (navigation, search, and recommendation) and an application scenario (mobile portals, Web search, and e-commerce), to describe how user profiling, personalization, and adaptive interface design can be combined to produce a more efficient and effective information service.

The first case-study will focus on navigation in mobile portals and highlight how today's mobile users are faced with a significant navigation hurdle when it comes to accessing mobile content. We will describe recent research that speaks to the scale of this problem and describe an effective solution in the form of a technique that automatically adapts portal structure in response to user behaviour. Moreover, this particular solution has now been commercialised by *ChangingWorlds Ltd.* and is used by leading mobile operators to reduce portal navigation times by 50%, resulting in a significant improvement in the overall user experience and an increase in mobile portal usage by up to 30%.

The second case-study will focus on a critical challenge in Web search, namely how to help existing search engines cope more efficiently with the vague queries that are commonplace in Web search. We will describe a *community-based* search solution that works in concert with an underlying search engine, to adapt a result-list according to the learned preferences of a community of like-minded searchers. We will describe how this solution can identify and promote results that are likely to be more relevant to a given community of searchers. We will also outline the results of a recent trial in a corporate search scenario, which highlight how this form of promotion can lead to more successful search sessions when compared to a leading search engine.

Our final case-study will focus on recommender systems in an e-commerce setting. While recommendation technologies have been exploited to good effect when it comes to suggesting simple products, such as books or DVDs, we will argue the need for more sophisticated strategies when it comes to helping users in more complex product-spaces, where individual products are represented in terms of a set of features and where different users will be willing to make different compromises over these features. In particular we will look at the issue of harvesting feedback from users as a way to inform recommendation, and describe how recommendation techniques can be used not only to make product suggestions but also to offer users different feedback options with which to refine their recommendations. We will describe the development of a recommender system for selling digital cameras online and present the results of a recent trial, which highlight how our approach can produce more efficient recommendation sessions that lead to more satisfied consumers.

CASE-STUDY 1: INTELLIGENT NAVIGATION IN MOBILE PORTALS

Today the vast majority of mobile Internet content is accessed via the portals of mobile operators. For example, recent research (Church, Smyth, Cotter, & Bradley, 2007) has highlighted how more than 90% of mobile subscribers use their operator's portal as their primary source of content. Less than 10% of users avail themselves of search engines to locate off-portal content, despite the recent introduction of the leading Web search players (e.g., Google and Yahoo!) into the mobile arena. At the same time, mobile Internet usage has remained at relatively low levels with accessibility cited as one of the most critical barriers impacting user satisfaction and usage. In this case-study we describe and evaluate how the usability of mobile portals can be significantly enhanced by automatically adapting the structure of a mobile portal according to the needs and preferences of individual users.

The Click-Distance Problem in Portal Navigation

Mobile portals are examples of hierarchical menu systems (HMS) (Marsden & Jones, 2001), and long before the arrival of the mobile Internet different forms of hierarchical menu systems were studied extensively with respect to their general usability and navigation characteristics (Larson & Czerwinski, 1998; Miller, 1981; Zaphirs, 2000). Certainly the scale of the usability and navigation problems associated with mobile portals today, and the mismatch between user expectations and realities, has been highlighted by a number of recent studies (Chittaro & Cin, 2002; Ramsey & Nielsen, 2000), especially when it comes to the average length of time that it takes mobile users to navigate to content services within a typical mobile portal.

One way to measure the navigation effort required by users of a portal is to consider the number of navigation interactions that are needed from the user to access a typical item of content or service. The so-called *click-distance* model (Smyth & Cotter, 2002a, 2002b) assumes two basic types of navigation interaction–a menu select, where the user selects a specific menu option on a portal page and a menu scroll where the user scrolls up or down through a number of options on a portal page–and computes the click-distance of an item of content as the total number of menu selects and scrolls needed to access this item from the portal home page; see Equation 1.

$$ClickDistance(i) = Selects(i) + Scrolls(i) \quad (1)$$

Thus, large click-distances are indicative of protracted navigation times and recent studies illustrate the extent of the click-distance problem among modern mobile portals. For example, an analysis of 20 European mobile portals reported an average click-distance in excess of 16 (Smyth, 2002). Large click-distances are a fundamental feature of a one-size-fits-all approach to portal design and the only sustainable solution to the usability problem that this entails is to break with this tradition. Ultimately, portal click-distance can be greatly minimised by tailoring the portal for the needs of an individual user, so that content and services that are of interest to a particular user are near to the portal home page, and thus accessible with a minimum number of clicks. Less relevant content and services can be relegated to the outskirts of the portal.

Figure 1. The menu hierarchy (a) and hit-table entries (b) corresponding to a sequence of visits by a given user. (c) menu tree corresponding to the static, default portal structure

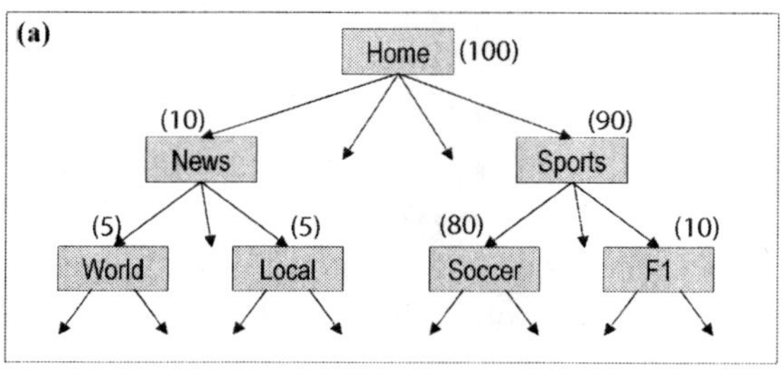

(b)

Home	(News 10), (Sports 90),...
News	(World 5), (Local 5), ...
Sports	(Soccer 80), (F1 10),...
...	....

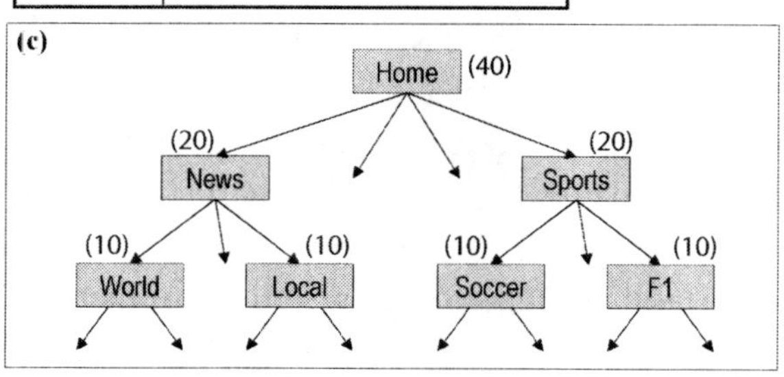

Recent research has made it possible to use *user profiling* and *personalization* techniques to learn about the preferences of individual users and this information can be used to automatically adapt the structure of the portal on a user-by-user basis. For example, if a given user regularly accesses her local cinema's listings then this content service can be made available from the portal home page (or at least nearby to the home page) rather than languishing deep with the portal structure. In general, personalization research seeks to develop techniques for learning and exploiting user preferences, to deliver the right content to the right user at the right time–see (Billsus, Pazzani, & Chen, 2000; Fu, Budzik, & Hammond, 2000; Perkowitz, 2001; Perkowitz & Etzioni, 2000; Reiken, 2000; Smyth & Cotter, 2000)–and in the next section we will describe how these ideas can be applied to the personalization of a portal structure to aid navigation effort; see also (Anderson, Domingos, & Weld, 2001; Smyth & Cotter, 2002b, 2002a).

Personalizing Mobile Portals

As users access a portal over time they build up a navigation history and this history can be very revealing with respect to their content preferences and information needs. By recording these access patterns–that is, by recording each sequence of menu options that are accessed–it is possible to construct an accurate picture of an individual user's navigation history (see also (Herder, 2003)) as the basis for a comprehensive user profile. The so-called *hit-table* data-structure is used to store this information for a given user; see Figure 1(a

& b) for an example of a partial menu tree and corresponding hit-table entries. A hit-table can be thought of as a simple hash-table, keyed according to the menu identifier, and storing the number of accesses made by that user to options within that particular menu. For example, Figure 1(a & b) reflects how one particular user has accessed the *News* section of their portal's home page 10 times and the *Sports* section 90 times, over a series of sessions. The hit-table entries can be used directly to compute the basic probabilities that a given menu option will be accessed within the portal. In fact, there are two important types of hit-table. The *user hit-tables* reflect the access patterns for each individual user. In addition, as shown in Figure 1(c) there is also a *static hit-table* that is maintained to reflect the portal's default structure. This static hit-table makes it possible to deliver the standard (default) menu structure (as developed by the portal designer) early on, but this will eventually be over-ridden by the personalized portals as the access probabilities build.

The core idea behind our *personalized navigation* technique is to use the access frequency data in the hit-table to generate a probabilistic model of user navigation preferences. This model can be used to predict the likelihood that some portal/menu option o will be selected by a user *u*, given that they are currently in menu *m*, and based on their past navigation history. Thus, we wish to compute $P_u(o|m)$, the access probability of *o* given *m* for user *u*, for all options o accessible from *m* (either directly or indirectly, through descendant menus). Put simply, when a user arrives at portal's menu page m, we do not just return its default options, $o_1,...,o_n$, which have essentially been hard-coded by the portal editor/designer. Instead, we compute the options, $o_1,...,o_k$, that are most likely to be accessed by the user from *m*; that is, the *k* menu options, accessible from *m*, which have the highest access probabilities. This can mean promoting certain menu options into *m*, options that by default belong to descendants of *m*. The size of the final personalized menu is constrained by some maximum number of options, *k*, and the constituent options of *m* are ordered according to their access probabilities.

This approach to personalization has been implemented and deployed as a core component of the *ClixSmart Navigator* mobile portal platform developed by ChangingWorlds Ltd. The basic process model to achieve this is presented as Figure 2 and includes the following sequence of steps:

1. The user requests a menu page from their mobile handset.
2. The request is forwarded by the WAP Gateway with the user's unique ID (MSISDN number) to the Device Manager, which

Figure 2. Constructing a personalized portal page

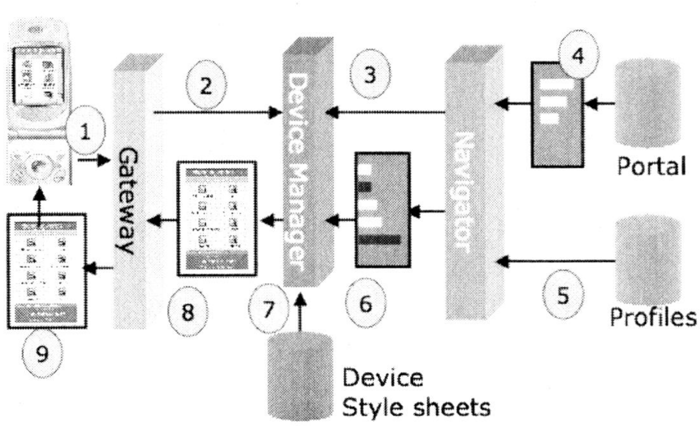

ultimately optimizes the content according to the features of the target handset.

3. The Device Manager recognises the device type and then forwards the request to the Navigator Server.
4. The Navigator Server examines the portal and requests the default menu content.
5. The Navigator Server examines the user profile database and requests the user's current profile if it has not already been downloaded.
6. The Navigator Server is responsible for the portal personalization and combines the static portal with the user's profile in order to construct the personalized portal menu by reordering and/or promoting content links.
7. The Device Manager reads the device style sheet for the user's device.
8. The Device Manager formats the personalized menu for the appropriate device and sends the response to the WAP Gateway.
9. The WAP Gateway forwards the personalized page to the user.

Obviously step 6 is the critical part of the process from a portal personalization standpoint: it is here that the personalized version of the particular menu, *m*, is generated. The Navigator Server component must determine how the default options of m should be ordered, and whether any of the menu options that appear below *m* merit promotion. Since portal style guides usually limit menu size, a means of ordering eligible options is required. One solution is to compute the *k* most probable options from *m*; that is the *k* options with the highest $P_u(o|m)$. Thus, the *k* options that are most likely to be accessed, given that the user is currently accessing menu *m*, are added to *m*. To do this we take account of the hit values listed for each option in both the static and user hit-tables, by using the recorded access frequencies as a way to estimate the necessary access probabilities. For example, given the data shown in Figure 1, $P_u(News|Home)$ is calculated as the combined relative access frequencies, taking actual user accesses and default static hit values into account. Thus, $P_u(News|Home) = (20 + 10)/(40 + 100) = 0.214$. Similarly, $P_u(World|Home)$ is calculated by chaining access probabilities so that $P_u(News|Home)P(World|News) = (20 + 10)/(40 + 100)(5 + 10)/(10 + 20) = 0.107$.

According to the above it is possible to calculate the access probabilities for all of the menu options that are accessible from *m* (in this case *m* is the portal home page). For the current example, in descending order of access probability we have *Sports, Soccer, News, F1, World,* and *Local*. And for $k = 3$, *Sports, Soccer,* and *News* are selected, in this order, for addition to the requested *Home* menu.

By way of an example, Figure 3(a) presents a series of portal pages leading the user to their local cinema listings via a number of intermediate menu options. Assuming that this becomes a well-traveled path for the user in question then we can expect the portal to promote the *Ster Century* cinema service to a more prominent position in the portal for that user. An example promotion scenario is presented in Figure 3(b) to illustrate this. The *Ster Century* option has been promoted to the top position within the Entertainment menu, reducing its click-distance significantly, by eliminating a number of intermediate portal levels. In addition, the *Entertainment* menu, within the portal Home page, has been reordered from position 5 to position 1.

In this way menu reorderings and promotions (and conversely demotions) are side effects of the access probability calculations and provide a fluid personalization scheme that gracefully adapts the navigation structure of a portal in response to a user's access patterns. The examples here have been kept simple for reasons of clarity, focusing on the promotion of single items, for example. Of course in reality there may be a number of content services competing for a limited number of promotion slots. In theory options can be promoted from anywhere deep within the portal structure

Figure 3. (a) An example sequence of navigation steps through a series of portal pages leading the user to their local cinema listings (Ster Century) via a number of intermediate menu options. (b) An example personalization scenario is presented in which the Ster Century service has been promoted to the top position within the Entertainment menu. In addition, the Entertainment menu has been promoted within the portal Home page, from position 5 to position 1

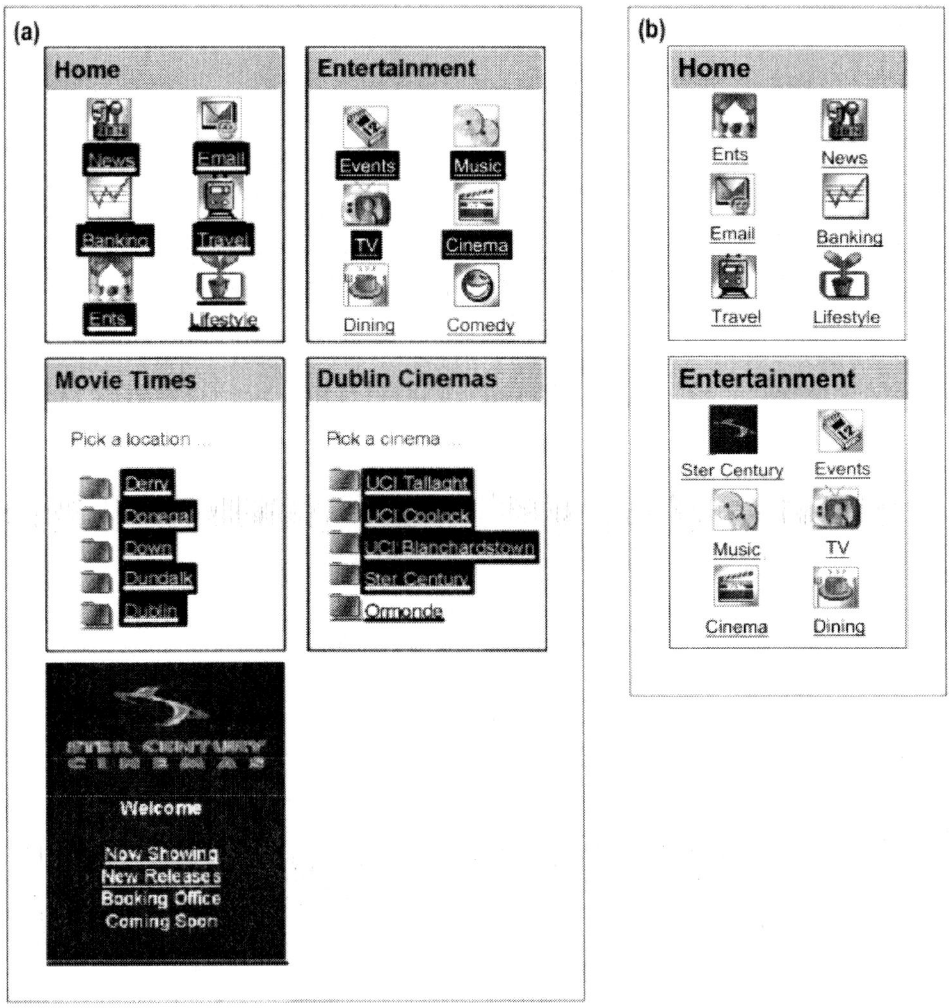

once their probabilities build sufficiently, although in practice certain limits may be necessary to control the speed and scope of personalization; see (Smyth, Cotter, & Oman, 2007). It is worth noting that the above focuses solely on the issue of menu reordering as a basic form of user interface adaptation. However, it remains silent with respect to other more ambitious forms of interface adaptation that might, for example, involve the adaptation of mobile content itself.

Evaluation

The personalization technology described in this case-study has been deployed widely by many of the world's leading mobile operators. One of the benefits of this activity has been the ability to carefully evaluate the impact of personalization on live-users in realistic usage scenarios. The evaluation results presented in this section are drawn from one recent trial with a major

European operator. For the purpose of the trial, a mirror of the standard operator portal was managed by the ClixSmart platform, offering portal personalization to a group of almost 900 test users, who were selected at random. The usage patterns of these test users were tracked during an 8-week trial period and compared to the usage of the remaining subscriber-base, which served as a control group.

The usage results are presented in Figures 4(a-d) and show very significant benefits associated with the activity levels of the test group, relative to the control. For example, in Figure 4(a) we see how the test group enjoys a gradual decline in their average session click-distance over the trial period. To begin with the typical user required an average of 8.7 clicks to access content but by the end of the trial this had dropped by more than 30% to 5.9; indeed our studies indicate that on average click-distance will typically fall by about 50% over a 3 month period.

Figures 4(b-d) highlight certain key activity indicators of particular interest to mobile operators. In this instance we have graphed the average increase in activity for each group of users during the 8-week trial period compared to the previous 8-weeks pre-trial. For example, in Figure 4(b) we compare the change in the average number of users accessing the portal during a typical week. The results show that the test group using the personalized portal increased their activity levels by more than 100% between the 8-week pre-trial period and the 8-weeks during the trial; during the 8-week pre-trial period an average of

Figure 4. Key evaluation metrics: (a) average session click-distance for test users during each of the 8 trial weeks; (b) average comparative increase in the number of users accessing the portal on a weekly basis; (c) average comparative increase in the number of user sessions; (d) average comparative increase in the number of page requests

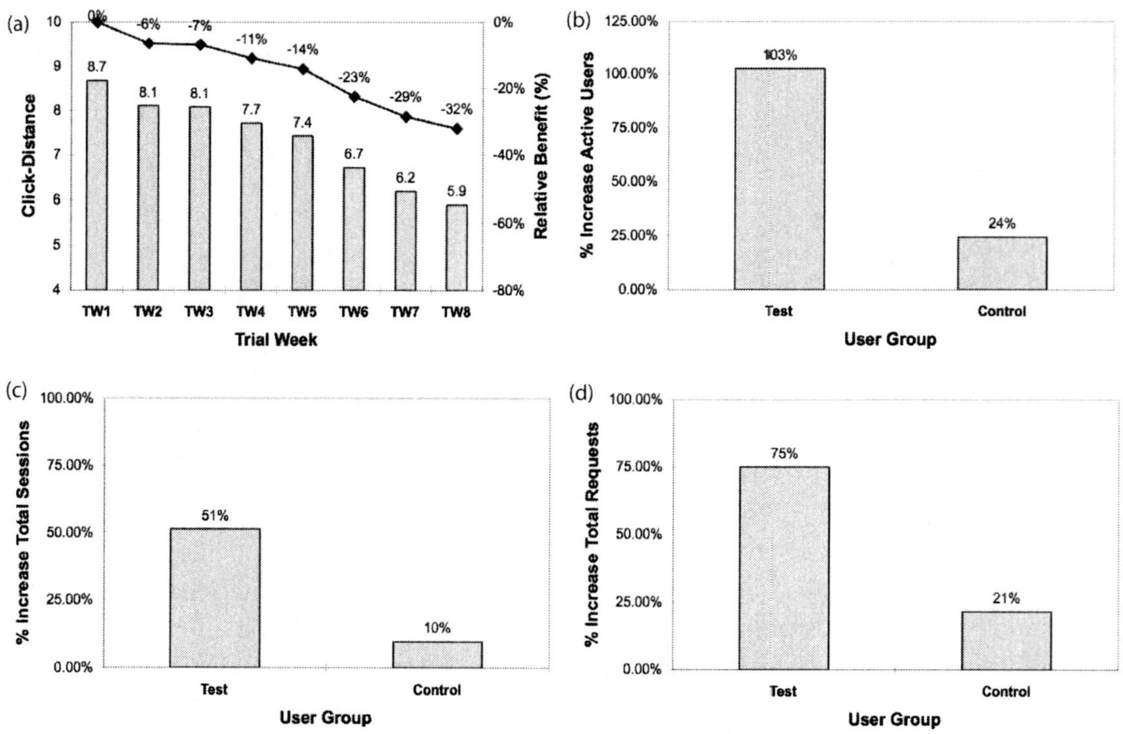

just over 140 of the test users access the portal on a weekly basis and this rose to just under 290 users during the trial period. In contrast, during the same period of time the average increase in the activity of the control group increased by only 24%.

Similar increases are seen across other key metrics such as number of sessions (Figure 4(c)) and total requests (Figure 4(d)). For instance, we see a 54% (75%-21%) relative increase in the average total weekly requests generated by the test users compared to the control group. In other words, despite the fact that click-distance was falling for the test users during the trial–so they were generating fewer navigation requests–these users were generating an increased proportion of content requests. It is worth noting that at the time of this trial the operator in question employed a request-based charging model, whereby users were charged on the basis of requests. Therefore this benefit can be linked directly to an expected uplift in revenue for the operator.

CASE-STUDY 2: COMMUNITY-BASED PERSONALIZATION FOR WEB SEARCH

While navigation dominates information access on mobile devices, query-based search has come to play the dominant role in the more traditional Web. Web search is especially challenging for a variety of reasons. For a start the sheer scale and heterogeneity of the Web represents a significant information access challenge in and of itself. Recent estimates of the Web's current size speak about a rapidly growing, distributed, and diverse repository of 10s of billions of publicly accessible information items, from the largely text-based content of HTML Web pages, PDFs and blogs to less structured content such as photos, video and podcasts; see (Lyman & Varian, 2003; Roush, 2004).

Web search is made all the more difficult because of the nature of Web searchers and their queries. Today's typical Web searcher is a far cry from the information retrieval (IR) expert contemplated by the IR engines that lie at the core of modern search engines. Web searchers cannot be relied upon to produce high quality queries: typically they are vague and ambiguous, with the average query containing only about 2 query terms (Lawrence & Giles, 1998). Moreover, people use a wide variety of terms to refer to the same types of information (Furnas, Landauer, Gomez, & Dumais, 1987) and as a result there is often a mismatch between the terms found in search queries and the terms found within the documents being sought.

This case-study will focus on our recent work on these so-called vague query and vocabulary gap problems. Our approach has been to re-cast the traditional document-centric view of Web search to emphasize instead the vital role that Web searchers themselves can play in solving the search problem. In short, we argue that it is useful to think of Web search as a social activity in which ad-hoc communities of like-minded searchers tend to search for similar types of information in similar ways. And we demonstrate that by capturing the search experience of such communities it is possible to adapt traditional (general-purpose) search engines so that they can respond more effectively to the needs of different communities of searchers, even in the face of vague queries. For example, when a member of a motoring community is searching for "jordan pictures" he/she is likely to select results related to the Formula One racing team, instead of alternative interpretations such as pictures of the Middle Eastern state or the UK fashion model, and the past search behaviour of other community members should support this.

In the following sections we outline our work on a community-based approach to Web search known as *Collaborative Web Search* (CWS); see (Smyth et al., 2005, 2004). CWS is a post-processing search technique that maintains a profile of the search patterns and preferences of separate communities of searchers. When responding to a new query by some community member, CWS uses the host community's profile to enrich the results returned by an underlying search engine(s) by identifying and promoting results that have been previously selected by community members in response to similar queries. We summarise recent results which highlight the potential for CWS to significantly improve the precision of the results returned by traditional search engines.

The Case for Community-Based Web Search

Collaborative Web search is motivated by regularity and repetition that is inherent in Web search, especially among the searches of communities of like-minded individuals: similar queries tend to recur and similar pages tend to be selected for these queries (Smyth et al., 2005, 2004). CWS proposes to exploit these regularities when responding to new queries by reusing the result selections from similar past queries. But just how commonplace is community-based search and how regular are community search patterns?

Even though most searches are conducted through generic search engines, many are examples of community-based searches. For instance, the use of a Google search box on a specialised Web site (e.g. a motoring enthusiast's site) suggests that its searches are likely to be initiated by users with some common (motoring) interest. Alternatively, searches originating from a computer laboratory assigned to 2nd year students are likely to share certain characteristics related to their studies (courses, projects etc.) and social lives (societies, gigs etc.).

Previous analyses of search engine logs have shown how query repetition and selection regularity is prevalent in community oriented search scenarios. For example, (Smyth et al., 2004) report how up to 70% of search queries from community searches share at least 50% of their query terms with other queries. Moreover, they show that there is a strong regularity between the selections of community members in response to similar queries: similar queries lead to similar selections. CWS takes advantage of this repetition and regularity by recording community searches (queries and result selections) and then promoting results that have been regularly selected in the past, by community members, in response to queries that are similar to the target query.

Collaborative Web Search

Figure 5 presents the basic architecture of collaborative Web search. Briefly, a proxy-based approach is adopted to intercept queries on their way to the underlying search engine and to manipulate the results that are returned from this engine back to the searcher. In this way users get to use their favourite search engine in the normal way, but with CWS promotions incorporated into the result-lists directly via the proxy. For example, consider a user U_i submitting query q_T to Google. This request is redirected to the CWS system whereupon two things happen. First, the query is passed on to Google and the result-list RS is returned in the normal way. Second, in parallel the query is also used to access a local store of the search activity for U_i's community–the CWS hit-matrix–to generate a ranked set of promotion candidates, R_P, as outlined below. These promotion candidates are annotated by the explanation engine to present the searcher with a graphical representation of their community history. Result lists R_P and R_s are merged and the resulting list R_{final} is returned to the user; typically this merge involves promoting the k (e.g., $k = 3$) most relevant promotions to the head of the result-list.

Thus for a target search query, CWS combines a default result-list, R_S, from a standard search engine, with a set of recommended (promoted) results, R_p, drawn from the community's past search history. To do this the search histories of a

Figure 5. Proxy architecture for a CWS system

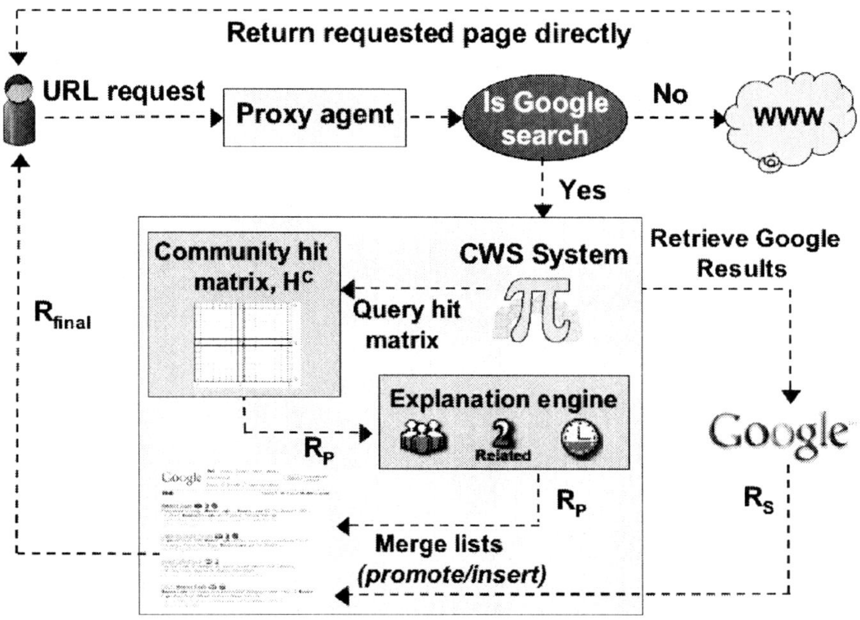

given community, C, of users ($C = \{U_1, ..., U_n\}$) are stored in a *hit-matrix*, H^C, such that each row corresponds C to some query qi and each column to some selected result page p_j. The value stored in H^C_{ij} refers to the number of times that page p_j has been selected for query q_i by members of C. In this way, each hit-matrix acts as a repository of community search experiences: the results that the community members have found to be relevant for their queries.

$$Relevance(p_j, q_i) = \frac{H_{ij}}{\sum_{\forall j} H_{ij}} \quad (2)$$

$$Sim(q, q') = \frac{|q \cap q'|}{|q \cup q'|} \quad (3)$$

$$W\,Rel(p_j, q_T, q_1, ..., q_n) = \frac{\sum_{i=1...n} Relevance(p_j, q_i) \bullet Sim(q_T, q_i)}{\sum_{i=1...n} Exists(p_j, q_i) \bullet Sim(q_T, q_i)} \quad (4)$$

When responding to a new target query, q_T, H^C is used to identify and rank results that have been regularly selected in the past. The relevance of a result pj in relation to a query *qi* can be estimated by the relative frequency that p_j has been selected for q_i in the past, as shown in Equation 2. More generally, we can pool the results that have been selected for queries that are similar to q_T (see Equation 3) and rank each result according to the weighted model of relevance shown in Figure 4, which weights each individual result's relevance by the similarity of the associated query to q_T.

Figures 6 and 7 present sample screenshots of the result-list returned by Google for the query '*Michael Jordan*'. In the case of Figure 6 we see the default Google result-list, with results for the basketball star clearly dominating. In Figure 7, however, we see a result-list that has been modified by our proxy-based version of CWS, trained by (in this example) a community of computer science researchers. The results are presented through the standard Google interface but we see that the top 3 results are promotions for the well-known Berkeley professor, which are more

Figure 6. The result list returned by a search engine in response to the query 'Michael Jordan'

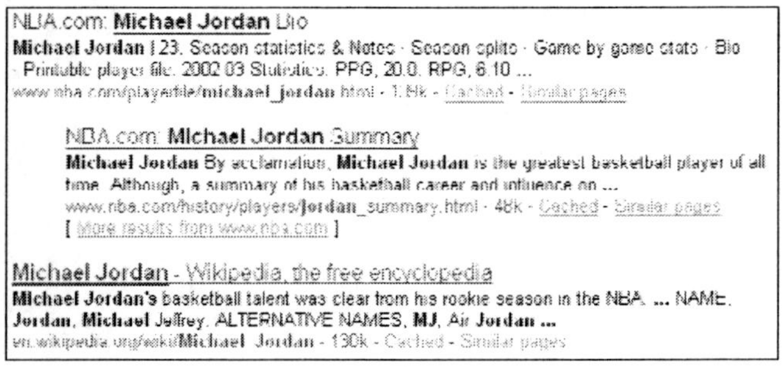

Figure 7. The result list returned by CWS in response to the query `michael jordan' issued within a community with a shared interest in computer science. The extra explanation information available by mousing-over each promoted result icon type is also shown

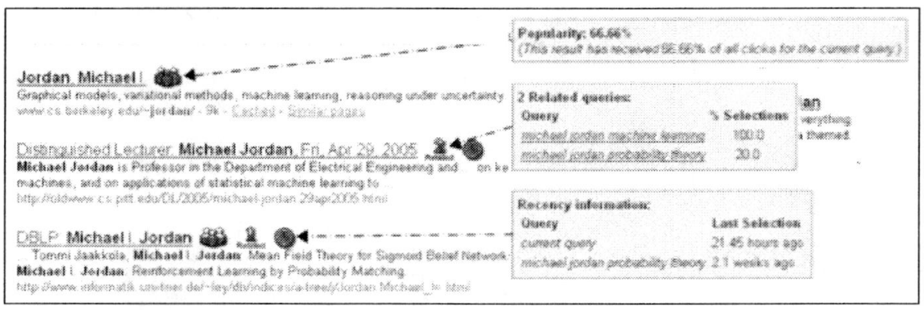

relevant to this particular community of searchers. In addition, promoted results are annotated with explanation icons that have been designed to capture different aspects of the result's community history. These include icons that capture the popularity of the result among community members, information about how recently it has been selected, and information about the other queries that have led to its selection.

It is worth highlighting here that the above approach, while community-based, has remained relatively silent on the origin of communities or the precise mechanisms by which community membership, for a searcher, are determined. In this research we have focused on a number of straightforward ways to associate users with communities. For example, in the evaluation that follows we will discuss a well-defined community of people who are employed by the same company. Other community types, referred to above, include the visitors to a themed web-site. Going forward there is an interesting research challenge to be addressed, involving the identification and discovery of dynamic communities of Web users, which we shall briefly discuss in a future section.

Evaluation

The current proxy-based architecture has been used as the basis of a long-term trial of the CWS approach in a corporate search scenario. In this section we will describe some recent results drawn from this trial, which speak to the value of the community-based promotions offered by CWS.

The trial participants included the 70+ employees of a local Dublin software company where the CWS architecture was configured to work with the standard Google search engine so that all Google requests were redirected through the CWS system. The search experience was based on the standard Google interface with a maximum of 3 results promoted (and annotated with explanations) in any session; if more than 3 promotions were available then non-promoted results were annotated with explanation icons but left in their default Google position. The results presented here are drawn from just over 10 weeks of usage and cover a total of 12,621 individual search sessions.

One of the challenges in evaluating new search technologies in a natural setting is how to evaluate the quality of individual search sessions. Ideally we would like to capture direct relevance feedback from users as they search. While it would be relatively straightforward to ask users to provide such feedback during each session or as they selected specific results, this was not feasible in the current trial because participants were eager to ensure that their search experience did not deviate from the norm, and were unwilling to accept pop-ups, form-filling or any other type of additional feedback. As an alternative, in this evaluation, we used a less direct measure of relevance based on the concept of a successful session (see also (Smyth et al., 2004, 2005)). We define a *successful session* to be one where at least one search result has been selected,

Figure 8. The success rates for sessions containing promotions compared to those without promotions

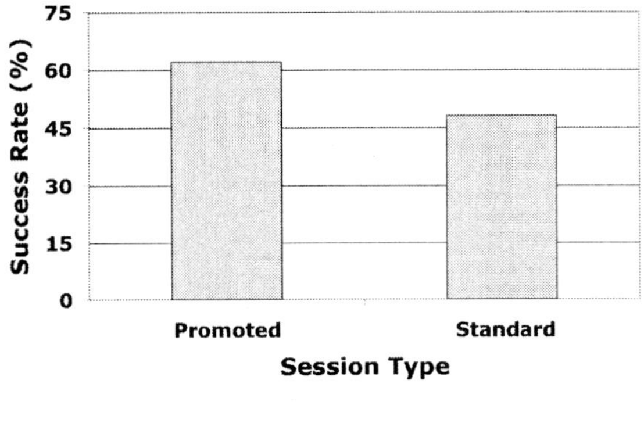

indicating that the searcher has found at least one (partially) relevant result. In contrast, search sessions where the user does not select any results (so-called *failed sessions*) are considered to be unsuccessful, in the sense that the searcher has found no relevant results. While this is a relatively crude measure of overall search performance it at least allows us to compare search sessions in a systematic way.

A comparison of success rates between sessions with promotions (promoted sessions) and search sessions without promotions (standard sessions) is presented as Figure 8. The results show that during the course of the 10-week trial, on average, sessions with promotions are more likely to be successful (62%) than standard sessions (48%) containing only Google results, a relative benefit of almost 30% due to the community-based promotion of results. In other words, during the course of the trial we found that for more than half of the standard Google search sessions users failed to find any results worth selecting. In contrast, during the same period, the same searchers experienced a significantly greater success rate for sessions that contained community promotions, with less than 40% of these sessions failing to attract user selections. Within an enterprise these results can have an important impact when it comes to overall search productivity because there are significant savings to be made by eliminating failed search sessions in many knowledge-intensive business scenarios. For example, a recent report (Feldman & Sherman, 2000) by the International Data Corporation (IDC) found that, on average, knowledge workers spend 25% of their time searching for information and an enterprise employing 1,000 knowledge workers will waste nearly \$2.5 million per year (at an opportunity cost of \$15 million) due to an inability to locate and retrieve information. In this context any significant reduction in the percentage of failed search sessions can play an important role on improving enterprise productivity, especially in larger organisations.

CASE-STUDY 3: DYNAMIC CRITIQUING IN PRODUCT RECOMMENDATION

So far we have described two case-studies focusing on very traditional forms of information access, namely navigation and search. Both are reactive information access techniques that respond to explicit requests from the user for information. Recommendation techniques provide a third alternative, promising a more proactive approach to information access by pushing suggestions to users without the need for an explicit information request or query. For example, Amazon (www.amazon.com) famously uses recommendation techniques to make product suggestions based on a user's purchasing history. Recommender systems, such as those used by Amazon, rely on single-shot recommendation techniques in the sense that the user is presented with a single set of suggestions. In this section we will focus on an alternative mode of recommendation in which users are engaged in an extended dialog with the user. Such conversational recommender systems are designed to help users navigate through complex information or product spaces. Typically they guide a user through a sequence of iterations, recommending specific items (or products), and using feedback from users to refine their suggestions in subsequent iterations (Burke, Hammond, & Young, 1997; McGinty & Smyth, 2002, 2003a, 2003b). For example, when shopping for a new digital camera a conversational recommender system will present a sequence of suggestions and ask the user to provide feedback on each suggestion; for instance, the user might be asked to rate each suggested camera or they might be given the opportunity to provide feedback on a particular feature of a suggested camera. This feedback is then used to inform the next recommendation cycle.

One common form of feedback is called *critiquing*: the user indicates a preference over a particular feature of a recommended item. For example, when shopping for a PC a user might indicate that they like the current suggestion but they are looking for something "*cheaper*"; "*cheaper*" is a critique over the price feature of the PC case. Critiques were originally proposed by the well-known FindMe recommender systems (Burke et al., 1997) and we will focus on the use of critiquing in this case-study. Normally, critiquing-based recommender systems rely on unit critiques (that is, critiques over individual product features), but sometimes it is useful to be able to critique multiple features simultaneously. Such multiple-feature critiques are called compound critiques and they potentially allow the user to navigate more efficiently through a complex product space. For example, a PC shopper may ask for a "*more powerful*" model if they are looking for a faster processor, more memory and a larger hard-disk; in this case the user can provide feedback on 3 features (processor speed, memory, hard-disk) simultaneously. In the past, some recommender systems have attempted to harness the power of compound critiques by pre-defining a fixed set of critiques to offer to the user. However, such an approach lacks flexibility and in complex product domains it may be useful to create more relevant compound critiques on the fly to avail of the additional feedback information that they offer. Thus, in this case-study we describe recent work investigating how a recommender can help a user to more effectively navigate a complex product space by automatically generating and suggesting novel feedback options to the user based on their current *recommendation session*. We will describe how data mining techniques can be used to automatically discover useful compound critiques during a recommendation session and how these critiques can lead to improved recommendation efficiency in practical recommendation scenarios.

Figure 9. A digital camera recommender system that implements unit and compound critiquing

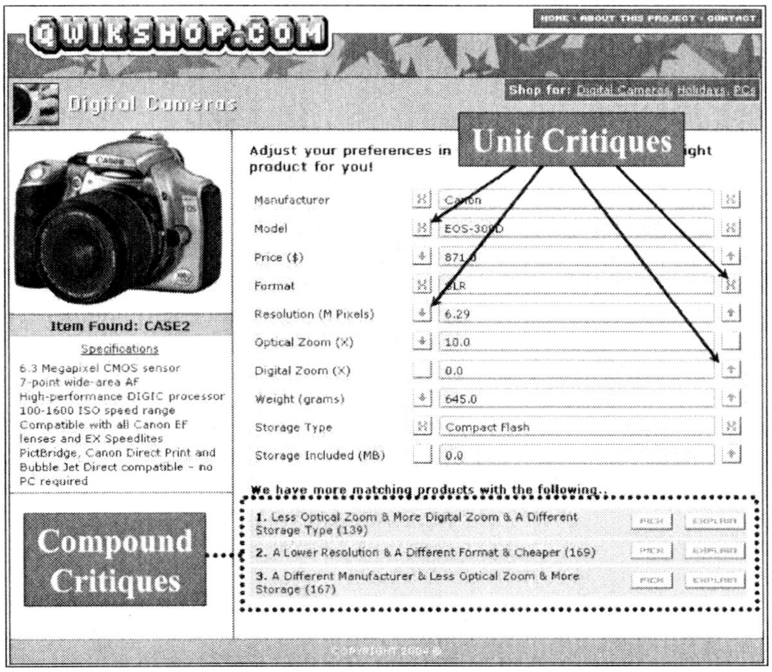

Dynamically Generating Compound Critiques

The research behind this case-study is motivated by the need to develop a more dynamic approach to critiquing, one in which compound critiques are generated, on-the-fly, during each recommendation cycle (Reilly, McCarthy, McGinty, & Smyth, 2004). Figure 9 shows a screenshot of a conversational recommender system that we have developed to showcase and evaluate this *dynamic critiquing* approach. This screenshot shows a snapshot of a particular recommendation cycle as part of a larger recommendation session. At this point in the session the user has been presented with a suggestion for a particular Canon camera and the camera's features are shown in the main panel along with their corresponding unit critiques; in what follows we will often refer to an individual product as product *case* and the set of products as a *case-base*, adopting terminology from the case-based reasoning and case-based recommendation literature (see for example, Smyth, 2007). The interface also includes a set of 3 compound critiques, which have been dynamically generated by analysing the features present among the cases that remain to be considered at this point in the recommendation session. In this case-study our focus is on the generation of compound critiques that are appropriate for the particular recommendation cycle and in this section we will describe how data-mining techniques are used to discovery, select, and rank interesting compound critiques that are designed to help the user to navigate more efficiently.

The first step in critique discovery is to generate a set of so-called critique patterns from the cases that remain in the current recommendation cycle. Each critique pattern reflects the differences between a remaining case and the current recommended case as a set of unit critiques. Figure 10 illustrates what we mean with the aid of an example. It shows the current case that has been selected for recommendation to the user as part of the current cycle and also a case, *c*, from the case-base. The resulting critique pattern reflects how case *c* differs from current case in terms of individual feature critiques. For example, the critique pattern shown includes a "<" critique for resolution–we will refer to this as *[Resolution <]*–because the comparison case has a lower resolution than the current recommendation.

Recurring sets of unit critiques within the critique patterns are candidates for compound critiques; for example, we might find that many of the remaining product cases are for cameras with a higher resolution and a lower price than the current recommendation. Discovering these recurring subsets is equivalent to the so-called market-basket analysis problem, where the task is to find regularities in the shopping behaviour of customers (Hu, Chin, & Takeichi, 2000) by identifying sets of products that tend to be purchased together: each critique pattern is equivalent to the shopping basket for a single customer, and the individual critiques correspond to the items in this basket. The combinatorics of a typical task domain–thousands of products and customers–make this a challenging problem, leading to an explosion in the number of possible groups of recurring items. However, it is not so acute in our critiquing scenario because there are only a limited number of possible critiques. For instance, each numeric feature can have a < or a > critique and each nominal feature can have a = or a *!=* critique, so there are only *2n* possible critiques in a product case-base where the product cases are made up of n individual features.

Previously (McCarthy, Reilly, McGinty, & Smyth, 2004a, 2004b; Reilly et al., 2004) we have shown how the well-known *Apriori* algorithm (Agrawal, Mannila, Srikant, Toivonen, & Verkamo., 1996; Hu et al., 2000) can be used to efficiently discover compound critiques as association rules of the form *A*→*B*: from the presence of a certain set of critiques (*A*) one can infer the presence of certain other critiques (*B*). For example, one might learn that from the presence of the critique, [Price <], we can infer the presence of *[Memory <]* with a high degree of probability; in other words the pattern *{[Price <],[Memory <]}* is commonplace. We use *Apriori*, during each recommendation cycle, to generate a collection of compound critiques (frequent itemsets over the pattern-base), and then select a small subset of the best of these compound critiques for presentation to the user to complement the standard unit critiques.

We can expect a large number of compound critiques, of different sizes, to be generated during a typical recommendation cycle. From a user interface and availability viewpoint it is obviously not practical to present large numbers of different compound critiques, as feedback options, to the

Figure 10. Illustration of how a sample critique pattern may be generated in the digital camera

	Current Case	Case c from CB	Critique Pattern
Manufacturer	Canon	Sony	!=
Model	Powershot S500	DSC-V1	!=
Format	Ultra Compact	Ultra Compact	=
Resolution (M Pixels)	5.1	5.0	<
Optical Zoom (X)	3	4	>
Digital Zoom (X)	4.1	4	<
Weight (grams)	215	298	>
Storage Type	Compact Flash	Memory Stick	!=
Storage Included (MB)	32	16	<
Price (Euro)	443.00	455.00	>

user during each cycle. For this reason a filtering strategy is needed so that we can select the most useful critiques, say the top 3, for presentation purposes. We have previously shown how the support values that *Apriori* generates can be used to select a subset of these compound critiques for presentation to the user (McCarthy et al., 2004a; Reilly et al., 2004). Very briefly, "support" is the percentage of patterns for which the rule is correct; that is, the number of patterns that contain both A and B divided by the total number of patterns. For instance, we would find that the rule *[Resolution >]→[Memory >]* has a support of 0.2 if there are a total of 100 critique patterns but only 20 of them contain *[Resolution >]* and *[Memory >]*.

Apriori is a multi-pass algorithm, where, in the *kth* pass, all large itemsets of cardinality *k* are computed. Initially frequent itemsets are determined. These are sets of items that have at least a predefined minimum support. Then, during each iteration those itemsets that exceed the minimum support threshold are extended. We have shown that presenting critiques with low support values provides a good balance between their likely applicability to the user and their ability to narrow the search (see (McCarthy et al., 2004a; Reilly et al., 2004) for further details).

Evaluation

In this section we describe the results of a recent live-user trial using our digital camera recommender previewed in Figure 9. We asked 38 postgraduate students to use the system and locate a digital camera that they would be prepared to purchase. They were provided with a brief description of the recommender interface, highlighting the use of unit and compound critiques during product navigation. During the trial the full selection and critiquing behaviour of each participant was recorded and at the end of the trial participants were asked to rate their level of satisfaction with the camera they decided to `purchase'.

To better understand the concrete benefits of compound critiquing, after the trial we divided the usage data into two groups of users, based on how frequently they availed themselves of compound critiques. The low-frequency group refers to those users who selected compound critiques less than 25% of the time (25% was the median compound critique application frequency) where as the high-frequency users are those who selected compound critiques 25% or more of the time. The average session length for each of these user groups is presented in Figure 11 and shows a clear and significant advantage for those users who tended to select proportionally more compound critiques. The low-frequency users used compound critiques just under 9% of the time on average and required almost 28 cycles per session before they found a satisfactory camera. In contrast, the high-frequency group used compound critiques 44% of the time and located a satisfactory camera with an average of less than 9 cycles. This represents an reduction in average cycle length, for the high-frequency compound critique users, of approximately 70% relative to the low-frequency users.

Figure 11. Average session length for low-frequency and high-frequency users

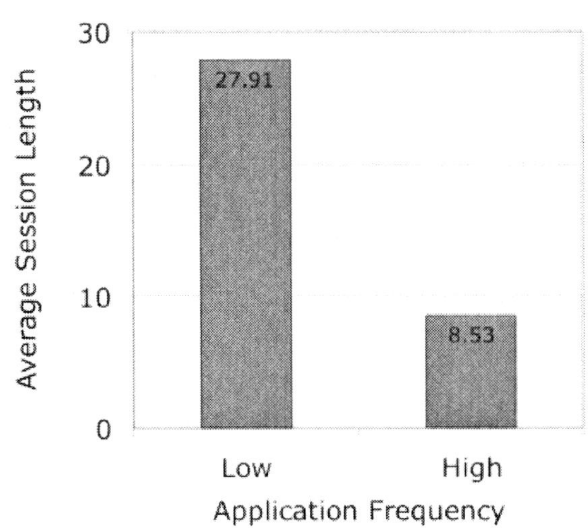

Figure 12. Average satisfaction rating for low-frequency and high-frequency users

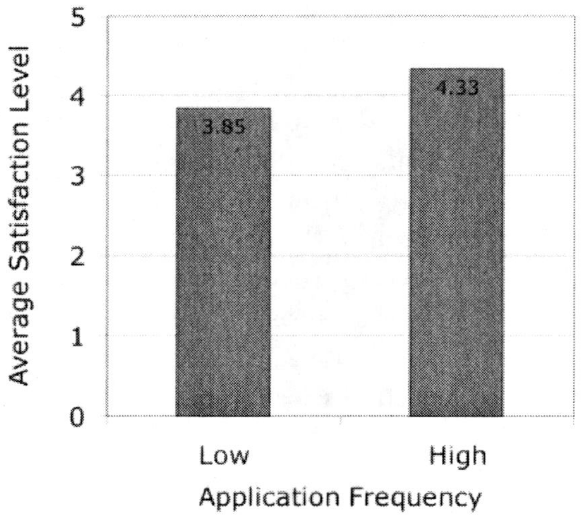

While these efficiency results are striking one might reasonably question whether it is fair to compare these user groups in such a direct manner. For example, it may be the case that the low-frequency users are simply more difficult to satisfy, or that longer sessions might result in more satisfied users. To investigate this issue we compared the two groups according to their average satisfaction rating, provided as part of a post-trial questionnaire. The results are presented in Figure 12 and clearly show that not only are the high-frequency users every bit as satisfied with their target cameras as the low-frequency users, they actually appear to be marginally more satisfied. The high-frequency users reported a 13% improvement in their satisfaction levels compared to the low-frequency users.

CONCLUSION

Helping people to access information more easily and reliably is an important challenge in today's information age especially as the demographics of Internet users broaden to accommodate a diverse range of user types and skill levels. Recent work in the area of personalization and adaptive user interface design has demonstrated how many traditionally one-size-fits-all information access paradigms can be adapted for the needs of individual users, and in this chapter we have described three case-studies as exemplars of this type of work in the areas of navigation, search, and recommendation. In each case-study we have described how a particular information access interface can adapt to the needs of its users in three different application domain scenarios: the mobile Internet, Web search, and e-commerce. And in each case-study we have evaluated the benefits of these approaches. It is worth noting how these 3 different case-studies also serve to highlight three very different types of "personalization" approaches. For example, in the first case-study on mobile portal personalization, long-term profiles were maintained at the level of individual users. The benefits of this approach included a more detailed understanding of an individual's long-term preferences with which to make personalization decisions. However, one of the potential disadvantages of such an approach relates to the privacy implications arising out of the profiling of individual users. In our experience mobile subscribers appear to be quite willing to "trade" their navigation preferences for an improved portal experience. However the same might not be true in other applications where personal information may be more sensitive. Web search is a good example of this–our search queries and result selections can be very revealing, much more so than our browsing patterns–and so in Web search, in an effort to protect the privacy of the individual searcher, we chose to profile at the community level. This community-based personalization of search results still offers significant benefits to the end user but at the same time allowed individual searchers to remain anonymous. Our final case-study adopted an even more privacy-sensitive approach to personalization by maintaining short-term (session-based) profiles of users only.

This allowed our product recommender system to adapt to the user within a particular session without the need to maintain persistent profiles in the long-term. Looking to the future it seems certain that personalization technologies will have an important role to play in providing users with more intuitive and proactive access to the right information at the right time. In only a few short years, for example, personalized recommendation technologies have helped companies like Amazon to significantly improve the accessibility of vast product catalogs. At the same time, related technologies have allowed mobile operators to greatly improve the usability of mobile portals. As the ability to access the right information at the right time will continue to dominate our personal and professional lives, the future of these technologies looks bright. However, in practice these technologies must be developed and deployed in a manner that gives due consideration to the privacy of the end-user. And so in every deployment we must consider the economics of personalization from a user perspective if we are to fully understand their willingness to trade a degree of personal information in return for an improved service. Getting this wrong, or ignoring it completely, will likely greatly limit the impact of personalization technologies going forward. Getting it right, on the other hand, has the potential to fundamentally change the way that users will access information online far into the future.

FUTURE RESEARCH DIRECTIONS

So far in this chapter we have described three important modes of information access–navigation, search, and recommendation–and three different examples of how these approaches can be adapted for the needs of individuals or groups of users. In each case we have highlighted the practical benefits of such personalization techniques. Of course these case-studies represents just three point examples of a diverse array of research in this general area of personalization. While many practical advances have been made over the past few years, many open problems and challenges still remain. In this section we will highlight some of the challenges as they relate to the particular case-studies presented in this chapter.

The case-study on collaborative web search highlighted the importance of communities of like-minded individuals and showed how the activities of these communities could be harnessed to improve search quality. This approach relies on the availability of concrete search communities. Sometimes identifying these communities is relatively straightforward; for example, a community of students in a class, a community of work colleagues, the members of a special interest group, or even just the visitors to a themed web-site. However, other times it is more challenging to identify online communities and today there is considerable research being invested in the development of a wide range of techniques for identifying potentially nebulous groups of related users online; see for example, (Dourisboure, Geraci, & Pellegrini, 2007; Goggins, Laffey, & Tsai, 2007; Zhang, Ackerman, & Adamic, 2007; Zhou, Manavoglu, Li, Giles, & Zha, 2006). Obviously this particular strand of research is especially interesting in the context of the collaborative web search technique but many open problems remain and recognising disparate groups of users who behave as a community remains a challenging task.

Groups of related users have always played an important role when it comes to the generation of recommendations; for example, collaborative filtering techniques generate recommendations from the ratings of groups of related users (e.g. (Konstan et al., 1997; Rafter, Bradley, & Smyth, 2000)). Recently, however, researchers have begun to look at the issue of how best to make recommendations for groups of users, as opposed to recommendations for single users; see (Jameson & Smyth, 2007). Generating recommendations for groups of users introduces a new set of problems because group members may have conflicting interests; for example consider the many competing needs of a group of friends trying to plan a group vacation. In response researchers have started to look at the different ways that group recommender systems can understand the trade-offs that might exist between competing recommendations with a view to encouraging compromise between group members where appropriate; see for example, (McCarthy, Salam¥, Coyle, McGinty, & Nion, 2006). This o work is still in its early stages but provides a rich new set of problems for recommender systems research, especially when it comes to the management of these trade-offs and compromises (see for example, (McSherry, 2003b, 2003a, 2004)and the complex interface issues that are introduced when groups of users must collaborate in the recommendation process.

Staying with recommender systems, it is worth highlighting another important strand of recent research activity on the importance of explaining recommendations to users; see for example, (Doyle, Cunningham, Bridge, & Rahman, 2004; Herlocker, Konstan, & Riedl, 2000; Reilly, McCarthy, McGinty, & Smyth, 2005). The basic premise is that it is not sufficient for a recommender system to simply propose a recommendation in isolation. Some attempt should be made to justify and explain these recommendations if users are to come to accept them as good suggestions. Researchers have now started to experiment with different types of explanation techniques and interfacing options with a view to better understanding how users respond to different types of explanation information. For example, the early work of (Herlocker et al., 2000) look at the use of a variety of different explanation types in the context of a collaborative filtering recommender system. Similarly, the work of (Coyle & Smyth, 2005, 2007a, 2007b) evaluate different forms of explanation information in the context of Web search. One interesting perspective to take on this line of research is that it emphasises the important role that the user interface can play in a recommender system. In the past the lion's share of recommender systems research has focused on the development of new and improved recommendation algorithms, with the primary goal being to improve the quality of the recommendations being made. More recently however researchers have started to consider the vital support role that the user interface can and should play in recommender systems.

On this issue of recommender interfaces it is worthwhile highlighting related work that focuses on how different styles of information access techniques might be integrated to provide a unified interface for recommendation, search, and navigation. For example, the work of (Farzan, Coyle, Freyne, Brusilovsky, & Smyth, 2007) look in particular at how search, navigation and recommendation techniques can be combined in the context of of a digital library and how users can benefit from different forms of recommendation support as they browser and search for information. This particular piece of work also touches on how this type of support can be delivered to the user in terms of the interfacing features needed to support the recommendation process.

In this section we have touched on a number of areas of recent research that remain early-stage but that highlight some interesting avenues for future research. These areas introduce new challenges and provide many new opportunities for significant developments in the coming years as we consider how information access technologies can be better adapted for the needs of individuals and groups of users.

ACKNOWLEDGMENT

This material is based on works supported by the Science Foundation Ireland under Grant No. 03/IN.3/I361. The author also gratefully acknowledges the support of ChangingWorlds Ltd and the assistance of Evelyn Balfe, Oisin Boydell, Keith Bradley, Paul Cotter, Maurice Coyle, Jill

Freyne, Kevin McCarthy, Lorraine McGinty, and James Reilly.

REFERENCES

Agrawal, R., Mannila, H., Srikant, R., Toivonen, H., & Verkamo., A. I. (1996). Fast Discovery of Association Rules in Large Databases. *Advances in knowledge discovery and data mining,* (pp. 307-328) MIT Press.

Anderson, C., Domingos, P., & Weld, D. (2001). Adaptive Web Navigation for Wireless Devices. In *Proceedings of the 17th international joint conference on artificial intelligence (IJCAI'01)* (pp. 879-884).

Billsus, D., Pazzani, M., & Chen, J. (2000). A learning agent for wireless news access. In Proceedings of the ACM conference on intelligent user interfaces (pp. 33-36).

Burke, R., Hammond, K., & Young, B. (1997). The FindMe Approach to Assisted Browsing. *Journal of IEEE Expert,* 12(4), 32-40.

Chittaro, L., & Cin, P. D. (2002). Evaluating interface design choices on wap phones: Navigation and selection. *Personal and ubiquitous computing,* 6 (4), 237–244.

Church, K., Smyth, B., Cotter, P., & Bradley, K. (2007). Mobile Information Access: A Study of Emerging Search behaviour on the Mobile Internet. ACM Transactions on the Web, 1 (1).

Coyle, M., & Smyth, B. (2005). Explaining Search Results. In *Proceedings of the 19th international joint conference on artificial intelligence (IJCAI '05)* (pp. 1553-1555). Edinburgh, Scotland.

Coyle, M., & Smyth, B. (2007a). On the community-based explanation of search results. In D. N. Chin, M. X. Zhou, T. A. Lau, & A. R. Puerta (Eds.), *Proceedings of the ACM conference on Intelligent user interfaces* (pp. 282-285). ACM.

Coyle, M., & Smyth, B. (2007b). Supporting intelligent navigation in web search. ACM Transactions on Internet Technology (TOIT). Dourisboure, Y., Geraci, F., & Pellegrini, M. (2007). Extraction and classification of dense communities in the web. In *WWW '07: Proceedings of the 16th international conference on world wide web* (pp. 461–470). New York, NY, USA: ACM.

Doyle, D., Cunningham, P., Bridge, D., & Rahman, Y. (2004). Explanation Oriented Retrieval. In P. A. G. Calero & P. Funk (Eds.), *Proceedings of the European conference on case-based reasoning (ECCBR-04).* Springer. (Madrid, Spain)

Farzan, R., Coyle, M., Freyne, J., Brusilovsky, P., & Smyth, B. (2007). Assist: adaptive social support for information space traversal. In S. Harper et al. (Eds.), *Proceedings of International conference on hypertext* (pp. 199-208). ACM.

Feldman, S., & Sherman, C. (2000). The High Cost of Not Finding Information. In (IDC White Paper). IDC Group. Fu, X., Budzik, J., & Hammond, K. (2000). Mining Navigation History for Recommendation. In *Proceedings of conference on intelligent user interfaces* (pp. 106-112).

Furnas, G. W., Landauer, T. K., Gomez, L. M., & Dumais, S. T. (1987). The vocabulary problem in human-system communication. *Communications of the ACM,* 30(11), 964-971.

Goggins, S. P., Laffey, J., & Tsai, I.-C. (2007). Cooperation and groupness: community formation in small online collaborative groups. In *Group '07: Proceedings of the 2007 International ACM conference on conference on supporting group work* (pp. 207–216). New York, NY, USA: ACM.

Herder, E. (2003). Modelling User Navigation. In *Proceedings of the 9th International Conference on User Modelling* (pp. 417-419). Springer-Verlag.

Herlocker, J. L., Konstan, J. A., & Riedl, J. (2000). Explaining collaborative filtering recommendations. In *Proceedings of the International conference on computer supported cooperative work*. 241–250.

Hu, Z., Chin, W., & Takeichi, M. (2000). Calculating a New Data Mining Algorithm for Market Basket Analysis. *Lecture Notes in Computer Science*, (Vol. 1753, pp.169–175) Springer-Verlag.

Jameson, A., & Smyth, B. (2007). Recommendation to groups. In P. Brusilovsky, A. Kobsa, & W. Nejdl (Eds.), *The adaptive web* (Vol. 4321, pp. 596-627). Springer-Verlag.

Konstan, J., Miller, B., Maltz, D., Herlocker, J., Gorgan, L., & Riedl, J. (1997). GroupLens: Applying collaborative filtering to usenet news. *Communications of the ACM*, 40(3), 77-87.

Larson, K., & Czerwinski, M. (1998). Web Page Design: Implications of memory, structure and scent for information retrieval. In *Proceedings of the CHI'98 human factors in computer systems* (pp. 25-32). ACM Press.

Lawrence, S., & Giles, C. L. (1998). Context and page analysis for improved web search. *IEEE Internet Computing*, July-August, 38-46.

Lyman, P., & Varian, H. R. (2003). How much information. Retrieved from http://www.sims.berkeley.edu/how-much-info-2003 on January 14th, 2005.

Marsden, G., & Jones, M. (2001). Ubiquitous computing and cellular handset interfaces are menus the best way forward? In *Proceedings of the south african institute of computer scientists and information technologists annual conference (SAICSIT)* (pp. 111–119).

McCarthy, K., Reilly, J., McGinty, L., & Smyth, B. (2004a). On the Dynamic Generation of Compound Critiques in Conversational Recommender Systems. In *P. D. Bra (Ed.), Proceedings of the 3rd International conference on adaptive hypermedia and adaptive web-based systems (AH-04).* (Eindhoven, The Netherlands)

McCarthy, K., Reilly, J., McGinty, L., & Smyth, B. (2004b). Thinking Positively–Explanatory Feedback for Conversational Recommender Systems. In P. Cunningham & D. McSherry (Eds.), *Proceedings of the European conference on case-based reasoning (ECCBR-04): Explanation workshop* (pp. 115-124). (Madrid, Spain)

McCarthy, K., Salamo, M., Coyle, L., McGinty, L., & Nion, B. S. . P. (2006). Group Recommender o Systems: A Critiquing Based Approach. In *Proceedings of the FLAIRS 2006 Conference* (pp. 1-16). Springer Verlag. (Florida, USA.)

McGinty, L., & Smyth, B. (2002). Comparison-Based Recommendation. In S. Craw (Ed.), *Proceedings of the th European conference on case-based reasoning (ECCBR-02)* (pp. 575-589). Springer. (Aberdeen, Scotland.)

McGinty, L., & Smyth, B. (2003a). The Role of Diversity in Conversational Systems. In D. Bridge & K. Ashley (Eds.), *Proceedings of the 5th International conference on case-based reasoning (ICCBR-03).* Springer-Verlag. (Trondheim, Norway.)

McGinty, L., & Smyth, B. (2003b). Tweaking critiquing. In *Proceedings of the workshop on personalization and web techniques at the International joint conference on artificial intelligence (IJCAI-03).* Morgan-Kaufmann. (Acapulco, Mexico)

McSherry, D. (2003a). Explanation in case-based reasoning: An evidential approach. . In B. Lees (Ed.), *Proceedings of the 8th UK workshop on case-based reasoning.* (Cambridge, UK)

McSherry, D. (2003b). Similarity and compromise. In K. D. Ashley & D. G. Bridge (Eds.), *Proceedings of the 5th International conference on case-based reasoning* (pp. 291-305). SpringerVerlag.

McSherry, D. (2004). Explaining the pros and cons of conclusions in CBR. . In P. A. G. Calero & P. Funk (Eds.), *Proceedings of the European Con-*

ference on Case-Based Reasoning (ECCBR04). Springer. (Madrid, Spain)

Miller, D. (1981). The depth/breadth tradeoff in hierarchical computer menus. In *Proceedings of the 25th annual meeting of the human factors and ergonomics society* (pp. 296-300).

Perkowitz, M. (2001). Adaptive web sites: Cluster mining and conceptual clustering for index page synthesis. PhD Thesis, Department of Computer Science and Engineering. University of Washington.

Perkowitz, M., & Etzioni, O. (2000). Towards adaptive web sites: Conceptual framework and case study. *Journal of Artificial Intelligence*, 18(1-2), 245-275.

Rafter, R., Bradley, K., & Smyth, B. (2000). Automatic collaborative filtering applications for online recruitment services. *In O. S. P. Brusilovsky & C. Strapparava (Eds.), Proceedings of the International conference on adaptive hypermedia and adaptive web-based systems* (pp. 363-368). Springer-Verlag.

Ramsey, M., & Nielsen, J. (2000). The wap usability report. Neilsen Norman Group. Reiken, D. (2000). Special issue on personalization. Communications of the ACM, 43(8).

Reilly, J., McCarthy, K., McGinty, L., & Smyth, B. (2004). Dynamic Critiquing. In P. G. Calero & P. Funk (Eds.), *Proceedings of the European conference on case-based reasoning (ECCBR04).* Springer-Verlag. (Madrid, Spain)

Reilly, J., McCarthy, K., McGinty, L., & Smyth, B. (2005). Explaining compound critiques. *Artificial Intelligence Rev*iew, 24 (2), 199-220. Roush, W. (2004). Search Beyond Google. MIT Technology Review, 34–45.

Smyth, B. (2002). The plight of the mobile navigator. MobileMetrix.

Smyth, B. (2007). Case-based recommendation. In P. Brusilovsky, A. Kobsa, & W. Nejdl (Eds.), *The adaptive web* (Vol. 4321, pp. 342-376). Springer.

Smyth, B., Balfe, E., Boydell, O., Bradley, K., Briggs, P., Coyle, M., et al. (2005). A live-user evaluation of collaborative web search. In *Proceedings of the 19th International joint conference on artificial intelligence (IJCAI '05)* (pp. 1419–1424). Morgan Kaufmann. (Edinburgh, Scotland)

Smyth, B., Balfe, E., Freyne, J., Briggs, P., Coyle, M., & Boydell, O. (2004). Exploiting query repetition and regularity in an adaptive community-based web search engine. *User Modeling and User-Adapted Interaction: The Journal of Personalization Research,* 14 (5), 383-423.

Smyth, B., & Cotter, C. (2000). Wapping the Web: A Case-Study in Content Personalization for WAP-enabled Devices. *In Proceedings of the International conference on adaptive hypermedia and adaptive web-based systems (AH'00)* (pp. 98-108). Springer-Verlag

Smyth, B., & Cotter, P. (2002a). Personalized adaptive navigation for mobile portals. In *Proceedings of the 15th European conference on artificial intelligence - prestigious applications of artificial intelligence.* IOS Press.

Smyth, B., & Cotter, P. (2002b). The Plight of the Navigator: Solving the Navigation Problem for Wireless Portals. In *Proceedings of the 2nd International Conference on Adaptive Hypermedia and Adaptive Web-Based Systems (AH'02)* (pp. 328-337). Springer-Verlag.

Smyth, B., Cotter, P., & Oman, S. (2007). Enabling intelligent content discovery on the mobile internet. In *Proceedings of the conference on innovative applications of artificial intelligence (IAAI/AAAI)* (pp. 1744-1751).

Zaphirs, P. (2000). Depth vs. breadth in the arrangement of web links. In *Proceedings of 44th annual meeting of the human factors and ergonomics society* (pp. 139-144).

Zhang, J., Ackerman, M. S., & Adamic, L. (2007). Expertise networks in online communities: structure and algorithms. In *WWW '07: Proceedings of the 16th international conference on world wide web* (pp. 221–230). New York, NY, USA: ACM.

Zhou, D., Manavoglu, E., Li, J., Giles, C. L., & Zha, H. (2006). Probabilistic models for discovering e-communities. In *WWW '06: Proceedings of the 15th international conference on world wide* web (pp. 173–182). New York, NY, USA: ACM.

ADDITIONAL READING

Burke, R. D. (2007). Hybrid web recommender systems. In P. Brusilovsky, A. Kobsa, & W. Nejdl (Eds.), *The adaptive web* (Vol. 4321, pp.. 377-408). Springer.

Chellappa, R. K., & Sin, R. G. (2005). Personalization versus privacy: An empirical examination of the online consumer's dilemma. *Inf. Tech. and Management*, 6 (2-3), 181-202.

Dou, Z., Song, R., & Wen, J.-R. (2007). A large-scale evaluation and analysis of personalized search strategies. In *WWW '07: Proceedings of the 16th international conference on world wide web* (pp. 581-590). New York, NY, USA: ACM.

Eirinaki, M., & Vazirgiannis, M. (2007). Web site personalization based on link analysis and navigational patterns. *ACM Trans. Inter. Tech.*, 7 (4), 21.

Flesca, S., Greco, S., Tagarelli, A., & Zumpano, E. (2005). Mining user preferences, page content and usage to personalize website navigation. *World Wide Web*, 8 (3), 317-345.

Gauch, S., Speretta, M., Chandramouli, A., & Micarelli, A. (2007). User profiles for personalized information access. In P. Brusilovsky, A. Kobsa, & W. Nejdl (Eds.), *The adaptive web* (Vol. 4321, pp. 54-89). Springer.

Goy, A., Ardissono, L., & Petrone, G. (2007). Personalization in e-commerce applications. In P. Brusilovsky, A. Kobsa, & W. Nejdl (Eds.), *The adaptive web* (Vol. 4321, pp. 485-520). Springer.

Gretzel, U., & Fesenmaier, D. (06-7). Persuasion in recommender systems. *Int. J. Electron. Commerce,* 11 (2), 81-100.

Kobsa, A. (2007). Privacy-enhanced personalization. *Commun. ACM,* 50 (8), 24-33. Lawrence,

S., & Giles, C. L. (2000). Accessibility of information on the web. *Intelligence*, 11 (1), 32-39.

Liang, T.-P., Lai, H.-J., & Ku, Y.-C. (06-7). Personalized content recommendation and user satisfaction: Theoretical synthesis and empirical findings. *J. Manage. Inf. Syst.*, 23 (3), 45-70.

Marchionini, G. (2006). Exploratory search: from finding to understanding. *Commun. ACM,* 49 (4), 41-46.

Massa, P., & Avesani, P. (2007). Trust-aware recommender systems. In *Recsys '07: Proceedings of the 2007 acm conference on recommender systems* (pp. 17-24). New York, NY, USA: ACM.

Micarelli, A., Gasparetti, F., Sciarrone, F., & Gauch, S. (2007). Personalized search on the world wide web. In P. Brusilovsky, A. Kobsa, & W. Nejdl (Eds.), *The adaptive web* (Vol. 4321, pp. 195-230). Springer.

Mobasher, B., Burke, R., Bhaumik, R., & Williams, C. (2007). Toward trustworthy recommender systems: An analysis of attack models and algorithm robustness. *ACM Trans. Inter. Tech.*, 7 (4), 23.

Pierrakos, D., Paliouras, G., Papatheodorou, C., & Spyropoulos, C. D. (2003). Web usage mining as a tool for personalization: A survey. *User Modeling and User-Adapted Interaction*, 13 (4), 311-372.

Recsys '07: Proceedings of the 2007 acm conference on recommender systems. (2007). New York, NY, USA: ACM. (General Chair-Joseph A. Konstan and Program Chair-John Riedl and Program Chair-Barry Smyth)

Resnick, P., & Varian, H. R. (1997). Recommender systems. Commun. ACM, 40 (3), 56-58.

Schafer, J. B., Frankowski, D., Herlocker, J. L., & Sen, S. (2007). Collaborative filtering recommender systems. In P. Brusilovsky, A. Kobsa, & W. Nejdl (Eds.), The adaptive web (Vol. 4321, p. 291-324). Springer.

Smyth, B. (2007). A community-based approach to personalizing web search. *Computer*, 40 (8), 42-50.

White, R. W., Kules, B., & Bederson, B. (2005). Exploratory search interfaces: categorization, clustering and beyond: Report on the XSI 2005 workshop at the human-computer interaction laboratory, University of Maryland. *SIGIR Forum*, 39 (2), 52-56.

Chapter III
The Effects of Human Factors on the Use of Web-Based Instruction

Sherry Y. Chen
Brunel University, Middlesex, UK

ABSTRACT

Web-based instruction is prevalent in educational settings. However, many issues still remain to be investigated. In particular, it is still open about how human factors influence learners' performance and perception in Web-based instruction. In this vein, the study presented in this chapter investigates this issue in a Web-based instructional program, which was applied to teach students how to use HyperText Markup Language (HTML) in a United Kingdom (UK) university. Sixty-one master's degree students participated in this study. There were a number of interesting findings. Students' task achievements were affected by the levels of their previous system experience. On the other hand, the Post-Test and Gain scores were positively influenced by their perceptions and attitudes toward the Web-based instructional program. The implications of these findings are discussed.

INTRODUCTION

Web-based instruction is prevalent in educational settings. The value of Web-based instruction lies in the capabilities of hypermedia, which permit significant flexibility in the delivery of non-linear course material (Khalifa & Lam, 2002). Students are allowed to learn in their own way—to determine their own path through the material available (Barua, 2001)—and to learn things at their own pace (Chen, 2002). However, the freedom offered by Web-based instructional programs may come with a problem, because flexibility increases complexity (Ellis & Kurniawan, 2000). Learners are forced to determine their own learning strategies and, therefore, will differ in their perceptions and approaches to learning. In particular, some learners who lack the skills of independent learning may find this difficult and become confused (Last, O'Donnell, & Kelly, 2001), so they may forget what they have already covered, and miss important information (McDonald, Stodel, Farres, Breithaupt, & Gabriel, 2001). This suggests that not all students will appreciate the flexibility and freedom offered by the Web and that human factors, therefore, are important issues to be considered in the development of Web-based instruction programs.

In this vein, the study reported in this chapter aims to investigate how human factors influence students' reactions to a Web-based instruction program. The chapter begins by building a theoretical framework to present the relationships between Web-based instructional programs and individual differences. It then describes an empirical study of students' learning experiences in a Web-based instructional program. Subsequently, the design implications are discussed based on the findings of this empirical study.

THEORECTICAL FRAMEWORK

Web-Based Instruction

Over recent years, the World Wide Web (Web) has been becoming a useful tool for information distribution (Sridharan, 2004). In particular, there is an increase in use of the Web for instruction (Evans, 2004). Web-based instruction provides a number of advantages, among which dynamic interaction and flexible schedule are two key items. In terms of dynamic interaction, Web-based instruction presents an enormous amount of information through various interconnections that offer students a rich exploration environment. The development of Web-based instruction provides learners with many opportunities to explore, discover and learn in theory according to their individual needs. Students can create individualized learning paths to reach the desired goals, move at their own speed and retrieve additional information as needed (Hui & Cheung, 1999). There is a shift away from didactic instruction to discovery of information (Smaldino, 1999). This approach is in line with the constructivist philosophy of learning, where the learner is encouraged to interact with the environment to construct individual knowledge structure (McDonald et al., 2001).

With regard to flexible schedule, Web-based instruction allows learners to read course content through a computer network at any time and at different places (Chang, Henriquez, Honey, Light, Moeller, & Ross, 1998). Burton and Goldsmith (2002) found that such a flexible schedule makes Web-based instruction appealing to students, including the convenience of not having to be on campus during the week, to easily arrange personal commitments and to take courses around work schedules. This type of learning may be particularly beneficial to individuals who live in remote places (Daugherty, 1998). Individuals living in remote areas can have access to the same course content as those living in big cities. This is why many educators have tried to develop a distance learning program on the Web. As pointed out by Clark and Lyon (1999), Web-based instruction has been predicted to be the future of all types of distance learning programs.

However, these advantages may come with a price. Power and Roth (1999) reported that Web-based instruction is more dynamic and flexible than other learning material, but it creates new challenges related to the effect on learners' comprehension. Ng and Gunstrone (2002) indicated that although students had positive perceptions to self-based learning provided by Web-based instruction, the unstructured nature of the Web made some students need more time to search information. Quintana (1996) stated that while students gained the advantage of flexibility in time, pace and distance with Web-based instruction, many students, on the other hand, felt isolated, lack of motivation, or lack of support and feedback consequently to drop out of the course. Hedberg, Harper, and Corrent-Agostinho (1998) indicated that some students are still working to come to grips with a new and difficult way of learning. They exemplify the concern by asking for more incentive, more time, more structure and more guidance. These studies provide evidence that not all types of students appreciate being given freedom in their learning processes. In particular, students who need more guidance through the learning process may meet an increased number of problems in using Web-based instructional programs. To address this limitation, Web-based instruction should be developed to support the unique needs of each individual learner (Carter, 2002). Only when their needs are identified can developers of programs effectively enhance functionality and increase learners' satisfaction (Ke, Kwakkelaarb, Taic, & Chenc, 2002). Therefore, understanding of learners' individual differences arguably becomes an important consideration in the development of Web-based instruction programs.

Human Factors

Human factors play an important role in learning. Individuals differ in traits such as skills, aptitudes and preferences for processing information, constructing meaning from information and applying it to real-world situations (Jonassen & Grabowski, 1993). The effects of human factors on students' task performance in a computer-based learning environment have been a growing research area (Wang & Jonassen, 1993; Ke et al., 2002). Among all human factors, gender differences (Ford & Miller 1996), domain knowledge (Mitchell, Chen, & Macredie, 2005) and system experience (Reed &Oughton, 1997; Chen & Ford, 1998) have been recognized as especially relevant factors to users' interaction with the Web. In terms of gender differences, previous research indicates that gender differences influence users' navigation strategies in Web-based instruction. Schwarz (2001) found that females and males request different kinds of support when locating particular information. Male users need a larger frame of reference, while female users ask procedural directions. The other study by Roy and Chi (2003) indicated that males tended to navigate in a broader way than females. They also found that males tended to perform more page jumps per minute, which indicates that they navigate the information space in a nonlinear way.

In respect of domain knowledge, research suggested that less knowledgeable users experienced more disorientation problems in Web-based instruction (Last et al., 2001). This may be due to the fact that they are unfamiliar with the subject matter of the text, so they cannot rely on prior knowledge to help them structure it. On the other hand, more knowledgeable users may experience fewer navigation problems because their greater grasp of the conceptual structure of the subject matter can enable them to impose structure on the Web (McDonald et al., 2001). In regard to system experience, novices and experts demonstrate different attitudes toward the use of Web-based instruction. Liaw (2002) found students' experience using the Internet to be a good predictor of their computer and Web attitudes. Furthermore, Torkzadeh and Van Dyke (2002) found the transition from low experience to high experience could improve Internet self-efficacy.

Results from these studies suggest that human factors play an important role in the use of Web-based instruction programs. These studies also indicate that further empirical works are needed to identify the learners' different preferences, and their results may help to guide the development and evaluation of Web-based instructional programs. This chapter presents such a study, which aims to examine how human factors influence students' reactions to a Web-based instructional program.

RESEARCH DESIGN

Web-Based Instruction Program

The Web-based instructional program, which was used to give an HTML tutorial, began by giving an introduction to the learning objectives and explaining the available navigation approaches provided in the instructional program. The contents were divided into three sections: (1) What is HTML? (2) Working with HTML, and (3) Relations with Standard Generalized Markup Language (SGML) and the Web. Section 2 is the key element of the Web-based instructional program, which covers 12 sub-topics of HTML authoring. Each sub-topic was further split into five parts, comprising (a) overview, (b) detailed techniques, (c) examples, (d) related skills, and (e) references. Information was presented in 82 pages using texts, tables, an index and maps.

As shown in Figure 1, the screen was divided using frames. In the top frame was a title bar showing the section name being viewed and the other available section buttons. In the left frame were the Main Menu, Index, Map and Quit buttons. The right frame displayed the main content for each section, including topic buttons and text-based hypertext links.

In terms of navigation control, the Web-based instruction program took advantage of the features of non-linear learning and provided students with freedom of navigation. Topics and sub-topics could be studied in any order. In other words, students were allowed to decide their own navigational routes through the subject matter. Three types of navigation control were available in this tutorial, as shown in Table 1.

Pre-Test and Post-Test

Examining students' learning outcome in theoretical knowledge was conducted by using a Pre-Test and Post-Test methodology. The students were evaluated with the Pre-Test to examine their levels of prior HTML knowledge, and with the Post-Test for assessing learning achievement. Both tests were presented in paper-based formats and included 20 multiple-choice questions. Only one

Figure 1. Screen design of the HTML tutorial

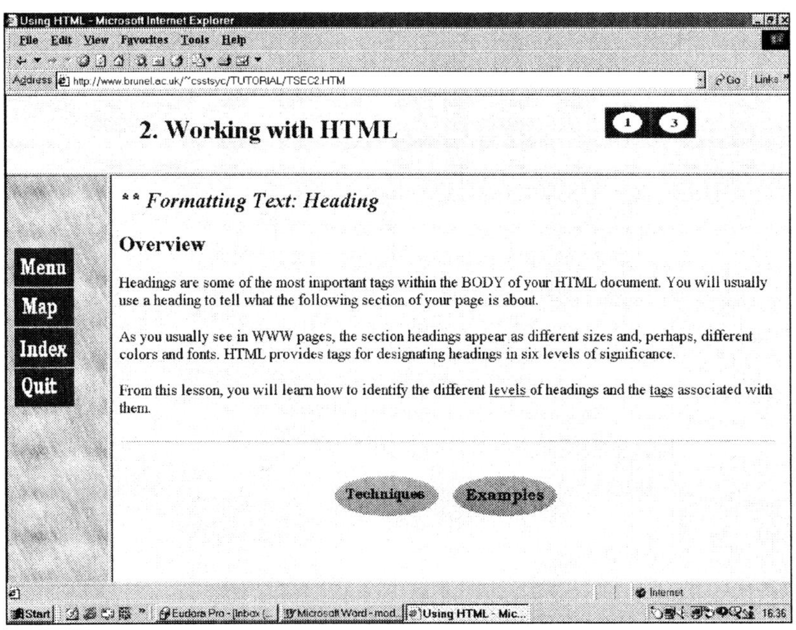

Table 1. Three types of navigation control

Control	Purposes	Tools
Sequence Control	To allow students to decide the sequence of subjects to be learned	• *Subject Maps*: to show all topics and subtopics in a hierarchical way • *Keyword Index*: to list keywords in an alphabetical way • *Back/Forward*: to see the page previously visited
Content Control	To allow students to control the selection of the contents they wish to learn	• *Section Buttons*: to choose three sections of the main content • *Main Menu:* to present main topics • *Hypertext Links*: to connect relevant concepts
Display Control	To allow students to choose one of several display options that cover the same concept	• *Display Options*: to include overview, examples and detailed techniques, and so forth

correct answer was provided among the multiple choices provided in each question. The formats of the questions were similar, with only the specific subject of the question being modified. The questions covered all three sections of the Web-based instruction program, from basic concepts to advance topics.

Students were allotted 20 minutes to answer each test and were not allowed to examine the content presented in the program at the same time. Students' learning outcome was assessed by:

- **Post-Test score:** Each student's score on the Post-Test, ranging from 0 to 20 to identify general learning performance
- **Gain score:** Score difference between the Pre-Test and Post-Test, to measure improved learning performance by taking the HTML tutorial.

Task Sheet

Students were assigned to do a practical task, which involved constructing a Web page using Notepad to measure learning outcome on the real skills that they had learned. The practical task entailed 10 key areas (e.g., creating hypertext links, changing background colors, formatting text, etc.). A printed task sheet was given to the students that described the detailed features of the Web page to be completed. The students were allowed to decide the order in which they attempted to complete the task activities on the sheet, and could look at the content of the HTML tutorial simultaneously.

One and a half hours were allocated for each student to complete the task. The starting and end times for each student were recorded. Students' task achievement was evaluated by:

- **Task score:** A score consisting of summing items successfully completed, on a 0-10 scale
- **Task time:** The total time spent for completing the tasks.

Exit Questionnaire

The questionnaire was divided into two parts. The first part sought information regarding biographical data relating to the student and his or her experience of using computers, the Internet and HTML. The second, which was the main focus, consisted of three open-ended questions and 47 closed statements to collect students' responses to the Web-based instructional program. It took students approximately 20 minutes to respond to all questions.

The open-ended questions were related to students' opinions about the strengths and weaknesses of the HTML tutorial and the barriers that they met. Students were requested to express their opinions in their own words. Enough space was provided for them to write down their opinions. The closed statements were designed to collect information about students' comprehension, preferences, and satisfaction or dissatisfaction with the Web-based instructional program. It included five sections: (1) level of understanding; (2) content presentation; (3) interaction styles; (4) functionality and usability; and (5) difficulties and problems.

Each closed statement could be classed as either "in favor" or "not in favor" of the program. The number of 'favored' statements was almost equal to the 'not-favored' statements (20 favored statements and 27 not-favored statements), in an attempt to reduce bias in the questionnaire. All statements used a five-point Likert Scale consisting of: 'strongly agree'; 'agree'; 'neutral'; 'disagree'; and 'strongly disagree.' Students were required to indicate agreement or disagreement with each statement by placing a check mark at the response alternative that most closely reflected their opinion. Their perceptions and attitudes were measured by:

- **Positive perceptions:** the total score for all favored statements of the Exit Questionnaire with the same Likert Scale
- **Negative attitudes:** The total score for all not-favored statements of the Exit Questionnaire with the same Likert Scale.

Procedure

All participants took part in the study in the same room at the same time, and they all interacted with the Web-based instructional program accessed using Microsoft's Internet Explorer. The participants were asked to do the following activities:

1. Take the Pre-Test to ascertain levels of prior knowledge of HTML
2. Interact with the Web-based instructional program (i.e., HTML Tutorial)
3. Do a practical task, which involved constructing a Web page using HTML
4. Complete the Post-Test to identify learning performance
5. Fill out a paper-based exit questionnaire to describe their personal details and reflect on their opinions of the Web-based instructional program.

Data Analyses

To investigate how human factors influence student learning in the Web-based instructional program, the data obtained from Pre- and Post-Tests, practical tasks and the exit questionnaire were used to conduct statistical analyses to identify students' learning experience. T-test was applied to examine the gender differences, and ANOVA was used to identify the differences among different levels of prior knowledge. In addition, Pearson's correlation was employed to find the relationships between students' learning performance and their perceptions and attitude. A significance level of $P<.05$ was adopted for the study. In addition, the mean scores are employed to describe the learning outcome for each individual group.

DISCUSSION RESULTS

The participants (N=61) consisted of master's students at Brunel University's Department of Information Systems and Computing. Despite the fact that the participants volunteered to take part in the experiment, the sample is evenly distributed in terms of gender and system experience. There were 32 males and 29 females. The computer experience and Internet experience reported by the participants ranged from average to excellent on a five-point scale. Their familiarity with the subject content, *HTML authoring*, ranged from none to good. As shown in Table 2, there is the similar proportion of computer and Internet experience and HTML authoring in both male and female groups.

Table 3 describes the students' overall learning performance. In terms of perceptions and attitudes, a majority of students (78%) felt that the Web-based instruction program was useful and they liked the Web treatment of the content.

Table 2. Distribution of participants

	Male (N=32)	Female (N=29)	Total (N=61)
Computer Experience			
None	0	0	0
Little	0	0	0
Average	9	11	20
Good	12	10	22
Excellent	10	9	19
Internet Experience			
None	0	0	0
Little	0	0	0
Average	12	10	22
Good	9	12	21
Excellent	10	8	18
HTML Authoring			
None	8	7	15
Little	9	11	20
Average	6	7	13
Good	8	5	13
Excellent	0	0	0

Table 3. Overall learning outcomes

	Post Test	Gain Score	Task Score	Task Time
Mean	10.4	7.7	6.5	46.5
SD	1.8	0.9	1.6	6.8

Tasks vs. Tests

As indicated in Section 3, students needed to be assessed by both practical task and paper-based tests. It is important to note that both task and tests were markedly different. The distinctions between them are similar to those between open-book examination and closed-book examination. The practical task was completed in "open-book" examination style, with the students building their Web pages while being guided by the task sheet. The practical task could be completed successfully without recourse to memory by applying knowledge read from the screen at the particular time it was needed. On the other hand, the Post-Test looked like a closed-book examination, as it was a multiple-choice factual test that entailed recalling knowledge from memory and was completed after learning using the Web-based instructional program. These differences can also be associated with those between *procedural knowledge* and *declarative knowledge*. Derry (1990) distinguishes between these two, procedural being "knowledge how," and declarative being "knowledge that." Procedural refers to knowledge of how to do things, while declarative refers to knowledge about the world and its properties (McGilly, 1994). Practical tasks refer to procedure knowledge of how to use HTML, while paper-based tests refer to declarative knowledge about the properties of HTML.

Another interesting finding is that the students' task scores were affected by the levels of their previous Internet experience and HTML authoring (Table 4). On the other hand, there were positive relationships between the students' perceptions and attitudes and their Post-Test ($P<.05$) and Gain scores ($P<.01$). In other words, the students who had more positive perceptions toward the Web-based instructional program could obtain better Post-Test and Gain scores than those who had more negative attitudes toward the program.

Table 4. Task score and prior knowledge

Internet Experience	Excellent	Good	Average	Little	None
Mean	8.2	6.9	4.3	N/A	N/A
SD	1.9	1.6	0.7	N/A	N/A
Significance	P<.01				
HTML Authoring	Excellent	Good	Average	Little	None
Mean	N/A	8.4	7.2	6.0	4.2
SD	N/A	1.8	1.3	0.7	0.3
Significance	P<.05				

This implied that performance on the practical task of applying procedural knowledge could be promoted by prior system experience in using the Internet and HTML authoring, but it would not be affected by the matching or mismatching of instruction with students' preferences. Conversely, the ability to recall declarative knowledge appears to have been facilitated mainly by matching instructional presentation with learners' preferences, but it is not influenced by prior system experience of using the Internet and HTML authoring.

Gender Differences

There were interesting correlations between the students' learning performance and their gender differences. Female students performed better than male students in the Post-Test. Conversely, the male students outperformed the female students in the practical task (Table 5). As indicated earlier, the differences between the Post-Test and practical task can be related with those between *declarative knowledge* and *procedural knowledge*. It implies that female students are better at acquiring declarative knowledge rather than procedural knowledge. Conversely, male students are skilled at gaining procedural knowledge instead of declarative knowledge.

For learning attitudes, the male students were patient in completing the task. On the other hand, the female students felt nervous doing the tasks, and some of them (N = 10) gave up doing the tasks within 15 minutes. In addition, the female students needed more guidance than the male students did. The female students tended to ask for instruction from the tutor, instead of trying to correct errors by themselves. These findings are in line with some previous studies, which found that males showed more interest in using and learning about computers while females reported fear of using computers and feeling helpless around them (Shashaani, 1994; Koch, 1994). For this phenomenon, educators should help female students build their confidence in facing the challenge of using computers, instead of giving too detailed instructions. In addition, educational settings should ensure that instructional programs should not place any students at a disadvantage due to their gender differences (Owen & Liles, 1998).

Table 5. Gender differences in learning outcomes

	Post Test	Gain Score	Task Score	Task Time
Gender Differences				
Female				
Means	12.4	9.3	4.5	35 .5
SD	1.9	1.1	0.6	3.8
Male				
Means	8.5	6.2	8.6	56.4
SD	0.8	0.7	1.8	7.8
Significance	P<.01	P<.05	P<.01	P<.01

Prior Knowledge

Through analyzing students' prior knowledge, one thing seems evident: For doing practical task, students who had greater experience of using the Internet or HTML authoring seemed able to look for relevant information in an efficient way. Conversely, students who were lacking prior knowledge of the subject content needed more time to decide the learning paths for completing the task (Table 6). It seemed that students' existing knowledge did influence their interaction with the Web-based instructional program. These findings arguably supported results from previous studies (Shih & Gamon, 1999; Gay, 1986), which found there was a positive relationship between learner control and prior knowledge.

Expert learners who had an adequate amount of prior knowledge on the subject felt familiar with the interface and the contents of the Web-based instructional program, so they were confident about being more active when navigating the Web-based instructional system. On the other hand, novice learners might not be aware of the best order to read the material or what the most important information was. Therefore, it is important to provide novice learners with an initial phase of orientation relating to both interface and domain contents (Linard & Zeillger, 1995). One way to do this is by providing visual paths, which can be displayed by means of cues to indicate how far students are along a path or by giving some conceptual description for the possible sequences. An alternative method is to provide good labels for the pages. Labels that clearly indicate the role of a particular page may help novices successfully tdecide the appropriate coherent path (Lewis & Polson, 1990).

Learning by Doing

In this Web-based instruction program, students were asked to do a practical task (i.e., designing a Web page with HTML). A significant number of students (44%) reported that doing the task was a useful way of helping them to set a focus in the Web-based instructional program. From this 44% of students, 52% of them obtained Post-Test scores above the average (=10.4) and 63% of them demonstrated more positive perceptions to the Web-based instructional program. These results implied that "learning by doing" could assist some students to set their effective learning strategies. As indicated by Smith and Parks (1997), tasks serve to simulate "goal directed" browsing in such a way that learning performance can be enhanced.

On the other hand, a few students (30%) reported that doing the task hindered their learning. They found that they lost other important information they needed to learn because they were concentrating on doing the task. From these

Table 6. Prior knowledge and task time

Task Time					
Internet Experience	Excellent	Good	Average	Little	None
Mean	39.2	44.5	54.4	N/A	N/A
SD	5.5	6.1	8.1	N/A	N/A
Significance	P<.05				
HTML Authoring	Excellent	Good	Average	Little	None
Mean	N/A	31.4	41.9	50.5	61.2
SD	N/A	3.2	4.3	5.9	7.3
Significance	P<.05				

30% of students, 58% of them obtained Post-Test scores below the average and 54% of them showed more negative attitudes toward the Web-based instructional program. This raises some interesting questions for further studies: (a) whether task activities can facilitate promoting students' learning performance in a Web-based instructional program; and (b) what the relationships are between students' attitudes and their learning patterns as reflected in a Web-based instructional program with and/or without setting tasks.

CONCLUSION

The aforementioned findings provide evidence that Web-based instructional programs may not be suitable for all learners as an instructional methodology. Instructors must be aware of individual differences, such as gender and levels of prior knowledge possessed. Some learners—for example, novice learners—may need greater support and guidance from instructors, while others may be able to follow Web-based instructional programs relatively independently. Thus, instructors should not assume that every student would benefit equally from Web-based instructional programs in educational settings. There remains the need for guidance to ensure that all learners attain their learning potential.

Implementing Web-based instructional programs is a complex process composed of interactions among students, instructional content and the features of Web-based instructional programs. It is important for educational settings to have a good plan in advance. Instructors should remain cautious about making a sweeping decision to convert entire curricula onto Web-based instructional programs. The goals of such a process should be weighed against potential problems (e.g., alienating certain learners). To avoid alienating a certain group, instructors should continue to incorporate a number of different teaching strategies into their lectures. In addition, this transition requires time for the student and time in the classroom to acquaint students with Web-based instructional programs. This is especially the case for students who have difficulties in independent learning; there is a need to let them have a longer time for this shift. With this issue in mind, such innovation in teaching and learning will be more meaningful and valuable.

This study has shown the importance of understanding individual differences in the development of Web-based instructional programs, but it was only a small-scale study. Further studies need to be undertaken with a larger sample to provide additional evidence. The other limitation is that this study adopted self-developed Pre- and Post-Tests, so the reliability and validity of these tests are questionable. Therefore, testing and modification of the tests are needed in the future. There is a need to conduct future research that would examine the impact of other individual differences, such as cognitive styles, cultural background or domain knowledge. Such research should also be conducted within a more sophisticated multimedia Web-based instructional program, including the presentation of animation and video. It would be interesting to see how individual differences influence student learning in multimedia Web-based instructional programs. The findings of such studies could be integrated to build robust user models for the development of personalized Web-based instructional programs that can accommodate individual differences.

REFERENCES

Barua, S. (2001). An interactive multimedia system on "Computer Architecture, Organization, and Design." *IEEE Transactions on Education, 44,* 41-46.

Burton, L., & Goldsmith, D. (2002). *Students' experience in online course: A study using asychronous online focus groups.* Newington: Connecticut Distance Learning Consortium.

Carter, E. W. (2002). Doing the best you can with what you have: Lessons learned from outcomes assessment. *Journal of Academic Librarianship 28*, 36-41.

Chang, H.H., Henriquez, A., Honey, M., Light, D., Moeller, B., & Ross, N. (1998). *The Union City story: Education reform and technology students' performance on standardized tests.* New York: Center for Children and Technology.

Chen, S.Y. (2002). A cognitive model for non-linear learning in hypermedia programmes. *British Journal of Educational Technology, 33*, 449-460.

Chen, S.Y., & Ford, N.J. (1998). Modelling user navigation behaviours in a hypermedia-based learning system: An individual differences approach. *International Journal of Knowledge Organization, 25*(3), 67-78.

Clark, R., & Lyons, C. (1999). Using Web-based training wisely. *Training, 36*(7), 51-61.

Daugherty, M., & Funke, B.L. (1998). University faculty and student perceptions of Web-based instruction. *Journal of Distance Education, 13*(1), 21-39.

Derry, S. J. (1990). Learning strategies for acquiring useful knowledge. In B.F. Jones & L. Idol (Eds.), *Dimensions of thinking and cognitive instruction* (pp. 347-379). Hillsdale: Lawrence Erlbaum Associates.

Ellis, R. D., & Kurniawan, S.H. (2000). Increasing the usability of online information for older users. A case study in participatory design. *International Journal of Human-Computer Interaction, 12*(2), 263-276.

Evans, C., Gibbons, N.J., Shah, K., & Griffin, D.K. (2004). Virtual learning in the biological sciences: Pitfalls of simply putting notes on the Web. *Computers and Education, 43*, 49-61.

Ford, N., & Miller, D. (1996). Gender differences in Internet perceptions and use. *Aslib Proceedings, 48*, 183-192.

Gay, G. (1986). Interaction of learner control and prior understanding in computer-assisted video instruction. *Journal of Educational Psychology, 78*(3), 225-227.

Hedberg, J.G., & Corrent-Agostinho, S. (2000). Creating a postgraduate virtual community: Assessment drives learning. *Educational Media International, 37*(2), 83-90.

Hui, S., & Cheung, K.P. (1999). Developing a Web-based learning environment for building energy efficiency and solar design in Hong Kong. *Solar Energy, 67*(1-3), 151-159.

Jonassen, D.H., & Grabowski, B.L. (1993). *Handbook of individual differences, learning, and instruction.* Hillsdale: Lawrence Erlbaum Associates.

Ke, H., Kwakkelaarb, R., Taic, Y., & Chenc, L. (2002) Exploring behavior of e-journal users in science and technology: Transaction log analysis of Elsevier's ScienceDirect OnSite in Taiwan. *Library & Information Science Research, 24*(3), 265-291.

Khalifa, M., & Lam R. (2002). Web-based learning: Effects on learning process and outcome. *IEEE Transactions on Education, 45*, 350-356.

Koch, M. (1994). No girls allowed! *Technos, 3,* 14-19.

Last, D.A., O'Donnell, A.M., & Kelly, A.E. (2001). The effects of prior knowledge and goal strength on the use of hypermedia. *Journal of Educational Multimedia and Hypermedia, 10*(1), 3-25.

Lewis, C., & Polson, P.G. (1990). Theory-based design for easily learned interfaces. *HCI, 5,* 191-220.

Liaw, S.-S. (2002). An Internet survey for perceptions of computers and the World Wide Web: Relationship, prediction, and difference. *Computers in Human Behavior, 18,* 17-35.

Linard, M., & Zeillger, G. (1995). Designing navigational support for educational software. *Proceedings of Human Computer Interactions* (pp. 63-78).

McDonald, C. J., Stodel, E. J., Farres, L. G., Breithaupt, K., & Gabriel, M. A. (2001). The demand-driven learning model: A framework for Web-based learning, the Internet and higher education, *4*(1), 9-30.

McGilly, K. (1994). *Classroom lesson: Integrating cognitive theory and classroom practice.* Cambridge: MIT.

Mitchell, T. J. F., Chen, S. Y., & Macredie, R. D. (2005). Hypermedia learning and prior knowledge: Domain expertise vs. system expertise. *Journal of Computer Assisted Learning, 21,* 53-64.

Ng, W., & Gunstone, R. (2002). Students' perceptions of the effectiveness of the World Wide Web as a research and teaching tool in science learning. *Research in Science Education, 32*(4), 489-510.

Owen, M. B., & Liles, R. (1998). *Factors contributing to the use of Internet by educators.* Retrieved from http://outreach.missouri.edu/netc98/manuscripts/owen-liles.html

Power, D. J., & Roth, R. M. (1999). Issues in designing and using Web-based teaching cases. *Proceedings of the Fifth Americas Conference on Information System (AMCIS 1999)* (pp. 936-938).

Quintana, Y. (1996). *Evaluating the value and effectiveness of Internet-based learning.* Retrieved from www.crim.ca/inet96/pa pers/c1/c1_4.htm

Reed, W. M., & Oughton, J. M. (1997). Computer experience and interval-based hypermedia navigation. *Journal of Research on Computing in Education, 30,* 38-52.

Roy, M., & Chi, M. T. C. (2003). Gender differences in patterns of searching the Web. *Journal of Educational Computing Research, 29,* 335-348.

Schwarz, J. (2001). *Lost in virtual space: Gender differences are magnified.* Retrieved October 15, 2002, from www.washington.edu/newsroom/news/2001archive/06-01archive/k061301.html

Shashaani, L. (1994). Gender differences in computer experience and its influence on computer attitudes. *Journal of Educational Computing Research, 11*(4), 347-367.

Shih, C., & Gamon, J. (1999). *Student learning styles, motivation, learning strategies, and achievement in Web-based courses.* Retrieved from http://iccel.wfu.edu/publications/journals/jcel/jcel990305/ccshih.htm

Smaldino, S. (1999). Instructional design for distance education. *Techtrends, 43*(5), 9-13.

Smith, & Parks. (1997). *Virtual hierarchies and virtual networks: Some lessons from hypermedia usability research applied to the World Wide Web.* Retrieved December 4, 1998, from http://ijhcs.open.ac.uk/smith/smith-nf.html

Sridharan, K. (2004). A course on Web languages and Web-based applications. *IEEE Transactions on Education, 47*(2), 254-260.

Torkzadeh, G., & Van Dyke, T.P. (2002). Effects of training on Internet self-efficacy and computer user attitudes. *Computers in Human Behavior, 18,* 479-494.

Wang, S. R., & Jonassen, D. H. (1993, April). *Investigating the effects of individual differences on performance in cognitive flexibility hypertexts.* Annual Meeting of the American Educational Research Association. Atlanta, GA.

This work was previously published in Integrating Information & Communications Technologies into the Classroom, edited by L.Tomei, pp. 19-35, copyright 2007 by Information Science Publishing (an imprint of IGI Global).

Chapter IV
The Next Generation of Personalization Techniques

Gulden Uchyigit
Imperial College London, UK

ABSTRACT

Coping with today's unprecedented information overload problem necessitates the deployment of personalization services. Typical personalization approaches model user preferences and store them in user profiles, used to deliver personalized content. A traditional method for profile representation is the so called keyword-based representation, where the user interests are modelled using keywords which are selected from the contents of the items which the user has rated. Although, keyword based approaches are simple and are extensively used for profile representation they fail to represent semantic-based information, this information is lost during the pre-processing phase. Future trends in personalization systems necessitate more innovative personalization techniques that are able to capture rich semantic-based information during the representation, modelling and learning phases. In recent years ontologies (key concepts and along with their interrelationships) to express semantic-based information have been very popular in domain knowledge representation. The primary goal of this chapter is to present an overview of the state-of-the art techniques and methodologies which aim to integrate personalization technologies with semantic-based information.

INTRODUCTION

The advent of the Internet, personal computer networks and interactive television networks has lead to an explosion of information available online from thousands of new sources, a situation which is overwhelming to the end-user and is likely to worsen in the future. Personalization technologies have emerged as specialized tools in assisting users with their information needs. Personalization can be defined as the process of enabling a system to tailor information to its user's needs and preferences.

Personalization technologies became popular in the early 90's, soon after the Web first came into existence. As the number of services and the volume of content continues to grow personalization technologies are more than ever in demand. Over the years they have been deployed in several different domains including entertainment and e-commerce domains, their applications ranging from electronic newspapers to online shops. As a general rule, personalization systems acquire *domain knowledge* along with user's *information need* before they are able to deliver any personalized information to the user.

In recent years developments into extending the Web with semantic knowledge in an attempt to gain a deeper insight into the meaning of the data being created, stored and exchanged has taken the Web to a different level. This has lead to developments of semantically rich descriptions to achieve improvements in the area of personalization technologies (Pretschner and Gauch, 2004).

Traditional approaches to personalization include the *content-based* method ((Armstrong et al., 1995), (Balabanovic and Shoham, 1997), (Liberman, 1995), (Mladenic, 1996), (Pazzani and Billsus, 1997), (Lang, 1995)). These systems generally infer a user's profile from the contents of the items the user previously seen and rated. Incoming information is then compared with the user's profile and those items which are similar to the user's profile are assumed to be of interest to the user and are recommended. To be successful the content-based method needs to be capable of accurately predicting interest from the contents of other items. A traditional method for determining whether information matches a user's interests is through *keyword matching* (Smyth & Cotter, 2000). If a user's interests are described by certain keywords then the assumption is made that information containing those keywords should be of relevant and interest to the user. Such methods may match lots of irrelevant information as well as relevant information, mainly because any item which matches the selected keywords will be assumed interesting regardless of its existing context. For instance, if the word *learning* exists in a paper about *student learning* (from the educational literature) then a paper on *machine learning* (from artificial intelligence literature) will also be recommended. In order to overcome such problems, it is important to model the semantic meaning of the data in the domain. In recent years ontologies have been very popular in achieving this.

Ontologies are formal explicit descriptions of concepts and their relationships within a domain. Ontology-based representations are richer, more precise and less ambiguous than ordinary keyword based or item based approaches (Middleton et al., 2002). For instance they can overcome the problem of *similar* concepts by helping the system understand the relationship between the different concepts within the domain. For example to find a job as a *doct*or an ontology may suggest relevant related terms such as *clinician* and *medicine*. Utilising such semantic information provides a more precise understanding of the application domain, and provides a better means to define the user's needs, preferences and activities with regard to the system, hence improving the personalization process.

The primary challenge of next generation of personalization systems is to effectively integrate semantic knowledge from domain ontologies into the various parts of the personalization method, including data preparation, user modelling and recommendation phases (Mobasher, 2005). This chapter will present a comprehensive overview in the following areas:

- **Data preparation:** *Ontology learning, extraction and pre-processing* - This combines research from natural language processing, statistical analysis and machine learning. Challenging aspects of this research is to automatically extract and learn domain ontologies and automatically define domain concept hierarchies for richer representation of the data found in the domain.

- **User modelling with semantic based information:** Challenging aspects of this research is to automatically model user preferences utilising semantic information for richer representation of the user models.
- **Ontology-based recommender systems:** Challenging aspects of this research is to incorporate the ontological representations into the recommendation phase for better, well defined recommendations.

BACKGROUND

For many years, the fields of information retrieval and information filtering have worked to apply software technology to information overload problems. As a result, personalization techniques have emerged utilising many of the techniques from these fields. In (Oard, 1997), a generic information filtering model is described as having four components: a method for representing the documents within the domain; a method for representing the user's information need; a method for making the comparison; and a method for utilising the results of the comparison process. According to (Oard 1997) an ideal text filtering system is described by:

$c(p(\text{info need}), d(doc)) = j(\text{info need}, doc)$, $\forall$ info need $\in I$, $\forall\ doc \in$ D

where, j is the user's judgment of some relationship between an interest and a document, c is the comparison method used for comparing the user's information need and a given document and p and d are the representation techniques used to represent the user's information need and the documents of the domain, respectively. The goal of the text filtering model is to automate this process, so that the results of the automated comparison process are equal to the user's judge-

Figure 1. A general framework for content-based filtering

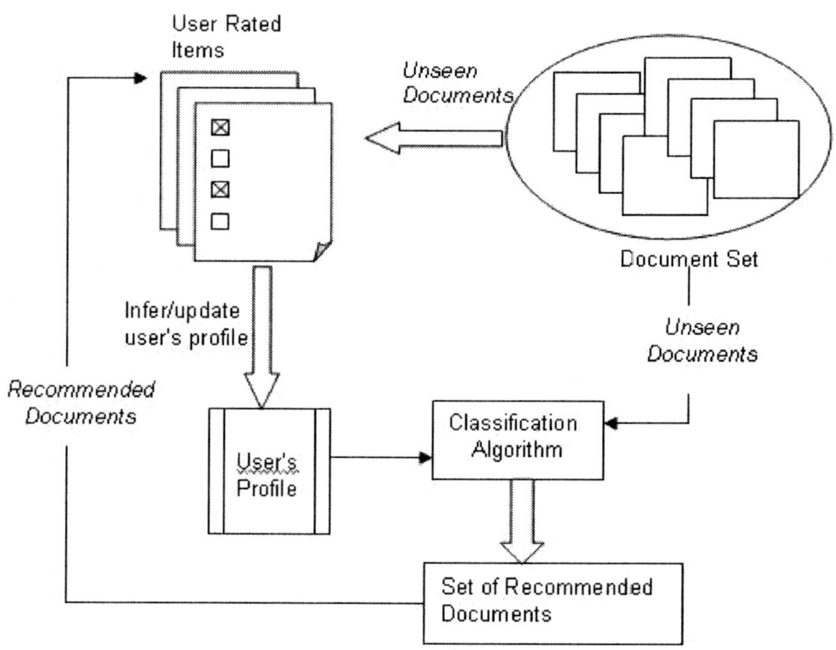

ment of the documents.

The content-based method was developed based on the text filtering model described by (Oard 1997). Figure 1, shows a general framework of the content-based method.

In general, content based systems automatically infer the user's profile from the contents of the document the user has previously seen and rated. These profiles are then used as input to a classification algorithm along with the new unseen documents from the domain. Those documents which are similar in content to the user's profile are assumed to be interesting and recommended to the user.

A popular and extensively used document and profile representation method employed by many information filtering methods, including the content based method is the so called *vector space representation* (Chen and Sycara, 1998), (Mladenic, 1996), (Lang, 1995), (Moukas, 1996), (Liberman, 1995), (T. Kamba and Koseki, 1997), (Armstrong et al., 1995)). The vector space method (Baeza-Yates and Ribeiro-Neto, 1999) consider that each document (profile) is described as a set of keywords. The text document is viewed as a vector in n dimensional space, n being the number of different words in the document set. Such a representation is often referred to as *bag-of-words*, because of the loss of word ordering and text structure (see Figure 2). The tuple of weights associated with each word, reflecting the significance of that word for a given document, give the document's position in the vector space. The weights are related to the number of occurrences of each word within the document. The word weights in the vector space method are ultimately used to compute the *degree of similarity* between two feature vectors. This method can be used to decide whether a document represented as a weighted feature vector, and a profile are similar. If they are similar then an assumption is made that the document is relevant to the user. The vector space model evaluates the similarity of the document d_j with regard to a profile p as the correlation between the vectors d_j and p.

This correlation can be quantified by the cosine of the angle between these two vectors. That is,

$$sim(d_j, p) = \frac{d_j \bullet p}{|d_j| \times |p|} = \frac{\sum_{i=1}^{t} w_{i,j} \times w_{i,p}}{\sqrt{\sum_{i=1}^{t} w_{i,p}^2 \times \sum_{i=1}^{t} w_{i,j}^2}}$$

In (Pazzani and Billsus, 1997), the Naïve Bayesian probabilistic classifier is used for classification of user's profile with new pages browsed by the user on the web. Here, the Naïve Bayesian probabilistic classifier is used to determine the

Figure 2. Illustration of the bag-of-words document representation using word frequency

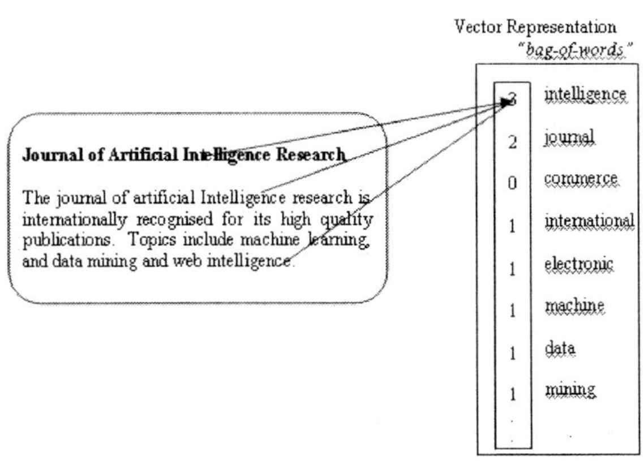

probability that a given page will belong to the set of pages liked or disliked, given the presence or absence of the words found within the user's profile. In this example the Naïve Bayesian probabilistic classifier is computed using the equation below:

$$c^* \equiv \arg\max P(v_j | d_j) \equiv P(v_j) \prod_i P(k_i | v_j)$$

Here, c* denotes the target value of the naive Bayesian probabilistic classifier, $v_j \in$ *{likes, dislikes}* represent the pages which have been liked and disliked by the user and $P(k_i | v_j)$ is the probability that a page contains the word k_i given that it was *liked* or *disliked.*

Table 1 shows a summary of some well known content-based recommender systems.

Collaborative-based systems (Terveen et al., 1997), (Breese et al., 1998), (Knostan et al., 1997), (Balabanovic and Shoham, 1997) are an alternative to the content-based methods. The basic idea is to move beyond the experience of an individual user profile and instead draw on the experiences of a population or community of users. Collaborative-based systems (Herlocker et al., 1999), (Knostan et al., 1997), (Terveen et al., 1997), (Kautz et al., 1997), (Resnick and Varian, 1997) are built on the assumption that a good way to find interesting content is to find other people who have similar tastes, and recommend the items that those users like. Typically, each target user is associated with a set of nearest neighbour users by comparing the profile information provided by the target user to the profiles of other users. These users then act as recommendation partners for the target user, and items that occur in their profiles can be recommended to the target user (Smyth & Cotter, 2000). In this way, items are recommended on the basis of user similarity rather than item similarity (see Figure 3). Content-based systems suffer from shortcomings in the way they select items for recommendations. Items are recommended if the user has seen and liked similar items in the past.

A user profile effectively delimits a region of the item space from which future recommendations will be drawn. Therefore, future recommendations will display limited diversity (Smyth & Cotter, 2000). This is particularly problematic for new users since their recommendations will be based on a very limited set of items represented in their immature profiles. Items relevant to a user, but bearing little resemblance to the snapshot of items the user has looked at in the past, will never be recommended in the future (Smyth & Cotter, 2000). Collaborative filtering techniques try to overcome these shortcomings presented by content-based systems. However, collaborative filtering alone can prove ineffective for several reasons (Claypool et al., 1999). For instance, *the early rater problem*, arises when a prediction can

Table 1. Summary of existing content-based systems

Reference	*Goal*	*Profile Representation*	*Classification Algorithm*
(Mladenic, 1996)	Web Browsing	Feature Vector	Naïve Bayes
SIFT	News Filtering	Feature Vector	Cosine Similarity
(Pazzani and Billsus, 1997),	Web Browsing	Feature Vector	Naïve Bayes
(Chen and Sycara, 1998)	Web Browsing	Feature Vector	Cosine Similarity
(Liberman, 1995)	Web Browsing	Feature Vector	Cosine Similarity
(Balabanovic and Shoham, 1997)	Web Browsing	Feature Vector	Cosine Similarity

Figure 3. Content vs. Collaborative-based methods

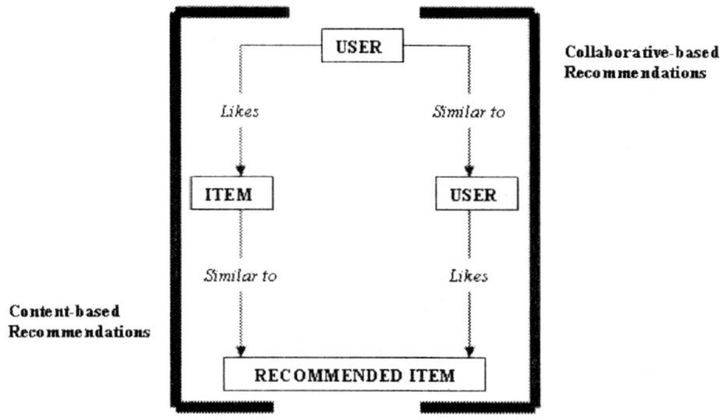

not be provided for a given item because it's new and therefore it has not been rated and it can not be recommended, *the sparsity problem* which arises due to sparse nature of the ratings within the information matrices making the recommendations inaccurate, *the grey sheep problem* which arises when there are individuals who do not benefit from the collaborative recommendations because their opinions do not consistently agree or disagree with other people in the community.

To overcome, the problems posed by pure content and collaborative based recommender systems, hybrid recommender systems have been proposed. Hybrid systems combine two or more recommendation techniques to overcome the shortcomings of each individual technique (Balabanovic, 1998), (Balabanovic and Shoham, 1997), (Burke, 2002), (Claypool et al., 1999). These systems generally, use the content-based component to overcome the new item start up problem, if a new item is present then it can still be recommended regardless if it was seen and rated. The collaboration component overcomes the problem of over specialization as is the case with pure content based systems.

DATA PREPERATION: ONTOLOGY LEARNING, EXTRACTION AND PRE-PROCESSING

As previously described personalization techniques such as the content-based method extensively employ the vector space representation. This data representation technique is popular because of it's simplicity and efficiency. However, it has the disadvantage that a lot of useful information is lost during the representation phase since the sentence structure is broken down to the individual words. In an attempt to minimise the loss of information during the representation phase it is important to retain the relationships between the words. One popular technique in doing this is to use conceptual hierarchies. In this section we present an overview of the existing techniques, algorithms and methodologies which have been employed for ontology learning.

The main component of ontology learning is the construction of the concept hierarchy. Concept hierarchies are useful because they are an intuitive way to describe information (Lawrie and Croft, 2000). Generally hierarchies are manually created by domain experts. This is a very cumbersome process and requires specialised knowledge from domain experts. This therefore necessitates tools for their automatic generation. Research into automatically constructing a hierarchy of concepts directly from data is extensive and includes work from a number of research groups including, machine learning, natural language processing and statistical analysis. One approach is to attempt to induce word categories directly from a corpus based on statistical co-occurrence (Evans et al., 1991), (Finch and Chater, 1994), (McMahon and Smith, 1996), (Nanas et al., 2003a). Another approach is to merge existing linguistic resources such as dictionaries and thesauri (Klavans et al., 1992), (Knight and Luk, 1994) or tuning a thesaurus (e.g WordNet) using a corpus (Miller et al., 1990a). Other methods include using natural language processing (NLP) methods to extract phrases and keywords from text (Sanderson and Croft, 1999), or to use an already constructed hierarchy such as yahoo and map the concepts onto this hierarchy.

Subsequent parts of this section include machine learning approaches and natural language processing approaches used for ontology learning.

Machine Learning Approaches

Learning ontologies from unstructured text is not an easy task. The system needs to automatically extract the concepts within the domain as well as extracting the relationships between the discovered concepts. Machine learning approaches in particular clustering techniques, rule based techniques, fuzzy logic and formal concept analysis techniques have been very popular for this purpose. This section presents an overview of the machine learning approaches which have been popular in discovering ontologies from unstructured text.

Clustering Algorithms

Clustering algorithms are very popular in ontology learning. They function by clustering the instances together based on their similarity. The clustering algorithms can be divided into *hierarchical* and *non hierarchical* methods. Hierarchical methods construct a tree where each node represents a subset of the input items (documents), where the root of the tree represents all the items in the item set. Hierarchical methods can be divided into the *divisive* and *agglomerative* methods. Divisive methods begin with the entire set of items and partition the set until only an individual item remains. Agglomerative methods work in the opposite way, beginning with individual items, each item is represented as a cluster and merging these clusters until a single cluster remains. At the first step of *hierarchical agglomerative clustering* (HAC) algorithm, when each instance represents its own cluster, the similarities between each cluster are simply defined by the chosen similarity method rule to determine the similarity of these new clusters to each other. There are various rules which can be applied depending on the data, some of the measures are described below:

- **Single-Link:** In this method the similarity of two clusters is determined by the similarity of the two closest (most similar) instances in the different clusters. So for each pair of clusters S_i and S_j,

  $$sim(S_{i,}S_j) = \max\{\cos(d_i, d_j) | d_i \in S_i, d_j \in S_j\}$$

- **Complete-Link:** In this method the similarity of two clusters is determined by the similarity of the two least similar instances of both clusters. This approach can be performed well in cases where the data forms the natural distinct categories, since it tends to produce tight (cohesive) spherical clusters. This is calculated as:

  $$sim(S_{i,}S_j) = \min\{\cos(d_i, d_j)\}$$

- **Average-Link or Group Average:** In this method, the similarity between two clusters is calculated as the average distance between all pairs of objects in both clusters, i.e. it's an intermediate solution between complete link and single-link. This is unweighted, or weighted by the size of the clusters. The weighted form is calculated as:

$$sim(S_i, S_j) = \frac{1}{n_i n_j} \sum \cos(d_i, d_j)$$

where n_i and n_j refer to the size of S_i and S_j *respectively.*

Hierarchical clustering methods are popular for ontology learning because they are able to naturally discover the concept hierarchy during the clustering process. Scatter/Gather (Lin and Pantel, 2001) is one of the earlier methods in which clustering is used to create document hierarchies. Recently new types of hierarchies have been introduced which rely on the terms used by a set of documents to expose some structure of the document collection. One such technique is lexical modification and another is subsumption.

Rule Learning Algorithms

These are algorithms that learn *association* rules or other attribute based rules. The algorithms are generally based on a *greedy search* of the attribute-value tests that can be added to the rule preserving its consistency with the training instances. Apriori algorithm is a simple algorithm which learns association rules between objects. Apriori is designed to operate on databases containing transactions (for example, the collections of items bought by customers). As is common in association rule mining, given a set of item sets (for instance, sets of retail transactions each listing individual item's purchased), the algorithm attempts to find subsets which are common to at least a minimum number S_c (the cutoff, or confidence threshold) of the item sets. Apriori uses a bottom up approach, where frequent subsets are extended one item at a time (a step known as candidate generation, and groups of candidates are tested against the data. The algorithm terminates when no further successful extensions are found. One example of an ontology learning tool is OntoEdit (Maedche and Staab, 2001), which is used to assist the ontology engineer during the ontology creation process. The algorithm semi automatically learns to construct an ontology from unstructured text. The algorithm uses a method for discovering *generalized* association rules. The input data for the learner is a set of transactions, each of which consists of set of items that appear together in the transaction. The algorithm extracts association rules represented by sets of items that occur together sufficiently often and presents the rules to the knowledge engineer. For example a shopping transaction may include the items purchased together. The generalized association rule may say that snacks are purchased together with drinks rather than crisps are purchased with beer.

Fuzzy Logic

Fuzzy logic provide the opportunity to model systems that are inherently imprecisely defined. Fuzzy logic is popular in modelling of textual data because of the uncertainty which is present in textual data. Fuzzy logic is built on theories of fuzzy sets. Fuzzy set theory deals with representation of classes whose boundaries are not well defined. The key idea is to associate a membership function with the elements of a class. The function takes values in the interval (0, 1) with 0 corresponding to no membership and 1 corresponding to full membership. Membership values between 0 and 1 indicate marginal elements in the class. In (Tho et al., 2006) fuzzy logic has also been used in generating of ontologies. Fuzzy logic is incorporated into ontologies to handle uncertainty in data.

Formal Concept Analysis

Formal Concept Analysis (FCA) is a method for deriving conceptual structures out of data. These structures can be graphically represented as conceptual hierarchies, allowing the analysis of complex structures and the discovery of dependencies within the data. FCA is increasingly applied in conceptual clustering, data analysis, information retrieval, knowledge discovery, and ontology engineering. Formal Concept Analysis is based on the philosophical understanding that a concept is constituted by two parts: its extension which consists of all objects belonging to the concept, and its intension which comprises all attributes shared by those objects. This understanding allows to derive all concepts from a given context (data table) and to introduce a subsumption hierarchy. The source data can be reconstructed at any given time, so that the interpretation of the data remains controllable. A data table is created with the objects as a left hand column and the attributes along the top. The relationships between each of the objects and their attributes are marked in the table. The set of objects which share the same attributes are determined. Each one of these pairs are then known as a formal concept. The sub-concept and super-concept are also determined form this which shows the hierarchy. A concept lattice is then determined using all the dependencies which is then determined as an ontology hierarchy.

Use of FCA methods in ontology learning have been popular in recent years (P.Cimiano et al., 2005), (Quan et al., 2004). In (Quan et al., 2004) FOGA (Fuzzy ontology generation framework) fuzzy logic is incorporated with formal concept analysis (FCA) as fuzzy formal concept analysis in which uncertainty information is directly represented by a real number of membership value in the range of (0, 1). These membership values are also used to cluster the concepts. The framework proposed in FOGA can automatically generate a fuzzy ontology. First a fuzzy formal context is represented as a data table as shown in Table 1 (a). In this example the context has three objects representing three documents, namely D1, D2 and D3. In addition it also has three attributes "Machine Learning (ML)", "Bayesian Networks (BN)" and "Fuzzy Logic" (FL) representing three research topics. The relationship between an object and an attribute is represented by a membership value between 0 and 1. A Confidence Threshold (T) is set to eliminate relations that have low membership values. Table 1(b) shows the cross table of the fuzzy formal context given in Table 1 (a) with T=0.5.

The concept lattice is then generated from the fuzzy formal context presented in Table 1(b).

The concepts are then clustered according to their similarity. Conceptual clusters are generated based on the premise if a formal concept

Table 1(a). A cross-table of a fuzzy formal concept (adapted from Quan et al., 2004)

	ML	BN	FL
D1	0.9	0.7	0.13
D2	0.8	0.4	0.75
D3	0.2	0.9	0.1

Table 1(b). fuzzy formal context in Table 1(a) with T=0.5 (adapted from Quan et al., 2004)

	ML	BN	FL
D1	0.9	0.7	–
D2	0.8	–	0.75
D3	–	0.9	–

A belongs to a conceptual cluster R, then its subconcept B also belongs to R if B is similar to A. A similarity threshold Ts is used to determine whether two concepts are similar. Figure 5, shows the conceptual clusters that are generated from the concept lattice given in figure 4. Figure 6, shows the corresponding concept hierarchy, in which each concept is represented by a set of attributes of

objects from the corresponding cluster. Following this is the construction of the fuzzy ontology, both the intentional and extensional information of FCA concepts needs to be converted into the corresponding classes and relations of the ontology.

NATURAL LANGUAGE PROCESSING (NLP)

NLP techniques have been used in (Lin and Pantel, 2001) to determine classes, where each concept is

Figure 4. A fuzzy concept lattice generated from FCA (adapted from Quan et al., 2004)

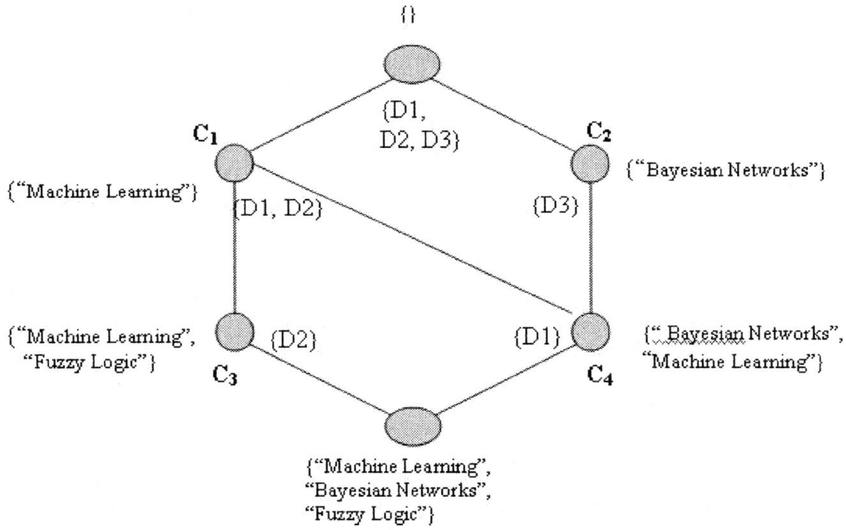

Figure 5. Conceptual Clusters (adapted from Quan et al., 2004)

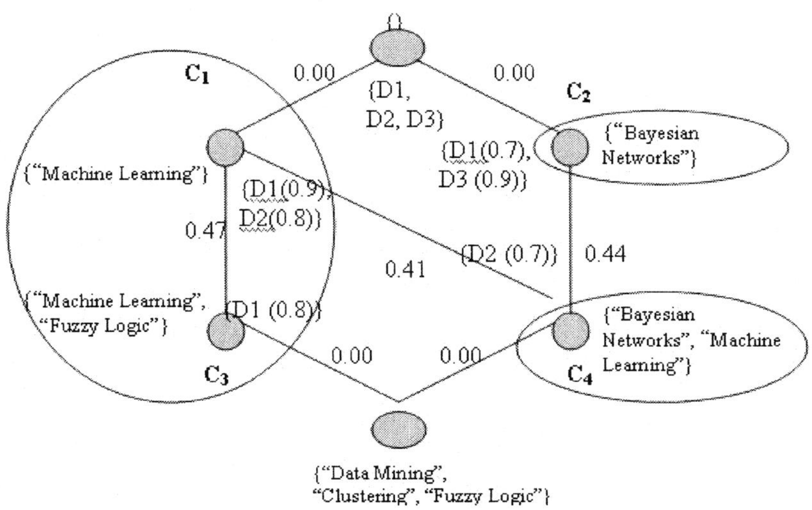

Figure 6. Concept Hierarchy (adapted from Quan et al., 2004)

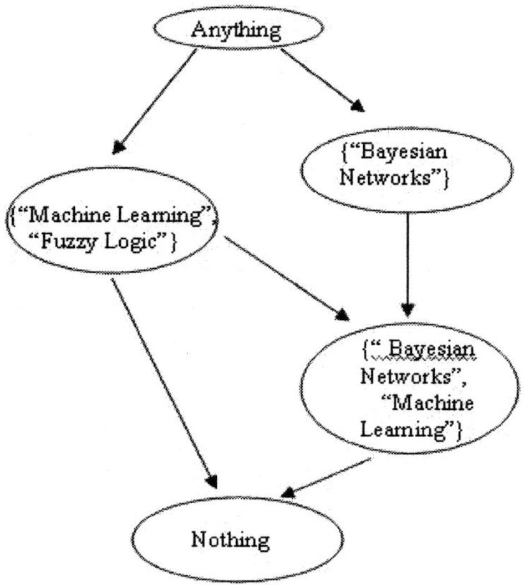

a cluster of words. Artequkt (Alani et al., 2003), which operates in the music domain, utalises NLP techniques in order to extract information about the artists. Artequkt uses WordNet and GATE (Bontcheva et al., 2004), an entity recognizing tool as the tools for identifying the information fragments. Relations between concepts are extracted by matching a *verb* with the entity pairs found in each sentence. The extracted information is then used to populate the ontology. The system in (Agirre et al., 2004) uses textual content from the web to enhance the concepts found in WordNet. The proposed method constructs a set of topically related words for each concept found in WordNet, where each word sense has an associated set of words. For example the word bank has the two sense: *river bank*: estuary, stream and as a *fiscal institute*: finance, money, credit, loan. The system queries the web for the documents related to each concept from WordNet and builds a set of words associated with each topic. The documents are retrieved by querying the web using a search engine and by asking for the documents that contain the words that are related to a particular sense and not contain words related to another sense. In (Sanchez and Moreno, 2005) the hierarchy construction algorithm is based on analyzing the neighbourhood of an initial keyword that characterizes the desired search domain. In English the immediate anterior word for a keyword is the one frequently classifying it (expressing a semantic specialization of the meaning), whereas the immediate posterior one represents the domain where it is being applied. The previous word for a specific keyword is used for obtaining the taxonomical hierarchy of terms (e.g breast cancer will be subclass of cancer). The process is repeated recursively in order to create a deeper-level subclass (e.g metastatic breast cancer will be a subclass of breast cancer). On the other hand, the posterior word for the specific keyword is used to categorize the web resource considered as a tag that expresses the context in where the search domain is applied (e.g colon cancer research will be an application domain where colon cancer is applied). Following this is a polysemy detection algorithm is performed in order to disambiguate polysemic domains. Using this algorithm the agents construct a concept hierarchy of the domain.

The use of semantic techniques in personalization of the information search process has been very popular in recent years. It generally makes use of the user's context during the search process. Typical search engines retrieve information based on keywords given by users and return the information found as a list of search results. A problem with keyword-based search is that often they return a large list of search results with many of them irrelevant to the user. This problem can be avoided if users know exactly the right query terms to use. Such query terms are often hard to find by the user. Refining the query during the searching process can improve the search results. Ontology enhanced searching tools that map a user query onto an ontology ((Parry, 2004)) has been very popular. In (Widyantoro and Yen, 2002) a strategy for query refinement is presented. This approach is based on fuzzy ontology of term associations. The system uses its knowledge about term associations, which it determines using statistical co-occurrence of terms, to suggest a list of broader and narrower terms in addition to providing the results based on the original query term. The broader and narrower terms referring to whether the semantic meaning of one subsumes or covers the semantic meaning of the other. The narrower than terms are then used to narrow down the search results by focusing to the more specific context while still remaining in the context of the original query. The broader than is used to broaden the search results. The definition that term t_i is narrower-than term t_j is the ratio between the number of co-occurrences of both terms and the number of occurrences of term t_i. Therefore the more frequent term t_i and t_j co-occur and less frequent term t_i occurs in documents, t_i is narrower-than t_j. A membership value of 1.0 is obtained when a term always co-occurs with another term. In contrast, the membership value of narrower term relation between two terms that never co-occur will be 0. In (Gong et al., 2005) a search query expansion method which makes use of WordNet is proposed. It creates a collection-based term semantic network (TSN) using word co-occurrences in the collection. The query is expanded in three dimensions using WordNet to get the hypernym, hyponym and synonym of the relation (Miller et al., 1990b). To extract the TSN from the collection, Apriori association rule mining algorithm is used to mine out the association rules between the words. TSN is also used to filter out some of the noise words from WordNet. This is because WordNet can expand a query with too many words. This adds noise and detracts from the retrieval performance, thus leading to low precision. Each page is assigned with a combined weight depending on how the frequency of the original query, expanded hypernym, synonyms and hyponym. Each one of these weights is multiplied with a factor (α,β,γ) that are experimentally determined using the precision recall, the retrieval performance based on the expansion word. For

Table 2. Ontology learning systems and their techniques. (i.e C= Clustering, RL= Rule Learning, FL= Fuzzy Logic, FCA = Formal Concept Analysis, NLP= Natural Language Processing, SM=Statistical method)

	Reference	C	RL	FL	FCA	NLP	SM
Ontology learning	(Lin and Pantel, 2001)	✓				✓	
	(Maedche and Staab 2001)		✓				
	(Tho et al. 2006)			✓			
	(P. Cimiano et al, 2005)				✓		
	(Quan et al 2004)			✓	✓		
	(Bontcheva et al, 2004)					✓	
	(Agirre et al, 2004)					✓	
	(Alani et al, 2003)					✓	
	(Sanchez and Moreno 2005)					✓	
	(Widyantoro and Yen 2002)			✓		✓	✓
	(Gong et al., 2005)					✓	✓
	(Miller et al 1990b)		✓			✓	

instance hypernyms relation has less significant impart than hyponyms and synonym relation, hyponyms may bring more noise so its factor is less than the others.

Table 2 summarises all systems and the techniques employed for the ontology learning process.

USER MODELLING WITH SEMANTIC DATA

Integrating semantic information into the personalization process requires for this information to be integrated in all stages of the personalization stage including the user modelling process. Using conceptual hierarchies to represent the user's model has its advantages including determining the user's context. A hierarchical view of user interests enhances the semantics of the user's profile, as it is much closer to the human conception of a set of resources (Godoy and Amandi, 2006). Recent developments have integrated semantic knowledge with the user model to model context. Automatically constructing the user's model into a conceptual hierarchy allows the modelling of contextual information. In (Nanas et al., 2003b), a method of automatically constructing the user profile into a concept hierarchy is presented. The system starts by extracting the concepts from the domain and employing statistical feature selection methods. The concepts are then associated by defining the links between them. The extracted terms are linked using a sort of a "*sliding window*" The size of window defines the kind of associations that are taken into consideration. A small window of few words defines the *Local Context*, whereas, a larger window defines a *Topical Context*. The goal of topical context is to identify semantic relations between terms that are repeatedly used in discussing the topic. To identify topical correlations a window of 20 words are chosen, 10 words at either side of the term. Weights are assigned to the links between extracted terms. For instance to assign a weight w_{ij} to the link between the terms t_i and t_j the below formula is used:

$$w_{i,j} = \frac{fr_{ij}^{\;2}}{fr_i \cdot fr_j} \cdot \frac{1}{d}$$

where, fr_{ij} is the number of times term t_i and t_j appear within the sliding window, fr_i and fr_j are respectively the number of occurrences of t_i and t_j in documents rated by the user, and d is the average distance between the two linked terms. Two extracted terms next to each other has a distance of 1, while if there are n words between two extracted terms then the distance is n+1. The hierarchy is identified by using topic subtopic relations between terms. The more documents that a term appears in the more general the term is assumed to be. Some of the profile terms will broadly define the underlying topic, while the others co-occur with a general term and provide its attributes, specialization and related concepts. Based on this hypothesis, the terms are ordered into a hierarchy according to frequency count in different documents.

Concept hierarchies can also be constructed by making use of a pre-constructed hierarchy such as yahoo (Sieg et al., 2005), (Pretschner and Gauch, 2004). In (Pretschner and Gauch, 2004) the user profile is created automatically while the user is browsing. The profile is essentially a reference ontology in which each concept has a weight indicating the user's perceived interests in that concept. Profiles are generated by analyzing the surfing behavior of the user, especially the content, length and the time spent on the page. For the reference ontologies existing hierarchies from yahoo.com are used. This process involves extracting the contents of documents which are linked from the hierarchy. Each concept in the yahoo hierarchy is represented as a feature vector. The contents of the links which are stored in the user's browsing cache are also represented as feature vectors. To determine user's profile these feature vectors and the concept feature vectors are compared using the cosine similarity, those concepts which are similar are inserted into the user profile. The concepts in the user profile is updated as the user continues to browse and search for information. A popular application of semantic information at present is in the area of education. Personalization techniques are the next new thing in e-learning systems (Gomes et al., 2006). Several approaches have been proposed to collect information about users such as preferences, following clicking behavior to collect likes and dislikes, and questionnaires asking for specific information to assess learner features (e.g tests, learner assessment dialogs, and preference forms). Ontologies can be used in defining course concepts (Gomes et al., 2006). In (Gomes et al., 2006) the system traces and learns which concepts the learner has understood, for instance number of correct or wrong answers associated with each concept. also associated with each concept is well learned or known etc. Representing learner profiles using ontologies is also a popular method (Dolog and Schafer, 2005) . The advantages of this is that they can be exchanged which makes learner profiles interoperable. (Carmagnola et al., 2005) present a multidimensional matrix whose different planes contain the ontological representation of different types of knowledge. Each of these planes represent user actions, user model, domain, context adaptation goals and adaptation methods. The framework uses semantic rules for representation. The knowledge in each plane is represented in the form of a taxonomy, they are application independent and modular and can be used in different domains and application. Each domain is defined at different levels: at the first level there is the definition of general concepts. For example, for domain taxonomy, the first level includes macro domain such as: tourist information, financial domain, e-learning domain etc; for the adaptation goals-taxonomy, the first level specifies general goals such as: inducing/pushing; informing/explaining; suggesting/recommending, guiding/helping and so on for all the ontologies. At the following levels there are specialized concepts. For example for the tourist domain, the next level can include tourist categories (travel, food etc.) while the adaptation-goals taxonomy can include more specific goals such as explaining to support learning or clarify or to teach a new concept or correct mistakes. User modelling and adaptation rules can be applied at the points of intersection within the matrix. In (Mylonas et al., 2006) a fuzzy ontology framework for personalization of multimedia content is presented. The main idea here is to extract context and make use of the context within the personalization process. The user context is extracted from using fuzzy ontology. In the fuzzy ontology framework the concept link relationships are assigned a value (0, 1) which determines the degree to which each concept is related to each other. One concept can be related with some degree and the same concept can be related with another concept another degree. The user preference model is a representation of concepts. During the searching process the user's context stored in the preference model is combined with the document retrieved using the query alone. Developing user models which are generic which can be used in many different application areas can be very advantageous. In (Tchienehom, 2005) a generic profile model is presented which encapsulates the use of semantic information in the profile. The generic profile model is subdivided into four levels: the profile logical structure, the profile contents, the profile logical structure semantics and the content semantics.

ONTOLOGY-BASED RECOMMENDER SYSTEMS

In recent years, web trends expressing semantics about people and their relationships have gained a lot of interest. The friend of a friend (FOAF) project is a good example of one of the most popular ontologies. The FOAF project is an ontology which describes people and their friends (Middleton et al., 2002). Such ontologies are advantageous in that they are able provide an easy way of defining user groups based on their interests (Mori et al., 2005). Utilising ontologies this way allows for groups of users with similar interests to be identified, hence, making the recommendation process more accurate. OntoCapi (Alani et al., 2002) is a system which helps to identify communities of people based on specific features which they have in common, for instance who attended same events, who co-authored same papers and who worked on same projects etc. OntoCapi uses a fixed ontology for identifying groups of users. OntoCapi is developed for the research domain, researchers are recommended papers depending on their research interests. Papers are recommended based on the similarity of the profiles of different researchers. An interesting aspect of the OntoCapis is that it is able to identify communities of interests using relations such as conference attendance, supervision, authorship, and research interest and project membership. In essence, OntoCapi uses all this information to develop the communities of interest. QuickStep(Middleton et al., 2002) is also a recommender system which heavily relies on a pre-defined ontology. The ontology used here is for the research domain and is computed by domain experts. The ontology contains usual information such as "*interface agents*" is-a "*agents*" paper. The concepts defined in the ontology hierarchy are represented by weighted feature vectors of example papers found in the domain. The system uses a kind of bootstrapping technique which uses each user's list of publications. It represents the user's papers as feature vectors and maps them to the concept hierarchy using the nearest neighbour algorithm. It then uses those concepts to generate a profile for the user. Each concept is assigned with an interest value determined from the topics which the papers belong. The interest value is partly determined from the number of papers that belong to this topic and the user's interest in them. The recommendations are then formulated from the correlation between the user's current topics of interest and papers that are classified as belonging to those topics. The recommendation algorithm also makes use of the classification confidence, which is the classification measure of topic with the document. In (Mobasher et al., 2004), semantic attribute information and the user ratings given to the objects are used in providing the user with collaborative recommendations. Semantic information is extracted from the objects in the domain this semantic information is then aggregated. The aggregation reveals the semantic information which all the objects have in common. For instance, if the objects in the domain are descriptions of romantic movies and comedy movies, aggregating the extracted semantic information for these objects may reveal romantic comedies. As for making predictions whether the user will like certain items the combine the semantic similarity along with the ratings that the users have given to these individual items.

Context representation in mobile environments has also become popular in recent years. Representing context for these environments is usually multi-faceted, giving the user situation in terms of location, time, contacts, agenda, presence, device and application usage, personal profile and so on. The most important advantage of using an ontological description of these entities is that they can be augmented, enriched and synthesized using suitable reasoning mechanisms, with different goals. In (Buriano et al., 2006) a framework is presented which utalises ontologies to define dimensions such as "moving" or "alone/accompanied", "leisure/business" and so on. User's mood can also be represented in this way, all this can used in computing the recommendation. In (Cantador and Castells, 2006) a pre-defined ontology is used which is represented using semantic networks. User profiles are represented as concepts, where a weight represents the user's interest in a particular concept. Users are then clustered using Hierarchical agglomerative clustering, where concepts are clustered. The concepts and user clusters are then used to find emergent, focused semantic social networks. Several other recommender systems exist which utilise pre-defined ontologies to reason about the classes which exist in the ontology (Aroyo et al., 2006), (Blanco-Fernndez et al., 2004) and to base their recommendations on. In the recommendation process the system is very reliant on the data which is available for it to extract the user's interests. Recently free textual reviews have become popular for extracting opinion. In (Aciar et al., 2006) present an interesting framework for extracting semantic information from unstructured textual consumer reviews. To do this a pre-defined domain ontology is utilised where important concepts are identified from the textual review. These are the combined with a set of measures such as opinion quality, feature quality and overall assessment to select the relevant reviews and provide a recommendations to the user.

CONCLUSION AND FUTURE WORK

Integrating of semantic information with the personalization process brings countless advantages to the personalization process. Most recently the use of ontologies have shown very promising results and have taken the personalization process to another level. Ontologies provide interoperability and enable reasoning about the knowledge in the domain as well as user's needs. Other advantages include in the way information is returned to the user. Using an ontology to represent the recommended output can be used for the explanation process (i.e giving reasons as to why certain recommendations were made). Explanations such as this are important for trust building between the user and the system. In this chapter we presented an overview of some of the techniques, algorithms, methodologies along with challenges of using semantic information in representation of domain knowledge, user needs and the recommendation algorithms.

Future Research Directions

Future trends in personalization systems will continue with the theme of improved user and domain representations. In particular systems will dynamically model the domain by extracting richer more precise knowledge from the domain and to be integrated in all stages of the personalization process. Software agents integrated with such personalization systems can be an interesting research direction, where the agents can autonomously and dynamically learn domain ontologies and share these ontologies with other agents.

Another interesting dimension of personalization technologies is their use with ubiquitous mobile applications. Improved personalization techniques which are able to model user's context can advance the personalized applications embedded on these devices.

Future research directions in application of personalization technologies will be increasingly popular as the basis of applications areas such as e-learning, e-business and e-health.

REFERENCES

Aciar, S., Zhang, D., Simoff, S., and Debenham, J. (2006). *Recommender system based on consumer product reviews.* In Proceedings of the IEEE/WIC/ACM International Conference on Web Intelligence.

Agirre, E., Alfonseca, E., and de Lacalle, O. L. (2004). *Approximating hierarchy-based similarity for wordnet nominal synsets using topic signatures.*

Alani, H., Kim, S., Weal, D. M. M., Hall, P. L. W., and Shadbolt, N. (2003). *Automatic extraction of knowledge from web documents.* In Proceedings of 2nd International Semantic Web Conference

- Workshop on Human Language Technology for the Semantic Web abd Web Service.

Alani, H., O'Hara, K., and Shadbolt, N. (2002). *Ontocopi: Methods and tools for identifying communities of practice.*

Armstrong, R., Freitag, D., Joachims, T., and Mitchel, T. (1995). Webwatcher: *A learning apprentice for the world wide web.* In AAAI Spring Synopsium on Information Gathering from Heterogenous, Distributed Environments.

Aroyo, L., Bellekens, P., Bjorkman, M., Broekstra, J., and Houben,G. (2006). *Ontology-based personalisation in user adaptive systems.* In 2nd International Workshop on Web Personalisation Recommender Systems and Intelligent User Interfaces in Conjunction with 7th International Conference in Adaptive Hypermedia.

Baeza-Yates, R. and Ribeiro-Neto, B. (1999). *Modern Information Retrieval.* Addison Wesley.

Balabanovic, M. (1998). *Learning to Surf: Multiagent Systems for Adaptive Web Page Recommendation.* PhD thesis, Department of Computer Science, Stanford University.

Balabanovic, M. and Shoham, Y. (1997*). Fab: Content-based, collaborative recommendation.* Communications of the ACM, 40(3):6672.

Blanco-Fernndez, Y., Gil-Solla, J. J. P.-A. A., Ramos-Cabrer, M., Barragns-Martnez, B., Garca-Duque, M. L.-N. J., FernndezVilasl, A., and Daz-Redondo, R. P. (2004). *Avatar: An advanced multi-agent recommender system of personalized TV contents by semantic reasoning.* In Web Information Systems WISE 2004, Springer-Verlag.

Bontcheva, K., Tablan, V., Maynard, D., and Cunningham, H. (2004). *Evolving gate to meet new challenges in language engineering.* Natural Language Engineering, 10.

Breese, J., Heckerman, D., and Kadie, C. (1998). *Empherical analysis of predictive algorithms for collaborative filtering.* In Proceedings of the Fourteenth Conference on Uncertainty in Artificial Intelligence. Morgan Kaufmann Publisher.

Buriano, L., Marchetti, M., Carmagnola, F., Cena, F., Gena, C., and Torre, I. (2006). *The role of ontologies in context-aware recommender systems.* In 7th International Conference on Mobile Data Management.

Burke, R. (2002). *Hybrid recommender systems: Survey and experiments.* User Modeling and User-Adapted Interaction, 12(4).

Cantador, I. and Castells, P. (2006). *A multilayered ontology-based user profiles and semantic social networks for recommender systems.* In 2nd International Workshop on Web Personalisation Recommender Systems and Intelligent User Interfaces in Conjunction with 7th International Conference in Adaptive Hypermedia.

Carmagnola, F., Cena, F., Gena, C., and Torre, I. (2005). *A multidimensional approach for the semantic representation of taxonomies and rules in adaptive hypermedia systems.* In PerSWeb05 Workshop on Personalization on the Semantic Web in conjunction with UM05.

Chen, L. and Sycara, K. (1998). *Webmate: A personal agent for browsing and searching.* In 2nd International Conference on Autonomous Agents, Minneapolis MN USA.

Claypool, M., Gokhale, A., Miranda, T., Murnikov, P., Netes, D., and Sartin, M. (1999). *Combining content-based and collaborative filters in an online newspaper.* In SIGIR'99 Workshop on Recommender Systems: Algorithms and Evaluation, Berkeley, CA.

Dolog, P. and Schafer, M. (*2005). Learner modelling on the semantic web.* In PerSWeb05 Workshop on Personalization on the Semantic Web in conjunction with UM05.

Evans, D., W.Hersh, Monarch, I., Lefferts, R., and Henderson, S. (1991). *Automatic indexing of abstracts via natural-language processing using a simple thesaurus*. Medical Decision Making, 11(3):108-115.

Finch, S. and Chater, N. (1994). *Learning syntactic categories: A statistical approach*. In Oaksford, M. and Brown, G., editors, Neurodynamics and Psychology. Academic Press.

Godoy, D. and Amandi, A. (2006). *Modeling user interests by conceptual clustering*. Information Systems. Elsevier Science, 31(4):247265.

Gomes, P., B. Antunes, L. R., Santos, A., Barbeira, J., and Carvalho, R. (2006). *Using ontologies for elearning personalization*. In eLearning Conference.

Gong, Z., Cheang, C. W., and U, L. H. (2005). *Web query expansion by wordnet*. In Database and Expert Systems Applications, Springer Verlag, pages 166-175.

Herlocker, J., Konstan, J., Borchers, A., and Reidl, J. (1999). *An algorithmic framework for performing collaborative filtering*. In Proceedings of the Conference on Research and Development in Information Retrieval.

Kautz, H., Selman, B., and Shah, M. (1997). *Referral web: Combining social networks and collaborative filtering*. Communications of the ACM, 40(3):6365.

Klavans, J., Chodrow, M., and Wacholder, N. (1992). *Building a knowledge base from parsed definitions*. In Jansen, K., Heidorn, G., and Richardson, S., editors, Natural Language Processing: The PLNLP Approach. Kluwer Academic Publishers.

Knight, K. and Luk, S. (1994). *Building a large scale knowledge base for machine translation*. In Proceedings of the Thirteenth National Conference on Artificial Intelligence, pages 773-778. AAAI Press.

Knostan, J., Miller, B., D.Maltz, Herlocker, J., Gordon, L., and Riedl, J. (1997). *Grouplens: Applying collaborative filtering to Usenet news*. Communications of the ACM, 40(3):7787.

Lang, K. (1995). *Newsweeder: Learning to filter Netnews*. In 12th International Conference on Machine Learning.

Lawrie, D. and Croft, W. (2000). *Discovering and comparing topic hierarchies*. In Proceedings of RIAO.

Liberman, H. (1995). *Letzia: An agent that assists in web browsing*. In Proceedings of the 1995 International Joint Conference on Artificial Intelligence, Montreal, Canada.

Lin, D. and Pantel, P. (2001). *Induction of semantic classes from natural language text*. In Knowledge Discovery and Data Mining, pages 317-322.

Maedche, A. and Staab, S. (2001). *Ontology learning for the semantic web*. IEEE Intelligent Systems, 18(2):72-79.

McMahon, J. and Smith, F. (1996). *Improving statistical language model with performance with automatically generated word hierarchies*. Computational Linguistics, 2(22):217-247.

Middleton, S., Alani, H., Shadbolt, N., and Roure, D. D. (2002). *Exploiting synergy between ontologies and recommender systems*. In Semantic Web Workshop.

Miller, G., Beckwith, R., Fellbaum, C., Gross, D., and Miller, K. (1990a). *Introduction to wordnet: An online lexical database*. Journal of Lexicography, 3(4):235-244.

Miller, G. A., Beckwith, R., Fellbaum, C., Gross, D., and Miller, K. J. (1990b). *Introduction to wordnet: An on-line lexical database*. International Journal of Lexicography, 3(4):235-244.

Mladenic, D. (1996). *Personal WebWatcher: design and implementation*. Technical report,

Department for Intelligent Systems, J. Stefan Institute, Jamova 39, 11000 Ljubljana, Slovenia.

Mobasher, B. (2005). Web usage mining and Personalization. In Munindar P. Singh (ed.) *The Practical Handbook of Internet Computing*. CRC Press.

Mobasher, B., Jin, X., and Zhou, Y. (2004). *Semantically enhanced collaborative filtering on the web.* In Web Mining: FromWeb to SemanticWeb: First EuropeanWeb Mining Forum, pages 57-76.

Mori, J., Matsuo, Y., and Ishizuka, M. (2005). *Finding user semantics on the web using word co-occurrence information.* In PerSWeb05 Workshop on Personalization on the Semantic Web in conjunction with UM05.

Moukas, A. (1996). *Amalthaea: Information discovery and filtering using a multi-agent evolving ecosystem.* In Proc. 1st Intl. Conf. on the Practical Application of Intelligent Agents and Multi Agent Technology, London.

Mylonas, P., Vallet, D., Fernndez, M., Castells, P., and Avrithis, Y. (2006). *Ontology-based personalization for multimedia content.* In 3rd European Semantic Web Conference - Semantic Web Personalization Workshop.

Nanas, N., Uren, V., and Roeck, A. D. (2003a). *Building and applying a concept hierarchy representation of a user profile.* In Proceedings of the 26th annual international ACM SIGIR conference on Research and development in information retrieval, pages 198-204. ACM Press New York, NY, USA.

Nanas, N., Uren, V., and Roeck, A. D. (2003b). *Building and applying a concept hierarchy representation of a user profile.* In Annual ACM Conference on Research and Development in Information Retrieval archive Proceedings of the 26th annual international ACM SIGIR conference on Research and development in information retrieval.

Oard, D. (1997). *The state of the art in text filtering.* User Modeling and User-Adapted Interaction, 7.

Parry, D. (2004). *A fuzzy ontology for medical document retrieval.* In ACSW Frontiers '04: Proceedings of the second workshop on Australasian information security, Data Mining and Web Intelligence, and Software Internationalisation, pages 121-126, Darlinghurst, Australia, Australia. Australian Computer Society, Inc.

Pazzani, M. and Billsus, D. (1997). *Learning and revising user profiles: The identification of interesting web sites.* Machine Learning, 27:313-331.

P.Cimiano, Hotho, A., and Staab, S. (2005). *Learning concept hierarchies from text corpa using formal concept hierarchies.* Journal of Artificial Intelligence Research, (24):305-339.

Pretschner, A. and Gauch, S. (2004). *Ontology based personalized search and browsing.* Web Intelligence and Agent Systems, 1(4):219-234.

Quan, T. T., Hui, S. C., and Cao, T. H. (2004). Foga: A fuzzy ontology generation framework for scholarly semantic web. In Workshop on Knowledge Discovery and Ontologies In conjunction with ECML/PKDD.

Resnick, P. and Varian, H. (1997). Recommender systems. Communications of the ACM., 40(3):56-58.

Sanchez, D. and Moreno, A. (2005). A multi-agent system for distributed ontology learning. In EUMAS, pages 504-505.

Sanderson, M. and Croft, W. B. (1999). *Deriving concept hierarchies from text.* In Research and Development in Information Retrieval, pages 206-213.

Sieg, A., Mobasher, B., Burke, R., Prabu, G., and Lytinen, S. (2005). *Representing user information context with ontologies.* In Proceedings of the 3rd International Conference on Universal Access in Human-Computer Interaction.

Smyth, B. and Cotter, P. (2000). A personalised television listings service. *Communications of the ACM, 43*(8).

T. Kamba, H. S. and Koseki, Y. (1997). *Antagonomy: A personalised newspaper on the world wide web.* International Journal of Human Computer Studies, 46(6):789-803.

Tchienehom, P. L. (2005). Profiles semantics for personalized information access. In PerSWeb05 Workshop on Personalization on the Semantic Web in conjunction with UM05.

Terveen, L., Hill, W., Amento, B., McDonald, D., and Creter, J. (1997). Phoaks: A system for sharing recommendations. Communications of the ACM, 40(3):5962.

Tho, Q. T., Hui, S. C., Fong, A., and Cao, T. H. (2006). Automatic fuzzy ontology generation for semantic web. IEEE Transactions on Knowledge and Data Engineering, 18(6):842856.

Widyantoro, D. H. and Yen, J. (2002). Using fuzzy ontology for query refinement in a personalized abstract search engine. In 10th IEEE International Conference on Fuzzy Systems, pages 705-708.

ADDITIONAL READING

Web-mining Applications and techniques Anthony Scime Published 2005 Idea Group Inc (IGI)

What Is Personalization? Perspectives on the Design and Implementation of Personalization in Information Systems Haiyan Fan Journal of Organizational Computing and Electronic Commerce 2006, Vol. 16, No. 3&4, Pages 179-202

Personalization in E-Commerce Applications A. Goy and L. Ardissono and G. Petrone in Advances in Mass Customization and personalization. Springer-Verlag, New York/Berlin (2003)

The Adaptive Web Brusilovsky, Peter Kobsa, Alfred; Nejdl, Wolfgang (Eds.) Lecture Notes in Computer Science Springer Verlag 2007 ISBN 978-3-540-72078-2

Intelligent Techniques for Web Personalization IJCAI 2003 Workshop, ITWP 2003 Lecture Notes in Computer Science , Vol. 3169 Mobasher, Bamshad; Anand, Sarabjot Singh (Eds.) 2005, ISBN: 978-3-540-29846-5

Content-based Recommendation Systems Michael J. Pazzani, and Daniel Billsus Book chapter in "The Adaptive Web: Methods and Strategies of Web Personalization" (Springer, LNCS #4321), 2007

Adaptive News Access Daniel Billsus, and Michael J. Pazzani Book chapter in "The Adaptive Web: Methods and Strategies of Web Personalization" (Springer, LNCS #4321), February 1, 2007

Data Mining for Personalization. In The Adaptive Web: Methods and Strategies of Web Personalization, Brusilovsky, P., Kobsa, A., Nejdl, W. (eds.). Brusilovsky, P., Kobsa, A., Nejdl, W. (eds.). Lecture Notes in Computer Science, Vol. 4321, PP. 90-135, Springer, Berlin-Heidelberg, 2007

Ontological User Profiles for Personalized Web Search. A. Sieg, B. Mobasher, R. Burke. Proceedings of AAAI Workshop on Intelligent Techniques for Web Personalization. B. Mobasher, S. Anand, A. Kobsa, and D. Jannach (Eds.), AAAI Press Technical Report WS-07-08, PP. 84-91, July 2007

Contextual Recommendation. Sarabjot Singh Anand and Bamshad Mobasher. In From Web to Social Web: Discovering and Deploying User and Content Profiles. B. Berendt, A. Hotho, D. Mladenic, G. Semeraro (Eds.), Lecture Notes in Computer Science (LNCS 4737), PP. 142-160, Springer Berlin-Heidelberg, 2007

A Comparative Analysis of Personalization Techniques for a Mobile Application Nurmi, Petteri; Hassinen, Marja; Lee, Kun Chang Advanced Information Networking and Applications Workshops, 2007 IEEE

Evaluation of online personalization systems: A survey of evaluation schemes and a knowledge-based approach Y. Yang and B. Padmanabhan Journal of Electronic Research, Vol 6, No 2, 2005

Section II
Adaptive Content and Services

Chapter V
Advanced Middleware Architectural Aspects for Personalised Leading-Edge Services

Nancy Alonistioti
National & Kapodistrian University of Athens, Greece

Costas Polychronopoulos
National & Kapodistrian University of Athens, Greece

Makis Stamatelatos
National & Kapodistrian University of Athens, Greece

ABSTRACT

This chapter introduces context-driven personalisation of service provision based on a middleware architectural approach. It describes the emerging environment on service provision, outlining the increasing requirements for personalisation as well as the state-of-the-art approaches in personalisation. A novel information space is presented to introduce the middleware architectures for personalisation in service provision. Technology enablers for context and knowledge management as well as service adaptation are also introduced, and an architectural model for the personalisation functionality is presented. The study also touches upon advanced concepts based on autonomic computing and communications to introduce future research directions.

INTRODUCTION

In the context of future mobile communications users will be able to access an abundance of services that will be typically developed by many co-operating entities. Moreover, the diversity of service access contexts, which is inevitable in the era of pervasive, "anywhere" computing, and the co-existence of different technologies caused by the evolutionary character of the transition to next generation systems, will lead to the heterogeneity of the networks and systems that support end-user application provision. This creates the requirement for applications to be optimally delivered and executed over a large diversity of infrastructures and configurations, as well as for dynamic adaptability of services to changing conditions and contexts.

The current mobile communications paradigm was not built to support this evolution. The requirements deriving from the service and access methods diversity and heterogeneity are new to the traditionally vertically integrated and closed telecommunications environment thus disallowing an open service access, which would lead to a larger variety of choice and better quality of service for the user. Traditional architectures have, therefore, not taken under consideration the multiple capabilities that unfold in favour of the end-user. Considering that it would not be feasible to develop separate versions for different execution contexts, applications should be to a large extent agnostic of the environment they run on. Intelligent mechanisms should exist for identifying the context and the particular high-level requirements of an application and mapping them to appropriate reconfiguration operations on the underlying hardware and software infrastructure. To this end, context management, knowledge building and the respective decision making process are key factors for the service personalisation and system adaptation in future mobile communications. A need for middleware platforms, that will abstract this management load and complexity and enable an end-user seamless service experience, emerges.

In order to address these requirements this chapter is organised as follows: The first section ("Personalisation aspects and evolution from state of the art") includes state-of-the-art and beyond on personalisation aspects. More specifically, the first subsection provides information about the notion of personalisation in the 3G world as well as basic concepts that compose the current approach in personalisation. It also introduces the terms of user context, user profile, profile management and context awareness. The next subsection ("Personalisation aspects—State of The Art") presents in more details specific personalisation aspects: profile and context awareness, information representation and information repositories. The following subsection outlines the corresponding progress beyond-state-of-the-art: a novel information space for personalisation and the ontological representation of contextual information in the vision of reconfigurable and autonomic systems.

The next section discusses solutions for personalised service provision through middleware architectures. More specifically, several object-oriented architectures together with relevant standardisation activities are presented in the first subsection. In the same sense, a number of personalisation aspects are discussed in the following subsection focusing on functional issues ("Functional Issues for Personalisation"); profile, context and knowledge management mechanisms, as well as service adaptation issues are therein included. Furthermore, the next subsection presents an integrated middleware framework for personalised service provision support.

The section that follows initiates a discussion about advanced concepts in personalised service provision such as situation awareness, autonomic features in service management (service provision, service adaptation etc) as well as the corresponding evolution of middleware solutions. More specifically, it comprises two subsections which present characteristic features on autonomic computing and communications as well as a discussion on personalised service provision and adaptation in the context of autonomic communications.

Finally, this chapter concludes on the innovative approaches and differentiations of current approaches in service personalisation aspects. Points to future research directions have been added to further guide the interested user.

PERSONALISATION ASPECTS AND EVOLUTION FROM STATE OF THE ART

This section will deal with the notion of personalisation and, in specific, the way it is defined and considered in the relevant literature on one hand, and, on the other hand, the way it has been captured in concrete systems and applications. Thereafter follows a presentation on the relevant standards and state of the art results stemming out of research projects, while, in the end of this section, an evolution path based on new concepts is laid forward.

Concepts on Personalisation

In the 3G world, various definitions of service personalisation can be found in research activities and literature; generally, personalisation of a service is to **adapt services** in order to fit the needs and requirements of a user (Jørstad et al, 2006a); furthermore personalisation should be applied on a service provider agnostic basis. (Blom, 2000) considers personalisation of a service as the **ability** to allow a user to adapt, or produce, a service to fit user's particular needs. Alike, personalisation is considered as the **process** where services are adapted to fit each individual user's requirements (needs and preferences) (Jørstad et al, 2006b). In the same approach, (Kellerer et al, 2003a) refers to personalisation as aiming at supporting users in selecting their favourite services from the rapidly increasing diversity of mobile services and adjusting selected services to their individual needs. A bit more extended scope is stated by (Kellerer et al, 2003b) where personalisation is considered as the matchmaking of a user's preferences and demands to the available services under the constraints of a given situation or environment.

The above presented definitions identify a common approach for service personalisation: a service's value/functionality is provided to a user according to user's requirements and needs. Extending this approach, service personalisation is performed based on specific information about the environment within which is to be provided. Currently, as presented in the definitions, the "environment" spans, mainly, across user's requirements and needs. More specifically, user context, being central in the current approach, includes the user, the device that is being utilised and the service that is to be provided and consumed.

A number of personalisation aspects may be derived by the definition and the features/capabilities that are therein implied to be supported in a service personalisation eco-system. Such aspects are mainly related to the information that is needed to drive each personalisation process. The vision of personalised service provision is mainly based on advanced profiling concepts and mechanisms as well as context awareness in service provision and adaptation (Wagner et al, 2003). Contextual and profile information itself needs to be identified together with the framework for collecting, storing and interpreting such information. More specifically, the information representation is an important aspect; the representation must be performed in interpretable ways that will facilitate the next steps in personalisation. Finally, the information interpretation itself should be elaborated. In the next sections such aspects will be presented with regards to the state-of-the-art impact—literature; additionally, specific points of novelty will be outlined.

Personalisation Aspects: State Of The Art

In this section, the state of the art in specific identified aspects is presented in order to pave the way beyond. Current approaches will be presented; such approaches include mainly research activities and achievements as presented in the related literature, international conferences, journals and magazines. The objective of this section is to provide fundamental reference on issues related to the service personalisation area.

Profile and Context Awareness

An essential field in service personalisation is linked to the information that is necessary to perform service personalisation; in the current approaches, as already presented, such information includes the user, the utilised device and the service to be consumed. In other words, personalisation in the state-of-the-art includes user preferences, device capabilities and service requirements. (Jørstad et al, 2006a) considers the information space of service personalisation and identifies the User, Service and Device as the actors whose information has to be taken into account towards performing personalisation; additionally a modelled approach of the actors' relationship is proposed. Such an information space is depicted in Figure 1 as a typical one that reflects the current approach for personalisation information space. Alike, for (Kellerer et al, 2006a; "The Operators Vision", 2003) the common view of personalisation is referred to as the combined use of knowledge about the user, his context and the available services to select and tailor services to his individual needs.

Figure 1. Current information space for service personalisation

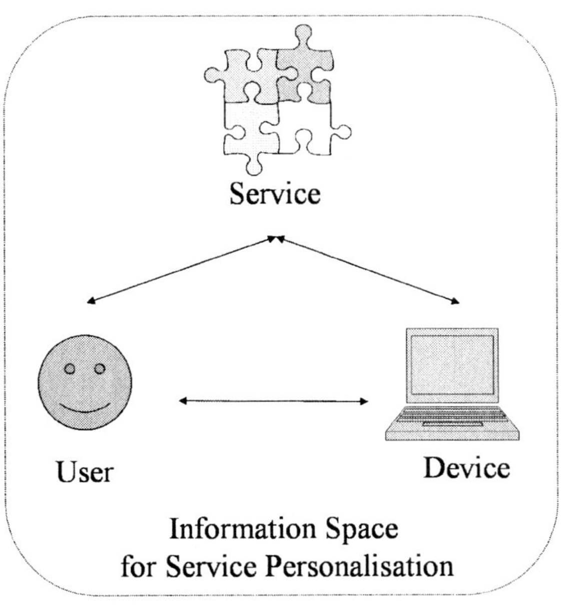

Such an approach is depicted in Figure 1; the Personalisation Information Model is presented as proposed by (Jørstad et al, 2006b). Again, such a model includes service personalisation information (service data, content, usage and profile) as well as user information and preferences. According to this model, profiling heterogeneous environments is reflected to the different types of user devices; such devices have different capabilities and configurations/settings. Additionally, user profiling is a highly differentiated concept: users with different needs, preferences and context request and consume application services.

On top of profile information, user context is a yet critical domain in personalisation. In heterogeneous environments context awareness is to ensure optimum service provision as well as enhance user quality of service and experience. (Arbanowski et al, 2004) approaches user context as including many aspects, such as, user's needs and preferences, history and behaviour as well as location related information.

In general, context awareness enables a service behaviour adaptation according to information and knowledge about the service provision environment. In the same sense as with the profiling issue, the aforementioned environment information needs to be available; in a heterogeneous environment this is not a trivial task. In the literature, contextual information about the service provision environment includes network connectivity information, temporal context and user location information. Additionally, the environment changes in a dynamic fashion, in an unpredictable manner. (Kellerer et al, 2003b) identifies three main domains of interest to be taken into account, namely, user context including, user profile and preferences, available services' features, and the capabilities and constraints of the employed network. On the other hand, even the network information is tailored to the individual user; being referred to as the employed network; this means that the scope is more or less the same: such information can be considered as part of the user context.

The next section presents the current activities/ approaches in profile and contextual information representation.

Context and Profile Management Information Representation and Information Repositories

This section provides a brief overview on profile and context information representation approaches as identified, mainly, in the standardisation domain.

3GPP Generic User Profile (GUP) ("3GPP Generic User Profile", 2005) is the collection of user related data which affects the way in which an individual user experiences services and which may be accessed in a standardised manner as described in this specification. The objective of specifying the 3GPP Generic User Profile is to provide a means to enable harmonised usage of the user-related information originating from different entities. The specification of the GUP shall also allow extensibility to cater for future developments. GUP will be accessed by different stakeholders and managed either by one (centralised) or by different stakeholders (decentralised) such as the user, subscriber, value added service provider and network operator by a standardised access mechanism. GUP allows intra-network usage (i.e. data exchange between applications within a mobile operator's network) and inter-network usage (between mobile operator's network and value added service providers). The objective of the Generic User Profile as developed within 3GPP is to provide a conceptual description for harmonised usage of user-related information located in different entities ([U]SIM, user devices, network nodes, application servers etc). GUP provides architecture, data description method as well as interface for accessing and manipulating user-related data for suppliers and consumers. GUP is structured in a component-based approach. A composite data type is used to define the structure of the whole GUP Component. The structure includes the definition about what kind of Data Element Groups and/or which Data Elements belong to the defined GUP Component as well as the data types and valid values of the data (Figure 3).

3GPP Virtual Home Environment (VHE) ("The Virtual Home Environment", 2006) is defined as a concept for personal service environment portability across network boundaries and between terminals. Within VHE concept users are consistently presented with the same personalised features, User Interface customisation and services in a network and terminal independent basis regarding the corresponding terminal and network capabilities wherever the user may be located. In a VHE a user profile consists of general user-related information and subscribed services related information; such information include individual user information regarding user preferences about personalised services provision and presentation. A single user may have different multiple profiles due to differentiated roles/preferences according to different situations/needs (for instance a user being at home, abroad, at work, etc). Figure 2 depicts the logical components of 3GPP's VHE vision and their relationships' from user's point of view.

W3C Composite Capabilities/Preferences Profile (CC/PP) ("Composite Capability", 2007) defines a high-level structured framework for describing device capabilities and user preferences information. CC/PP framework utilizes the Resource Description Framework (RDF) ("Resource Description Framework", 2007), a semantic web language that is used to represent metadata about web resources in a machine understandable format. The CC/PP framework communicates information about the capabilities and characteristics of a device and of the network bearer to web servers and gateways/proxies, so that an adaptation process may be performed on the server side and the content can be rendered to the device. CC/PP defines a general-purpose structure for a profile, which contains a set of

Figure 2. The Logical Components of the VHE from User's Point of View ("The Virtual Home Environment", 2006)©2002. 3GPP™ TSs and TRs are the property of ARIB, ATIS, CCSA, ETSI, TTA and TTC who jointly own the copyright in them. There are subject to further modifications and are therefore provided to you "as is" for information purposes only. Further use is strictly prohibited.

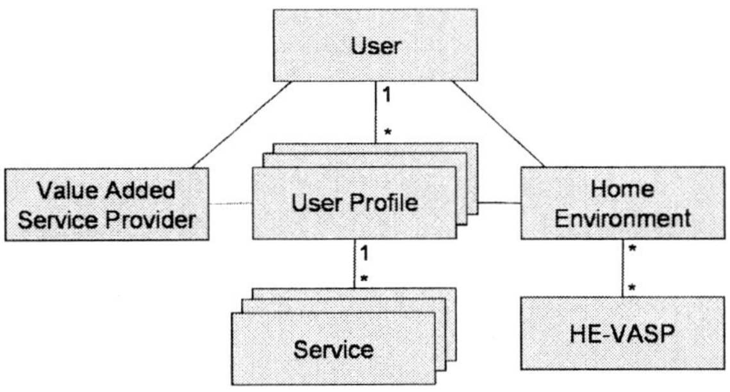

Figure 3. The main parts of GUP©2004. 3GPP™ TSs and TRs are the property of ARIB, ATIS, CCSA, ETSI, TTA and TTC who jointly own the copyright in them. They are subject to further modifications and are therefore provided to you "as is" for information purposes only. Further use is strictly prohibited.

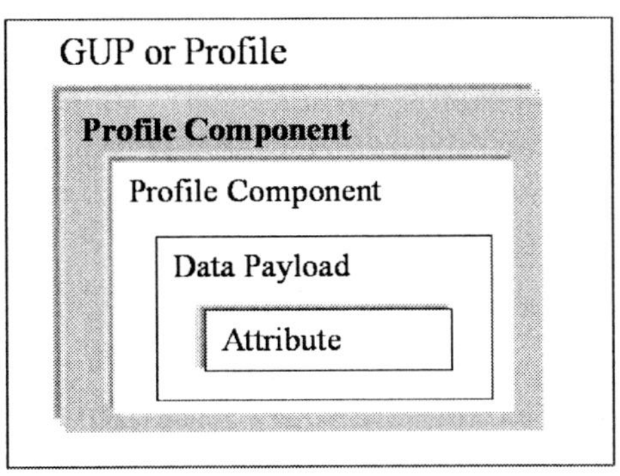

attributes about the device capabilities and user preferences of a device, but it does not define any specific attributes. CC/PP provides the rules of how to construct a vocabulary that describes capabilities and preferences, but does not specify the actual attribute names and values. The work on CC/PP 2.0 started in the Device Independence Working Group (DIWG) and is now carried out by the Ubiquitous Web Applications Working Group (UWAWG) ("Ubiquitous Web", 2007).

The **User Agent Profile (UAProf)** is a specific variant of CC/PP proposed by the Open Mobile Alliance (**OMA**) ("Device Management", 2007). It is an application of CC/PP and therefore it inherits the syntax and semantics of CC/PP. The UAProf specification is concerned with capturing classes of device capabilities and preference information. These classes include (but are not restricted to) the hardware and software characteristics of the device as well as information about the network to which the device is connected.

At this point, it must be noted that although the above presented profiling languages provide a basis for meta-data descriptions of profile information, based on XML and/or RDF, such languages are missing a step forward for advanced profiling requirements. As it will be shown in next subsections, knowledge engineering concepts are able to push forward the profile representation and interpretation providing a high level of expressiveness.

Context-Based Personalised Services Generation

The generation of personalised services has also been addressed, based on the presented approaches for personalisation information. This section lists a number of context-based approaches for personalised service generation:

- (Ralph et al, 2006) presents a framework for on-line personalisation which is based on the division of the information to be utilized into two domains, namely, the User Space that contains user-provided/derived information and the Provider Space that includes all of the information, systems and objects that comprise the website. In this framework several personalisation scenarios are defined to resolve corresponding problems: "Given a user interacting with a website and some user data (from the User Space), reconfigure the Provider Space to maximize expected user satisfaction".

- In the framework of IST MOBIVAS project a distributed software platform has been developed that provides an advanced and flexible solution for the deployment and management of value-added services offered to 3G mobile users. The entire framework comprises specific functionalities which include automatic service registration and deployment by third party service providers including reconfiguration actions on the underlying network for optimal service provision. Moreover, it provides end user a mobile portal for personalised and service discovery. Special care has been given to accounting, charging and billing issues that have been included in the core functionality of MOBIVAS platform (Houssos et al, 2002).
- In (Williams et al, 2005) a framework for personalisation in a pervasive environment is presented, that has been developed as part of IST Daidalos project. Daidalos architecture incorporates the so-called Pervasive Service Platform (PSP) at the top level and the underlying Service Provisioning Platforms. The main objective is the provision of pervasive services to the end user and is achieved though the collaborative operation of the mentioned platform that incorporate specific functionalities such as Context Management, Personalisation, Rule Management, Event Management, Pervasive Service Management, and Security & Privacy Management. Its architecture has been detailed in (Williams et al., 2005).
- Within the IST E^2R (phase I & II) project the concept of personalised service provision has also been captured in project's prototyping activities; a reconfiguration management and control platform has been developed that reflects projects achievements in the system architecture domain. Such a software platform has incorporated personalised service provision scenarios that are based on mechanisms for context and knowledge management, policy management and cognitive/self-* features, such as self-configuration, self-optimization and self-healing (Patouni et al., 2006).
- In (Mostefaoui et al, 2004) a generic approach is presented that combines service-oriented and context-aware computing in order to provide users with more tailored composite services in pervasive computing environments. The general architecture, called CB-sec is formed in a layered approach. In this sense, the physical entities layer represents a federation of physical computing devices and sensors, the application layer supports users to implement context-aware services, and the context management layer facilitates the retrieval, classification and storage of contextual information for hardware and software sensors retrieval, classification and storage, whereas, the service provisioning layer caters for the discovery, composition, execution and caching of the requested services ("Composite Capability", 2007).
- In (Kellerer et al, 2003a) a concept for a personalised service provisioning environment is outlined that is based on key features such as profiling, context-awareness, multi-agent technology, proactive service discovery, dynamic service and dynamic service adaptation.
- Finally, (Maamar et al, 2004) presents an approach for personalising Web services

composition and provisioning using context information. Composition addresses the situation of a user's request that cannot be satisfied by any available service, and thus requires the combination of several Web services whereas provisioning focuses on the deployment of Web services according to his/her preferences. Such an approach is based on three types of context, namely, User context, Web-Service context and Resource context; further, Web services engage in *conversations* when they are subject to personalisation. Finally, different types of *policies* are developed to manage the integration of personalisation into Web services composition and provisioning. The use of these policies guarantees that Web services' provided functionality is not affected by the personalisation procedure.

Evolution Paths Based on New Concepts and Requirements

The future communication world, already referred to as the Beyond-3G (**B3G**) telecommunications environment will be characterized by the co-existence of multiple systems, including cellular, wireless local area, metropolitan area and broadcast; such a heterogeneity results to an increased overall complexity. Furthermore, such systems will consist of distributed components that will be configured in a dynamic fashion. The presented heterogeneity in terms of the coexistence of diverse wireless communications technologies raises the reconfigurability concept. Reconfigurability provides to terminals and network elements the mechanisms for dynamically setting/altering parameter values of a single radio access technology, dynamically allocating resources to and among radio access technologies and distributing radio access technologies to network elements.

Reconfigurability is considered as the collection of software and cognitive radio technologies that aim to differentiate user perception in volatile radio conditions while optimising the use of network resources. Autonomic computing emerges as a new paradigm for managing increasingly complex tasks at the business, system, and device level without human intervention.

Such a telecommunications environment results in a novel service provision framework; service provision aspects will be impacted and facilitated in the context of cognitive reconfigurable systems; within the communication space formed by these technologies, the users will be provided the required services, at affordable cost, in different heterogeneous contexts, using diverse equipment and through the different available technologies. In such an environment the user will use heterogeneous devices in varied environments and contexts (including the home, office, transportation, on the move, etc.) and through heterogeneous access systems (such as fixed, wireless local area networks, cellular and broadcast technologies).

Based on the above presented new concepts and requirements it is expected that the essential issue of information to drive the personalisation will also be affected. In the following paragraphs the emerging approaches are outlined. The work on information space, the personalisation information model as well as new entries in the context and knowledge management and representation in standards working groups and bodies is depicted in the next section.

Personalisation Information Model

Based on the novel approaches within research projects in reconfigurability and autonomic communications, contextual information seems to move towards a more dynamic nature. In the presented state of the art, the user profile includes preferences and personal information, the service profile includes mainly service requirements and the device profile includes mainly device capabilities; each of such profile instances includes more or less static information. But things are changing rapidly: in the reconfigurability vision, a device can change functionality in a dynamic fashion thus changing configurations and even its capabilities. This means that the former static profile information may be considered as dynamic in nature thus being included into the composite notion of context. Alike, a user device is concerned and aware not only of the employed network type but also of the available ones and this in a dynamic fashion: a UE may connect to a network after a reconfiguration, thus after a configuration/capabilities change. Additionally, multi-homing devices are expected to further impact the device capabilities information model as well as the corresponding representation. In the same sense, service personalisation is highly differentiated after an individual reconfiguration action: service requirements are to be fulfilled in a different level, according to the current configuration of a device, user preferences may be turned on after a reconfiguration process, a connection to a different RAT may also activate a number of differentiations accordingly. A novel approach for the information space takes into account multiple types of information; as depicted in Figure 4 the

Figure 4. Novel information space for service personalisation

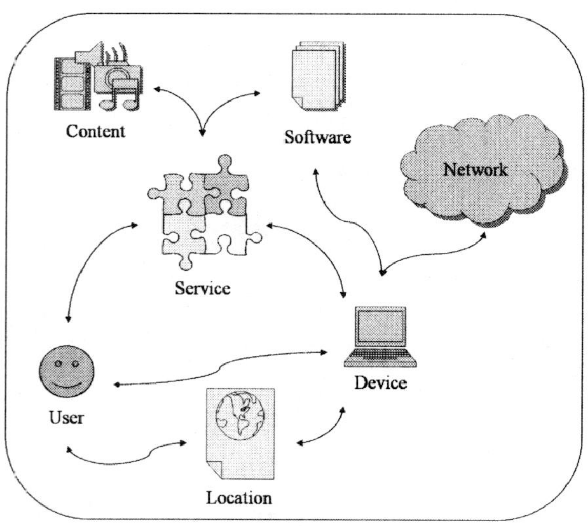

information space for service personalisation is to include user, service, device, network, content, software and location related information. As already mentioned, such information will be mainly dynamic in fashion due to the new concepts and requirements. Additionally, the storage of the information will be performed on a distributed approach; multiple copies may need to be maintained thus increasing the need for synchronisation among the different repositories.

The importance of ontology-based context representation and knowledge management in heterogeneous systems with reconfigurable devices exploiting also autonomic features is considerable. An ontology is a data model that represents a domain and is used to reason about the objects in that domain and the relations between them. Figure 5 provides an example ontology schema for a telecommunications environment depicting both the objects (user, service, RAT, operator, etc) as well as the corresponding relations. Ontologies provide a means to represent any type of knowledge in a standard way; this includes information by reference that is to be provided by stakeholders (profiles, static information) or collected in a dynamic way (profile, dynamic information, and context) as well as information by inference that is based on contextual information representation. An interesting approach to this direction is presented by (Lewis et al, 2004), which states that ontologies will provide a strong mechanism for addressing the heterogeneity in user task requirements, managed resources, services and context. It also presents two complimentary approaches that exploit ontology-based knowledge in support of autonomic communications: service-oriented models for policy engineering and dynamic semantic queries using content-based networks. The work performed by (Laukkanen, 2004) studies the role of Semantic Web Technologies in Context-Aware systems. It also describes the role of context ontologies for service adaptation and presents a simplified network ontology and among others a Network QoS Ontology.

Figure 5. Example ontology schema

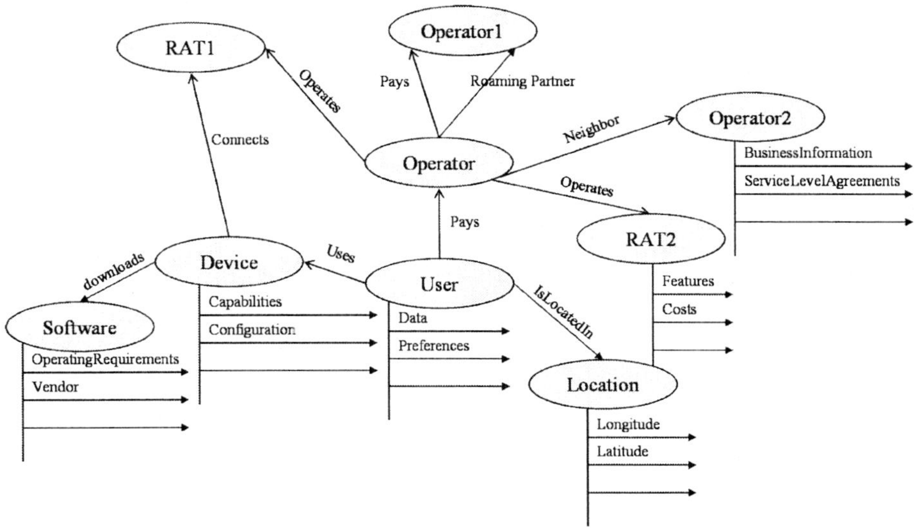

MIDDLEWARE ARCHITECTURES AND SOLUTIONS FOR PERSONALISED SERVICE OFFERING

The modern mobile communications environment has witnessed the introduction and gradual proliferation of the Internet technologies, which have assisted in bringing the same freedom-of-choice feeling enjoyed in the Internet to the traditional cellular technologies. High data rate mobile multimedia applications, the request for seamless communication across heterogeneous access and networking technologies, as well as the introduction of pervasive computing have greatly increased the requirements on service platforms and middleware. Nevertheless, the mobile user—even more than the internet user—will increasingly request services that are tailored to his/ her personal needs and preferences and well aligned with his surroundings and the situation he/ she is in. A personalised service offering in this diverse environment can only be catered by flexible middleware architectures that will combine the open internet paradigm with the mobile communications one.

This section will present existing architectural solutions featuring object oriented technologies and will discuss the interesting functional issues that emerge in the process to a personalised service offering. An integrated framework which addresses these challenges is presented thereafter.

Object Oriented Architectures for Service Provision

Legacy mobile service provision platforms have focused on vertically integrating components on a per-service basis trying to achieve the optimum individual service delivery but overlooking the emergent needs for service composition and reusability. This monolithic approach has been the cause for high integration and implementation efforts on the application developer side, especially in cases where individual service composition was required to provide a comprehensive service offering. On top of that, from an end-user perspective, the service experience became fragmented because of the inconsistent use of user information and context among the various services and the mobility requirements.

A successful service provision platform needs to be able to handle contextual and profile information about the user in an integrated manner for all services, providing open interfaces to the application developers but at the same time ensuring that the mobile operators' resources exposure is controlled and protected from arbitrary and unauthorized use. Integration of resources, interoperability and scalability are important assets for the operator and the application developer, whereas security, usability and privacy are always important for the end-user.

Object Oriented Architectures have emerged as a promising concept in order to deal with these overwhelming issues. The list of these architectures' inherent features, which includes (among others) encapsulation, inheritance and polymorphism fits right into the mobile service platforms requirements description. Encapsulation takes care that the internal resources are protected from external unauthorised access, while at the same time the object's behaviour is publicly exposed and available for use. Inheritance is the key enabler for the extension and reusability of already available services in the direction of building more complex and sophisticated ones. Finally, polymorphism is the feature that enables practically the same functionality to be experienced as a service's different behaviour according to the service offering's context/ parameters.

The discussion above shows that it is with solid foundation that several standardisation bodies have chosen the object-oriented model to describe their architectures for an open mobile communications service environment. The Open Mobile Alliance (OMA) has proposed the Open Service Environment (OSE), which attempts to answer to all the modern requirements on providing a personalised service offering ("OMA Service Environment", 2007). The Parlay Group has defined the Parlay specification of open, technology independent interfaces forming an architecture that has also been adopted by ETSI & 3GPP standardisation bodies as the Open Service Access architecture for third generation mobile networks ("Parlay/ OSA", 2007; "ETSI OSA", 2007; "OSA API", 2007).

Service Oriented Architectures (SOA), a promising paradigm which follows the object orientation paradigm success and adopts its main features, has emerged as a compelling technology in service management architectures. SOA focuses on distributed, loosely coupled capabilities—named services, which may reside under the control of different ownership domains, and can be described, published and invoked in a

Figure 6. OMA open service environment

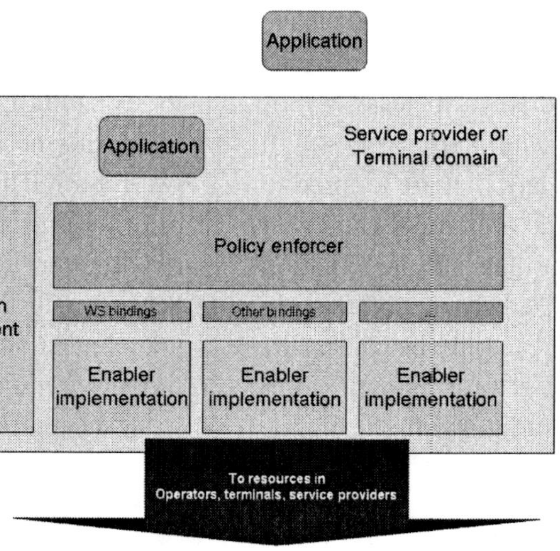

Figure 7. Relationship between Parlay X and Parlay APIs ("Parlay X", 2002)

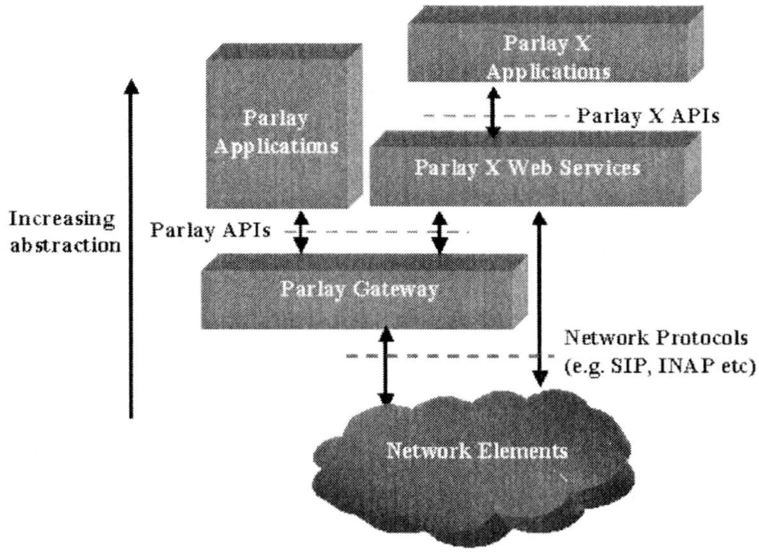

standardised way. In this sense, SOA adds greater flexibility and addresses in a more comprehensive way the service composition requirement, while maintaining the advantages of object-oriented architectures. Again, the Parlay Group has moved forward into standardising part of its specification following the SOA paradigm, namely the Parlay X web services.

Functional Issues for Personalisation

Delving more into details about the necessary functionality offered by a middleware with the aim to support personalised service provision, one needs to discern four main functional domains, i.e. profile, context management, knowledge management and service adaptation. Although for the purposes of this study, context and contextual information are considered broader terms that encompass profile information, a separate section is dedicated on profile management to denote the importance of profile information handling for the purposes of a personalised service offering.

Context Management

Driving a car seems to wake up one's eagerness for learning. It is not rare that one wonders about this and that right when being behind the steering wheel. This information can prove extremely valuable for the driver and could lead him/ her to take the one way or the other or just simply satisfy his/ her curiosity. Therefore, it is important to present this info in a timely and proper manner. In case that this is traffic information, it's important to know whether the driver is currently on the move or just staying still on the side of the road. Knowing that, the traffic info service can adapt to the driver's situation and offer voice instructions when he/ she is on the move and augment the service experience with visual map or textual information when he/ she has stopped. Getting the service tailored to the situation the user is in really makes the customer satisfied.

But to be able to adapt the provided service according to the user's environment and situation, one needs to know the context that surrounds him/ her. In the situation above, a speed sensor would have sufficed to clarify whether the user is on the move or not. In general, context can be retrieved with multiple and diverse ways but sensors technology evolution has really assisted in retrieving a plethora of contextual information in a cheap and timely way. Services can benefit from information about the user and the surrounding environment, e.g. location, speed, noise, temperature, lighting conditions etc.; information that can be gathered by the respective sensors, a database, a profile repository or even a separate service that is able to aggregate contextual information out of other context information objects (van Kranenburg et al, 2006). Context retrieval can therefore be considered the first and elementary step in order to be able to tailor a service to the user's personal situation.

Nevertheless, contextual information cannot be of great value to applications unless it goes through a pre-processing stage. Due to its raw state, it is subject to various error sources such as temporary unavailability (e.g. due to the sensor's ephemeral malfunctioning or high CPU load), physical constraints or temporary effects that can limit the sensors' precision, low "freshness" (because of outdated and no longer applicable to the situation information) etc. To address this issue, the term Quality of Context (QoC) (in analogy to Quality of Service) has been introduced in order to describe the quality/ value of the information that is used as context. QoC is deduced by metrics like precision, probability of correctness, trust-worthiness, resolution, age etc. and can determine the worth of contextual information for a specific application (Krause et al, 2005). Context pre-processing can be expected to enhance QoC, since "odd", non-contiguous, old and/ or non-trustworthy data values, which were erroneously accounted for, can be dropped and/ or filled in, thus "smoothing" the data value set. This important filtering process is followed by a reformatting step in order to feed more efficiently and in an acceptable format the next step in the context management process, context composition (Sigg et al, 2006).

Context Composition is the process, where raw contextual data is aggregated from different context sources and compiled into a more abstract context description. Challenges in this step include the combination of information coming from multiple sources into meaningful higher level derived context information. In the above example, a high speed measurement (coming from the speed sensor) combined with infrequent changes of the vehicle's bearing (measured by a compass) might point to the direction that the user is driving on a highway, which is the derived contextual information that will pose a strict response time requirement on the service provision process. Suppose though that, after juxtaposing the location of the car on the region road map, there seems to be no highway around the user's location. What conclusion can we draw from that? Which of the measurements are better to trust? During the context composition phase, the challenge of resolving contradicting measurements in order to provide a trustworthy context description can be resolved with the use of the QoC metric and the application of trust policies on context sources.

Knowledge Management

Inferring user situation by using contextual information at hand can prove to be a lengthy process resulting in sometimes dubious user situation descriptions. To alleviate this fact and produce reliable implicit knowledge from explicit contextual information, one turns to the use of additional information like semantics, context history and machine learning approaches.

Semantic information, as expressed usually through ontologies, is the means to integrate machine-interpretable contextual information with human reasoning, as depicted in the ontologies, and transform context info to knowledge. This further step in context interpretation can facilitate more accurate and relevant to the user situation decisions towards a personalised service offering based on knowledge deriving from the relationships among terms in an ontology. Going back to our example, driving at a high speed with frequent changes of direction, combined with our knowledge of real-world situations, might result in a decision that it is actually *dangerous* to distract the driver's attention with any kind of service information and point to a temporary pause in the service offering. This can be achieved with the reasoning of the current contextual information on a *Mobility* ontology, describing the relationships between dangerous driving and the factors speed, change of bearing, time of day etc. While this process of producing knowledge still remains lengthy but, indeed, adds reliability to the end result, taking advantage of historical information about the user can improve the process efficiency.

Historical information on a user's behaviour can be considered a key enabler in order to avoid going through all computational steps of transforming raw contextual information into knowledge, thus making context-aware service platforms more efficient. The idea is simple. If, for the past 2 months, our user has been driving on weekdays along the same road and this movement bears similar features through all the monitoring period, then one can deduce a pattern behaviour that can be summarised as such: "David tends to request traffic information while commuting on Mondays and Fridays right before he goes over crossing X65". This probabilistic pattern extraction process can be used to predict a user's behaviour and tailor the service offering to his/her needs, which are now predicted well in advance, thus being able to efficiently address each user's needs without adding too much computational load for on-the-fly context interpretation processing. Machine learning approaches, such as the Bayesian networks, can assist in building these high-level user behaviours (Devitt et al, 2006).

Profile Management

The importance of profile information in providing a service offering has been pinpointed above, as well as the various kinds of profiles that have been recognised in order to capture the necessary information. This section will present some challenges related to a service platform's profile management functionality, namely the profile storage and retrieval.

The composite heterogeneous mobile communications environment in the B3G era poses some new requirements on the profile storage mechanisms. The variety of interworking networks (e.g. 2G, 2.5G, 3G cellular systems, WLAN, WiMax etc) and their evolution requires a distributed approach on profile storage. It is far beyond any reality the argument that all profile information can be kept in a single point to facilitate a "one-stop-shop" approach for profile retrieval thus easily resolving synchronisation and security issues. Instead, the new environment calls for a decentralised approach, where each interworking partner reserves the right to manage information that lies under its royalty and control access to it. To present an example, the terminal profile main storage is expected to be inside the terminal under the control of the terminal manufacturer and the user, e.g. the OMA DM approach ("Device Management", 2007) but, nevertheless, a synchronised copy would be useful for the network's service delivery platform in order to adapt a service to a terminal's capabilities. Accordingly, the service profile is to be mainly stored within the control of the service provider but is expected to be handed over to the terminal, the user and possibly the network at a given time. In any case, the synchronisation challenge emerges with a growing significance, since multiple copies might be kept in different places and profile information will be modified on a more frequent basis. Profile database synchronisation could be the solution, in cases where computational resources are not scarce—after all, service profiles have been successfully synchronised so far in UDDI registries ("Universal Description", 2005)– but this cannot be the case for low-end terminals not supporting database mechanisms.

On the opposite side, with regards to profile information retrieval, it is clear that the above considerations on storage mechanisms have to be taken into account in order to facilitate efficient and timely information retrieval. On top of that, the B3G mobile communications era features the openness of the telecommunication environment to third parties (e.g. VASPs, content providers etc.), who were previously not directly related to the service offering. Therefore, it becomes critical to restrict access to information residing within each partner's responsibility domain to entities that have been authorised for this purpose. A security framework that will provide reliable and flexible (e.g. supporting multiple security schemes) profile access mechanisms and will facilitate the authorisation requirement without "overloading" the links with overhead information transporting credentials back and forth would be the key to address the profile retrieval security requirement.

Service Adaptation

Service adaptation is the final step in the service provision chain that will actually enable a personalised service offering. It's the lever which turns all the gathered contextual information and inferred knowledge into added value for the user and the service experience he/ she will enjoy. The underlying middleware is of good use only if, after monitoring the context, it "acts" appropriately without the need for human intervention in the control loop (Erickson, 2002). These "actions" include *modality control* and *flexible offering*.

The term "modality control" refers to the means that the service is presented to the user. This functionality answers to the "*How* is it more appropriate to present the service results to the user?" question. Deciding on whether to offer the service in video, audio, text (or even not at all) according to the situation context and actually performing the relevant adaptation is the element that will be appreciated by the user and considered actually "intelligent". In our driving example, sensing high levels of noise in the car can mean that the user is enjoying his/ her favourite music loud, so it might be better to present the audio information in a text format or, alternatively, lower the car stereo volume, should there be such a possibility, risking though going against the user's wishes. This would naturally require on the underlying middleware side to support the transition among all three modes, which in some cases is not obvious. In extreme situations, a service could also be adapted, so as to be paused, delayed, or not offered at all, if this is dictated by safety reasons (as indicated above in the driving fast scenario).

Of equal importance for the end result is the service content transcoding issue. It's not uncommon (even in the pc world) for users to actually have access to the desired content but to be unable to play it back due to the lack of the necessary codecs. The case becomes even stronger in the mobile world's restricted environment. It's of great importance, therefore, for the user to have access to the content in the right format, or, in other words, in a format adapted to his/ her device. The transcoding functionality can utilize contextual information about the user's terminal and, in specific, about the supported video and audio formats and employ the relevant algorithms. These algorithms usually decode the original data to a raw intermediate format and then re-encode it in the target format in order to adapt it to the terminal capabilities. The same approach would be also useful in order to change the bit rate of a downloadable stream or file, also known as transrate. In this case, monitoring information on the network a device is camped on could drive the transrating process in order to improve the user experience by saving bandwidth, time and/ or money (Chandra et al, 2000).

Service adaptation entails also a flexible service offering capability. The ability to dynamically add/remove/replace/compose service components in order to provide a personalised service enables a much more rich and flexible service set to be provided to the user (Houssos et al, 2005). In this case, adapting a service could mean a more personalised and user friendly result or even prove the lever to open a whole new service set for the user. While converting the results of a location based service from miles to kilometres would just prove convenient for a user accustomed to the metric system when in the UK, translating the service results into e.g. the handset's selected language could enable a roaming user to have access to all kind of services the serving mobile operator offers. This can be easily achieved if the underlying middleware draws contextual information about e.g. the user's country of origin or selected language and uses it to feed e.g. the results of a weather service into a translation engine. In this way, dynamic service composition, as a constituent functionality inside the service adaptation functionality block, can facilitate a more personalised service offering.

Middleware and Solutions for Personalised Service Provision

To give a unified view on the issues presented above, Context, Knowledge, Profile Management and Service Adaptation are integrated into a common middleware framework to support personalised service provision. The framework presented in Figure 8 (in UML notation) comprises contextual information, knowledge engineering concepts such as ontologies, as well as the corresponding distributed repositories utilizing access management mechanisms such as authentication. Furthermore, profile management includes component based profile information forming as well as notifications of profile updates through a notification service. Resource monitoring is performed in a dynamic fashion through the identification of the most appropriate reporting type. Finally, the resource monitoring reports support the estimation of the performance measures.

Starting from the upper right on the figure, *rawProfileData* inside *Profile Access Management* represents profile information that is to be retrieved from a profile repository (either external

Figure 8. Integrated middleware framework for personalised service support

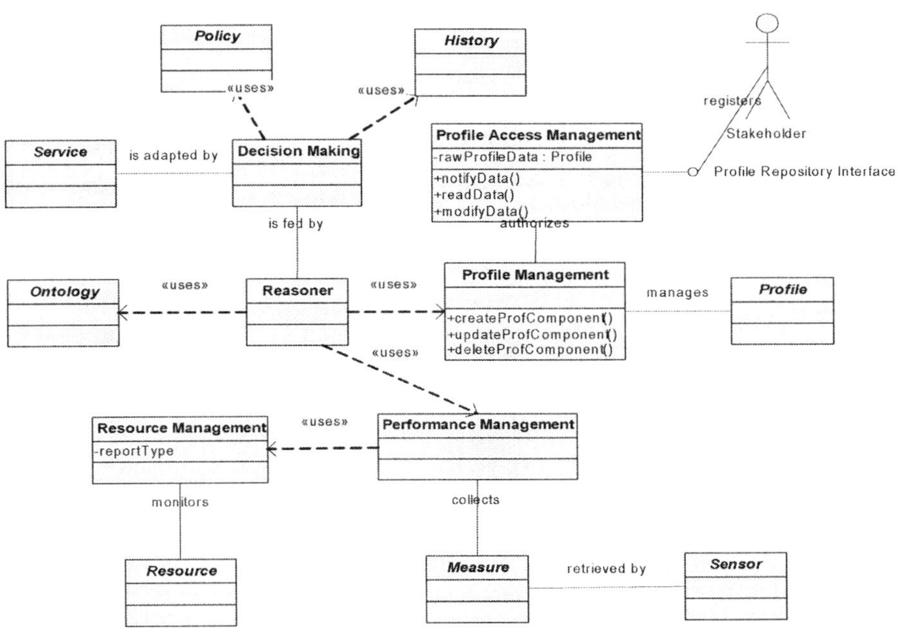

or internal) in any possible form. For instance, a Manufacturer *(Stakeholder)* may provide a user terminal's profile (capabilities and default configuration) in an xml-based format. *Profile* stands for an abstract class that represents profile information in the platform specific operational form (e.g. made up of profile components, like CC/PP (Composite Capability, 2007). In realisation terms, a *Profile* instance may be one of the defined specialisations (*User Profile, Device Profile, Service Profile and Network Profile*).

Profile information is maintained in profile repositories and made available to the system via a *Profile Repository Interface*. This interface is to provide the *notifyData()* method that notifies involved entities about profile information updates. *Profile Access Management* realizes profile retrieval and update functions through the *readData*() and *modifyData*() operations. The retrieved value forms the *rawProfileData*. Its main functionality includes authorisation mechanisms that are to control access in the aforementioned profile repositories. *Profile Management* class has the responsibility to map/ transform the retrieved *rawProfileData* to the adopted profile representation scheme (e.g. in terms of profile components and attribute value pairs) as well as to update the profile instances utilising the *createComponent(), updateComponent() and deleteComponent()* operations.

The *Resource* class (bottom left) represents a resource of the system (e.g. available device memory, power information etc.), whereas the *Measure* class stands for a specific measure that has been identified (e.g. location, speed etc.). *Resource Management* will monitor a set of identified *Resources* and collect the monitoring records. Such records will be used by the *Performance Management* class in order to evaluate/ estimate the value of the identified *Measures*.

The *Reasoner* will aggregate the required profile, resource and performance information from the *Profile Management, Resource Management* and *Performance Management* classes, respectively, and will reason on them utilising the relevant *Ontology*. The results will be fed to the *Decision Making* class in the form of a high-level, abstract contextual description. The impact of *Policy* and *History* classes on the contextual description will be evaluated by the *Decision Making* class and will drive the *Service* adaptation procedure.

The above described framework claims to propose a solution to address the challenges highlighted above, both in terms of advanced context and knowledge management mechanisms as well as the important profile management issues in order to drive the service adaptation functionality.

ADVANCED CONCEPTS IN PERSONALISED SERVICE PROVISION

Situation aware service provision over self-managed cognitive systems becomes an important issue in order to exploit the advanced autonomic capabilities of the underlying communication environment. It is thus related to the detection, identification and organisation of the communication context, the respective autonomic capabilities available, as well as the compilation of pervasive services resulting in an advanced service offering to the user. Autonomous adaptation and reconfiguration of the service and communication characteristics to existing and emerging situations will support a dynamic and tailored to user and surrounding conditions practice of service provision. The aforementioned service adaptation enables the minimization of adverse and unstable network conditions impact by using self adjustment/configuration techniques at high network layers based on information obtained from the network. It further enables to get the best of the network infrastructure and associated resources, being able to adaptively ensure sufficient quality of service, guarantee always best served for users, and tune to user needs and preferences, independently of the actual network characteristics.

In such systems, complex decisions and actions will have to be made in the direction of achieving optimal self-configuration and self-management of communication system elements and services. Moreover, distributed negotiation, policy exchange and prioritisation of domain policies for distributed decision making in such environments is an important aspect to achieve flexibility and manage complexity. The service space will have to establish an abstraction of the autonomic capabilities of the underlying communication and proactive negotiations will be triggered between or to the self-managed elements vicinity.

All the above, lead to the evolution of middleware solutions in order to support cognitive and autonomic system behaviour, autonomic personalisation of service provision and negotiations over heterogeneous systems for advanced service and application offerings.

Cognitive and Autonomic Concepts

The characteristic features of autonomic communications are the use of highly decentralized algorithms that have desirable emergent properties while retaining both a high level of global predictability and a close integration with cognitive and other contextual goals (Dobson et al, 2006). The autonomic systems operation follows a feedback cycle (Figure 9). The system monitors information from a variety of sources including traditional network sensors and management reporting streams but also including higher-level device and user contextual information. The respective observations form the basis of a knowledge model that is used to identify the current system situation and context. This model feeds the decision making process targeting context aware system adaptation. The decisions result to configuration actions, which are realized by the network and the autonomic systems. The impact of the decisions and implemented actions is the self-configuration and self-management of autonomic systems. A high profile use of autonomic techniques is provided by IBM's autonomic computing initiative (Kephart et al, 2003). The autonomic computing has been introduced as a way of reducing the total cost of ownership of complex IT systems by allowing dynamic reconfiguration and optimisation based on emerging context and ongoing system's behaviour. It combines a technological vision with a business rationale for increasing the coupling between business goals and IT services.

Autonomic communications address emerging research items from the autonomic computing field and their applicability on the communications field. The impact of these concepts in the services, communication, networking, and distributed computing paradigms is profound. The ultimate vision of autonomic communication research is that of a networked world in which networks and associated devices and services will be able to work in a totally unsupervised manner, able to self-configure, self-monitor, self-adapt, and self-heal—the so-called "*self-* properties*".

This evolution will accommodate new functionality in networks, services and devices, enabling the dynamic adaptation of the respective functional components to changing conditions and context, user requirements and preferences. Moreover, autonomic communications concepts are targeting to efficiently cope with the complexity and associated costs currently involved in the effective and reliable deployment of networks and communication services. This will result in highly manageable and reactive systems, incorporating advanced capabilities for dynamic adaptation and personalisation of services and communication system behaviour.

Technologies that play a significant role in the middleware solutions for personalised autonomic communications are related to context management, decision making and policy description (e.g., SWRL), ontologies, as well as reconfiguration management protocols and functional entities. An ontology can enable inferences to be made about

Figure 9. Autonomic and cognitive feedback cycle

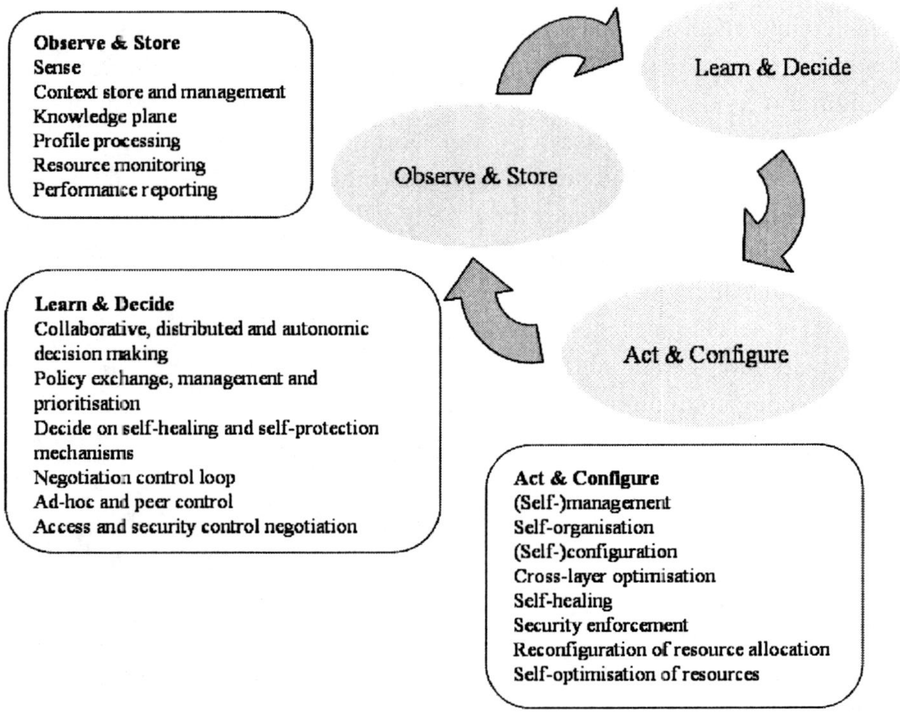

the knowledge that they contain (Fox et al, 1998). Moreover, based on the policies incorporated in the system, decisions can be derived and respective reconfiguration actions can be planned.

The implication of such concepts in the personalisation of services and systems lies on the rethinking of the user requirements and context fusion in a way that this will appear and captured by the autonomic system as part of the policies affecting the system's behaviour.

Personalisation in Autonomic Communications and Services

Personalisation and adaptation of service, infrastructure and content, will be a process encompassing variability of choices based on knowledge, proactiveness of autonomic elements and prediction of alternative situations. Tuning self-managed communication elements into varying service requirements and physical or domain policy related restrictions cut out notable research and market areas. Self-managed network and terminal elements may not belong to the same domains (e.g., operators etc.). Similarly services may not be deployed and offered by the same domains or actors. Therefore, the network status information has to be processed in order for the available network resources to be identified and presented in a uniform way enabling, on one hand, service provisioning over varying network conditions and, on the other hand, network scalability.

The personalisation aspects in an autonomic communications and services environment become an issue of user context fusion in this particular environment. As stated earlier in this chapter (static) profile information is now considered dynamic in nature and included into the composite notion of context. In this sense, by user context, it is meant:

- User requirements and preferences (preferred services, mode of operations, connections, preferred devices, preferred RATs etc.)

- User zones of activity (e.g., entertainment, home, office)
- User related context from sensors and other sources (e.g., location, activity status—in a meeting, in cinema, etc.)

The fundamental personalisation features will encompass all the above information as part of autonomic system self-awareness. The policy framework is in this way extended to capture the user context as part of the system policies and feed respectively the decision making. Based on the user related policies, the respective decisions will trigger the actuation of system and service adaptation in order to personalise accordingly the system behaviour and service provision (Figure 10).

An important evolution of the system personalisation capability is the enhancement of the knowledge plane of the autonomic and cognition loop. The knowledge plane elaborates on spatial and temporal context views and enriches the decision making process. It is therefore an asset for the dynamic personalisation that can be supported by the autonomic systems. Therefore, the personalisation of services in autonomic environments becomes more and more a dynamic feature incorporated in the self-awareness and self-adaptation process of the autonomic system. It is based on recursive context in order to capture ongoing behaviour, environment and user related information and preferences and match all these with existing and emerging user policies in order to achieve vigorous and self-motivated personalisation configurations.

Figure 10. Autonomic personalisation process

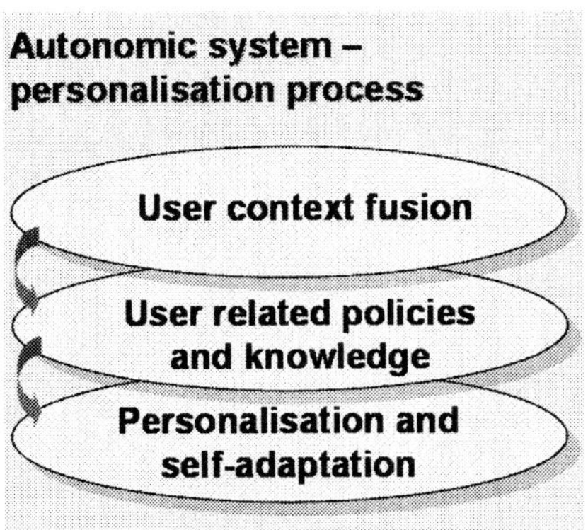

It is thus apparent that the autonomic and cognitive systems evolutions have a great impact on the notion of personalisation and on respective functionality and middleware solutions. Future systems will contain fundamental functional entities with integrated dynamic features resulting in highly advanced personalisation features.

CONCLUSION

Personalisation remains a challenging issue in the forthcoming mobile communications era. The provision of application and services that are aware of the individual preferences and characteristics of subscribers of mobile networks contributes in experiencing communication with personalised touch and feel while using the mobile devices. In that scope, user profiles and context-awareness have a critical role. The former contributes in collecting, concatenating and publishing various user-specific attributes, the latter in adapting service offering to the composite notion of user context. Additionally, object oriented design principles are very important in the introduction of middleware and service provision solutions.

The notion of context is defined as the combination of information relevant to the nearest environment of a user, such as the user location, the serving network, his terminal device, etc. The contextual information is encoded in various related profiles such as, the user preferences profile and the terminal, ambient network, and service profiles. The combination of all these profiles constitutes the user context. In situation–aware architectures, the notion of (user) context is composite in nature and dynamically composed since its constituting segments may be distributed. Contextual information affects significantly a service's deployment and execution, since context-aware services should adapt to context and related updates. A new dimension in personalisation aspects is also introduced with the emergence of autonomic systems. The notion of personalisation is extended to capture the dynamic context fusion in a way that this will appear and captured by the autonomic system as part of the policies and knowledge affecting the system's behaviour. Therefore, personalisation features become part of the knowledge plane, self-awareness and self-adaptation of the autonomic system.

FUTURE RESEARCH DIRECTIONS

Future middleware solutions will target the facilitation and abstraction of nice technologies, specifically focused on the migration of heterogeneous computing and telecommunication systems with cognitive and autonomic features. Personal awareness and situation awareness will have impact on service provision over self-managed cognitive systems evolution. In order to exploit the advanced autonomic capabilities of the underlying communication environment, new architectures and approaches will exploit the detection, identification and organisation of the communication context, the respective autonomic capabilities available, as well as the compilation of pervasive services resulting in an advanced service offering to the user. Encapsulation of novel features for autonomous adaptation and reconfiguration of the service and communication characteristics to existing and emerging situations will be targeted in order to support a dynamic and tailored to user and surrounding conditions practice of service provision. In such systems, complex decisions and actions will have to be made in the direction of achieving optimal self-configuration and self-management of communication system elements and services. Moreover, policy exchange and prioritisation of domain policies for distributed decision making in such environments is an important aspect to achieve flexibility and manage complexity. The service space will have to establish an abstraction of the autonomic capabilities of the underlying communication and proactive negotiations will be triggered between or to the self-managed elements vicinity. This will be impacting the service adaptation decisions.

The aforementioned service adaptation will enable the minimisation of adverse and unstable network conditions impact by using self adjustment/configuration techniques at high network layers based on information obtained from the network. The emergence of such middleware characteristics will further contribute to get the best of the network behaviour, facilities and associated resources, being able to adaptively ensure sufficient quality of service, guarantee always best served for users, and tune to user needs and preferences, independently of the actual network characteristics.

Therefore, the future research directions in this field will yield the evolution of middleware solutions in order to support cognitive and autonomic system behaviour, autonomic personalisation of service provision and negotiations over heterogeneous systems for advanced service and application offerings.

REFERENCES

3GPP Generic User Profile (GUP); Stage 3; Network (Release 6), V6.1.0, 3GPP TS 29.240 (2005). Retrieved from http://www.3gpp.org/

Arbanowski, S., Ballon, P., David., K., Droegehorn, O., Eetink, H., Kelleler, W., van Kranenburg, H., Raatikainen, K., & Popescu-Zeletin, R. (2004). I-centric Communications: Personalization, Ambient Awareness, and Adaptability for Future Mobile Services. *IEEE communications Magazine*, 42(9), 63-69

Blom, J. (2000) Personalization - a taxonomy. In *CHI 2000 Workshop on Designing Interactive*

Systems for 1-to-1 E-commerce (pp. 313-314). ACM Press

Chandra, S.; Ellis, C., S.; & Vahdat, A., (2000). Application-level differentiated multimedia Web services using quality aware transcoding. *IEEE Journal on Selected Areas in Communications,* 18(12), pp. 2544-2565.

Composite Capability/Preference Profiles (CC/PP): Structure and Vocabularies 2.0. The World Wide Web Consortium (W3C) (2007). Retrieved from http://www.w3.org/TR/2007/WD-CCPP-struct-vocab2-20070430/

Device Management Working Group. Open Mobile Alliance (2007). Retrieved from http://www.openmobilealliance.org/tech/wg_committees/dm.html

Devitt, A., Danev, B., & Matusikova, K. (2006, December). *Constructing Bayesian Networks Automatically using Ontologies.* Paper presented at the Second Workshop Formal Ontologies Meet Industry (FOMI), Trento, Italy

Dobson, S., Massacci, F., Denazis, S., Nixon, P., Fernandez, A., Saffre, F., Gaiti, D., Schmidt, N., Gelenbe, E., & Zambonelli, F., (2006). A Survey of Autonomic Communications. *ACM Transactions on Autonomous and Adaptive Systems*, 1(2), 223–259.

Erickson, T. (2002). Some problems with the notion of context-aware computing. *Communications of the ACM,* 45(2), pp. 102-104.

ETSI OSA Phase 4 (Draft Parlay 6.0 Specifications) (2007). ETSI Retrieved from http://portal.etsi.org/docbox/TISPAN/Open/OSA/Parlay60.html

Fox, M.S., Gruninger, M. (1998). Enterprise Modelling. *AI Magazine, American Association for AI,* pp. 109-121

Houssos, N., Gazis, E., Panagiotakis, S., Gessler, S., Schuelke, A., & Quesnel, S., (2002). *Value AddedService Management in 3G networks.* Paper presented at Network Operations and Management Symposium, Florence, Italy.

Houssos, N., Alonistioti, N., & Merakos, L. (2005). Specification and dynamic introduction of 3rd party, service-specific adaptation policies for mobile applications. *Mobile Networks and Applications*, 10(4), pp. 405-421.

Jørstad, I., Van Thanh, D., & Dustdar, D. (2006a). *Personalisation of Next Generation Mobile Services.* Paper presented at Ubiquitous Mobile Information and Collaboration Systems (UMICS2006), Luxembourg, June 5-6.

Jørstad, I., Van Thanh, D., (2006b). Service Personalisation in Mobile Heterogeneous Environmnents. In *Advanced International Conference on Telecommunications AICT-ICIW '06. International Conference on Internet and Web Applications and Services* (pp. 70-70). IEEE Computer Society

Kellerer, W., Hirschfeld, R., Tarlano, A. & Wagner, M. (2003a, June). *Towards a Personalized Service Provisioning Environment.* Paper presented at the IST Mobile Communications Summit Aveiro, Portugal.

Kellerer, W., Wagner, M., Balke, W., Schulzrinne H. (2003b). Preference-based Session Management for Personalized Services. *European Transactions on Telecommunications*, 15(4), pp. 415-427.

Krause, M., Hochstatter, I. (2005). Challenges in Modelling and Using Quality of Context (QoC). In *Mobility Aware Technologies and Applications, Second International Workshop, MATA* 17-19 October 2005, Montreal, Canada

Laukkanen, M. (2004). *Semantic Web Technologies in Context-Aware Systems* (Seminar Paper). Department of Computer Science, University of Helsinki.

Lewis, D., Feeney, K., Tiropanis, T., & Courtenage, S. (2004). Semantic-based Policy Engineering for Autonomic Systems. In: Smirnov, Michael, (Ed.), *Autonomic Communication: First International IFIP Workshop, WAC 2004: revised selected papers* (pp. 152-164). Lecture Notes in Computer Science (3457). Springer, Berlin, Germany.

Maamar, Z.,Al Khatib, G., Mostefaoui, S., K. (2004), *Context-based Personalization of Web Services Composition and Provisioning,* Paper presented at the Euromicro Conference, Rennes, France.

Mostefaoui, S., K., Hirsbrunner, B., (2004). *Context Aware Service Provisioning.* Paper presented at the International Conference on Pervasive Services ICPS, Beirut, Lebanon.

OMA Service Environment (Approved version 1.0.4) (2007). Open Mobile Alliance Retrieved from http://www.openmobilealliance.org/release_program/ose_v1_0.html

OSA Application Programming Interface (API) version 7 (2007). 3GPP TS 29.198-X. Retrieved from http://www.3gpp.org/ftp/Specs/html-info/29198.htm

Parlay X Web Services (2002). The Parlay Group white paper. Retrieved from http://www.parlay.org/imwp/idms/popups/pop_download.asp?contentID=7103

Parlay/ OSA specifications release 6 (2007). The Parlay Group Retrieved from http://www.parlay.org/en/specifications/apis.asp

Patouni E. et al. (2006). *E²R Scenario on Autonomic Communication Systems for Seamless Experience.* E²R II White Paper. Retrieved from http://e2r2.motlabs.com/whitepapers/E2RII_ScenarioAutonomic_White_Paper.pdf

Ralph, P., & Parsons, J., (2006). *A Framework for Automatic Online Personalization.* Paper presented at the 39th Hawaii International Conference on System Sciences—2006, Kauai, HI.

Resource Description Framework (RDF). The World Wide Web Consortium (W3C) (2007). Retrieved from http://www.w3.org/RDF/

Sigg, S., Haseloff, S., & David, K. (2006). The Impact of the Context Interpretation Error on the Context Prediction Accuracy. In *Third Annual International Conference on Mobile and Ubiquitous Systems: Networking & Services,* 17-21 July, San Jose, California

The Operators Vision on Systems Beyond 3G, (2003), EURESCOM Project P1203. http://www.eurescom.de

The Virtual Home Environment. 3GPP TR 22.121 V5.3.1 (2002-06). Retrieved from http://www.3gpp.org/

Ubiquitous Web Applications Working Group (UWAWG). The World Wide Web Consortium (W3C) (2007). Retrieved from http://www.w3.org/2007/uwa/

Universal Description, Discovery and Integration (UDDI) (2005) OASIS, v3.0.2, retrieved from http://www.oasis-open.org/specs/index.php#uddiv3.0.2

Wagner, M., Kellerer, W., Tarlano, A., & Hirschfeld R.(2003, October). *From Personal Mobility to Mobile Personality.* Paper presented at the Eurescom Summit, Heidelberg, Germany

van Kranenburg, H., Bargh, M.S., Iacob, S., Peddemors, A. (2006). A Context Management Framework for Supporting Context-Aware Distributed Applications. *IEEE Comunications. Magazine,* August 2006, vol. 44, no. 8, 67-74.

Williams, H., M., Roussaki, I., Strimpakou, M., Yang, Y., MacKinnon, L., Dewar, R., Milyaev, N., Pils, C., & Anagnostou, M., (2005). *Context-Awareness and Personalisation in the Daidalos Pervasive Environment.* Paper presented at International Conference on the International Conference on Pervasive Services, ICPS, Santorini, Greece.

ADDITIONAL READING

Chan A.T.S., Siu-Nam C. (2003). MobiPADS: a reflective middleware for context-aware mobile computing. *IEEE Transactions on Software Engineering*, 29(12), pp. 1072-1085.

Davies J.; Studer R.; Warren P. (Eds.) (2006). *Semantic Web Technologies: Trends and Research in Ontology-based Systems.* Wiley. July 2006. ISBN 0470025964.

Dillinger, M., Madami, K., & Alonistioti, N. (Eds.) (2003). *Software Defined Radio: Architectures, Systems and Functions.* Wiley. ISBN 0470851643

Farshchian B., Zoric J., et al. (2004, October). *Developing pervasive services for future telecommunication networks.* Paper presented at WWW/Internet 2004, Madrid, Spain.

Gomez-Perez, A., Fernandez-Lopez, M., Corcho, O. (2003), *Ontological engineering.* Springer-Verlag. ISBN 1852335513.

Jin Xiao; Boutaba, R. (2005). QoS-aware service composition and adaptation in autonomic communication. *IEEE Journal on Selected Areas in Communications*, 23(12), 2344-2360

Kephart, J. O. and Chess, D. M. (2003). The vision of autonomic computing. *Computer*, 36(1), pp. 41–50.

Korpipää P. et al. (2003). Bayesian Approach to Sensor-Based Context Awareness. *Personal and Ubiquitous Computing Journal*. 7(4).

Loke S. (2006), *Context-aware pervasive systems: architectures for a new breed of applications.* Auerbach. ISBN 0849372550.

Neely S.; Dobson S.; Nixon P. (2006). Adaptive middleware for autonomic systems, *Annals of Telecommunications*, 61(9–10), 1099-1118.

Ou S.; Georgalas N.; Azmoodeh M.; Yang K.; Sun X. (2006, July). *A Model Driven Integration Architecture for Ontology-Based Context Modelling and Context-Aware Application Development.* Paper presented at the Second European Conference on Model Driven Architecture - Foundations and Applications, ECMDA-FA 2006, Bilbao, Spain,.

Raz D.; Juhola A.-T.; Fernandez J.S.; Galis A. (2006). *Fast and Efficient Context-Aware Services*, Wiley. ISBN 047001668X.

Stojanovic, L., Schneider, J., Maedche, A., Libischer, S., Studer, R., Lumpp, Th, Abecker, A., Breiter, G. Dinger, J. (2004). The role of ontologies in autonomic computing systems, *IBM systems journal*, 43(3).

Chapter VI
Intelligent Information Personalization: From Issues to Strategies

Syed Sibte Raza Abidi
Dalhousie University, Canada

ABSTRACT

This chapter introduces intelligent information personalization as an approach to personalize the web-based information retrieval experiences based on an individual's interests, needs and goals. We present intelligent techniques to dynamically compose new personalized information by adapting existing web-based information in line with a dynamic user-model, whilst simultaneously addressing linguistic, factual and functional requirements. This chapter will highlight the different facets, tasks and issues concerning intelligent information personalization to guide researchers in designing intelligent information personalization applications. The chapter presents intelligent methods that address information personalization at the content level as opposed to the traditional approaches that focus on interface level information personalization. To assist researchers in designing intelligent information personalization applications we present our information personalization framework, named ***AdWISE*** *(**Ad**aptive **W**eb-mediated **I**nformation and **S**ervices **E**nvironment), to demonstrate how to systematically integrate various intelligent methods to achieve information personalization. We will conclude with a commentary on the future outlook for intelligent information personalization.*

INTRODUCTION: INFORMATION PERSONALIZATION

The access to and consumption of relevant, useful and correct information is paramount to Web users. However, the sheer volume of information available over the Web has led to the much-cited information overload problem; users are finding it cognitively stressful and difficult to find the 'right' and 'relevant' information. Notwithstanding the efficacy of information retrieval technologies, it is argued that solutions to tackle the information overload problem need to pursue a shift in focus—i.e. move from searching for information guided by the user's query towards personalizing the available information guided by the user's immediate needs and interests.

Information retrieval services such as Google, Yahoo, CiteSeer are now the preferred gateways or mediators to the vast information artefacts available over the Web (Shahabi et al. 2003). The term *information artifact* is used to broadly denote a document, image, media file and any other medium to represent information. Such information artifacts may either be structured, semi-structured, or unstructured. Functionally speaking, such information services aim to address the information overload problem by (a) finding a subset of information artifacts from a larger space of information artifacts (i.e. the Web) based on the user's search preferences; and (b) presenting a list of relevant information artifacts to the user—the user is required to subsequently choose from the list of retrieved information artifacts. Indeed, this alleviates the information overload problem to some extent but it does not fully solve the cognitive overload problem because the user is still required to *filter* the retrieved information based on contextual priorities, and then *adapt* it based on personal preferences.

Information users are different in nature—they manifest heterogeneous information seeking behaviours, needs and expectations. Yet, we note that most information retrieval services purport a *one size fits all* model whereby the same information is disseminated to a wide range of information users despite the individualistic nature of each user's needs, goals, interests, preferences, intellectual levels and information consumption capacity. We believe that this leads to a sub-optimal model because information seekers who are intrinsically distinct are not only compelled to experience a generic outcome but are further required to manually adjust and adapt the recommended information artifacts according to their immediate needs or preferences in order to achieve the desired results (Abidi et al, 2004a; Abidi et al, 2006). Therefore, we argue that there is both a case and the need to design information services that take into account the individuality of information seekers, and in turn aim to *personalize* their information seeking experiences and outcomes (Belkin et al, 1992; Abidi, 2002; Fink et al, 2002; Shahabi et al, 2003; Brusilovsky et al, 2006).

Intelligent Information Personalization can be defined as the dynamic and intelligent *adaptation* of generic information based on salient user characteristics—such as the user's demographics, knowledge, skills, persona, interests, taste, preferences, purpose, needs, goals, plans, behavioural attitudes and any other user-specific criteria—to effectuate a personalized information mediation experience for the user. Information Personalization (IP) activities aim to: (a) minimize the cognitive stress typically faced by users due to information overload; (b) improve the potential uptake of the information by the user; and (c) establish an implicit *trust* relationship between the user and the information service. IP involves two key activities: (i) a *user modelling* activity to develop a *user model* that characterizes the user in terms of a set of discernible characteristics or features. Each user is described in terms of feature values, such that the aggregation of feature-value pairs realizes a potentially unique user-model; and (ii) an *adaptation* activity that leverages a 'rich' user-model to personalize the information by dynamically modifying the information content, the information presentation style and/or the information composition structure. The adaptation algorithms perform an explicit mapping of the elements of a user model to specific adaptation directives—i.e. they determine that given the presence of certain user-defining features the following information artifacts are to be selected for adaptation, and what elements of the information artifact to adapt and how to adapt it. A key issue for IP is to ensure both the relevance and the utility of the personalized information in a manner that satisfies a priori defined completeness and consistency criterion.

IP is an emerging research area with a focus to develop criterion, methods, tools and evaluation metrics to develop IP applications and services. IP is largely pursued in the realm of adaptive hypermedia systems (Brusilovsky, 2001; Brusilovsky et al, 2006) that provide an umbrella framework incorporating hypermedia, artificial intelligence, information retrieval, databases and web technology to develop and deploy web-based IP systems (Brusilovsky, 2001; Brusilovsky et al, 2006). IP methods are largely based on (a) *information filtering* approaches involving content and collaborative filtering methods; (b) *artificial intelligence* approaches leveraging case-based reasoning, rule-based reasoning, natural language processing and planning methods; and (c) *adaptive hypermedia* approaches to adapt the presentation and link-structures of hypermedia documents. To date, an assortment of IP applications are available for tasks such as intelligent tutoring (Alrifai et al, 2006; Dolog et al, 2004, Brusilovsky, 1995; Calvin et al, 1997), customer relationships (Kosba et al, 2001), recommending music (Kuo et al, 2002), access to information sources (Andre et al., 1998; Ardissono et al, 2000; Arezki et al, 2004), electronic catalogues (Milosavljevic et al, 1998; Chittaro et al, 2000), health-care assistance (Bental et al., 2000; Abidi et al, 2001; Abidi, 2004b, Davis et al, 2006), information filtering and recommendations (Balabanovic, 1997; Billsus et al, 2000), tourist information (Fink et al., 2002; DeCarolis et al, 2005).

In this chapter, we present an Intelligent Information Personalization research program that seeks to personalize a user's web-based information mediation experience, guided by his/her dynamic user-model that entails the user's demographics, knowledge, interests, preferences, needs, goals and behavioural attitudes. Our IP approach extends beyond the prevailing techniques for personalizing the interface-level presentation of Web-based information. Instead, we address the more complex issue of personalizing the actual information content that is to be delivered to users. We approach IP as the problem of composing new information by adapting and synthesizing multiple existing information components, whilst satisfying a set of linguistic, factual and functional requirements. In addition, our IP approach is guided by the user's context to ensure that the information is relevant to the user's task(s) that mitigated the need for information.

In the forthcoming discussion, we present the different facets of IP (section 2), prominent issues that need to be considered when approaching IP (section 3) and an IP application framework that highlights the determinants, components and tasks pertinent to the design of intelligent IP applications (section 4). The latter half of the discussion will feature our intelligent information personalization framework termed ***AdWISE*** (**Ad**aptive **W**eb-mediated **I**nformation and **S**ervices **E**nvironment) that systematically integrates an assortment of intelligent methods to achieve IP. The AdWISE framework focuses on technical issues pertaining to intelligent content adaptation. We will present an overview of three intelligent IP applications within AdWISE—i.e. (i) the composition of personalized music playlists; (ii) the recommendation of user-specific news items; and (iii) the composition of personalized cardiovascular risk management recommendations. We will conclude with a short commentary on the future outlook for intelligent IP.

FACETS OF INFORMATION PERSONALIZATION

IP can be viewed as the problem of dynamically adapting three facets of an information artifact—i.e. *content*, *structure* and *presentation* of information based on a user-model (Brusilovsky, 2001; Brusilovsky et al, 1998).

- *Content adaptation* involves manipulating the *components* of an information artifact in response to a defined IP goal or a user-model. The information artifact subject to content adaptation is typically annotated and indexed accordingly. The granularity of content adaptation varies from words to sentences to paragraphs to page substitutions. Content adaptation is a non-trivial problem as it encompasses: (a) compositional personalization whereby the composition of the information is adapted by adding/deleting specific pages (Henze et al, 2000) or text fragments (Kosba et al, 1994). The idea is to design a personalized information artifact as a composite of multiple information fragments, where each information fragment is of direct relevance to the user. Composition of the personalized information artifact involves the systematic selection of a set of user-specific information fragments (potentially from different origins) and synthesizing them based on a specific presentation template; (b) linguistic changes whereby the language of the information content is systematically altered to meet the user's preferences, educational and skill levels (Boyle et al, 1994). The linguistic changes may involve the exclusion/inclusion of technical words to make the content more generic/specific, the inclusion of more personalized sentences directly addressing the user and asking the user to respond by performing certain actions; and (c) brevity changes whereby the amount of information provided to a user is moderated with respect to the users consumption capacity, for instance Adaptive stretchtext (Boyle et al, 1994).
  The IP systems developed so far provide a core document that is dynamically appended with pre-designed complementary information based on the user's profile (Ardissono et al, 2000; Brafman et al, 2004; Boyle et al, 1994)
- *Structure adaptation* involves the dynamic adaptation of the physical structure of an information artifact—i.e. re-aligning the order of the pages or hypermedia links based on the use-model (Smyth et al, 2002). Collateral structure adaptation (Ardissono et al, 2000), link sorting, link annotation, and link removal or addition (Oppermann et al, 2000) are some of the typical methods used to achieve structure adaptation.
- *Presentation adaptation* involves the presentation of the same information from different perspectives. Presentation adaptation approaches offer (a) changes to the physical layout or interface of the information artifact (Brusilovsky et al, 1998). Typically, this is achieved by text positioning (or focusing), graphics and multimedia inclusion/exclusion, background variations and GUI interface adaptation; (b) the inclusion of personal information such as the user's particulars at key points within personalized information artifact. This is achieved by generating a presentation template with placeholders for adding the user's particulars from external sources, such as a user interface or even a database. Current systems include the Anatom-Tutor (Beaumont 1994), Hypadapter (Hohl 1996) and Web systems, where these systems vary the length, presentation structure, language constructs and media type based on the user-model.

In conclusion, we will like to point out that content adaptation is the most interesting and challenging IP activity because it involves the dynamic selection of multiple information-fragments that correspond to a given user-model, and then synthesise them using a pre-defined presentation template to realise a personalized information artifact.

INTELLIGENT INFORMATION PERSONALIZATION ISSUES

Typically, information is created at a generic level for a wider audience, yet individuals use it with respect to their specific interests, needs, goals and consumption capacity. The automated transformation of generic information to personalized information is quite challenging, as it demands addressing a variety of issues. Some of these issues are highlighted below:

User-Model Compliance

The most basic, yet immensely paramount, IP issue is that the personalized information should be both *relevant* and *useful* to the user (Belkin et al, 1992; Palme, 1998). The user's relevancy and usefulness criterion are implicitly derived from his/her user model and explicitly obtained from the user's specification of the IP tasks.

Users are differentiated based on the feature-values (or dimensions) recorded in their user-models. For instance, two users may have different information preferences because they differ along the age dimension. Further differentiation between these two users is possible if they differ along the gender dimension as well. From an IP perspective both these distinct users should be provided with distinct information-mediation experiences.

User-model compliance can be achieved via information modelling—i.e. establish a direct correspondence between the information content and user-model dimensions. Here, the information content can be (i) classified into topics and/or genres; (ii) decomposed into text fragments or *snippets*, where each snippet is congruent with a set of user dimensions (or values of these dimensions); and (iii) annotated with linguistic variations suitable for specific user characteristics. An information modelling exercise will establish the relevance of the information content towards user-model values—i.e. mapping the user-model to the information model. Such user model—information model mapping implies that if the value of age feature equals 'young' then information content x and presentation style a should be used, whereas if the value of the age feature is 'adult' then information content y with presentation style b and structure type q is more relevant. Such mappings can be directly derived by domain experts or learnt based on the user information usage history.

Establishing Factual Consistency

IP methods dynamically adapt an information artifact based on a global scheme for content, structure and/or presentation adaptation. By putting an emphasis on just user-model compliance there is the potential that the adaptation process may inadvertently lead to factual inconsistencies within the personalized information artifact. Factual inconsistency can be at the (a) document's structural level whereby the synthesis of multiple information artifacts may realise a factually inconsistent page ordering which renders the personalized information artifact incoherent, or (b) document's content level whereby the synthesis of multiple information fragments might inadvertently lead to the generation of factually inconsistent information whereby one information-fragment is stating a certain fact/recommendation whilst the next information-fragment is contradicting the same fact/recommendation.

A common limitation of many IP methods is that they do not track and address the above-mentioned factual inconsistencies. Establishing factual consistency is an important issue for content adaptation, therefore IP methods should incorporate a high-level sanity checking mechanism based on some *apriori* defined criterion and rules, but without recourse to detailed content checking. IP methods should, therefore, additionally establish factual consistency of the personalized information beyond user-model compliance (Abidi et al, 2004a, Abidi et al, 2006).

Context Awareness

Information is sought in context. The context may predicate the salient aspects of the individual, environment, motivation and/or expected outcome associated with the information seeking activity. Context, therefore, implies a generalized set of intrinsic relationships between a set of perspectives believed in some way to help make clear and understand the current information-mediated task, event or discussion, and the corresponding information needed (Carmichael et al, 2005; Dilley, 1999; Lawrence et al, 1998). Typically, IP methods do not incorporate a rich context description within the adaptation algorithm, rather the user-model is deemed to represent context (Cheverst et al, 2002). This leads to a simplification of the IP problem specification and the eventual outcome may not necessarily be best adapted to the user's immediate needs. Context, for all intents and purposes, is a dynamic entity and therefore demands a richer representation that goes beyond the user-model.

We posit that an important issue for IP is context awareness whilst adapting information artifacts. A rich IP context should include:

1. A set of features describing the user—i.e. the user-model
2. A description of the task(s) that mitigate the need for information. Different tasks demand different information content and presentation style. This means that for a specific problem domain, the different tasks a user may potentially be engaged with should be explicitly characterized and then specific information requirements should be determined for each task type. For instance, in academia the different information-mediating tasks can be differentiated as writing or reviewing a research paper, preparing lectures or evaluation material, writing a report, critiquing or validating a viewpoint and so on. Each of these tasks may demand specific information, yet the information requirements for each task may differ in terms of the brevity, volume, factual consistency and presentation style. A potential solution is a *task-information* mapping matrix that encodes a mapping between information-mediating tasks and the corresponding information requirements.
3. A history of past (i) information seeking activities and experiences, (ii) rating of the information artifacts, and (iii) information uptake patterns
4. A global perspective vis-à-vis the opinions/ratings/experiences of past users for similar information artifacts.

In our view, IP methods should both incorporate and leverage a rich context—i.e. go beyond the typical user-model based characterization of the user—to ensure that the personalized information is adapted not only based on the user's characteristics but also takes into account the user's immediate activities and additional support information.

Behaviour Modelling

IP methods can benefit by leveraging the behavioural disposition of the user towards the information that is being personalized. For instance, IP for educational interventions can be guided by the taking into account the behavioural readiness of the individual to uptake the personalized educational content. As much as the user-model and the contextual model determine the overall relevancy of the personalized information content, behaviour modelling can enhance the acceptance and uptake of the personalized information by further tailoring the content along implicit behavioural attitudes. Behaviour modelling is an interesting issue for IP because if we are able to ascertain the user's behavioural attitude towards information-based interventions, then this knowledge can be utilized to guide the personalization process to better personalize the information (Davis et al, 2006).

Behaviour modelling is particularly relevant for activities that involve the recommendation of personalized information to users in anticipation of effectuating a positive behaviour change or to achieve learning—i.e. activities involving education, training, therapy, financial management and so on. For IP purposes, behaviour modelling can help determine how the user might potentially respond to the recommended information—if the user's response is deemed to be sub-optimal then the IP methods can re-adapt the information to improve the user's acceptance or readiness towards the information. For effective incorporation of behavioural modelling to streamline IP, it is important that IP systems incorporate a feedback mechanism to (a) gather and gauge the user's feedback about the personalized information; (b) either implicitly deduce or explicitly ask the user about the veracity of the behaviour model—the behaviour model has a temporal nature and is expected to modulate (either towards the desired outcomes or in the opposite direction); and (c) dynamically adjust the user's behaviour model, based on the observed or deduced feedback, to streamline the personalized information with respect to the current behaviour model.

A variety of behaviour modelling techniques exist, however for IP purposes we recommend the Trans-Theoretical Model of intentional behavior change as it matches the change principles and processes to each individual's current readiness to change in order to guide the user through the process of modifying problem behaviour(s) and acquiring positive behaviours (Sarkin et al, 2001; Spencer et al, 2002).

Social and Privacy Considerations

Social and privacy considerations are quite prevalent in our prevailing ubiquitous information sharing and access environments. Social considerations may involve the user's subjective predisposition towards certain information artifacts—i.e. whether such information artifacts are acceptable. Information privacy spans from hiding sensitive personal information to hiding information access and use behaviours to restricted information visualization preferences in shared workplaces/environments. In this regard, it is desirable that IP methods take into account the user's social and privacy concerns or preferences (Kobsa, 2001).

Information presentation can be streamlined with respect to the privacy level of the user's prevailing environment in which the information is to be viewed. For instance, if the user is within a public place then sensitive information should not be explicitly presented to the user. Depending on the sophistication of the IP framework the privacy level can be either determined automatically based on the user's activity behaviour or can be set manually. Likewise, social considerations can be recorded within the user-model and can guide the selection of information artifacts. We believe that addressing the user's social and privacy concerns or preferences as an IP constraint will lead to context-aware IP that is tuned to not only to the user-model but also to environmental elements (Carmichael et al, 2005).

Multi-Dimensional User Views

IP methods can provide a better personalized output if they have a richer description of the user's views on items that he/she may have rated for appropriateness, likeness and utility. Typically, the user-model may record discrete and absolute ratings of information artifacts, for instance whether the user liked or disliked, found useful or not useful a particular information artifact. We argue that such a mechanism for recording user's views is too rigid because (a) it does not provide a sense of why the user rated the information artifact as such; (b) were there any aspects of the artifact which the user likened (or even disliked) more than other aspects; and (c) whether the change in values for certain aspects of the information artifact might influence his/her rating of the artifact. To get a better sense of the user's attitude towards an information artifact (or type of information artifacts), it will be useful to provide the user an opportunity to rate an artifact along multiple dimensions and to allow him/her to describe his/her rating criterion. Take for instance, typically information services would ask whether the user likened or not a particular music album (i.e. CD), book, movie, article and so on. We argue that this presents a restricted user view; rather the user should be given a list of dimensions/aspects/features pertaining to the information artifact and then asked to rate each dimension of the information using a predefined range of rating values. For example, a music album can be rated along the dimensions of music quality, lyrics, singer performance, direction, rhythm, etc., where each dimension can be rated using a Likert scale.

IP methods can benefit from multi-dimensional user views on information artifacts, as opposed to discrete rating values, to provide personalized information artifacts that are more fine-grained and closer to the user's real opinion on the information artifacts (Chedrawy et al, 2006a; Chedrawy et al, 2006b).

Hybrid Personalization Approach

The choice of the right approach to achieve the desired personalized effect is an important design consideration for IP applications. Given that IP can be achieved through a variety of approaches, each with their own strengths and weakness, it is advantageous to pursue a hybrid approach whereby different approaches are synergized to yield a more effective IP output. For instance, in an information sharing parlance, IP can be guided by three elements: (a) the interests and experiences of the user seeking information for a particular task—i.e. the user model and the contextual model; (b) the ratings/recommendations of like-minded peers for information artifacts that can be potentially be provided to the user; and (c) the past responses and experiences of key users (or domain experts) pertaining to similar information personalization situations. In this case, the IP problem is characterized at three levels—i.e. personal, community of peers, and expert's experiences. An efficacious IP design should entail a specialized IP approach to best serve the issues and problems at each individual level of the IP problem, and then synergize these approaches to yield a more effective hybrid personalization approach.

Information Modelling

The extent of IP largely depends on the suitability of the information artifact for adaptation, yet there is nominal consideration to optimizing the design of the information artifact to achieve improved adaptation. From an IP perspective, information modelling includes (a) annotating the information artifact with semantic information, constraints or specific instructions that are useful for the IP method; (b) decomposing the information artifact into smaller more meaningful information fragments or snippets; (c) classifying the information artifacts into meaningful classes or genre; (d) indexing the information artifacts along a taxonomy of topics and sub-topics; creating a metadata specification of the information artifact design that can be used to for presentation and/or organization adaptation. We argue that information modelling—i.e. preparing the information artifacts for downstream IP—is an important IP issue and its proper treatment will help optimize the efficiency of the IP methods in terms of providing more informed and improved personalized information mediation experiences.

ADWISE: A FRAMEWORK FOR INTELLIGENT INFORMATION PERSONALIZATION

IP is an emerging area and the use of intelligent methods to achieve IP is an even more recent approach. The IP research area is experiencing both growth and maturity in terms of the emergence of interesting personalization approaches, applications and a far-reaching research agenda. However, despite a well-pronounced need for IP there do not yet exist formal techniques and/or frameworks that cover the entire spectrum of IP requirements.

We present our intelligent IP framework **AdWISE (Adaptive Web-based Information and Services Environment)** that features a confluence of IP approaches that realize an active synergy between methods drawn from artificial intelligence, information retrieval and adaptive hypermedia. AdWISE pursues IP at all three facets— (i) content adaptation through *compositional adaptation*—i.e. dynamically composing new information artifacts by selecting multiple information components that are individually relevant to the user-model, and then intelligently synthesizing them to compose a 'new' personalized information artifact; (ii) presentation adaptation by modifying the presentation template; and (iii) organizational adaptation by dynamically selecting the hypermedia links within the personalized document.

Determinants of Intelligent IP for Application Development

The AdWISE framework purports three main interacting determinants for intelligent IP, namely *Personalization context, Personalization constraints* and *Personalization methods* (shown in Figure 1).

Personalization Context

Understanding the context in which IP is being requested or is to be discharged is central to determining what to personalize? how to personalize? and on what basis? As much as the user-model guides the selection of the information artifacts relevant to the user, we argue that the context may further provide insights to assist in the selection, adaptation and presentation of the personalized content. In essence, the incorporation of context in IP activities adds a further level of sophistication to the IP output, ensuring that a user immersed in different contexts should get information that is

Figure 1. Determinants for intelligent IP

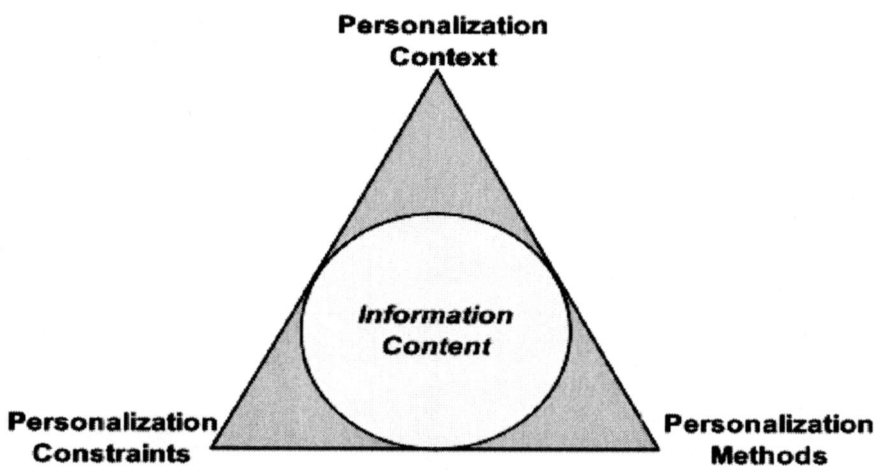

not just compliant to the user's model but is additionally personalized based on the user's prevailing context (Cheverst et al, 2002). Typically, the user-model is seen as the manifestation of context, however in our view this is rather a simplified interpretation of context because typically the user-model does not incorporate organizational and task-specific elements.

Context for IP encapsulates a variety of elements, such as the user-model, the tasks that mitigated the need for IP, the user's views on different types of information artifacts, privacy concerns with respect to different environment, user behaviour with respect to certain information, tasks or situations, information display modalities, inclusion and exclusion criteria and tolerance to noise together with input on the user's ability to filter noise. The personalization context can be determined through user feedback and/or questionnaire, passive observation of the user, intelligent software agents monitoring the user's activities and mining the log of user's activities over a network/website/system. Finally, it is important that context is represented using a functional representation scheme that allows for (a) dynamic context update based on environmental inputs and user-feedback; and (b) mapping the context descriptions to specific personalization recommendation/instructions—i.e. what to personalize in the presence of specific contextual elements.

Personalization Constraints

IP researchers seek to personalize every interaction, information artifact and service, but realistically speaking there are always limits to what can be functionally achieved as an acceptable personalized experience. From a user-level, personalization constraints determine the scope of the IP sought and hence specify the user's preferences and expectations. From an application-level, personalization constraints determine the various IP parameters that need to be set for the IP methods to produce the desired results—this implies that the IP methods should have the necessary functionality to modulate their IP logic and processes in response to dynamic personalization constraints. For an IP application, typical personalization constraints may determine the following: (a) level of confidence in selecting the information artifact to be used; (b) the user's tolerance levels to noise in the personalized output; (c) the user's expected/acceptable information coverage—i.e. whether the user will be satisfied if the personalized output partially covers the user's interests; (d) factual consistency considerations during compositional adaptation; (e) information presentation preferences; (f) how to deal with situations when viable choices may be available; (g) design of the information artifact; and (h) any other IP criteria that may make the IP output more relevant and useful to the user.

Functionally the personalization constraints are determined as a two-step process: (1) the IP application allows the user to set the user-level personalization constraints in terms of criterion that are understandable and meaningful to the user. Some of these constraints may be derived from the personalization context; and then (2) the user-specific personalization constraints are translated to operational parameters for the IP methods. This demands a clear mapping of user-specific constraints to IP method-specific functional parameters.

To achieve meaningful IP results, it is important that the IP application allows the user to specify a wide range of personalization constraints. The AdWISE framework stipulates an integral association between the three IP determinants such that the personalization context guides the setting of the personalization constraints that are finally modelled and executed by the personalization methods.

Personalization Methods

IP is executed through personalization methods that constitute a discernible IP strategy implemented in terms of IP algorithms. The IP strategy stipulates the constituent IP tasks and the input/output for each individual task. The IP algorithms encapsulate the IP logic for each IP task. The personalization method, therefore, combines the strategy with its technical implementation to yield personalized information. It may be noted that IP cannot be realistically executed without having both the strategy and the algorithms; therefore personalization methods are integral to any IP activity. The IP strategy needs to be application specific therefore it is expected to vary for different IP applications. However, the IP algorithms can be developed as standard modules—with the provision for some parameter level adjustments to meet both the application and user requirements—and also to re-use the method in different applications. Functionally, the personalization methods incorporate both the personalization context to help formulate the IP strategy and the personalization constraints to help set-up the parameters for the IP algorithms.

Personalization methods are unique to each IP application and need to be designed based on the objectives of the IP exercise—i.e. personalization methods for educational content adaptation will be different from the personalization methods for recommending news. Personalization methods may be grounded in different research areas—such as information retrieval, artificial intelligence, adaptive hypermedia and pervasive computing. The design of personalization methods should be predicated by a clear understanding of the underlying IP principles used by each research area, as both information retrieval and artificial intelligence methods may approach user modelling or information composition in different ways.

In AdWISE, our approach is to develop hybrid personalization methods. Hybridization is achieved through (a) the systematic synergy of different IP approaches to formulate the IP strategy, for instance combining information filtering based on collaborative filtering (an IR method) with case based reasoning (an AI method) for compositional content adaptation; and (b) a modular system development approach that involves the implementation of task-specific modules that are systematically integrated to formulate the IP strategy. Each module may implement a particular IP task using a specific IP algorithm—it is possible to have multiple modules for the same task, each based on different research approach. The design objective for an IP application is therefore the selection of the most efficient personalization methods for the IP task at hand.

Figure 2. Components of an IP application

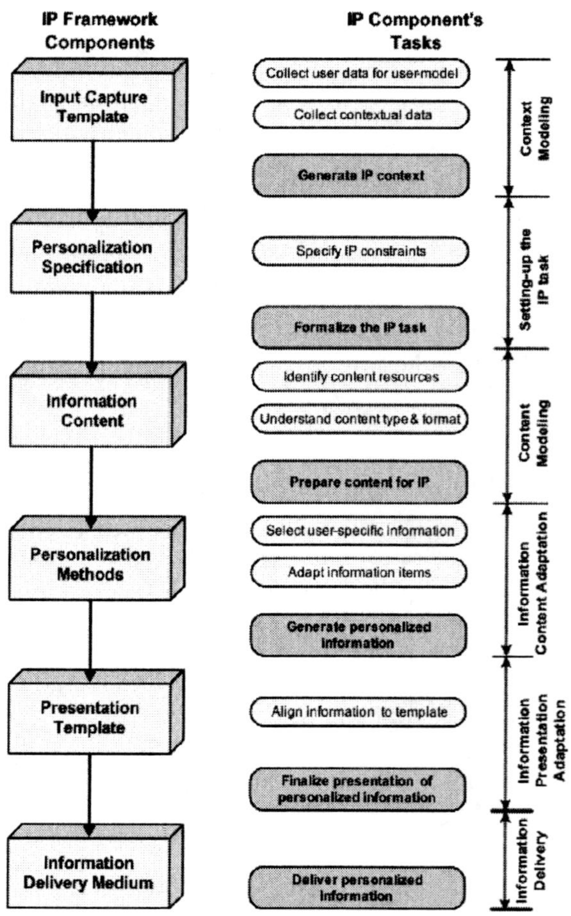

Components of an IP Application within AdWISE

The AdWISE framework proposes the following components (as shown in Figure 2) for developing an IP application.

Input Capture Template

This component serves as the user-interface to capture (a) user data pertinent for developing the user-model and for establishing the personalization context; (b) user's IP preferences that lead to the formulation of the personalization constraints.

Personalization Specification

This component comprises the personalization context—i.e. the user-model and additional environmental elements—and the personalization constraints. The personalization specification also entails a description—i.e. format and type—of the information content targeted for adaptation. The personalization specification is expected to serve as the blueprint for an IP exercise.

Information Content

This component represents the actual information content that is the object of the personalization exercise. The information content—for compositional adaptation this will be a set of snippets or text fragments—can either be stored in a content library using a pre-defined indexing scheme that guides the information selection process or it may be dynamically sourced from an information portal. Knowledge of the information model of the candidate information content is extremely important in determining the degree of personalization that is feasible with it, and this in turn guides the design of the personalization methods.

Personalization Methods

This constitutes the suite of personalization methods—comprising the personalization strategy and the algorithms—that will take the personalization context, personalization specification and information content as input and generate a personalized information artifact as output. Much of the IP research and resulting innovation is geared towards the development of personalization methods.

Presentation Template

This component determines how the personalized information is to be presented to the user. This may entail a pre-defined template/map to which user-specific information content is systematically added to compose personalized information. The presentation template can also be represented as a personalization strategy—i.e. as a set of rules/instructions eliciting the presentation logic—that determines the composition of the personalized output based on various factors, such as user-model, user context or presentation device. An IP application can have multiple pre-designed presentation templates, and the presentation logic may select the more relevant presentation template based on the specification of the IP task.

Information Delivery Medium

This component establishes how the personalized information is to be delivered to the user. The delivery medium determines (i) the device through which the information is to be viewed/consumed by the user, such as computer screen, hand-held device, mobile phone screen, printer and so on; and (b) the dissemination medium—such as a printed document, web page viewed through a browser, electronic document viewed through an application or sent through email (either as attachment or in the body of the email).

In the forthcoming discussion we introduce three exemplar intelligent IP projects that demonstrate different types of IP achieved within AdWISE. The exemplar applications pursue *Compositional Adaptation* in terms of the dynamic composition of a new document based on multiple components either from a specialized document repository or from Web resources. The complete details of these featured works can be found through their respective publications.

PERSONALIZING MUSIC PLAYLISTS: A COMPOSITIONAL ADAPTATION APPROACH

We introduce a novel IP approach for content adaptation—in particular compositional information personalization whereby a new personalized information artifact is composed by selecting and amalgamating individual components (from a set of user-specific information artifacts) that are deemed relevant to the user. The IP issues addressed in this approach were *user-model compliance, context awareness, multi-dimensional user views* and *hybrid models*. The approach is used to generate personalized music playlists by selecting individual music compilations (information components) from multiple music albums (information artifacts) that are deemed of interest and relevant to the user. We developed an IP application, namely ***PRECiSE-Personalized Recommendations in a Context-Sensitive Environment*** (Chedrawy et al 2006a, Chedrawy et al 2006b), as shown in Figure 3.

PRECiSE features a two-phase IP strategy that is a hybrid of information retrieval viz. CF methods (stage 1) and artificial intelligence viz. CBR based compositional adaptation (stage 2) methods. Phase 1 uses item-based Collaborative Filtering (CF) to identify the information artifacts that are relevant to the user-model; and Phase 2 applies compositional adaptation, in the realm of Case-Based Reasoning (CBR), to select the most salient information components from the set of relevant information artifacts found in phase 1. PRECiSE amalgamates the selected information components, after phase 2, to realise a composite personalized information artifact for the user. Note that PRECiSE does not use any additional planning mechanism for composing the information components. We explain below PRECiSE's IP strategy.

Phase 1: Context Sensitive Information Selection

This phase involves *context-sensitive information selection, whereby* a user-defined context is used to retrieve relevant information artifacts. Traditional collaborative filtering approaches compare items along a single dimension—i.e. whether the item was likened or not by the user—which in our view is insufficient to give a deeper sense of the context in which a recommendation is sought, processed and offered. In our approach, we create a 'rich'

Figure 3. PRECiSE Framework

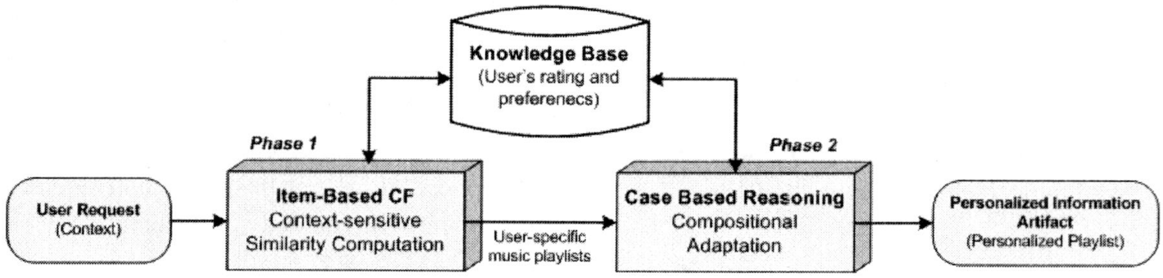

context for IP, such that a user can rate an item along multiple dimensions—the rating on these dimensions is subsequently used to recommend relevant information artifacts to similar users. For instance, for our music playlist compilation problem the potential dimensions to differentiate between music compilations were lyrics, song tunes, band, vocals, direction, video, etc.

In our work, we extended the item-based collaborative filtering method proposed by (Sarwar et al, 2001 such that instead of having one similarity value for two items ***i*** and ***j***, a similarity vector of dimension ***P*** is generated (***P*** is the total number of dimensions available for rating an item). The components of this vector are the individual similarities calculated based on the dimensions selected by a user. Based on the user's context—i.e. a set of selected dimensions—we compare music compilations that have been previously rated by other users and compute the degree of similarity between them with respect to the user's preferred dimensions. Our context-based collaborative filtering algorithm is described below:

- The user chooses multiple dimensions along which similarity between items is desired. A separate rating matrix $M_d(u,i)$ is generated for each selected dimension. $M_d(u,i)$ is the rating of user u on item i for dimension d.
- Identify users that have rated both items and then apply the similarity technique proposed by Sarwar (2001). Let $DS_d(i,j)$ be the *Dimensional Similarity* between two co-rated items i and j with respect to perspective d, calculated using the equation shown in Box 1.
- The *Contextual Similarity* $CS(i,j)$ between items i and j is computed as:

$$CS(i,j) = \frac{\sum_{d=1}^{D} W_d * PS_d(i,j)}{W_d}$$

Note that, similarity computation is achieved only over the dimensions selected by the user.

- Let the set I_u contains all items that have been rated by user u. For every item $i \in I_u$, find the set of k most similar items (K_u). The set K_u excludes any item that has been rated/preferred by u and hence belong to the set I_u.
- For every item $i \in K_u$, compute its similarity $S\text{-}set(i,I_u)$ to the set I_u. This similarity is the sum of the similarities (calculated in *Step 2*) between all items rated by user u and item i.

$$S-set(i \in K_u, I_u) = \sum_{j \in I_u} CS(i,j)$$

- Sort the set K_u by the similarity $S\text{-}set(i,I_u)$ in decreasing order and select the top N items.
- The selected N items are deemed as being the most relevant to the user.

Phase II: Compositional Information Personalization

This phase involves *compositional information personalization* whereby the most salient informa-

Box 1.

$$DS_d(i,j) = \frac{\sum_{u \in U} (M_d(u,i) - \bar{M}_d(u))(M_d(u,j) - \bar{M}_d(u))}{\sqrt{\sum_{u \in U} (M_d(u,i) - \bar{M}_d(u))^2} \sqrt{\sum_{u \in U} (M_d(u,j) - \bar{M}_d(u))^2}}$$

where $\bar{M}_d(u)$ is the average rating of user u on all rated items. U is the set of all users in the CF knowledge base. Let W_d the weight assigned to dimension d, reflecting the importance of the said dimension to the user tion components from the information artifacts selected in phase I are systematically selected to formulate a new composite personalized information artifact (Abidi, 2002). A systematic compilation of individual information components, originating from different, yet relevant information artifacts, yields a fine-grained personalized information artifact that is much closer to the user-model as opposed to the original information artifacts that may have some components that are not necessary of interest to the user. We apply our compositional adaptation technique to select the most salient information components from an information artifact. The basis for our compositional adaptation strategy is defined by (a) the frequency of occurrence of an information component in the set of relevant information artifacts; and (b) the degree of similarity between the user's request and the retrieved information artifact (measured in terms of the *appropriateness degree*). Compositional adaptation is achieved as follows:

- In phase I we computed the similarity between a retrieved information artifact I and an user u as $S(u,I)=S\text{-}set(i,I_u)$.
- For every selected information artifact I_i (as determined in phase I), calculate the normalized similarity (NS) of I_i for the user u over the entire set of retrieved information artifacts (RI) as follows:

$$Temp = \sum_{k=1}^{RI} 1/S(u,I_k)$$

$$NS(u, I_k) = 1 - 1/(S(u, I_k) * Temp)$$

- Make a set of all the available information components across all the retrieved information artifacts. Let $Comp_{I_k}$ be an information component and AD^{Comp_I} be the AD for $Comp_I$. In order to compute the Appropriateness Degree (AD) of each component, the normalized similarities (NS) of the similar information artifacts that contain this component are added to one another. Calculate the *Appropriateness* Degree (AD) for each information component based on the AD of its parent information artifact as follows:

For I = 1 to *number of available information components*
If $Comp_I$ exists within a retrieved information artifact I_k then

$$AD_u^{Comp_I} = AD_u^{Comp_I} + NS(u, I_k)$$

- Sort the distinct components of the N items by their AD, and select the M top components—i.e. the components that are most similar to the user. The value for M can be specified by the user.

The M selected components are amalgamated for form a composite personalized information artifact that is recommended to the user.

Working Example

We present a working example for recommending personalized music playlists. The user with ID 130 has previously rated a set of music compilations (i.e. information artifacts) where each compilation consists of 10 songs (i.e. information components). Now we apply our IP approach to generate a personalized playlist as follows:

Output from Phase I: CF is applied with a context comprising 3 perspectives results in the recommendation of 10 music compilations (see Table 1). The appropriateness degree (AD)—a measure of how much the information artifacts are compliant to the user-model—is averaged over the 10 recommended compilations and found to be 1.134. The F1-metric with a context (i.e. 0.34) is found to be significantly better than the F1-metric without context (i.e. 0.76), thus emphasizing the role of context in enhancing the relevance of the recommended information.

Table 1. N Recommended music compilations (Phase I), where N=10

User ID	Compilations (Information Artifacts)					F1 Metric	AD
130	47	92	295	331	332	0.34	1.134
	348	379	876	1012	1197		

Table 2. A sample of the 10 recommended compilations and their constituent songs. Shaded songs are the most relevant to the user

User ID	Item ID	Songs (Components)					AD
130	332	2	26	46	63	88	1.801
	348	22	35	104	125	187	
	379	2	20	41	110	128	
	876	20	25	125	196	198	
	1012	24	35	113	161	198	

Table 3. New composite recommendation comprising the 10 most relevant songs for user ID '130'

User ID	Personalized Music Playlist				
130	2	20	22	25	46
	71	104	125	187	198

Output from Phase II: We apply compositional adaptation to the recommended compilations (in Table 1). Table 2, shows a sample of the recommended music playlists together with their components. Table 3 shows the final personalized recommended music playlist.

We note an improvement in the quality of the final personalized recommendation in terms of the *F1-metric*, and the *appropriateness degree* that has increased significantly by 58.8%. The personalized music playlist, originating from different items, will be presented to the user as being most relevant to his/her interest.

Discussion

In this project we introduced a new IP approach featuring a unique hybrid of item-based collaborative filtering and case based reasoning, that realized IP at a fine-grained level. The approach was vindicated by our empirical results that indicate that the usage of context as well as the compositional adaptation has provided more precise personalized information as per the user-model. An interesting future research direction is to explore quantifying the users' ratings based on the Multi-Attribute Utility Theory.

PERSONALIZING RECOMMENDATION OF NEWS ITEMS: A CONSTRAINT SATISFACTION APPROACH

This project involves the selection of news items based on the user-model that entails a list of news topics that are of interest to the user (Abidi et al, 2006b). The IP issues addressed in this approach are *User-model compliance*, *factual consistency*, *information modelling* and *hybrid models*. The IP requirements were as follows:

1. The personalized information should be relevant to the interests of the user. The user may choose the degree of relevance to include either all or a partial list of topics of interest in the final personalized information.
2. The personalized information should be factually consistent—i.e. the set of information artifacts being presented to the user should mutually satisfy the factual consistency constraints specified by the user.
3. The personalized information should offer maximum information coverage—i.e. present to the user the largest possible number of information artifacts that meet both the user's interests and are also mutually factually consistent.

Intuitively speaking, the problem of IP entails the satisfaction of two different constraints for each information artifact: (a) *relevancy constraints* to establish the relevance of the information to the user; and (b) *factual consistency constraints* to establish the factual consistency between the selected information artifacts (Abidi et al, 2006a). IP is achieved without deep content analysis, rather by leveraging the pre-defined classification of information artifacts in terms of topics to determine both the relevance of the information towards the user and the factual compatibility between multiple information artifacts.

This IP approach is applied for news item selection for a personalized news delivery service using the Reuters-21578, Distribution 1.0 data-set. We developed an intelligent IP system that addressed two main tasks:

1. Automatic acquisition of factual consistency constraints from the corpus of information artifacts. The idea is to eliminate the need for acquiring factual consistency constraints from domain experts. The constraint acquisition method is designed based on association rule mining concepts, and it leverages the topic-based indexing scheme for the information artifacts.
2. Constraint satisfaction based IP that involves three main stages: (1) Find all the information artifacts relevant to the user-model—i.e. finding the *user-relevant set*; (2) From the user-relevant set, find a simplified solution whereby each user interest is accounted for by a single information artifact, whilst ensuring factual consistency between the selected information artifacts—i.e. finding the *basic information set*. The basic information set is the baseline solution meeting all Personalization constraints and can be presented to the user if no further optimization is possible; (3) Build on the basic information set to maximize the coverage of the personalized information by including additional information artifacts from the user-relevant set whilst maintaining factual consistency between all the selected information artifacts—this will lead to the *optimal personalized set* that is the final IP solution.

We developed an intelligent IP system that features a hybrid of constraint satisfaction methods to satisfy a variety of constraints to personalize information as per the user model (see Figure 4). In addition, we provided a user preference setting mechanism whereby users can set the personalization constraints, such as tolerance to inconsistency or degree of information coverage and comprehensiveness in line with their information needs.

Elements of the Constraint Satisfaction Based IP System

Personalization Context: The context comprises the user-model that characterizes (a) user's *interests* represented as a list of topics, (b) user's *toler-*

Figure 4. The functional steps and the corresponding methods

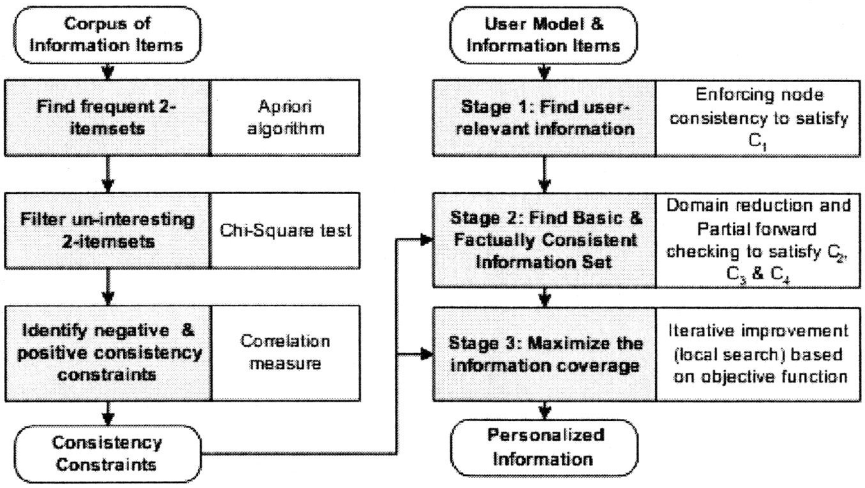

ance towards inter-document inconsistency, and (c) user's *preference* towards the coverage of the solution—i.e. whether the solution should satisfy all user-interests or instead it should satisfy all consistency constraints.

Information Artifacts: The information artifacts (i.e. documents) comprise two sections: (a) *Content* section that contains the actual information; and (b) *Context* section that contains a list of topics categorizing the document.

Information Personalization Constraints: IP is achieved by satisfying two types of constraints: (a) *Relevancy constraints* to ensure that the selected documents are relevant to the user's interest as specified in the user-model; and (b) *Consistency constraints* to (i) ensure that the personalized information is factually consistent. This is achieved through *negative consistency constraints,* which define what pairs of topics cannot co-exist together. Negative consistency constraints are represented as the tuple *nc* (*topic1, topic2, degree*), where *degree* is the degree of inconsistency between the two topics. Two documents cannot be simultaneously presented to the user if the topics they represent cannot coexist; and (ii) to maximize the coverage of the personalized information. This is achieved through *positive consistency constraints*, which define what topics' if simultaneously presented would likely be of interest to the user. Positive consistency constraints are represented as the tuple *pc* (*topic1, topic2, degree*), where *degree* is the degree of similarity between the two topics. For example, recently in the news the topics *athletics* and *Olympics2008* appear quite frequently, thus suggesting a positive consistency constraint between *Olympics2008* and *athletics.* Such a constraint can be used to recommend additional information about *Olympics2008* if the user is interested in *athletics* and vice versa.

Constraint Satisfaction Specification for IP: In our constraint satisfaction approach for IP, the topics representing the user's interest are viewed as variables, and domains of the variables comprise any combination of available information artifacts. Requirement 1 was solved as a unary constraint to the variables and represented by constraint c_1. Requirement 2 was represented by a unary constraint c_2 and a binary constraint c_3. Requirement 3 was addressed through an objective function O. c_1, c_2, c_3 and O are explained below.

We define our IP problem as $P\ (V, D, C, O)$.

- Variable set $V = \{v_1, v_2, \ldots, v_n\}$, where n is the number of topics of a user's interest; v_i, $1 \leq i \leq n$, represents the ith topic of a user's interest.

- Domain set $D = \{d_1, d_2, \ldots, d_n\}$; d_i, $1 \leq i \leq n$, represents the domain of v_i. Suppose $s = \{t_1, t_2, \ldots, t_m\}$ is a set consisting of all information artifacts, then d_i is the power set of s without the empty set ø. E.g. If $\{t_1, t_2\}$ is the set of information artifacts, the domain of the variable will be $\{\{t_1\}, \{t_2\}, \{t_1, t_2\}\}$.
- Constraint set $C = \{c_1, c_2, c_3\}$; $c_1 = rel(v_i)$, where $1 \leq i \leq n$, is a unary constraint, and means the value of v_i must be relevant to users' interest (Requirement 1). Suppose v_i represents the ith topic of a user's interest, and the domain of v_i is $\{\{t_1\}, \{t_2\}, \{t_1, t_2\}\}$. By checking the topics of t_1 and t_2, we know t_1 is relevant to the ith topic of the user's interest, but t_2 is not. To satisfy c_1, $\{t_2\}$ and $\{t_1, t_2\}$ will be removed from the domain of v_i. $c_2 = con1(v_i)$, where $1 \leq i \leq n$, is a unary constraint, and means the information artifacts assigned to v_i must be consistent to each other (Requirement 2). Suppose the system is trying to assign $\{t_1, t_2\}$ to v_1. To decide whether c_2 is satisfied or not, we can check the consistency between t_1 and t_2. Suppose t_1 presents topics 'acquisition' and 'stocks', and t_2 presents topics 'acquisition' and 'gold'. We take one topic from t_1 and t_2 respectively to form pairs of topics ordered alphabetically. Then we get four pairs - *(acquisition, acquisition)*, *(acquisition, gold)*, *(acquisition, stocks)* and *(gold, stocks)*. We check these four pairs against the effective negative consistency constraints, and find that *(acquisition, gold)* triggers a negative constraint. So we know c_2 is violated and the assignment fails. $c_3 = con2(v_k, v_j)$, where $k \neq j$ and $1 \leq k, j \leq n$, is a binary constraint, and means the value of v_k and v_j must be consistent to each other (Requirement 2). When checking c_3, we take an information artifact from the value of both variables to form pairs of information artifacts. If any pair is inconsistent, c_3 is violated.
- $O = \Sigma_i (n_i * weight_i)$ is the objective function, where i is a member of the set of satisfied positive consistency constraints—S. n_i is the time the constraint i is satisfied. $weight_i$ is the correlation value of the constraint i. The target is to find a complete valuation that maximizes the objective function. This function will be used in step3 (coverage maximization) of our CSP process solving.

Tasks of the Constraint Satisfaction Based IP System

We explain in detail the two main IP tasks.

Task 1: Finding the Factual Consistency Constraints

We acquire consistency constraints directly from the given corpus of information artifacts (with pre-assigned topics) by using the association rule-mining approach. The premise of the approach is that when information is composed it entails some inherent relationships between discussion topics that can meaningfully co-occur within a given document. We leverage these intrinsic relationships between topics to establish factual consistency constraints such that the frequency of co-occurrence of information topics may reflect the degree of consistency between the topics. We treat topics as items in the *Apriori* rule association method to find 2-itemsets. We select the 2-itemsets with high support value and calculate the correlation between the two items. The correlation value is then used to distinguish between positive and negative consistency constraints as follows:

- If $0 < \text{corr}(A, B) < 1$, A and B are correlated negatively it means these two topics are inconsistent to each other, so a negative consistency constraint can be established between these two topics.

- If corr(A, B) > 1, A and B are positively correlated, and they encourage the co-occurrence of each other, so a positive consistency constraint is found between these two topics.
- If *corr(A, B)* = 1, *A* and *B* are independent to each other.

After our experiments with the Reuters-21578 dataset, we acquired 913 frequent 2-itemsets We used the Chi-Square statistical significance test to measure the interestingness of the 2-itemsets, where the Chi-Square significance level was set to 95% and we acquired a smaller-sized but high quality set of 177 consistency constraints, which were sub-divided into 120 positive and 57 negative consistency constrains based on their correlation values.

Task 2: Constraint Satisfaction Based Information Personalization

Given a user-model as shown in Table 4, we briefly explain the three stages of our constraint satisfaction based IP approach:

Stage1-Filter user-relevant information: The first stage involves finding all the documents that correspond to the user's interest as per requirement 1. This involves the satisfaction of the relevancy constraint by enforcing node consistency to satisfy the unary constraint $c_1 = rel(v_i)$ by comparing the topics of the various documents against a user's interest as noted in the user-model. Functionally, if the variable v_{sports} has a value (i.e. news item) that

Table 4. An exemplar user-model, showing user interests and Personalization criteria

Component	Value
Interests	Acquisition, Gas, Income, Jobs
Tolerance	20% factual inconsistency
Preference	Satisfy all consistency constraints

Table 5. User relevant items for the variables

Variable	Retained Relevant item	Removed Relevant item
v_{acq}	t_1, t_2, t_3	t_{13}
v_{gas}	t_4, t_5, t_6, t_7	t_{14}
v_{income}	t_8	
v_{jobs}	$t_9, t_{10}, t_{11}, t_{12}$	t_{15}

is not equal to one of the interests of the user, then the value will be filtered out from v_{sports}'s domain. The outcome of this stage is the *user-relevant set* that contains user-relevant news items for each variable as shown in the second column of Table 5. For example, the relevant set of v_{acq} is found to be $\{t_1, t_2, t_3, t_{13}\}$ and for v_{gas} the user-relevant set is $\{t_4, t_5, t_6, t_7, t_{14}\}$.

Stage 2-Find the basic information set: At the end of stage 1, the size of the user-relevant set is typically quite large. We pursue to find the *basic information set* that satisfies all the constraints in the constraint set *C*. A solution is called *basic information set* if (i) each user interest is assigned at most one information artifact; and (ii) it violates the least number of consistency constraints; and (iii) least number of user-interests have no information artifact.

First, we use domain reduction methods to eliminate some elements from the domain of variables to make it feasible to search the solution space systematically. Next, we apply a variant of branch and bound method—i.e. Partial Forward Checking (PFC)—that systematically searches for the solutions by satisfying the constraints c_2, c_3 and c_4. Table 6 shows the two solutions for the basic information set.

Stage 3-Maximize information coverage: In this final step, we attempt to maximize the information coverage of the basic information set. Note that the solution at this stage contains at most one information artifact for every topic defined in the user's interest. This condition is in line with requirement 3 of our IP specification.

Table 6. Factually consistent basic information sets. Given the user's tolerance preference both solutions have an empty set for a single topic

Solution	Acquisition	gas	income	jobs
1	$\{t_1\}$	$\{t_4\}$	Ø	$\{t_9\}$
2	Ø	$\{t_4\}$	$\{t_8\}$	$\{t_9\}$

We use local search based optimization techniques to improve the solution by assigning values with more elements (information artifacts) to variables (topics of a user's interest) whilst maintaining the factual consistency. The iterative improvement method used here works as follows: It sets the solution at step 3 as the current solution and then searches the current solution's neighbourhood for a better solution. If there is such a solution, the current solution is set to this 'improved' solution, and the search goes on. Else, the current solution is returned as the result of optimization. Two criteria are used to determine which solution is better: (1) higher value of the objective function, i.e. a higher sum of degrees of the satisfied positive consistency constraints; and (2) higher number of information artifacts.

The optimization results (shown in Table 7) lead to two solutions—i.e. *solution3* and *solution4*. However, *solution4* has the higher objective function value and hence is designated as the final *optimal personalized set* that is presented to the user as personalized information.

Discussion

Viewing IP as a constraint satisfaction problem offers an interesting AI based perspective to the set of available IP approaches. We have demonstrated the successful application of a hybrid of constraint satisfaction methods to yield personalized information that is based on user's interests and Personalization constraints. In future we plan to analyse the content of the document, as opposed to meta-level topics, to establish richer consistency constraints using automated text categorization techniques involving learning mechanisms.

PERSONALIZING HEALTHCARE INFORMATION: A BEHAVIOURAL MODELLING APPROACH

For maximum impact, the delivery of healthcare information targeting lifestyle modification or therapy education for patients should take into account the behavioural readiness of the individual for undergoing change. We present a patient educational intervention approach that provides personalized information for the management of cardiovascular disease (CVD) risk based on the patient's CVD risk assessment and readiness to change his/her behaviour(s). We developed a unique IP approach for compositional information Personalization that addresses the IP issues of *user-model compliance, behavioural modelling* and *information modelling* (Davis et

Table 7. Final optimal presentation set

Solution	acquisition	gas	income	jobs	Objective function
3	$\{t_1\}$	$\{t_4, t_6\}$	NULL	$\{t_9, t_{10}, t_{12}\}$	45.28
4	**NULL**	$\{t_4, t_6\}$	$\{t_8\}$	$\{t_9, t_{10}, t_{11}, t_{12}\}$	**121.65**

al, 2006a; Davis, et al 2006b). The IP approach incorporates:

1. The selection of relevant information artifacts (or educational messages) based on both the patient's user-model and behaviour-model determining his/her readiness to behaviour change. The idea is not only to personalize the educational content based on the patient's imminent healthcare needs but also to tailor the information in accordance with the patient's predisposition to uptake the information vis-à-vis his/her current psychological state with regards to readiness to change lifestyle and behaviour in order to minimize CVD risk
2. The synthesis of the selected educational messages in accordance with a pre-defined educational template to realize personalized information that is consistent with the individual's change processes, decisional balance, and self-efficacy.

We developed a web-based patient educational system called PULSE (Personalization Using Linkages of SCORE and behaviour change readiness to web-based Education) that uses (a) Systematic COronary Risk Evaluation (SCORE) for assessing the patient's current CVD risk; and (b) the Trans-Theoretical Model (TTM) of intentional behaviour change to determine the patient's readiness to change. The Transtheoretical Model is a stage-based model that matches the change principles and processes to each individual's current stage of change, in order to guide them through the process of modifying problem behaviour(s) and acquiring positive behaviour(s). The IP logic is engineering from validated Canadian clinical guidelines and behaviour change literature, and is represented in terms of Medical Logic Modules (MLM). The educational information content, targeting both medical and psycho-social aspects of risk management, is modelled as information snippets derived from staged lifestyle modification materials and non-staged messages based on Canadian clinical guidelines to motivate personal risk management.

Design of PULSE

The PULSE system is developed along the lines of the IP application components proposed by AdWISE. We describe below the constituent IP components of PULSE.

User Model Data Capture Template: We use the commercially available Wellsource Coronary Risk Profile as the basis for our data capture model for collecting patients' demographic, behavioural, and clinical risk factor characteristics. The data capture template comprises 28 features to describe the patient and the disease evaluation.

User Model: The patient's user-model comprises three components: (1) the CVD Risk Profile component directs the selection of clinical guidelines for all risk factors based on the patient's risk; (2) the Staged Risk Factor Profile component directs the selection of TTM messages consistent with the patient's stage of change for specific modifiable risk factor behaviours; and (3) the Non-staged Risk Factor Profile component directs selection of messages for all non-staged risk factors.

Message Library: The messages library comprises three sections: (1) CVD Risk-matched Guidelines; (2) Staged Risk Factors; and (3) Non-staged Risk Factors. The various sourced materials are broken down into small tagged "snippets of information", <tagged>, and stored in an SQL (Standard Query Language) database. The CVD Risk-management Guidelines section contains risk-management target values and textual recommendations for the following risk factors – smoking, blood pressure (SBP and DBP), exercise, stress, depression, eating practices (as dietary recommendations), lipids (TC:HDL cholesterol, LDL cholesterol, and TG), glycemic control (FPG), alcohol, and weight management (Body Mass Index and waist circumference).

The target values and textual recommendations for all risk factors are based on the Canadian guidelines for cardiovascular rehabilitation and CVD prevention, diabetes, dyslipidemia, and hypertension.

The *Staged Risk Factors* section contains TTM (staged) educational documents addressing five risk factors – smoking, obesity, stress, depression, and physical inactivity. The *Non-staged Risk Factors* section contains non-staged risk management materials addressing two CVD risk conditions – age and gender – and five CVD risk factors – blood pressure, eating practices, lipid profile, glycemic control, and alcohol.

Decision Logic: Given a patient profile and a message library containing a vast collection of education interventions, the personalization mechanism involves the selection of the most relevant set of messages based on the patient's individual profile. Personalization is achieved through the processing of a set of symbolic rules based on decision logic—the decision logic maps the profile elements to specific messages. We develop a rule-based inferencing engine that incorporates the decision logic. To represent our medical knowledge we use MLMs, a standard for independent units composing a series of rules in health knowledge bases. Each MLM consists of four parts: an evoking event, logic, action, and data mapping. The logic contains "if-then" rules, where the IF part of the rules contains variables for one or more patient profile elements. The THEN part contains a list of messages that are selected as part of the patient's personalized educational material.

Display Template: We created a display template to systematically organize and present the messages chosen for each patient. The display template comprises four parts: (i) The Introductory Page provides a brief description about the personalized education document; (ii) The CVD Risk Profile offers a graphical display of this patient's risk, including a relative risk chart which displays the contribution of risk factors to total risk; (iii) The Progress Page provides a graphical display of changes in a patient's risk over time; and (iv) The Risk Factor Management section provides personalized information on each risk factor relevant to the patient. Each risk factor has its own section complete with an introductory brief, patient's current results, evidence-based target values, and lifestyle modification and risk management education.

Delivery Method: The PULSE system both collects patient data and delivers personalized educational information over the WWW.

Discussion

This project highlights the engineering of IP logic and interventional messages from validated knowledge resources, such as clinical practice guidelines and patient education material. Furthermore, the work exemplifies a novel IP approach for developing patient education programs that incorporate both patient physiological data and behavioural predisposition to lifestyle modifications, in order to design effective personalized healthcare interventions.

CONCLUSION

Personalization is now recognized as an important feature for Web applications. Survey results and market analysis have concluded that users prefer a personalized web experience, and one notes with interest the emergence of basic personalization features offered by popular websites, such as MY Yahoo, MY Google and My MSN. This chapter provides insights into issues that need to be considered when designing intelligent IP applications, and through our AdWISE framework we demonstrated some technical approaches and methods used to develop intelligent IP applications.

This chapter will be particularly useful for researchers in understanding the different facets of IP, and help them determine the kind of IP they need for their particular application (section 2). Next, we present a list of design and functional issues that need to be incorporated when designing intelligent IP applications (section 3). Typically, the central issue pursued by IP researchers is user-modelling, however we have attempted to introduce several additional key, yet usually ignored, issues that determine the functional and design specifications of any IP application. We believe that proper consideration to these issues will lead to more complete understanding of the problem and ensuing solutions to IP. We demonstrate a working intelligent IP framework—namely AdWISE—that highlights how the key design determinants of IP—i.e. personalization context, constraints and methods—are incorporated in designing specific intelligent IP applications. We also presented the main components of IP applications and associated tasks associated with each component. We anticipate that IP application developer will find the proposed road-map to IP application development useful as it will give a functional perspective to designing sophisticated and efficacious IP applications. The subsequent snapshot presentations of three IP applications will provide a sense of how these theoretical concepts are translated into actual intelligent IP applications.

FUTURE RESEARCH DIRECTIONS

The emergence of Web 2.0 will further amplify the need for intelligent IP given the growing trend for web-based social interactions and information sharing between users. We are witnessing a growing number of personal websites hosting information artifacts that are of interest to a wider community of users, and this is further contributing to the information deluge on the Web. The Web 2.0 concept aims to facilitate higher and open information sharing, but realistically speaking an increased demand for open information sharing need to be matched with improved methods to ensure that users are able to both sift through the information deluge and adapt the available information to their needs. This points to further developments in intelligent IP methods in tandem with Web 2.0 applications. We believe that future trends in intelligent IP will be driven by (a) developments in both the concepts and technologies around Web 2.0; (b) the changing demands and expectations of web users whereby they will be seeking not just personalized information but personalized services that are adapted to their needs; (c) ability to design reusable information artifacts and applications that can adapt such information artifacts towards a user-model; and (d) a 'new' set of user-satisfaction criterion involving efficiency, flexibility and trust. To meet the above, it is anticipated that future research in the core issues of IP will closely align with developments in the areas of adaptive web, semantic web, web services and semantic web services.

Next generation IP applications will be context-aware, proactive and pervasive; IP will be regarded as an enabling technology as opposed to a value-added feature. In line with these expectations, our research efforts concerning the future developments in ADWiSE will target the development of thin client-side applications that will provide runtime personalization on top of existing web applications, or server-side information retrieval applications that embed IP mechanisms within their algorithms. IP offered by ADWiSE will be (a) context-aware—i.e. applications will automatically sense the user's current task and then the underlying IP methods will deliver information that is directly relevant to the user's immediate information needs; (b) pervasive—i.e. the application will embed native personalization mechanisms on top of existing Web applications; and (c) proactive—i.e. applications will automatically invoke the appropriate personalization mechanisms whenever the user interacts with the Web. The proposed functionality of ADWiSE based applications will be such that the user at all times will have a personalized Web experience without the explicit need to find, set, invoke and apply personalization functions.

We note that one future trend is to approach IP applications as a Web Service. This will be a departure from traditional IP applications that are designed as specialized applications addressing a specific personalization target. Rather, the web service approach will promote the development of re-usable IP approaches and methods that can be dynamically applied within different operational environments to achieve a personalized experience. The use of Services Oriented Architectures (SOA) for dynamically composing IP services is an interesting research approach that is being pursued, though largely for specialized applications in E-learning, by the semantic web and adaptive web research communities. The underlying approach is to regard web-based information and web-services as a composite of individual, self-contained 'components' that are defined through a semantically rich representation formalism that also identifies the relationships between them. These components may vary in content topic and its coverage, functionality and complexity, yet they are and can be systematically synthesized based on a pre-defined document template, process plan or workflow to realize a personalized information artifact and/or service. Personalization in this case is pursued at the higher level of service composition and service orientation, whereby individual IP service components can be dynamically added or removed to develop customized IP applications that meet the personalization objectives. Orchestrating an active interplay between IP service components, based on the personalization specification and the metadata of the information content, will lead to dynamic IP applications. The use SOA may allow the provision of personalization services that are based on message exchange standards, information representation standards, pre-defined service behaviours, service planning models and well-defined information presentation interfaces/templates.

We believe that the next step ahead of the SOA approach to IP is the incorporation of the emerging Semantic Web (SW) technologies for intelligent IP. Through experience, we have learnt that personalization of information content is quite complex due to the present lack of semantic descriptions and standards for existing information resources. The SW supports standard semantic descriptions such as formal definitions of terms, ontological definitions of domain concepts, information resources and reasoning methods. Semantic web paradigm aims to provide both (a) a semantically rich explication and modelling of information; and (b) an intelligent information processing and access mechanism that takes into account the underlying semantic make-up of the information. We believe that the semantic description of the information is highly pertinent for personalizing it, and will lead to IP that is more validated, well-structured, standardized and with an associated trust value that will determine the relevance and utility of the personalized information towards the user-model. The semantic web stipulates standards, which currently are lacking in the IP domain, that will allow to achieve re-usability, shareability and interoperability of IP methods between different IP applications, thus leading to a IP applications that will offer (a) context-aware information discovery; and (b) component-level adaptation of information content composition.

Postscript: The way forward for intelligent IP will be powered by semantic web technologies. Guided by this belief, our future IP research, within the realm of the AdWISE framework, will be geared towards the development of next generation semantically powered reusable, shareable and interoperable IP methods and tools. Indeed, these are interesting times for IP research.

REFERENCES

Abidi, S. S. R., Chong, Y. H., & Zeng, Y. (2006). Generating customized yet factually consistent information: A constraint satisfaction approach. *Journal of Digital Libraries*, 6(3), 247-259.

Abidi, S. S. R., & Zeng Y. (2006). Intelligent information personalization leveraging constraint satisfaction and association rule methods. *19th Canadian Conference on Artificial Intelligence* (pp. 134-145), Berlin: Springer Verlag Press.

Abidi, S. S. R., & Chong, Y. H. (2004). An adaptive hypermedia system for information customization via content adaptation. *IADIS International Journal of WWW/Internet*, 2(1), 79-94.

Abidi, S. S. R., & Chong, Y. H. (2003). E-healthcare via personalized information services: Addressing the need for factually consistent information. In M.E. Orlowska, S. Weerawarana, M. Papazoglou, J. Yang (Ed.), *Lecture Notes in Computer Science 2910: 1st International Conference on Service Oriented Computing* (pp. 132-148). Berlin: Springer Verlag Press.

Abidi, S. S. R. (2002). Designing adaptive hypermedia for internet portals: A personalization strategy featuring case base reasoning with compositional adaptation. In F.J. Garijo, J.C. Riquelme & M Toro (Ed.) *Lecture Notes in Artificial Intelligence 2527: Advances in Artificial Intelligence* (60-69). Berlin: Springer Verlag Press.

Abidi, S. S. R., Han, C. Y., & Abidi, S. R. (2001). Patient empowerment via 'pushed' delivery of personalized healthcare educational content over the internet. *10th World Congress on Medical Informatics*. IOS Press.

Alrifai, M., Dolog, P., & Nejdl, W. (2006). Learner profile management for collaborative adaptive eLearning application. *Joint International Workshop on Adaptivity, Personalization and the Semantic Web at 17th ACM Hypertext'06 conference*. ACM Press.

Anderson, C., Domingos, P., & Weld, D. (2001). Personalizing web sites for mobile users. *10th International WWW Conference* (pp. 565-575). ACM Press.

André, E., Rist, T., & Müller, J. (1998) WebPersona: A lifelike presentation agent for the world-wide web. *Knowledge-Based Systems, 11*(1), 25-36.

Ardissono, L., & Goy, A. (2000). Tailoring the interaction with users in web stores, *User Modelling and User Adapted Interaction, 10*(4), 251-303.

Arezki, R., Poncelet, P., Dray, G., & Pearson, D. W. (2004) Web information retrieval based on user profile. *Third International Conference on Adaptive Hypermedia and Adaptive Web-Based Systems,* pp. 275-278.

Balabanovic, M. (1997) An adaptive web page recommendation service. *First International Conference on Autonomous Agents*. ACM Press, pp. 378-385.

Balabanovic, M.Bental, D., Cawsey, A., Pearson, J., & Jones, R. (2000) Adapting web-based information to the needs of patients with cancer. *Adaptive Hypermedia and Adaptive Web-based Systems*, Berlin: Springer-Verlag, pp. 27-37.

Beaumont I. (1994). User modeling in the interactive anatomy tutoring system ANATOM-TUTOR. *User Models and User Adapted Interaction, 4*(1), 21-45.

Belkin N.J., & Croft W.B. (1992). Information personalization and information retrieval: Two sides of the same coin? *Communications of the ACM, 35*(12), 29-38.

Berners-Lee, T., Hendler J., & Lassila JO. (2001). The semantic web. *Scientific American*, 2001, *284*(5), 34–43.

Billsus, D. & Pazzani, M. J. (2000) User modeling for adaptive news access. *User Modeling and User Adapted Interaction, 10*(2-3), 147-180.

Boyle, C., & Encarnacion A. O. (1994). MetaDoc: An adaptive hypertext reading system. *User Models and User Adapted Interaction, 4*(1), 1-19.

Brafman, R, Domshlak, C., & Shimony, S. (2004). Qualitative decision making in adaptive presentation of structured information. *ACM Transactions on Information Systems, 22*(4), 503-539.

Brusilovsky, P. (1995) Intelligent tutoring systems for World-Wide Web. Third International WWW Conference, pp. 42-45

Brusilovsky, P. (2001). Adaptive hypermedia. *User Modeling and User-Adapted Interaction, 11*, 87-110.

Brusilovsky, P., A. Kobsa & Nejdl, W. (Ed).(2006). The adaptive web: Methods and strategies of web personalization. Berlin: Springer Verlag Press.

Brusilovsky, P., Kobsa, A., & Vassileva, J. (Ed.) (1998). Adaptive hypermedia and hypertext. Dordrecht:Kluwer Academic Publishers.

Burke, R. (2000). Knowledge-based recommender systems. In A. Kent (Ed.), *Encyclopedia of Library and Information Systems*, 69(32), New York: Marcel Dekker.

Burke, R. (2002) Hybrid recommender systems: Survey and experiments. *User Modeling and User-Adapted Interaction, 12*(4), 331-370.

Carmichael, D. J., Kay, J. & Kummerfeld, B. (2005). Consistent modeling of users, devices and sensors in ubiquitious computing environment. *User Modeliing and User-Adapted Interaction, 15*, 197-234

Calvi, L. & Bra, P. D. (1997). Proficiency-adapted information browsing and filtering in hypermedia educational systems. *User Modeling and User Adapted Interaction, 7*(4), 257-277.

Chedrawy, Z. & Abidi, S. S. R. (2006). An adaptive personalization recommendation strategy featuring context-sensitive content adaptation. *International Conference on Adaptive Hypermedia and Adaptive Web-based Systems*, Springer Verlag Press.

Chedrawy, Z. & Abidi, S. S. R. (2006). Case based reasoning for information personalization: Using a context-sensitive case Adaptation Approach. *IEEE International Conference on Engineering of Intelligent Systems*, IEEE Press.

Cheverst, K., Mitchell, K., & Davies, N. (2002). The role of adaptive hypermedia in a context-aware tourist guide. *Communications of the ACM, 45*(5), 47-51.

Chittaro, L. and Ranon, R. (2000) Adding adaptive features to virtual reality interfaces for e-commerce. *Adaptive Hypermedia and Adaptive Web-based Systems*, Berlin: Springer-Verlag, pp. 86-91.

Davis, S., & Abidi, SSR (2006). Tailoring cardiovascular risk management educational interventions: A synergy of SCORE risk assessment and behavior change model. *11th International Symposium for Health Information Management Research*, pp. 66-78.

Davis, S., & Abidi, S. S. R. (2006). Adaptive patient education framework featuring personalized cardiovascular risk management interventions. *International Conference on Adaptive Hypermedia and Adaptive Web-based Systems,* Berlin: Springer Verlag Press.

Dolog, P, Henze, N, Nejdl, W., & Sintek, M. (2004). The personal reader: Personalizing and enriching learning resources using semantic web technologies. *International Conference on Adaptive Hypermedia and Adaptive Web-Based Systems*, Berlin: Springer Verlag.

De Carolis, B., Cozzolongo, G., & Pizzutilo, S. (2005). Generating personalized tourist map descriptions. In M. Ali and F. Esposito (Ed.): *Lecture Notes in Artificial Intelligence 3533*, Berlin: Springer Verlag, pp. 259–268.

Dilley, R. (1999). The Problem of Context. New York: Berghahn Books.

Fink, J., & Kobsa A. (2002). Putting personalization into practice, *Communications of the ACM, 45*(5), 41-42.

Fink, J. & Kobsa, A. (2002). User modeling in personalized city tours. *Artificial Intelligence Review, 18*, 33-74,

Hanani, U., Shapira, B., & Shoval, P. (2001). Information filtering: Overview of issues, research and systems. *User Modeling and User-Adapted Interaction, 11*, 203-259.

Hohl, H., Bocker, H., Gunzenhauser, R. (1996). HYPADAPTER: An adaptive hypertext system for exploratory learning and programming, *User Modelling & User Adapted Interaction, 6*(2), 131-156.

Kobsa, A., Koenemann, J., & Pohl, W. (2001). Personalized Hypermedia Presentation Techniques for Improving Online Customer Relationships. *The Knowledge Engineering Review, 16*(2), 111-155.

Kobsa, A. (2001) Tailoring privacy to user's needs. In: M. Bauer, P. J. Gmytrasiewicz, J. Vassileva (Ed.), *Lecture Notes on Artificial Intelligence 2109*, Berlin: Springer-Verlag, pp. 303-313.

Kobsa, A., Muller, D., & Nill, A. (1994). KN-AHS: An adaptive hypermedia client of the user modeling system BGP-MS. *Fourth International Conference on User Modeling*, pp. 99-105.

Kuo, F. F., & Shan, M. K. (2002). A personalized music filtering system based on melody style classification. *IEEE international Conference on Data Mining*, pp. 649–652.

Lawrence, S., & Giles, C. L. (1998). Context and Page analysis for improved web search. *IEEE Internet Computing*, pp. 38-46.

Milosavljevic, M., & Oberlander, J. (1998). Dynamic hypertext catalogues: Helping users to help themselves. *9th ACM International Hypertext Conference*, ACM Press, pp. 123-131.

Oppermann, R., & Specht, M. (2000). A context sensitive nomadic information system as an exhibition guide, *2nd International Symposium on Handheld and Ubiquitious Computing*, pp. 127-142.

Palme, J. (1998). Information filtering. *4th International Conference on Intelligent Tutoring Systems*. ACM Press.

Sarkin, J. A., Johnson, S. S., Prochaska, J. O. & Prochaska, J. M. (2001). Applying the transtheoretical model to regular moderate exercise in an overweight population: validation of a stages of change measure. *Preventive Medicine, 33*, 462-469.

Sarwar, B., Karypis, G., Konstan, J., & Riedl, J. (2001). Item-based collaborative filtering recommendation algorithms. *10th International World Wide Web Conference*, ACM Press, pp. 285-295.

Shahabi, C., & Chen, Y. S. (2003). Web information personalization: Challenges and approaches. *3rd International Workshop on Databases in Networked Information Systems (DNIS 2003)*, Berlin: Springer Verlag.

Smyth, B., & Cotter, P. (2002). Personalized adaptive navigation for mobile portals. *15th European Conference on Artificial Intelligence*, IOS Press, pp. 608-612.

Spencer, L., Pagell, F., Hallion, M. E. & Adams, T. B. (2002). Applying the transtheoretical model to tobacco cessation and prevention: a review of literature. *American Journal of Health Promotion, 17*, 7-71.

ADDITIONAL READING

Berners-Lee, T., Hendler, J., & Lassila, O. (2001). The semantic web. *Scientific American*, 284(5), 34–43.

Brafman, R., Domshlak, C., & Shimony. S. (2004). Qualitative decision making in adaptive presentation of structured information. *ACM Transactions on Information Systems*, 22(4), 503-539.

Fensel, D., Bussler, C., & Maedche, A. (2002). Semantic web enabled web services. *1st International Semantic Web Conference.*

Keidl, M., & Kemper, A.(2004). A framework for context-aware adaptable web services. *9th International Conference on Extending Database Technology.*

Masuoka, R., Parsia, B., & Labrou, Y. (2003). Task computing- The semantic web meets pervasive computing. *2nd International Semantic Web Conference.*

McIlraith, S., Son, T., & Zeng, H. (2001). Semantic web services. IEEE Intelligent Systems, Special Issue on the Semantic Web, 16(2), 46-53.

Mostafa, J. (2002). Introduction: Information Customization. *IEEE Intelligent Systems,* 17(6), 8-11.

Sirin, E., Parsia, B., & Hendler, J. (2004). Filtering and selecting semantic web services with interactive composition techniques. *IEEE Intelligent Systems*, 19(4), 42-49.

Chapter VII
A Semantically Adaptive Interface for Measuring Portal Quality in E-Government

Babis Magoutas
National Technical University of Athens, Greece.

Christos Chalaris
National Technical University of Athens, Greece.

Gregoris Mentzas
National Technical University of Athens, Greece.

ABSTRACT

This chapter introduces a semantically adaptive interface as a means of measuring the quality of e-government portals, based on user feedback. The interface is semantic as it uses ontologies in order to formalize well defined semantics about the adaptation criteria used. Furthermore it is adaptive as three axes of adaptation are applied: based on real-time feedback from users, based on problems encountered by the user and based on metadata of the pages visited by the user. The authors hope that applying the proposed adaptive interface as a means of measuring e-government portals' quality, will not only allow more focused and targeted assessment of quality, but will also increase users' response rates.

INTRODUCTION

E-government is the use of information technology to support government operations, engage citizens, and provide government services (Dawes, 2002). Many governments have created portal sites for their citizens. In the United States the main portal is USA.gov, in addition to portals developed for specific audiences such as DisabilityInfo.gov; in the United Kingdom the main portals are Directgov for citizens and businesslink.gov.uk for businesses (Wikipedia, 2007).

Citizens possess different access possibilities, skills, expectations and motivation, thus they face different problems during their navigation to an e-government portal while searching for a public e-service or during the actual service provision. This variety in citizens' skills, expectations and in problems they face has as consequence that each citizen has different perceptions concerning the quality of public e-services.

Another source of variation is the level of importance of each quality factor among users. For example, for some users without web experience—who are often lost in the information space of a portal - quality is related mostly with a clear and easy to follow portal structure, or the provision of help information related to the completion of submission forms. On the other hand, experienced users put more emphasis on advanced features like automatic recalling of user's personal data within portal's submission forms or on some technical characteristics of the portal.

Considering the aforementioned variations, it is apparent that a "one fits all" e-government services' assessment is not efficient. For example an experienced user must perform the evaluation without being bothered with irrelevant information. On the other hand an in depth examination of the various quality factors is needed by other groups of users that face problems. Besides citizens, an evaluation that is targeted to problems is very important also for the analysts, because such an approach supports them in the decision procedure about the planned actions for improvement.

For e-government services' assessment to be efficient, the evaluation should be organized in a way to serve every citizen individually. For the realization of such a customized and adaptive evaluation of e-government services, an intelligent, semantic-based platform is needed which allows each citizen to put emphasis in quality dimensions related with the problems he/she faces, depending on his/her skills and expectations (Magoutas, et. al, 2007). In that way quality assessment of e-government services will become more proactive offering more and better data that can be used as input for the support of decisions towards the improvement of services to citizens.

This chapter presents a semantically adaptive interface for measuring portal quality in e-Government. The chapter is structured in 5 sections. After this brief introduction, we present in section 2 the related work on the area, while in section 3 the motivation of this work is discussed. Sections 4 is the main section of the chapter and includes an overview of our approach, the ontologies that are responsible for providing the semantics upon which the adaptation is based, the functional description and technical specification of the system, as well as user scenarios and screenshots of the adaptive interface. Section 5 includes our conclusions and possible topics for further work, while section 6 describes future research directions and trends.

RELATED WORK

A research area which is very close to our work refers to adaptive hypermedia. An Adaptive Hypermedia System (AHS) tries to adapt information for a user based on a model of that particular user. Examples of adaptive hypermedia systems include AHA! (Bra et. al., 2003), ELM-ART (Brusilovsky et. al., 1996), and Adaptive Engine 3 - AE3 (Keeffe et. al., 2005). These systems use adaptive techniques in order to provide the adapted hypermedia for a user. There are four such techniques, which are adaptive navigation, adaptive presentation, structural adaptation, and historical adaptation (Tallon, 2005). Our approach uses the idea of adaptive presentation for quality measuring of e-government portals and services. Adaptive presentation is intuitively related to how the hypermedia is presented to the user. The hypermedia or content is adapted towards the user model provided. In our approach the adaptation is based on a user model that is constructed during runtime, using data mining on web server log and is modelled using semantic technologies (Apostolou et. al., 2006).

Adaptive systems have been developed for various application domains. In (Maneewatthana et. al., 2006) a system that brings together knowledge technologies and adaptive hypermedia in order to facilitate the reuse and sharing of information between knowledge workers is presented. This system helps employees of a modern organization or members of a community, to navigate large information spaces and browse information tailored to their needs, by using semantically structured information. Adaptive systems have been also deployed in educational settings, in order to offer the most appropriate resources to each learner, according to his/her knowledge and needs. There are several examples of multidisciplinary research concerning adaptive systems that support learning, including the systems presented in (Denaux et. al., 2004), (Dolog et. al., 2004) and (Razmerita and Gouarderes, 2004). The latter for example is combining research in grid computing, semantic web, e-learning and adaptation. Our approach tries to adopt adaptation techniques for the e-government application domain - and more specifically for the task of measuring e-government portal quality - by bringing together research related to portal quality, e-government services, semantics and adaptivity.

The research field of recommender systems is also very close to our work. Recommender systems take into account user's interests, either declared by the user or conjectured by the system, in order to rank or filter web pages. Some recommender systems make use of the domain semantics, such as relationships and entities in the domain, in order to build the user profile. An example of an ontology-based user-profiling approach that takes advantage of the knowledge contained in ontologies instead of attempting user-profile acquisition is described in (Middleton et al., 2004). In this research the authors describe the improvement of classical recommender systems with ontologies and show the benefits of ontologies for recommender systems. In our approach the ontological mappings of user interests to domain concepts, form also the basis of adaptation, but ontological modelling of common user problems is also been taken into account for the adaptation of the interface.

Related work concerning intelligent questionnaires has been done e.g. in (Brannen, 2001). The general aim of this work was to enable the creation and re-use of 'metadata' in the survey process and to innovate in the areas of the design and presentation of surveys. The metadata were captured into XML in this work. In our approach the metadata and semantics are captured in the more expressive OWL, allowing the definition of constraints for the domain model.

Our approach uses a quality ontology as the basis for the adaptation of the quality measurement interface. There are several ontologies in literature that are explicitly called QoS ontologies. The e-GovQoS, an Ontology for Quality of e-Government Services (Corradini et. al., 2006) takes into consideration dynamic aspects related to Quality of Services and their impact in the service composition, in particular when a large number of services are available to reach the same goal. The role of this Ontology is service discovery and composition based on their QoS characteristics. The emphasis is put on quality of web-services and low level quality metrics are mainly modelled.

A similar to e-GovQoS ontology is the one developed in Lancaster University (Dobson et. al., 2005). This ontology has been named QoSOnt, an ontology for Quality of Service and its role is service discovery and selection based upon QoS requirements. QoSOnt supports network and services as the type of system that QoS may refer to and the focus is given to its application in the field of service-centric systems.

Service discovery and composition is also the main role of the quality taxonomy developed in (Cappiello et. al., 2004). This taxonomy defines the quality characteristics of networks, channels of communication and access devices that can be used for the delivery of services and describes quality elements of a multi-channel environment.

An ontology for the specification of QoS metrics for tasks and Web services has been developed in (Cardoso et. al., 2002). The information formalized in the ontology allows the discovery of Web services based on operational metrics. The focus of this quality ontology is put on quality dimensions of time, cost and reliability.

All these ontologies focus on quality characteristics of web services that must be taken into account for a QoS–based service discovery and composition. They don't take into account quality characteristics related to user interaction with the portal. Their role is to enable a quality-aware service discovery, something that is meaningful only in case that are a large number of web-services are available to reach the same goal and quality is used as a criterion for their selection. However, they cannot be used for the subjective evaluation of a single public e-service and thus for a holistic and high level assessment of quality. Our work seeks to address these gaps by providing an openly available quality ontology and a relevant system that uses this ontology in order to enable an adaptive assessment of public e-services.

MOTIVATION

As most of the public administrations in Europe and developed countries recognised the need of e-government services the number of online Government to citizen (G2C) and Government to Business (G2B) services has substantially increased. For example according to Cap Gemini Report (Cap Gemini, 2006) for the 20 basic public services in the EU, the number of official service providers present online has crossed the 90% threshold in the EU-15 plus Norway, Iceland and Switzerland ('EU-18').

Although the number of e-government services increases, manifold problems related to quality of public e-services still exist; see e.g. the Top of the Web survey (eGovernment Unit, DG Information Society, European Commission, 2004). Some of the frequently reported usability problems include: not being able to find the needed service/information; difficult use of e-services; need for better help regarding the e-service provided on the website; language understandability; etc. (Papadomichelaki et. al., 2006).

The existence of these problems surfaces the need for a periodic, user-centric measurement of the quality of existing e-government services, as the basis of a continuous improvement process. In other words, we need to assess the quality level of the electronic services provided by public entities to citizens and business organizations.

The idea of a user-centric evaluation inheres the use of online questionnaires, as an efficient tool for collecting feedback. Questionnaires are used widely as data collection instruments, either in print form or online; see e.g. (Couper, 2001). The biggest advantage of online questionnaires is that they can provide real time feedback from the point of view of the user, while he/she is navigating at the portal. However, as in the offline world, users are not willing to answer a lot of questions, as they consider it a waste of time.

This fact leads often to a trade-off between the questionnaire's detail level and the anticipated response rates, at the design phase. Personalization techniques could be used for the dynamic composition of the online questionnaires in order to achieve the best compromise between the number of questions and completed questionnaires. Such a questionnaire is dynamically composed or adaptive, since the questions presented are not fixed, but their selection is based on specific criteria. For each user only a relevant set of questions is presented, thus reducing the time needed for filling-in the questionnaire. The dynamic composition of the questionnaire is based upon a quality ontology, which models explicitly and formally all quality aspects that must be taken into account for the assessment of public e-services delivered through an e-government portal, as well as their relationships.

The approach presented in this chapter can be used as well for measuring quality of private sector's web sites. The only difference in this case would be that a new ontology should be used, that would models the quality aspects of web sites with an emphasis on trading and commercial issues which we do not address in the following.

SOLUTION DESCRIPTION

In this section we discuss the proposed solution in order to deal with the issues presented previously. We start with a discussion about the conceptual approach, giving an overview of our proposed semantically adaptive interface for measuring portal quality in e-government. A description of the ontologies that enable the semantic adaptation, as well as their role, follows. This section continues with the functional description and technical architecture of the proposed system and finally user scenarios and screenshots of the adaptive interface are presented.

Conceptual Approach

As part of our previous work we have developed a quality model that allows the specification of quality dimensions and factors concerning the quality in e-services provided by public administrations (Papadomichelaki et. al., 2006). Factors and dimensions are both quality aspects that affect the perceived by users quality, but they examine quality in a different level of detail. Quality factors focus on high level quality aspects such as the usability of the portal/web site, the quality of information, while quality dimensions examine in more detail the relevant quality factor. Relevant quality dimensions for the aforementioned quality factors are for example the web site's structure and appearance, for portal's usability quality factor and information accuracy and freshness for information quality factor.

The quality model was constructed after a literature review of 36 European and international approaches on quality assessment of e-services, e-government services and traditional services; see (Papadomichelaki et. al., 2006). We model the quality factors and dimensions for e-government services explicitly with the quality ontology. An ontology represents an explicit specification of the conceptualisation of a domain of interest (Gruber, 1993). In fact, it structures and formalizes expert knowledge about the domain. That knowledge usually reflects a problem that has to be resolved in the domain. In other words, an ontology formalizes the procedural/operative knowledge needed to describe/resolve the given problem (Apostolou et. al., 2006). In our case the problem is the quality assessment of e-government services, while our proposed solution is the adoption of a semantic adaptive questionnaire addressed to users that visit the e-government portal.

Figure 1 gives an overview of our quality approach. We assume that a public organization incorporates into its e-services portal the adaptive questionnaire. Data about users' interactions with the e-government portal, obtained from click streams, are collected into the web log. User click streams are analyzed and depending on some pre-specified criteria the adaptive questionnaire is dynamically composed. An example of a criterion that is used for the questionnaire adaptation refers to the problems that users face during their navigation in the e-government portal. These problems are identified by a system component depicted as "user problem identification component" in Figure 1 and are stored into the problems ontology. Independently of the criterion that is used in order to decide which questions to incorporate into the adaptive questionnaire, the quality ontology is used for the questionnaire adaptation. Citizens

Figure 1. Overview of our approach

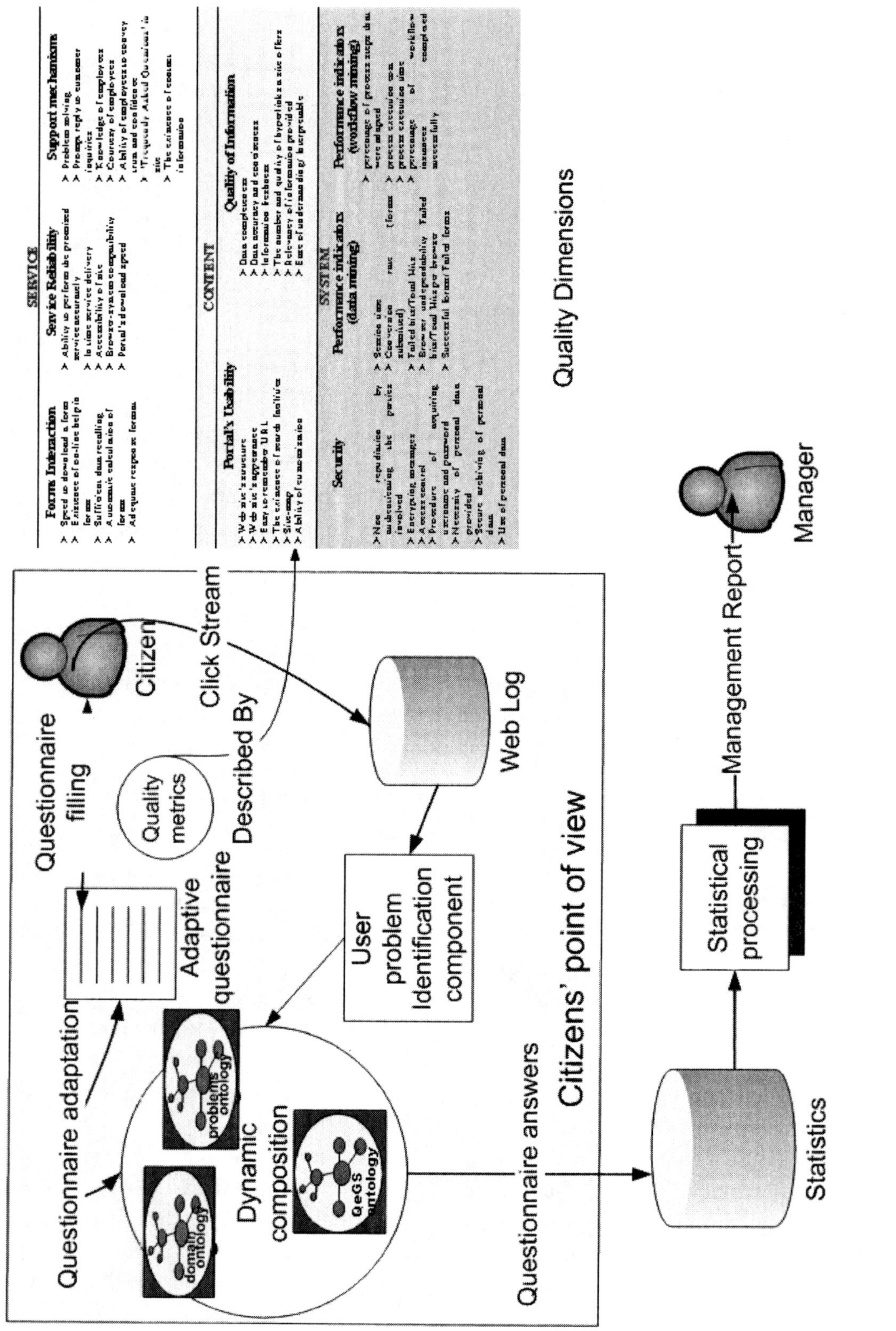

visiting the e-government portal fill the adaptive questionnaire, which is not the same for all users. Questionnaire's answers are stored into a database that is used as input for the statistical analysis of citizens' feedback.

Semantics of Quality Measuring Interface

It is apparent from the conceptual approach section, that quality measuring is based on ontologies that formalize well defined semantics about the adaptation criteria used for the dynamic composition of the appropriate for each case set of questions. The ontologies used by the semantic adaptive interface presented in this chapter are the Quality of e-Government services (QeGS) ontology, the problems ontology and the content or page types' ontology. We describe in this section the above mentioned ontologies and their role for interface adaptation.

The three ontologies are formalised using OWL (Guinness & Harmelen, 2003), since it is a standard language for representing ontologies on the web. They have been partially developed using open source ontology editor, namely Protégé and more specifically its OWL plug-in (Knublauch et. al., 2004) and has been successfully checked for inconsistencies using the trial version of the Description Logic Reasoner RacerPro (Haarslev & Möller, 2001).

Quality ontology concerns quality of e-government services and models quality aspects related to e-government services. Problems' ontology concerns common problems that users face while trying to consume an e-government service. Page types' ontology is responsible for modelling of common page types. The role of these ontologies is:

1. To enable the adaptivity and the customization of citizens' evaluation. The QeGS ontology models formally all factors and quality dimensions that affect the perceived by citizens quality during the e-government service provision. It targets specifically the relationships between "pieces" of domain knowledge, explaining how they contribute altogether to the overall quality. This knowledge is used in order to enable the dynamic composition of the presented questions that are used in order to obtain adaptively the citizens' feedback.
   Ontology-based queries are used for the match making between quality factors, dimensions and questions during adaptive questionnaire execution. For example, when a user rates low a first level question of the adaptive questionnaire, the ontology is queried to find out the relevant second level questions for the problematic first level question. In order to enable the adaptation process described above, questionnaire data are stored as concept's instances and the corresponding data/object properties of the QeGS ontology.
   Another criterion that is used for the adaptation of the questionnaire is the problems that the user faces during the navigation on the portal. If a problem has been identified from the click streams analysis, then only the second level questions that are related with this problem are presented. The combined use of QeGS Ontology together with problems ontology that models users' problems is necessary in order to enable this type of problem-based adaptation. Concerning the content based adaptation of the questionnaire some questions are presented only in case the user has visited some specific types of pages. Combined queries to QeGS ontology and content ontology which models the content of portal's pages, must be used for that.
2. To enable better communication (human to human). By defining a common-agreed vocabulary, the QeGS ontology ensures shared meaning regarding quality of e-government

services and supports better collaboration between various tasks of the assessment procedure. Similarly problems' ontology enables better communication concerning user problems and page types' ontology defines a common-agreed vocabulary for typical page types that e-government portals contain.

3. To enable sharing and benchmarking of knowledge regarding quality assessment gathered/learned in a web portal in other portals. By representing knowledge about quality of e-government services conceptually, in a machine-readable form, it is possible to distribute this knowledge without lost of its usability. It means that there will be possible to compare the quality assessments of a specific e-government portal, with the assessments of a second one. So, the QeGS ontology can serve as an enabler of benchmarking.

The QeGS ontology is based on a quality metrics system, which encapsulates all the quality aspects related to e-government services. This metric system allows the specification of quality dimensions, factors and constructs concerning the quality of e-services provided by public administrations (Apostolou et. al., 2006). Factors and dimensions are both quality aspects that affect the perceived by users quality, but they examine quality in a different level of detail. Quality factors focus on high level quality aspects such as the usability of the portal/web site, the quality of information, while quality dimensions examine in more detail the relevant quality factor. Relevant quality dimensions for the aforementioned quality factors are for example the web site's structure and appearance, for portal's usability quality factor and information accuracy and freshness for information quality factor.

Quality factors are categorized to quality constructs, in a way that each quality construct consists of one or more quality factors. Quality constructs are relevant with major quality areas affecting perceived quality, and are related with the way that an e-government portal is constructed. Examples of quality constructs are service quality construct, content quality construct and system quality construct.

There is a hierarchical relationship between constructs, factors and dimensions. Constructs are composed of quality factors, while factors consist of quality dimensions. Quality constructs, factors and dimensions as well as their hierarchical relationships are modelled with the QeGS ontology. We take advantage of these hierarchical relationships and their well defined semantics, for the specification of the adaptive quality evaluation by citizens.

Independently of the criterion that is used in order to decide which questions to incorporate into the adaptive questionnaire, the quality ontology is used for the questionnaire adaptation. Except of quality constructs, factors and dimensions the demographics of each citizen are modelled, because this information is very valuable for the analysis of their responses.

The Content or web portal or page types' ontology models different portal pages. There are some questions that are very strongly related with specific page types. Presentation of these questions is enabled or disabled according to the user behaviour in the portal. This means that in case the user hasn't visited some specific portal's sections, the relevant questions are not used during the dynamic composition of the questionnaire. QeGS ontology is interconnected with page types or content ontology, through the *hasRelatedContent* object property.

Similarly the link between QeGS and problem ontologies is the object property *hasRelatedQuestion*. Problem ontology models the most reported problems that user face during their navigation in an e-government portal in order to get public e-services.

Figure 2. Indicative concepts and relations of QeGS, problems and page types' ontologies

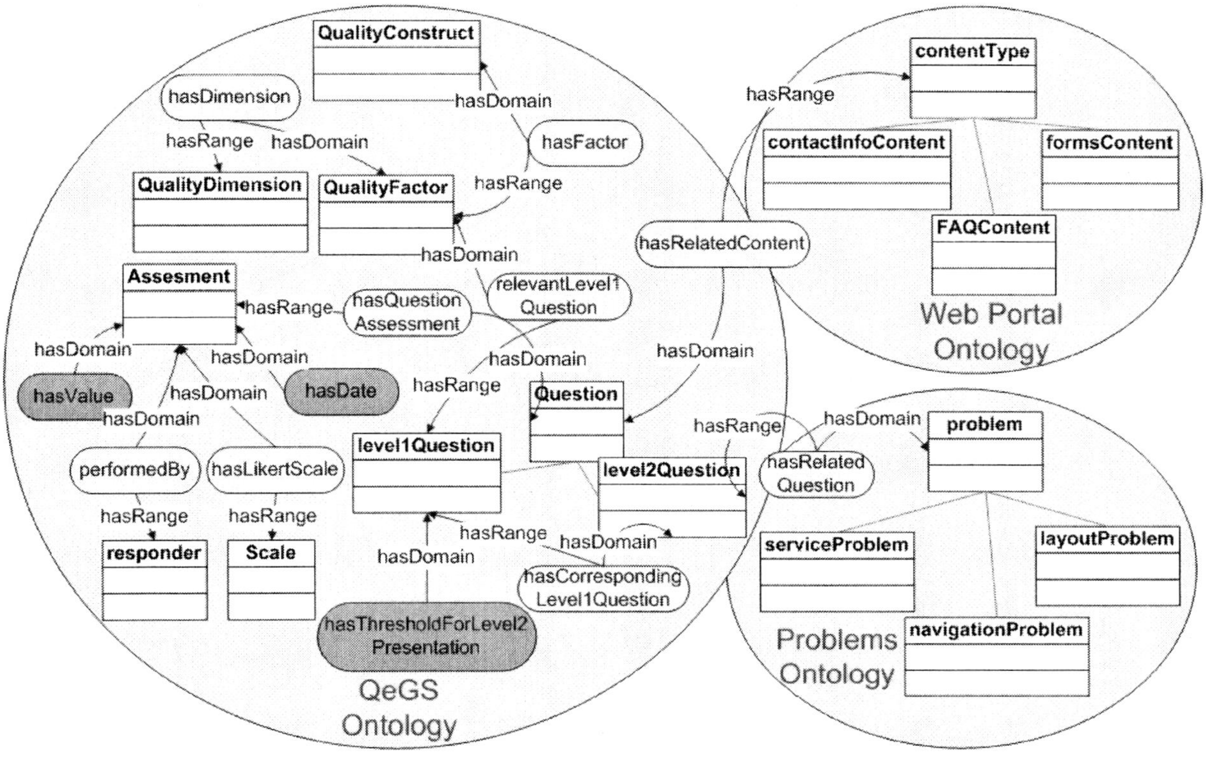

The major relationships between the concepts of the quality ontology as well as the major links between the three different ontologies are depicted in Figure 2. A quality construct has one or more quality factors. Each Quality factor is subsequently decomposed into its relevant quality dimensions and has a relevant first level question. The hierarchical relation between first and second level questions is represented by the object property *hasCorrespondingSecondLevelQuestion*. The concept of quality assessment has been modelled with the *Assessment* class. Each assessment is performed by a responder and has a specific value and date. The user rating threshold for a first level question, under which the second level questions are presented, is modelled with the *hasThresholdForLevel2Presentation* data type property.

Functional Description

The adaptive questionnaire is constituted of statements concerning the quality characteristics of the portal, represented by quality factors and dimensions, with which the user agrees or disagrees on a five point Likert scale (Likert, 1932). Quality statements or questions addressing the citizens are structured into two levels. First level questions measure the quality in a coarse-grained detail, while the second level questions examine in more detail (fine-grained) the relevant first level questions. This means that for each first level question a set of relevant second level questions exist. A similar relationship exists between quality factors and dimensions. Each factor affecting quality is related with a first level question, while each quality dimension is related with a second level question.

The questionnaire is presented at the end of the user session, as a pop up window. For the identification of the end of a user session, we use JavaScript techniques (Powell & Schneider, 2004). At this point, if no other criterion used for dynamic composition of questionnaire is met, only first level questions will be presented to citizens visiting the portal. Incorporation of level 2 questions will occur when a user grades low a quality factor, to examine in more detail the problematic quality factor. The idea of this mechanism is that a low grade for a first level question implies that the citizen has low perceived quality in the corresponding quality factor, but we are not aware which quality dimension is responsible for this poor quality. This problem is resolved by the introduction of the second level questions which refer to quality dimensions.

Figure 3 depicts an example of a first level question and some relevant second level ones. The first level question corresponds to portal's usability quality factor. The relevant quality dimensions for portal's usability that have been used for the construction of second level questions are portal's structure, portal's layout and the effectiveness of portal's search engine.

The dynamic composition of questionnaires is not based only on the answers of users to first level questions. A second criterion used for the selection of questions that will be presented to a user, is the user category he/she belongs. Users are categorized according to the problems they face during their navigation and their online behaviour at the e-government portal. A module that uses web log data to monitor users' actions and aims at real-time grouping of current users online is used for that purpose.

The idea here is that if a problem has been identified and the citizen is categorized into a specific user group along with other citizens facing similar problems, then the second level questions that are related with this problem are presented to citizen, at the end of his session. This mechanism implies a mapping of second level questions with possible user problems, which are being modelled in problems' ontology. For example a navigation problem is related with navigation questions, so if a navigation problem has been identified for a citizen, only second level questions relevant with navigation are presented. The purpose of this mechanism is to get user feedback for the problematic quality factor, reducing the need of many questions, as citizens answer only questions which relate to the specific problem. In this way the required time for answering questions is reduced, the questionnaire is adapted to the needs of the user and furthermore the user feedback is targeted to the problem. Examples of mappings

Figure 3. First and relevant second level questions example

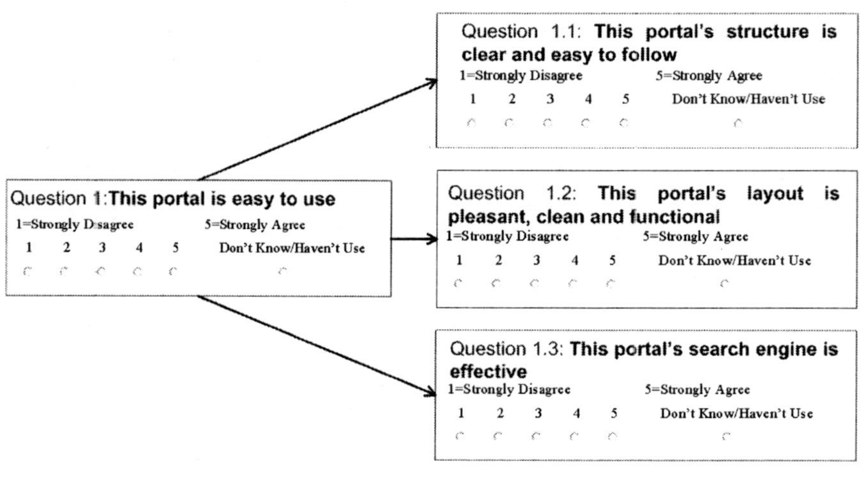

Table 1. Mappings of user problems with second level questions

Problem	Second Level Questions
Finding Service Problem	This portal's structure is clear and easy to follow.
	This portal's search engine is effective.
	This portal's site map is well organised
Forms Problem	Forms in this portal are downloaded in short time.
	Automatic recalling of user's personal data within portal's forms is satisfactory.
	The level of automatic calculation within portal's forms is satisfactory.
	Information about field's completion in this portal is enough.
	Submitted requests or results of the elaboration are easy to stored locally or printed
	This portal works properly with your default browser.
Layout Problem	This portal's layout is pleasant, clean and functional
	This portal is well customized to individual users' needs.
	This portal works properly with your default browser.
Links Problem	This portal offers enough and of high quality hyperlinks.
Navigation Problem	This portal's structure is clear and easy to follow.
	This portal's search engine is effective.
	This portal's site map is well organised
	This portal offers enough and of high quality hyperlinks.
Service Problem	This portal is well customized to individual users' needs.
	The information displayed in this portal is appropriate detailed.

between second level questions and user problems are depicted in Table 1.

A third criterion used for the selection of questions that will be presented to a user, is the content of the pages that the user has visited during the session. There are some questions of the questionnaire that are related with specific parts of portal. The majority of user sessions contain hits to a small portion of the portal's pages, so there is a high possibility that a user is asked about something that he hasn't met during his session. This is a big problem, as it discourages users to give their feedback through the questionnaire, the result being low response rates.

Examples of questions related with specific portal's parts, are questions concerning forms used for submission of information, and questions regarding support mechanisms. These questions are presented only in case of a user session that includes forms, or the FAQ page or the page with contact information, as long as these pages are used primarily for form submission or the initiation of the support process. For the categorization of portal's pages to the various page types, the web pages are annotated with semantic information, using an annotation editor, please refer to the Uren et. al., 2006 for a review of the most commonly used Annotation frameworks. Table 2 depicts some examples of question—content mappings.

A schematic representation of the adaptive interface's business logic is provided by the high level flow chart of Figure 4. As you can see in this flow chart the main adaptation axis of the presented interface is the user problems one. This means that problems that user has faced during her navigation in the e-government portal is the first think that is taken into account by the adaptation algorithm. If the problem identification component

Table 2. Mappings of visited content with first and second level questions

First Level Question	Second Level Questions	Related Content—page type
Portal's usability	This portal's structure is clear and easy to follow.	
	This portal's layout is pleasant, clean and functional	
	This portal's URL is easy to remember.	
	This portal's search engine is effective.	Search engine page
	This portal's site map is well organised	Site map page
	This portal is well customized to individual users' needs.	
Forms Interaction	Forms in this portal are downloaded in short time.	Forms Content
	Automatic recalling of user's personal data within portal's forms is satisfactory.	
	The level of automatic calculation within portal's forms is satisfactory.	
	Information about field's completion in this portal is enough.	
	Submitted requests or results of the elaboration are easy to stored locally or printed	
Support mechanisms	This portal provides contact information	Contact information
	Employees showed a sincere interest in solving users' problem.	Contact information
	Employees give prompt replies to users' inquiries.	Contact information
	Employees have the knowledge to answer users' questions.	Contact information
	The FAQ section of this portal covered completely the topic that you were interested in.	FAQ content
	Employees are courteous	Contact information
	Employees have the ability to convey trust and confidence	Contact information
Security	Acquisition of username and password in this portal is secure.	Login pages
	Only necessary personal data are provided for authentication on this portal.	Login page
	Data provided by users in this portal are archived securely	
	Data provided in this portal are used only for the reason submitted	

has identified at least one user problem, then the relevant with identified problems second level questions are presented. Otherwise the questionnaire is composed of first level questions. The second adaptation axis that is been taken into account in both cases, is the content that the user has visited on a per session basis. Questions that are relevant with non visited content are excluded from the displayed set of questions. User ratings' axis is been involved in the business logic only for first level questions and triggers the presentation of relevant to problematic factor second level questions.

Technical Architecture

The open source survey tool Web Survey Toolbox (Powers, 2006), developed by the Human Computer Interface (HCI) laboratory at the Carnegie Melon University, has been used for designing the survey, as it provides the required flexibility and security. A huge benefit of this survey tool is that using Java and JavaServer Pages (JSP), you can make your survey do almost anything. Branching, advanced branching, randomizing pages, and nearly anything you can think of the logic for is all possible when you edit web pages directly.

Figure 4. High level flowchart of adaptation logic. (AQ = Adaptive Questionnaire)

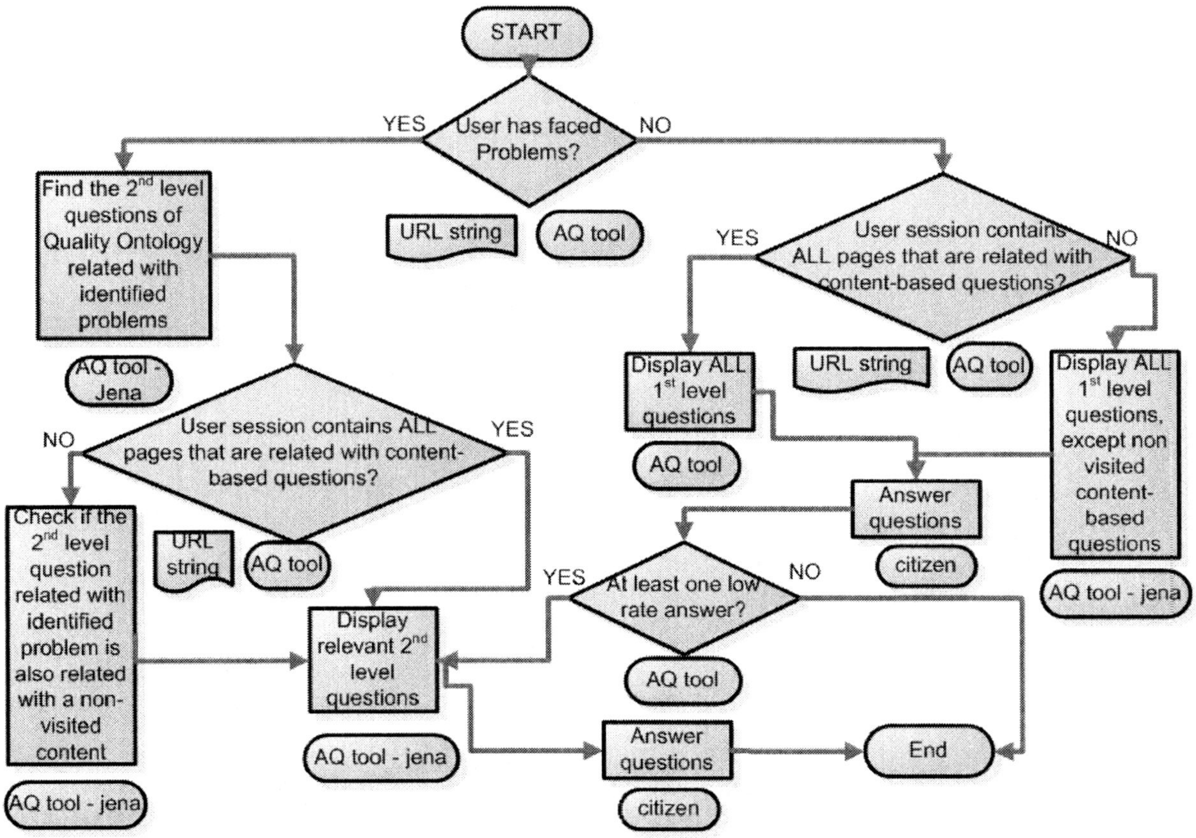

This open source tool interacts with mySQL database management system (DBMS) through Java Database Connectivity (JDBC) API (White et. al., 2001). A questionnaire repository is responsible for storing questions as well as users' answers. The system is hosted under apache tomcat web container. Apache Tomcat has been developed at the Apache Software Foundation (Chopra et. al., 2004) and implements the servlet and the JavaServer Pages (JSP) specifications from Sun Microsystems (Davidson & Coward, 1999), providing an environment for Java code to run in cooperation with a web server.

Web survey toolbox provides JSP tags as the main API that is used in order to encapsulate business logic in the questionnaire presentation. We have used the predefined JSP tags of the tool, and extended JSP pages in order to be able to communicate with the ontologies that are used by the adaptation business logic, i.e. the QeGS, pages types' and problems' ontologies. As a Semantic Web Framework we used Protégé OWL API (Knublauch & Horridge, 2005) which is an abstract layer above Jena.

The Protégé -OWL API provides classes and methods to load and save OWL files, to query and manipulate OWL data models, and to perform reasoning based on Description Logic engines. The API is built on top of a collection of Java interfaces from the model package which provide access to the OWL Model and its elements such as classes, properties and individuals. The OWL Model can be used to create, query, and delete resources of different types; and it provides objects to perform operations such as getting and setting resource property values, building relationships between

Figure 5. Technical architecture of the system

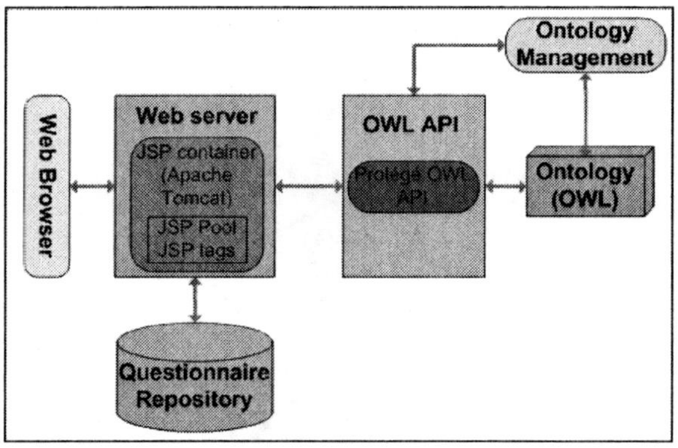

Figure 6. First page of the adaptive interface

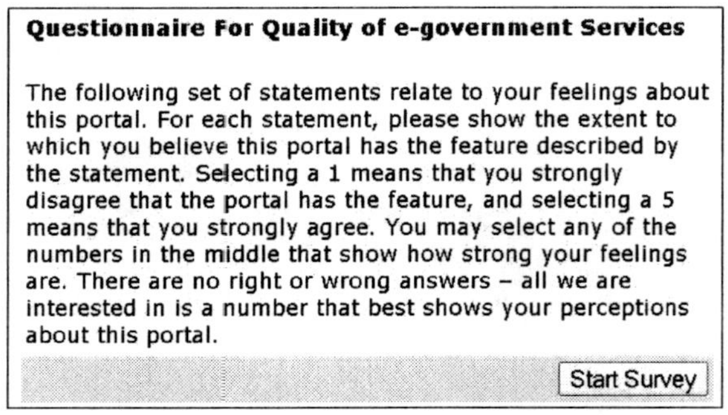

resources, and obtaining the set of restrictions for a property at a class. Other advanced features such as querying, and reacting to changes using listeners are also managed through this API. Figure 5 depicts the technical architecture of our system.

User Scenarios

We will now consider a user scenario in which we will provide the reader with a description of the functional performance of the system. The user scenario concerns a user that enters the e-government portal and visits some portal's pages, including a page that contains forms which are used for information submission. The user in this scenario has not visited any other portal content that is related with specific quality aspects, i.e. he has not visited any other page with concepts of Table 2, except of course from a forms page. In this scenario no problem has been identified by the component that monitors user click streams and actions. This component calls the adaptive questionnaire, by redirecting the user to the URL that corresponds to the questionnaire's start page which is depicted in Figure 6.

The URL that is called incorporates the query string, a part of the URL that contains data to be passed to web applications such as CGI programs or JSP pages. We make use of this feature of the HyperText Transfer Protocol (HTTP) in order to communicate data related with identified user problems and visited content, between the problem identification system component and the adaptive interface. Figure 7 depicts the Mozilla URL location bar showing an URL with the query string of this user scenario.

When the user pushes the "Start Survey" button the adaptation business logic is executed. In this use case, that the user hasn't faced any problem, first level questions that are related with visited content, as well as these first level questions that are content-independent, are displayed. Using the appropriate Protégé OWL API methods, references to all first level questions of the QeGS ontology are obtained by the system. For each first level question the value of the *hasRelatedContent* object property, which links the QeGS with the content ontology, is retrieved. If a question is related with a specific portal content and the user has visited this content, i.e. the query string includes this content as part of the content parameter; the specific first level question is displayed, otherwise not. Figure 8 depicts some first level questions that are presented in this use case, as well as a relevant code snip set. As you can see in the figure, the first level question related with forms is incorporated into the set of questions that are displayed, during the dynamic composition of the questionnaire. This is not the case however for the other content-related questions of Table 2, for example for the support mechanisms' question.

Figure 7. Query string of use case 1

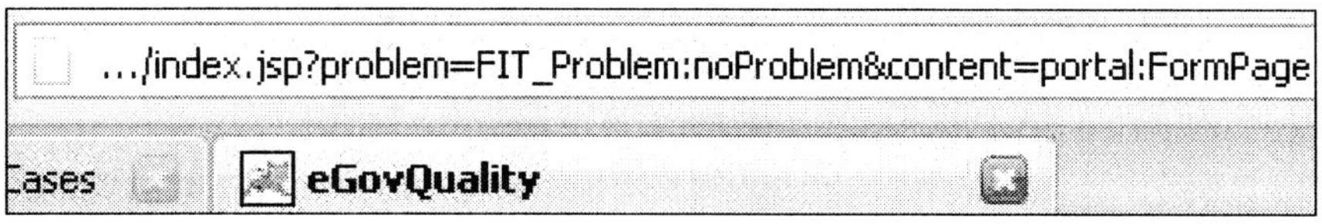

Figure 8. Part of interface for Step 2 of use case 1 and a relevant code snip set

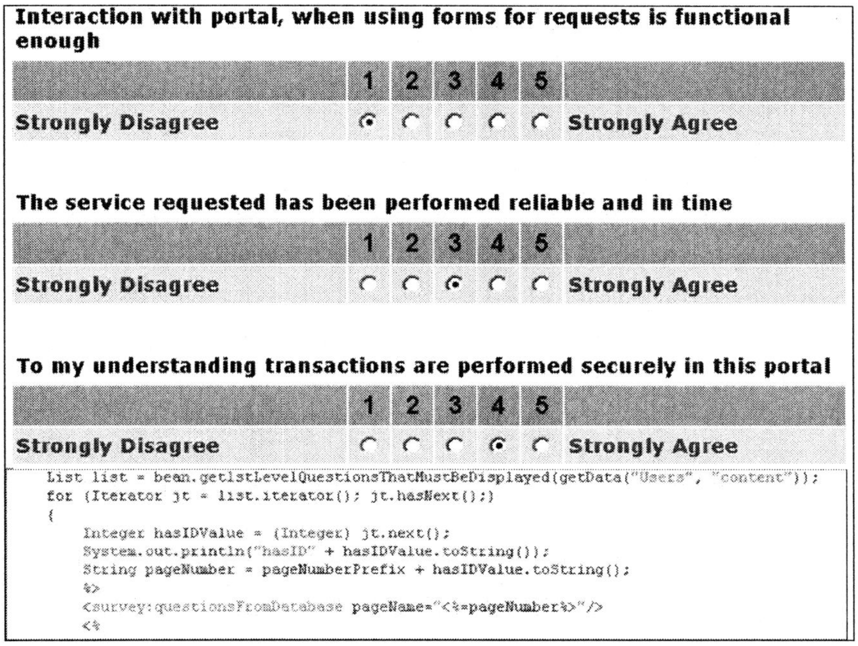

The next step of this user scenario is performed by the user actor, as he grades the presented first level questions using the five point Likert scale. In this scenario the user believes that interaction with portal when using forms for requests is not functional, thus he gives a low grade for the relevant question, as depicted in Figure 8.

After answering first level questions and clicking the NextPage button, a reference to each first level question of the QeGS ontology that the user has graded is obtained by the system. Furthermore the value of the property *hasThresholdForLevel2Presentation* of the *level1Question* concept is retrieved for each one of these questions. This property represents a threshold in the five point Likert scale, under which, second level questions should be presented. Depending on the value of this property and for all the questions that the given grade was below the threshold, relevant second level questions are displayed in the interface. The knowledge about corresponding second level questions for each first level one is modelled into the QeGS ontology through the object property *hasCorrespondingLevel2Question*. For this user scenario only the first level question concerning portal's forms was below the threshold, so a detailed examination of user's low perceptions is achieved with detailed questions about forms. Part of the user interface for this case is depicted in Figure 9, along with a relevant code snip set:

The scenario ends with the user grading second level questions, going to the next page and providing some demographic information (see Figure 10). Finally the system presents a thank you for filling out the survey message.

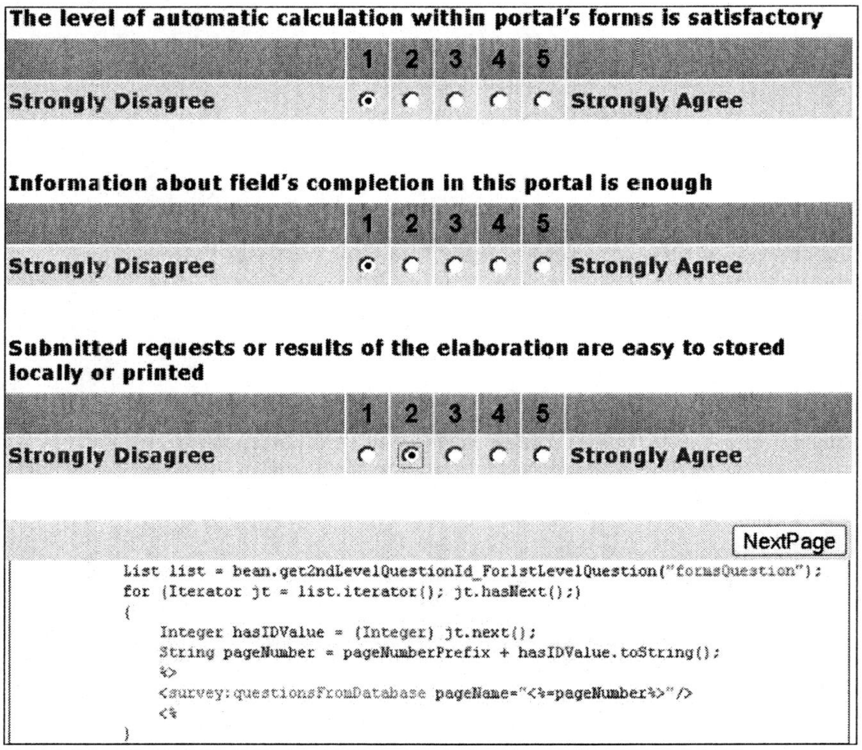

Figure 9. Part of interface for Step 3 of use case 1 and a relevant code snip set

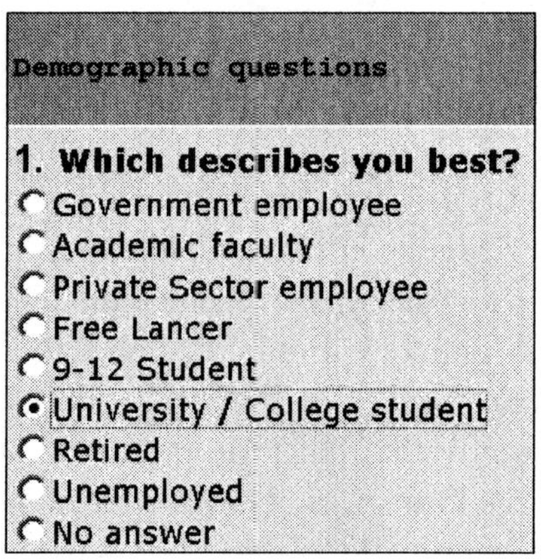

Figure 10. Part of the interface for Step 4 of use case 1

Let's consider briefly a second user scenario, putting focus on the main differences with the previous one. In the second user scenario the user has faced a links problem and a navigation problem during his session and he hasn't visited content related with quality aspects. The user monitoring and problem identification component calls the adaptive questionnaire, by redirecting the user to the URL depicted in Figure 11 that follows:

When the user pushes the "Start Survey" button of the first page, the adaptation business logic is executed once again by the system. In this use case, that the user has faced problems during his navigation, relevant to problems second level questions are presented in order to examine in detail these problems and their root cause. Using the problem query parameters and the appropriate Protégé OWL API methods, references to all identified problems of the problems' ontology are obtained. For each one of these problems, the values of the object property *hasRelatedQuestion*, which links the problems' with the QeGS ontology, are retrieved. For each problem the second level questions that are indicated by the aforementioned property, are presented except of course from those that are related with content which the user has not visited during his navigation. In our case, second level questions relevant with links and navigation are incorporated during the dynamic

Figure 11. Query string of use case 2

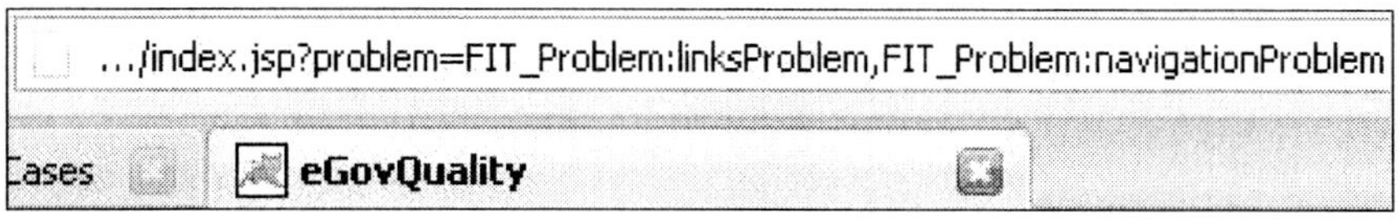

Figure 12. Part of interface for Step 2 of use case 2 and a relevant code snip set

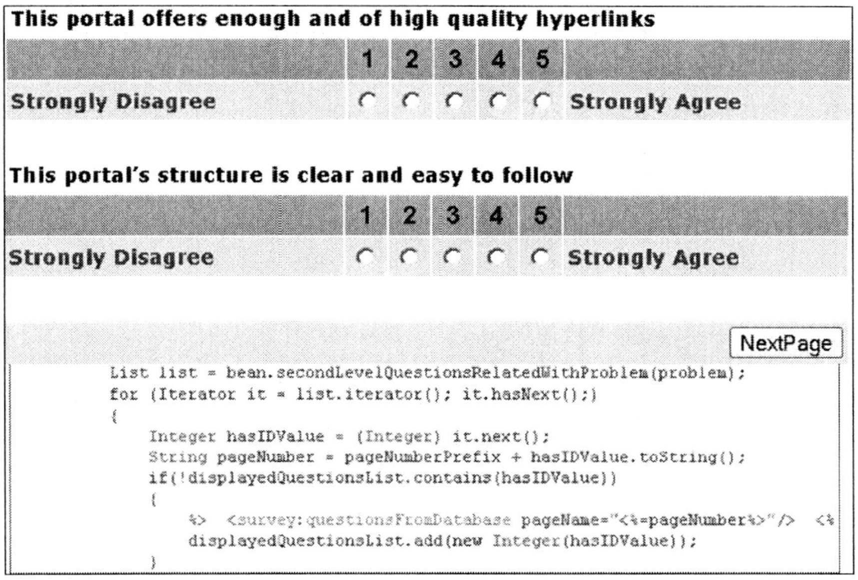

adaptation of the questionnaire. Figure 12 depicts second level navigation questions, along with a relevant code snip set.

Next steps of this scenario are very similar with the previous one, so we skip their description.

CONCLUSION AND FUTURE WORK

In this chapter we have provided a practical approach for the realization of a customized and adaptive evaluation of e-government services and presented a prototype ontology - based system that implements the aforementioned approach.

We have implemented a first prototype using the approach presented here and already had initial positive results. Currently we are testing our system in an e-government portal with more than 6000 daily users. Data collected in this environment will be used for further evaluating the system's effectiveness, as well as for measuring its added value in a productive environment. For this reason a comparison between static and adaptive evaluation will be made. This comparison will show if response rates are indeed improved using the adaptive option (quantitative evaluation) and furthermore if users are satisfied with the new approach, compared with the traditional one (qualitative evaluation). We intend to improve the system based on the pilot results and define new mappings between questions and user problems and also between questions and page types.

It is our belief that the use of the proposed semantically adaptive interface will allow more focused and targeted assessment of the quality of e-government services.

FUTURE RESEARCH DIRECTIONS

Adaptivity and personalization techniques imply the collection, either implicitly or explicitly, of users' data, which drive the adaptivity process. The process of gathering user data, raise big concerns about privacy issues. For example the learner model used by an adaptive tutoring system may include intellectual information about the learner; the user model of a recommender system may include the preferences and navigation habits of the user. Privacy laws enacted on various countries as well as users' attitude towards the provision of personal data are important factors that should be taken into account, during the design of an adaptive system. Kobsa, 2007 considers privacy protection in adaptive systems, analyzes the tension between them, and presents approaches to reconcile the both. Finding the appropriate balance in the trade-off between privacy and adaptivity is further complicated, by the fact that the privacy principals that are applied to legislation of different countries, or even to different states of the same country may vary. This implies that a thorough investigation of national privacy literature should be done before an adaptive system is used in a commercial or even in a research study context and furthermore that the privacy issues of adaptive systems is a research direction of interest.

In recent years there is a trend towards an on-the-move interaction of users with mobile computers, by making use of technologies like Wifi, GPS, GPRS and UMTS, enabling users to access services anytime, anywhere and by means of different types of mobile devices. In this new environment, the context can play an important role in the personalization experience. Context can be for example the location of the mobile device, the speed at which the user moves or the environmental conditions. Mobile device characteristics like limited resources and screen size, is an additional source of input for building user, environmental and device models that are subsequently used for a personalized service offering. Several applications of adaptive systems in mobile environments can be found in the literature, including applications like museum guides, navigation systems and shopping assistants (Krüger et. al., 2007). Since applications of adaptivity in a mobile context are in their early stage, models, frameworks and techniques addressing the peculiarities of this new environment are subject to future research.

REFERENCES

Apostolou, D., Feldkamp, D., Halaris, C., Hinkelmann, K., Magoutas, B., Papadomichelaki, X., Prackwieser, C., Probst, F., Schmidt, K.U., Stoiljkovic, B., Stoiljkovic, V., Stojanovic, L., Stojanovic, N., Thomas, S. M., Thönssen, B., Utz W., & Woitsch R. (2006). *Deliverable D2, framework for self-adaptive e-government of FIT IST Project.* Available at http://www.fit-project.org/Documents/D2.pdf

Bra, P. D., Aerts A., Berden, B., Lange, B., Rousseau, B., Santic, T., Smits, D., & Stash, N. (2003). *AHA! The Adaptive Hypermedia Architecture.* In Proceedings of the ACM Hypertext Conference, Nottingham, UK, pp 81-84

Brannen K. (2001). *Intelligent use of metadata in the questionnaire design process.* In Proceedings of the 2001 New Techniques and Technologies for Statistics Conference.

Brusilovsky, P., Schwarz, E., & Weber, G. (1996). *ELM-ART: An Intelligent Tutoring System on World Wide Web.* In Third International Conference on Intelligent Tutoring Systems, ITS-96, Montreal, 1996

Cap Gemini (2006). *Online Availability of Public Services: How is Europe Progressing?* Web-based Survey on Electronic Public Services, Report of the 6th Measurement

Cappiello, C., Missier, P., Pernici, B., Plebani, P., & Batini, C. (2004). *Qos in multichannel IS: the mais approach.* In Proceedings of the International Workshop on Web Quality (WQ'04), Munich, Germany, 2004

Cardoso, J., Sheth, A., Miller, J., Arnold, J., & Kochut, K. (2002). *Modeling quality of service for workflows and web service processes.* Journal of Web Semantics

Chopra, V., Bakore, A., Eaves, J., Galbraith, B., Li, S., & Wiggers, C. (2004). *Professional Apache Tomcat 5.* Published by Wrox, ISBN 0764559028, May 17, 2004

Corradini, F., Angelis, F. D., Polzonetti, A., Re, B., & Brugnoni, E. (2006). *e-GovQoS: an Ontology for Quality of e-Government Services.* In 5th International EGOV Conference 2006, DEXA, Krakow (Poland), pp. 171-178, September 2006.

Couper, M. (2001). *Web Surveys: The Questionnaire Design Challenge.* In Proceedings of the 53rd session of the ISI, http://134.75.100.178/isi2001/

Davidson, J., & Coward, D. (1999). *Java servlet specification v2.2.* Sun Press, 1999.

Dawes, S. (2002). *The Future of E-Governmen.t* Center for Technology in Government, Albany, NY: Center for Technology in Government.

Denaux, R., Dimitrova, V., & Aroyo, L. (2004). *Interactive Ontology-based User Modeling for Personalized Learning Content Management.* In Workshop on Applications of Semantic Web technologies for E-Learning (SWEL) held in conjunction with Adaptive Hypermedia 2004

Dobson, G., Lock, R., & Sommerville, I. (2005). *QoSOnt: a QoS ontology for service-centric systems.* In: EUROMICRO-SEAA'05.

Dolog, P., Henze, N., Nejdl, W., & Sintek, M., (2004). *Personalization in distributed e-learning environments.* In WWW Alt. '04: Proceedings of the 13th International World Wide Web Conference on Alternate Track Papers & Posters, New York, NY (pp. 170–179). New York, NY: ACMvPress.

eGovernment Unit, DG Information Society, European Commission, (2004). *Top of the web: user satisfaction and usage survey of egovernment services.* Available online from Europe's Information Society Thematic Portal Web site: http://europa.eu.int/information_society/activities/egovernment_research/doc/top_of_the_web_report_2004.pdf

Gruber T. (1993). *A Translation Approach to Portable Ontology Specifications.* Knowledge Acquisition, 5(2), 199-220.

Guinness, D. L. & Harmelen E. F. (2003). *OWL Web Ontology Language Overview.* W3C Proposed Recommendation, http://www.w3.org/TR/2003/PR-owl-ref-20031215/, December 15, 2003.

Haarslev, V., & Möller, R. (2001). *RACER System Description.* In: Goré R., Leitsch A., Nipkow T. (Eds.) International Joint Conference on Automated Reasoning (IJCAR 2001), Siena. Springer-Verlag, 2001, pp. 701–705.

Keeffe, I., Conlan, O., Dagger, D., & Wade V. (2005). *Dynamically Adapting Multimedia Content using Strategically-driven Generic Adaptive Services.* ACM Multimedia 2005, Singapore, November (Submitted)

Knublauch, H., Fergerson, R.W., Noy, N.F., & Musen, M.A. (2004). *The Protege OWL Plugin: An open development environment for Semantic Web applications.* Semantic Web - Iswc 2004, Proceedings 2004;3298:229-243.

Knublauch, H. & Horridge, M. (2005). *The Protégé-OWL API.* Available at http://protege.stanford.edu/plugins/owl/api/index.html

Kobsa, A. (2007). *Privacy-enhanced web personalisation.* In Brusilovsky P., Kobsa A., Nejdl W.

(Eds.): The Adaptive Web: Methods and Strategies of Web Personalisation, Springer-Verlag, Heidelberg, Germany, pp. 628-670

Krüger, A., Baus, J., Heckmann, D., Kruppa, M., & Wasinger, R. (2007). *Adaptive Mobile Guides*. In Brusilovsky P., Kobsa A., Nejdl W. (eds.): The Adaptive Web: Methods and Strategies of Web Personalization. Berlin, Heidelberg, New York: Springer (ISBN: 978-3540720782), 2007, pp. 521-549.

Likert, R. (1932). *A Technique for the Measurement of Attitudes*. Archives of Psychology 140, 55.

Magoutas, B., Halaris, C., & Mentzas, G. (2007). *An Ontology for the Multi-Perspective Evaluation of Quality in E-government Services*. In Sixth International EGOV Conference 2007, Regensburg (Germany), September 3-7, 2007.

Maneewatthana, T., Wills, G., & Hall W. (2006). *Adaptation in Adaptable Personal Information Environment*. In Adaptive Hypermedia and Adaptive Web-Based Systems, June 20th - June 23rd, 2006, Dublin, Ireland.

Middleton, S.E., Shadbolt, N.R., & Roure D.C.D. (2004). *Ontological user profiling in recommender systems*. ACM Transactions on Information Systems (TOIS) 22(1), 54–88.

Papadomichelaki, X., Magoutas, B., Halaris, C., Apostolou, D., & Mentzas, G. (2006). *A Review of Quality Dimensions in E-government Services*. In M.A. Wimmer et al. (Eds.): EGOV 2006, LNCS 4084, pp. 128–138, 2006.

Powell, T., & Schneider, F. (2004). *JavaScript: The Complete Reference*. McGraw Hill, 2004, iSBN: 0072253576

Powers, A. (2006). *Web Survey Toolbox Home Page*. Available online at: https://hciresearch.hcii.cs.cmu.edu/docs/display/wst/Home (accessed 01 June 2007).

Razmerita, L., & Gouarderes, G. (2004). *Ontology-based user modeling for personalization of grid learning services*. In Proceedings of ITS'04 GRID Learning Services Workshop, Maceio, Brazil.

Tallon, S. (2005). *Adaptive Ontology-Driven Personalised News Services*. A dissertation submitted to the University of Dublin, available at https://www.cs.tcd.ie/publications/tech-reports/reports.05/TCD-CS-2005-87.pdf

Uren, V., Cimiano, P., Iria, J., Handschuh, S., Vargas-Vera, M., Motta, E., & Ciravegna, F. (2006). *Semantic Annotation for Knowledge Management: Requirements and a Survey of the State of the Art*. Web Semantics, 4(1), pp. 14-28.

White, S., Fisher, M., Kattell, R., Hamilton, & G., Hapner, M. (2001). *JDBC API Tutorial and Reference, Second edition*. Addison Wesley, 2001

Wikipedia, (2007). *Web Portal*. Available at http:/en.wikipedia.org/wiki/Web_portal

ADDITIONAL READING

Adomavicius, G., & Tuzhilin A. (2005). *Toward the Next Generation of Recommender Systems: A Survey of the State-of-the-Art and Possible Extensions*. IEEE Transactions on Knowledge and Data Engineering, (2005) 17(6): p. 734-749

Baraglia, R., & Silvestri, F. (2007). *Dynamic Personalization of Web Sites Without User Intervention*. Comm. ACM, Vol. 50, 2, 63-67.

De Bra P., Aroyo, L., & Chepegin, V. (2004). *The Next Big Thing: Adaptive Web-Based Systems*. Journal of Digital Information, Vol. 5 Issue 1, Article No. 247, 2004-05-27

Halaris, C., Magoutas, B., Papadomichelaki, X., & Mentzas, G. (2007). *Classification and synthesis of quality approaches in e-government services*. Internet Research, Vol. 17, Issue: 4, Pages: 378-401

Chapter VIII
Ontology-Based Personalization of E-Government Services

Fabio Grandi
Università di Bologna, Italy

Federica Mandreoli
Università di Modena e Reggio Emilia, Italy

Riccardo Martoglia
Università di Modena e Reggio Emilia, Italy

Enrico Ronchetti
Università di Modena e Reggio Emilia, Italy

Maria Rita Scalas
Università di Bologna, Italy

Paolo Tiberio
Università di Modena e Reggio Emilia, Italy

ABSTRACT

While the World Wide Web user is suffering form the disease caused by information overload, for which personalization is one of the treatments which work, the citizen who gets ready to use the e-Government services which are made available on the Web is not immune from contagion. This seems a good reason to try to prescribe a personalization treatment also to the e-Government user. Hence, we introduce the design and implementation of Web information systems supporting personalized access to multi-version resources in an e-Government scenario. Personalization is supported by means of Semantic Web techniques and relies on an ontology-based profiling of users (citizens). Resources we consider are collections of norm documents (laws, decrees, regulations, etc.) in XML format but can also be generic Web pages and portals or e-Government transactional services. We introduce a reference infrastructure, describe the organization and present performance figures of a prototype system we have developed.

INTRODUCTION

In this Chapter, we present our research activities concerning the implementation of Web information systems supporting personalization for e-Government (**eGov**) applications (ECeGov, n.d.; USeGov, n.d.). More precisely, our work makes use of temporal database and Semantic Web techniques to provide *personalized* access to multi-version resources and services made available on the Web by the Public Administration (**PA**), aimed at improving and optimizing the involvement of citizens in the e-Governance process. The achievement of a high level of integration and involvement of the citizens in the eGov and e-Governance activities, the necessity to fairly deal with different categories of citizens (including disadvantaged ones, with a potential risk of increasing digital divide), the requirements to support flexible, user-friendly, precise, targeted and non-baffling services, all claim for the personalization of the services offered and of the information supplied. In this respect, eGov is suffering from a general problem due to the quick growth of information and services becoming available on the Internet, which makes the task of retrieving the resources of interest more and more difficult. Hence personalization based on user profiling is one of the most interesting solutions proposed to fulfill the needs of individual users and guide them towards a useful navigation.

In particular, we consider ontology-based user profiling and personalized access to online resources (internally available in multi-version format), which may range from guided browsing of PA informative Web sites and portals to selective querying collections of norm documents, and to enactment of customized services implementing administrative processes. Notice that, although all these kinds of resources are already available in existing eGov Web information systems, personalization is either completely absent or at most "predefined" in the Web site structure/contents or service definition/workflow, as for example in eGov portals organized according to the "*life events*" metaphor.

For instance, the Italian eGov portal (http://www.italia.gov.it), which is the main national portal to all the informational and transactional services provided by PAs, is composed of five main sections: "*I am...*", "*Life Events*", "*Thematic Areas*", "*Online Forms*", "*Online Services*". The main sections are further organized as hierarchical multi-level directories, which allow citizens to locate and access online resources. In this way, the paths to access specific resources of interests for an individual citizen have been hardwired in the portal structure by human experts and the citizen starting from the home page must follow, without any other kind of navigational aid, the right link sequence in order to locate and enjoy the desired resources. For example, in order to retrieve a norm concerning support to female entrepreneurship, one have to follow the link sequence:

"I am..." » "Woman" » "Women and Work" » "The Law for Female Entrepreneurship"

or, in order to find information on tax allowances for retired persons, the link sequence:

"Life Events" » "To Pay Taxes" » "Retired Person" » "Which Taxes on the Pension?" » "The Allowances"

Also other eGov portals usually show a similar organization and functionalities. For instance, the U.S. eGov portal (http://www.usa.gov), is organized into four main sections: "For Citizens", "For Businesses and Nonprofits", "For Government Employees" and "For Visitors to the U.S.", yet with a basically hierarchical multi-level structure. For example, an American citizen looking for recent norms ruling voting rights has to follow, starting from the home page, the link sequence:

"For Citizens" » "Voting and Elections" » "Learn about Elections and Voting" » "Help America Vote Act of 2002"

Another problem arises especially when a user is interested in locating norms of interest within official sources. For example a university professor could be looking for recently introduced changes in the management and fiscal treatment of research funds and could be directed by some search engine or predefined path to the latest State Budget Law. It could be the case that the norms of interest for him/her are contained in a couple of paragraphs of a few articles, but these are immersed in a several hundreds of articles making up the law. Hence, the norms of interest could be quite awkward to find within the retrieved document and having to go through the whole law text would result in a very time-consuming and daunting activity.

Therefore, personalization of (informational and transactional) eGov services would be desirable, in order to improve the involvement of citizens and the quality of their participation to the eGov process. As there are many "different kinds" of citizens before the law, there must correspondingly be many different kinds of services available but, if we consider an individual citizen, it would be desirable that only the services which are relevant to him/her be available when he/she accesses the eGov platform. Nonetheless, at the state-of-the-art, effective, automatic, flexible, on-demand, "intelligent" and, last but not least, efficient personalization facilities for delivery of adaptive contents and services are lacking.

In this work we present the results of a research started in 2003 (ECeG Project, 2003; Grandi et al., 2004) concerning the design and implementation of Web information systems for personalized access to norm and document repositories in XML format (XML, n.d.). Building upon previous work on temporal management of multi-version XML norm texts (Grandi et al., 2003; Grandi et al., 2005a; Mandreoli et al., 2006), we developed a platform for semantics-aware personalized access to the repository. Personalization is based on the maintenance of an *ontology* which classifies the citizens according to the limited applicability of norm provisions. Semantic information is then used to map the citizen's identity onto the applicable resources in the repository thanks to an intelligent and efficient retrieval system.

The Chapter is organized as follows. The second Section is devoted to the review of related works. The research activity will be described in the third Section, whereas prototype implementation and evaluation are the subject of the fourth Section. Finally, conclusions are drawn in fifth Section.

RELATED WORK

The problem of information overload when browsing and searching the Web becomes more and more crucial as the Web keeps growing exponentially. Web page filtering (Godoy & Amandi, 2005), personalized search (Micarelli et al., 2007), recommender systems (Resnick & Varian, 1997, Perugini et al., 2004) are all proposed solutions, built upon the concept of *user profile*, which have become necessary for most Web users to cope with this problem, by increasing the quality and reducing the quantity of retrieved information and speeding-up the search task.

In this context, *personalization* can be defined as the ways in which information and services can be tailored to match the unique and specific needs of an individual or a community (Callan et al., 2003). For instance, personalization is about building customer loyalty by creating a meaningful one-to-one relationship or, more in general, by understanding the needs of each individual and helping satisfy a goal that efficiently and knowledgeably addresses each individual's need in a given context (Riecken, 2000).

At the state-of-the-art, there is a quite large bibliography on user profiles, which can be defined according to different dimensions (Rich, 1999): canonical vs. individual, explicit vs. implicit, long-term vs. short-term. Another distinction, deriving from Artificial Intelligence research, can be made between knowledge-based and behavior-based user profiling. Knowledge-based approaches adopt static user models which are dynamically matched to users in order to find the best fit. Questionnaires and interviews are often used to obtain this kind of user knowledge. Behavior-based approaches involve the analysis of the user behavior during navigation and search activities to discover useful patterns and build individual or prototype user models, usually employing machine-learning techniques and using Web logs as data sources. Among others, Kobsa (2001), Cornelis (2003) and Frias-Martinez et al. (2006) produced good surveys on user modelling techniques and systems.

Ontologies (Gruber, 1993; Guarino, 1998), which are conceptualizations of a domain into a machine-understandable format, have recently become quite popular with the advent of the Semantic Web (Berners-Lee et al., 2001), where the introduction of common reference ontologies (OWL, 2004) becomes necessary to let information and its interpretation be shared by several agents (human users or automatic tools). However, ontologies had been already used either in the personalization field to represent user profiles and in the legal domain to support automatic reasoning.

In particular, ontologies have been diffusely exploited for either knowledge-based and behavior-based user profiling, as they can be used to model user interests and navigation contexts in a semantically rich form, including hierarchies of concepts with various properties of interest. The ontologies used for this purpose can either be hand-made, built and maintained by domain experts or by the users themselves possibly in a collaborative fashion, or engineered using (semi-)automatic methods, like analysis and mining of domain text documents and user activity logs. Ontologies can also be built dynamically or incrementally refined starting form an initial core, with or without explicit user intervention. Pretschner (1998) presents a thorough discussion of ontology-based user profiling techniques and systems. More recent proposals include (Gauch et al., 2003; Golemati et al., 2007, Middleton et al., 2004; Razmerita et al., 2003; Trajkova et al., 2004).

In the legal domain, the introduction of ontologies as a conceptualization tool for the purpose of legal knowledge systems dates back to the studies on Artificial Intelligence and Law in the late Eighties. Visser & Bench-Capon (1998) review the four main proposals produced by early research in this framework. More recent proposals can be found, for instance, in (Benjamins et al., 2005; Breuker et al., 2004; Casanovas et al., 2007; Lehman et al., 2005; LKIF-Core, n.d.).

Last but not least, one of the concerns of personalized search and management of user profiles is privacy protection (Shen et al., 2007), especially when personalization is done on the server side, since sensible data about users has to be processed and possibly stored.

PERSONALIZED ACCESS TO E-GOVERNMENT RESOURCES

In the framework of eGov, a large number of online resources including PA portals, informative websites, usable administrative services are progressively being made available to citizens. In particular, collections of norm texts and legal information presented to citizens (e.g. stored in large repositories in XML format, as in the "Norme in Rete" Web site (http://www.normeinrete.it)) are being made available and becoming popular on the internet owing to big investments and efforts made by governments and administrations. Such portals or websites are usually equipped with a keyword-based search engine or contain indexes and predefined navigation paths for user guidance (e.g. following the *life events* approach). In order to add personalization facilities, in this scenario found place our research activity entitled "Semantic web techniques for the management of digital identity and the access to norms", carried out as part of the Italian national project "European Citizen in eGovernance: Legal-philosophical, Legal, Information and Economical aspects" (ECeG Project, 2003).

The main objective of such activity has been the development of techniques enabling an effective and efficient personalized access to multi-version norm repositories. First of all, the fast dynamics involved in normative systems implies the coexistence of multiple *temporal versions* of the norm texts stored in a repository, since laws are continually subject to amendments and modifications (e.g. it is crucial to reconstruct the *consolidated version* of a norm as the one produced by the application of all the modifications it underwent so far). Moreover, another kind of versioning plays an important role, because some norms or some of their parts have or acquire a *limited applicability*. For example, a given norm defining tax treatment may contain some articles which are only applicable to particular classes of citizens: one article is applicable to unemployed persons, one article to self-employed persons, one article to public servants only and so on. Hence, a citizen accessing the repository may be interested in finding a *personalized version* of the norm, that is a version only containing articles which are applicable to his/her personal case. Notice that personalization avoids in some cases the user to have to go through a huge amount of irrelevant material to find out the relevant one and, thus, may help to make the search feasible.

In this work, in addition to norm documents, we will consider personalized access to general resources made available on eGov portals, which include informational and transactional PA services. In particular, we consider the design and implementation of an eGov Web information system with personalization facilities, deploying a knowledge-based user profiling which relies on a domain ontology maintained and certified by human experts.

Notice that such an approach to user profiling greatly alleviates the privacy concerns, as no behavior analysis is needed to build user models. Moreover, we will also adopt client-side execution of the dynamic match of users with the closest available model, which further reduces, if does not avoid at all, privacy issues, since sensible data are not processed outside the user's computer and there is no need to store the matching profile on the server at the end of the personalized search session.

Furthermore, the ambitious objective of our work is to design and implement personalization of (informational and transactional) services which can be certified as *legally valid*. In order to be legally valid, the personalization mechanism must use *exact* user profiling. This means that techniques usually adopted for user profiling involving approximate, probabilistic and/or incremental modelling (including usage mining, machine learning, preferences, etc.) cannot be used in this case. Moreover, the personalization system should embody two properties:

- **Consistency:** all the provided services are relevant to the user;
- **Completeness:** all the relevant services are provided to the user,

where "relevant" means ruled by norms which are all applicable to the user's case. As a first step, the aim of our implemented systems is to support consistency and, thus, all the non-relevant services among the available ones must be filtered out before delivery to the user. On the other hand, completeness will be reached only when all the possible PA services are made available online and, thus, depend on the global eGov implementation advancement.

Finally, differently from most other personalization approaches, we consider access to complex documents, such as semi-structured ones (e.g. official norm documents or service specifications), rather than unstructured documents such as simple Web pages. Indeed, the high flexibility that our approach provides, makes it possible to access individual fragments of the documents, returning all and only the ones that fit user needs and avoiding the retrieval of useless information as much as possible.

The Reference Infrastructure

In order to enhance the participation of citizens to an eGov procedure of interest through the provision of personalization facilities, their automatic and accurate positioning within the reference legal framework is needed. To this end, we first introduce the notion of citizen's *digital identity* as the total amount of information concerning him/her which is available online (Rodotà, 2001). The digital identity of the citizen contains all the information useful to determine *the profile of the user* accessing the eGov platform. In other words, profiles are built without user interaction, but by accessing information available in PA databases: date of birth, domicile, marital status and number of children from Registry databases, work status from Social Security databases, estate ownership from Cadastre databases, etc. For this reason, such information must be retrievable in an automatic, secure and reliable way from the PA databases through suitable services (*identification services*). For instance, in order to see whether a citizen is married, a simple query concerning his/her marital status can be issued to Registry databases. Notice that, unlike the classical notion of user profile, digital identity does not change together with the user behavior but either when the citizen's status changes (e.g. when (s)he gets married) or when the regulation concerning citizens requires additional information (as it may happen when a new law applicable to the citizen is enforced). When a citizen accesses the eGov platform supporting personalization, her/his automatic and accurate positioning within the reference legal framework relies on a domain ontology, called **civic ontology**. It corresponds to a representation

Figure 1. The complete personalization infrastructure

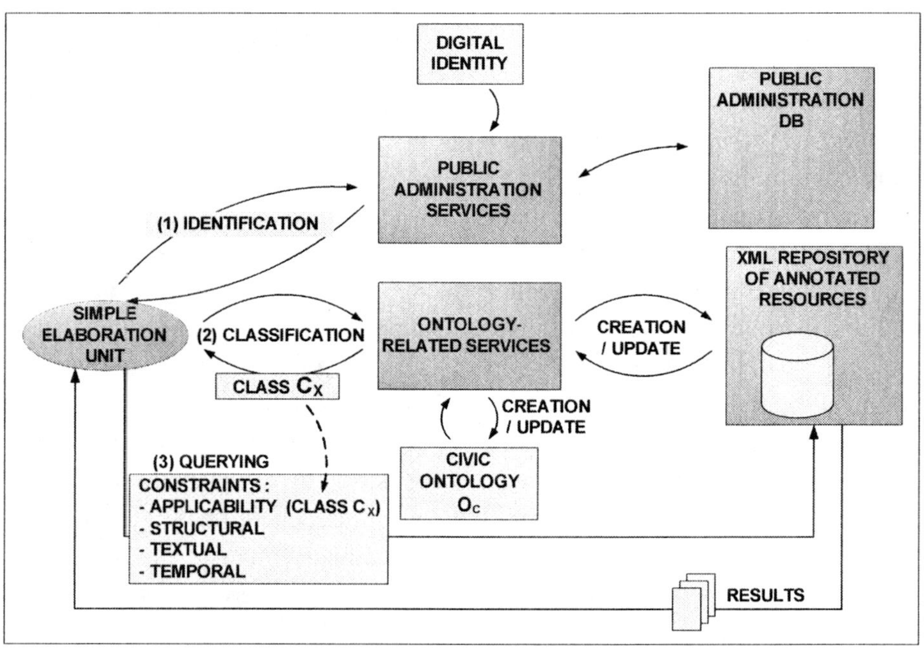

of citizens based on the distinctions introduced by subsequent norms which imply some limitation, total or partial, in law applicability. In the following, we refer to such norms as *founding acts*.

The resulting complete infrastructure is composed of various components that exchange information and cooperate to produce the final results as shown in Figure 1 through suitable support services implemented, for instance, as Web services (SOAP/XMLP, 2000). The collection of the resources which is put at the citizen disposal is stored in a repository encoded as multi-version XML documents. Each resource version is annotated with versioning coordinates, which conform to a data model supporting both timestamps and applicability attributes. The data model will be briefly described in Sec. 3.3.

We illustrate now the functioning of a user session in the eGov personalization system and describe the underlying infrastructure. Firstly, secure authentication[1] of the citizen accessing the infrastructure is ensured through a simple elaboration unit, running on the client side. This simple elaboration unit also acts as user interface, processes the citizen's requests and manages the results. Then, we can identify the following phases (Figure 1):

- the **identification phase** (step 1) consists of calls to identification services to reconstruct the digital identity of the authenticated user on-the-fly. In this phase the system collects pieces of information from all the involved PA databases and composes the identity of the citizen.
- the **classification phase** (step 2) in which the classification service uses the collected digital identity to classify the citizen with respect to the civic ontology ($\mathbf{O}_C$ in Figure 1), by means of an embedded reasoning service. In Figure 1, the most specific class C_X has been assigned to the citizen. Once the citizen has been classified, the class number C_X can then be used as a *surrogate* of his/her profile;
- finally, in the **querying phase** (step 3), the citizen's query is executed on the multi-version XML repository, by accessing and reconstructing the appropriate version of all and only resources which are applicable to the class C_X.

In order to supply the desired services, the digital identity is modeled and represented within the system in a format such that it can be translated into the same language used for the ontology (e.g. a Description Logic (Baader et al., 2002)). In this way, during the classification procedure, the matching between the civic ontology classes and the citizen's digital identity can be reduced to a standard reasoning task (e.g. *ontology entailment* for the underlying Description Logic (Horrocks & Patel-Schneider, 2003)).

Furthermore, the civic ontology used in steps 2 and 3 requires to be created and constantly maintained: each time a new founding act is enforced, the execution of a **creation/update phase** is needed. Notice that this process (and also the introduction of semantic annotations into the multi-version XML documents to maintain the mapping) is a delicate task which needs advice by human experts and "official validation" of the outcomes and, thus, it can only partially be automated. However, computer tools and graphic environments (e.g. based on the Protégé platform (Protégé, n.d.)) could be provided to assist the human experts to perform this task.

Notice also that personalization in an eGov framework *must* be based on an infrastructure like the one introduced here: only exact user profiling techniques must be used in order to offer services which are legally valid.

Exploiting Ontological Information for Semantic Annotation of Resources

The civic ontology introduced in the previous section is a legal domain ontology for the environment where the personalization system is active and, thus, must be built using as founding acts all the norms which are in force in such environment (e.g., for the Italian eGov portal, they are all the norms concerning citizens in the regulations of the Italian state). The resulting ontology, which is then used for knowledge-based user profiling of citizens accessing the personalization service, could be rather complex, including citizen classes, their relationships (e.g. IS-A links), properties/slots (possibly with restrictions), data types (defining the domain of some of the properties). In this respect, it does not differ from the ontologies usually considered for user profiling (e.g. in (Golemati et al., 2007)). The main difference is that citizens are not classified with respect to their interests, but only with respect to their position before the law.

However, despite the structural complexity of the civic ontology, the only ontological information which is relevant for semantic versioning and personalization of eGov resources are the citizen classes and their specialization/ generalization relationships (because of the IS-A semantics, all the norms which are applicable to a class are also applicable to its subclasses), that is the citizen class hierarchy. Hence, we will consider in the following only the class hierarchy extracted form the civic ontology. A fragment of such a hierarchy can be found in Figure 2, which corresponds to a classification of citizens according to a small corpus of norms ruling their status with respect to their work position.

At the current stage of the research, we consider a *tree-like* class hierarchy, that is a taxonomy of citizens induced by IS-A relationships like the one in Figure 2, without multiple inheritance. A tree-like hierarchy is sufficient to satisfy basic application requirements as to applicability constraints and personalization services, although more advanced application requirements may need a more sophisticated definition, including multiple inheritance, whose treatment which will be briefly discussed in the Future Research Directions section.

The multi-version XML data model we propose is an extension with applicability annotations of an XML data model supporting temporal versioning we developed in previous research (Grandi et al., 2003; Grandi et al., 2005a). Notice that, in the legal domain, temporal and limited applicability

Figure 2. A sample class hierarchy extracted from the civic ontology

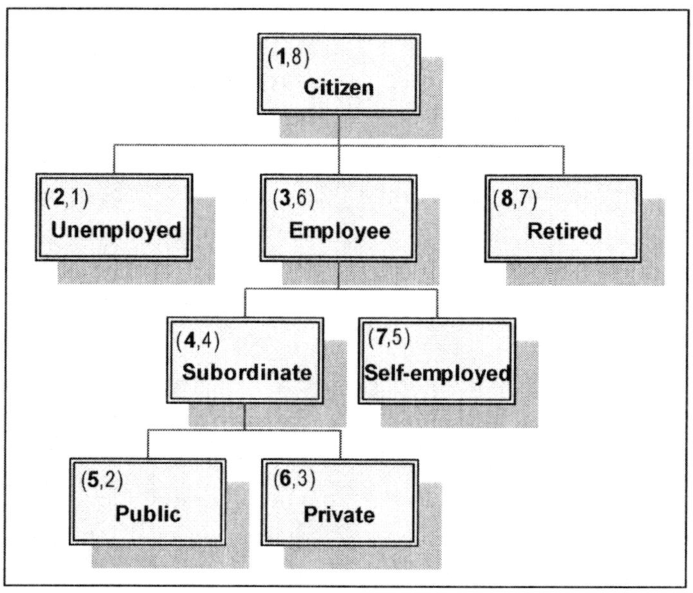

aspects may also interplay in the production and management of versions. For instance, a new norm might state a modification to a preexisting norm, where the modified norm becomes applicable to a limited category of citizens only (e.g. retired persons), whereas the rest of the citizens remain subject to the unmodified norm. However, since temporal and semantic versioning are treated in an orthogonal way in our model, also complex situations can be easily captured. More precisely, an independent semantic versioning dimension is introduced in the multi-version data model used for the representation and storage of the XML resources. In particular, in order to define a mapping between ontology classes and relevant norm parts, we add to the XML encoding of norms applicability annotations which reference the civic ontology classes. References are defined by means of the pre-order tree visit numbering scheme, which allows us to univocally identify each node in the citizen taxonomy. The pre-order values of the classes in Figure 2 are highlighted in boldface in the upper left corner of each node representation. Figure 3 shows a fragment of a multi-version XML norm text including semantic versioning, where the "*aa*" tag (**a**pplicability **a**nnotation) contains references to classes in the ontology[2]. The article in the XML fragment in Figure 3 is composed of two paragraphs and contains applicability annotations. In the XML node hierarchy, applicability is inherited by descendant nodes unless locally redefined. Hence, by means of redefinitions we can also introduce, for each part of a document, complex applicability properties including extensions or restrictions with respect to ancestors. For instance, the whole article in the Figure is applicable to civic class "3" (attribute *applies_to*) but the first paragraph whose applicability is limited to class "4" (applicability restriction). The second one, instead, is also applicable to class "8" (attribute *applies_also*), which is an extension. The representation of extensions and restrictions gives rise to high expressiveness and flexibility in an eGov scenario, where personalization requirements have to be met (i.e. even if we consider tree-like class hierarchies, there is actually no restriction in the shape of the mapping between pieces of an XML-encoded resource and the civic ontology structure).

The numbering scheme used for the applicability annotations is then extended with post-order numbers for query processing purposes, as the pre-order and post-order properties of trees allows us to quickly check ancestor-descendant relationships between the classes (Grust, 2002). This aspect is particularly important because when a portion of a document is annotated with reference to a class, it is also applicable to all its descendant classes. This means that, in order to access and reconstruct the appropriate version of all and only document portions which are applicable to the class C_X, it is necessary to check whether

Figure 3. A fragment of an XML norm with applicability annotations

```
<article num="1">
    <ver num="1">
        <aa applies_to="3"/> [... Temporal attributes ... ]
        <paragraph num="1">
            <ver num="1"> [ ... Text ... ]
                <aa applies_to="4"/> [... Temporal attributes ... ]
            </ver>
        </paragraph>
        <paragraph num="2">
            <ver num="1"> [ ... Text ... ]
                <aa applies_also="8"/> [... Temporal attributes ... ]
            </ver>
        </paragraph>
    </ver>
</article>
```

the version is annotated with a C_X's ancestor. The combination of the two codes are represented in the upper left corner of the ontology classes in Figure 2, in the form: (pre-order, post-order). For example, the class "Employee" has pre-order "3", which is also its identifier, whereas its post-order is "6". Hence, checking the ancestor-descendant relationship between nodes is reduced to a simple comparison between integer values: for example, the descendant classes of the class Employee are those classes that have pre-order value > 3 and post-order value < 6 (i.e. **D** region in Figure 4), whereas the ancestor classes have pre-order value < 3 and post-order value > 6 (i.e. **A** region in Figure 4).

The scheme explained above for semantic versioning of XML documents can be applied in a straightforward way to any kind of XML-encoded informational service available on an eGov platform (i.e. Web sites, portals, norm texts, data collections, etc.). Also locating transactional services, which is still an informational service, can be personalized in this way by adding semantic versioning, for example, to service registration databases accessible through the UDDI protocol (UDDI, n.d.).

As far as personalization of transactional services is concerned, the same technique we presented for norm documents can also be applied, provided that service workflows are specified using an XML-based definition language, like BPEL (WS-BPEL, n.d.) or XPDL (XPDL, n.d.). For instance, we can consider the eGov service for the "change of address" procedure, and assume that public servants are required by law to reside within a fixed distance from their workplace. Hence, the change-of-address service specification must include a variant part, which is executed for public servants only, requesting them to sign an electronic form where they declare that their new residence is within the prescribed distance. For example, Figure 5 shows a fragment of a multi-version BPEL specification for the change-of-address service to be executed on the Registry office server side. The fragment contains a variant part, corresponding to version 2 of the service specification, with an applicability annotation which references the public servants class ("5") in the ontology, where the citizen is supplied a declaration form and asked for a signed declaration. Hence, if the user of the personalization service has been classified as public servant, the query

Figure 4. Classes represented in terms of their pre-order and post-order numbers

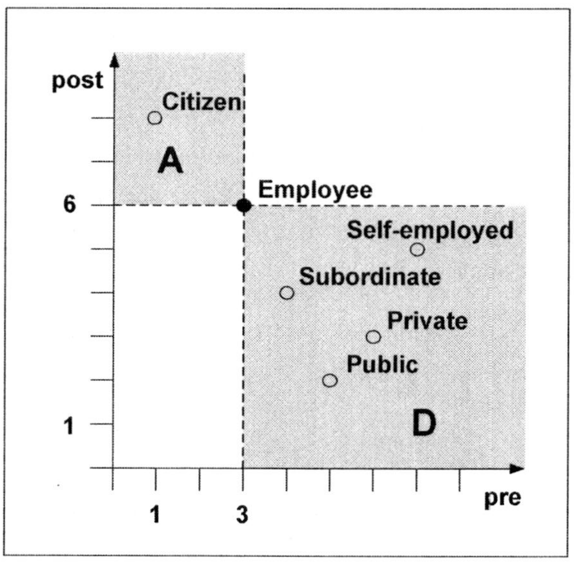

engine must reconstruct version 2 of the service, which is the one applicable to the citizen's case. Therefore, techniques very similar to the ones adopted in this work for semantic annotation of XML documents and for querying the multi-version repository can be used also in such a case. Notice that performance is not even an issue in this case, since the stored data required to represent the multi-version workflows is not large. For example, filtering of the multi-version XML specification with an XSL style-sheet (XSL, n.d.) on the server side would be sufficient to efficiently produce a valid BPEL (or XPDL) workflow specification, which embodies the appropriate service version to be executed on a BPEL-(or XPDL-)compliant enactment engine.

Hence, in the following, we focus on informational services and, in particular, on personalized access to large norm repositories only, which present critical performance issues and, thus, need special treatment.

Query Specification for Personalized Access to Resource Versions

The most complex queries that can be issued on our multi-version XML norm repositories can contain four types of constraints: temporal, structural, textual and applicability. The temporal, structural and textual constraints can be explicitly specified by the user through a suitable interface. The applicability constraint is implicit, since is automatically added by the system as part of the personalization mechanism and concerns the most specific class $\mathbf{O}_C$ assigned to the user by the classification service. The four type of constraints are completely orthogonal and enable a full support of multi-dimensional selection.

In order to understand the personalization mechanism, let us focus first on the applicability constraint. Consider again the ontology portion in Figure 2 and the norm fragment in Figure 3 and let John Smith be a "self-employed" citizen (i.e. belonging to class "7") willing to retrieve

Figure 5. A fragment of an XML-based service specification with applicability annotations

```
<flow>
...
      <ver num ="2">
            <aa applies _to="5" />

            <invoke  partner ="citizen"
                        portType ="changeAddressPT "
                        operation ="requestDeclaration "
                        inputContainer ="declaration _form" >
                  <target linkName ="request-to-citizen"/>
                  <source linkName ="citizen -to-office"/>
            </invoke>

            <receive  partner ="citizen"
                        portType ="acceptDeclarationPT "
                        operation ="sendDeclaration "
                        container ="declaration _signed" >
                  <target linkName ="citizen -to-office"/>
            </receive>

      </ver>
...
</flow>
```

that norm: hence, the sample article in the Figure will be selected as pertinent, but only the second paragraph will be actually presented as applicable. Then, we can consider the other constraints. For instance, the citizen John Smith could be interested in all the norms...

- which contain paragraphs (*structural constraint*), ...
- dealing with health care (*textual constraint*), ...
- which were valid between 2002 and 2004 (*temporal constraint*).

Such a query, including the implicit applicability constraint, is formalized within the simple elaboration unit in Fig. 1 and issued to the query processor using the standard XQuery FLWR syntax (XQuery, n.d.) as follows:

```
FOR $a IN path
WHERE textConstr ($a//paragraph//
text(), 'health AND care')
   AND tempConstr ('vTime OVERLAPS
PERIOD(2002-01-01,2004-12-31)')
   AND applConstr ('class _ 7')
   RETURN $a
```

where **textConstr**, **tempConstr** and **applConstr** are suitable functions allowing the specification of the textual, temporal and applicability constraints, respectively (the structural constraint is embedded in the XPath expressions used in the XQuery statement). The temporal constraints can involve four time dimensions: publication, validity, efficacy and transaction time (Grandi et al., 2003; Grandi et al., 2005a), allowing high flexibility in satisfying the information needs of citizens in the eGov scenario. In particular, by means of validity and efficacy time constraints, a user is able to extract consolidated current versions from the multi-version repository, or to access past versions of particular norm texts, all consistently reconstructed by the system on the basis of the user's needs and personalized on the basis of his/her identity.

IMPLEMENTATION AND PERFORMANCE EVALUATION

In order to test the efficacy and efficiency of the proposed personalized access solution, we built a prototype system supporting our data model. The system is based on a multi-version XML query processor designed on purpose, which is able to manage the XML data repository and to support all the temporal, structural, textual and applicability query features in a single component (Grandi et al., 2005b; Grandi et al., 2006; Mandreoli et al. 2007). It represents an extension of a previous work (Mandreoli et al., 2006), which follows an approach that was called "native" after its capability to manage the above features directly on the XML repository, without any other component. The Native approach is compared against a Stratum approach, where temporal and applicability constraints are processed by a module built on top of a commercial DBMS with XML storage and query support. The Stratum Approach prototype also represents an extension of a previous system we developed, only supporting temporal versioning (Grandi et al, 2003; Grandi et al, 2005a). In this Section, we will firstly describe the differences between the Stratum and the Native approach, and evaluate their performances.

Stratum versus Native Approach

Figure 6 outlines the architecture and functioning of the Stratum and Native approaches. The former approach, depicted in the left part of the Figure, relies on a XML engine offering XML data storage and management facilities including the application of structural and textual constraints and a software stratum, which is built on top, handling the additional temporal and applicability aspects. The documents are stored in the XML repository using the conventional XML data structures made available by the XML engine; typically, the chosen storage granularity is the whole document, although different options could be available. Then, the Stratum performs temporal and applicability filtering on the retrieved data in order to produce as output only the XML portions (paths and, more generally, twigs) satisfying all the user constraints. As to the temporal aspects, the initial experimental results obtained on the Stratum prototype show a post-processing behavior which is linear with the number of the documents involved in the results (see (Grandi et al., 2003; Grandi et al., 2005a) for further details). Moreover, since a standard XML engine is not aware of the temporal semantics, it makes it quite difficult to apply query optimization and indexing techniques especially suited for temporal XML documents. However, as we will show in the next section, the additional management of applicability constraints implies a limited performance overhead.

On the other hand, the Native approach, as shown in the right part of Figure 6, is based on a novel architecture. It is composed of a multi-version XML query processor designed on purpose, which is able to manage the XML data repository and to provide all the structural, textual, temporal and semantic query facilities in a single component. Differently from the Stratum approach, where temporal and applicability constraints are processed separately from the structural and textual constraints which are demanded to the XML engine, all the constraints are simultaneously handled by the multi-version XML query processor. Such a component stores the multi-version XML norms not as entire documents but after converting them into a collection of ad-hoc tuples, each representing one of its multi-version parts. The outcome is the XML fragment which is obtained by combining the relevant tuples and which, as for the Stratum, satisfies all the given constraints.

The Stratum is a software layer written in Java JDK 1.5, which uses the JDOM package for processing the entire documents which are retrieved by the underlying XML engine. The multi-version XML query processor is also implemented in Java JDK 1.5 and exploits ad-hoc data structures (relying on embedded "light" storage libraries) and algorithms, which allow users to store and reconstruct on-the-fly the XML norm versions satisfying the four types of constraints. Such a component stores the XML norms in a partitioned way, which is exploited, during query answering, in order to efficiently perform structural-join algorithms (Al-Khalifa et al., 2002) specifically adapted and tuned for the temporal/semantic multi-version context. Textual constraints are handled by means of an inverted index. Owing to the properties of the adopted pre- and post-order encoding of the civic ontology classes, the system is able to very efficiently deal with applicability constraints during query processing by means of simple comparisons involving class identifiers and semantic annotations.

The advantages of the Native approach over the Stratum one are manifold. By querying ad-hoc and temporally/semantically-enhanced structures (which have a finer granularity than entire documents), the Native system is able to access and fetch only the strictly necessary data (Mandreoli et al., 2006). Then, the retrieved XML portions which satisfy the temporal and semantic constraints can be directly assembled for the reconstruction of the retrieved documents, so that there is no need to retrieve whole XML documents and build space consuming structures such as DOM trees to manipulate them after retrieval, as the Stratum does.

Performance Evaluation

In order to evaluate the performance of our prototype systems, we defined a specific query benchmark and conducted a number of exploratory experiments to test its behavior under different

Figure 6. Stratum versus native approach

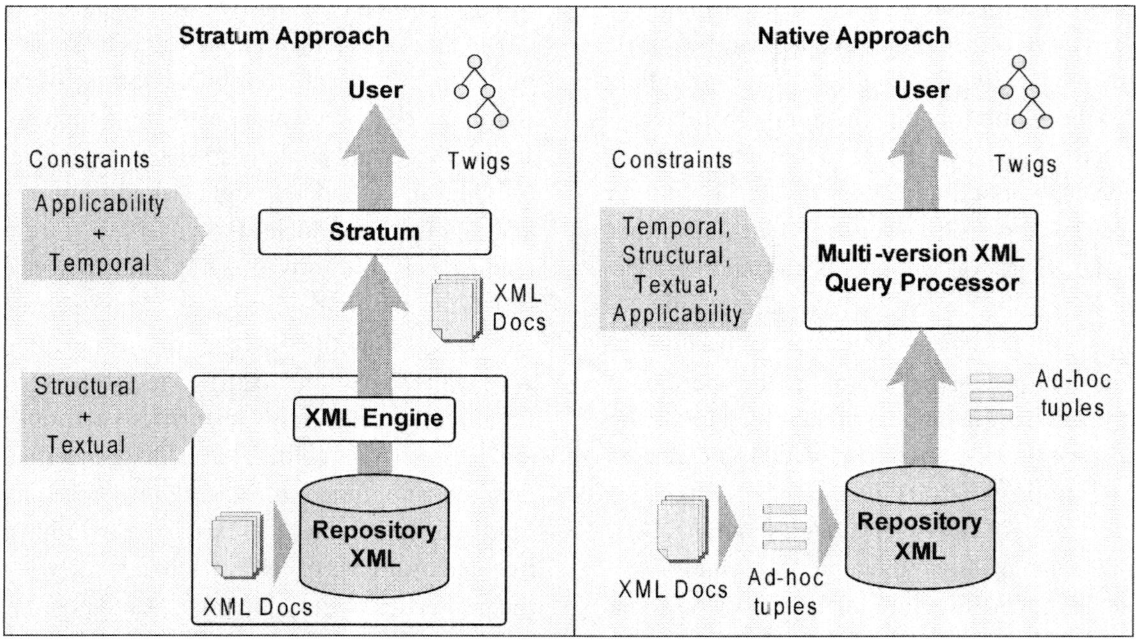

workloads. The experiments have been effected on a Pentium 4 2.5Ghz Windows XP Professional workstation, equipped with 512MB RAM and a RAID0 cluster of two 80GB EIDE disks with NT file system (NTFS). We performed the tests on three XML document sets of increasing size: collection C1 (5,000 XML normative text documents), C2 (10,000 documents) and C3 (20,000 documents). We will describe in detail only the results obtained on the collection C1, then we will briefly recall the scalability performance shown on the other two collections. The total size of the collections is 120MB, 240MB, and 480MB, respectively. In all the collections, the documents were synthetically generated by means of an ad-hoc XML generator, which is able to produce different kinds of documents compliant to our multi-version model. For each collection, the average, minimum and maximum document size is 24KB, 2KB and 125KB, respectively.

Experiments were conducted by submitting queries of five different types (Q1–Q5). Table 1 presents the features of the test queries and the query execution time for each of them. All the queries require structural support (St constraint); types Q1 and Q2 also involve textual search by keywords (Tx constraint); type Q3 contains temporal conditions (Tm constraint) on three time dimensions: transaction, valid and publication time; types Q4 and Q5 mix the previous ones, since they involve both keywords and temporal conditions. For each query type, we also present a personalized access variant involving an additional applicability constraint (Ap constraint), denoted as Qx-A in the first column of Table 1. Furthermore, for each query, the table displays its selectivity defined in two different ways: "Paths" indicates Path selectivity, that is the percentage of the relevant paths with respect to all the available paths, while "Docs" indicates Document selectivity, that is the percentage of relevant documents (i.e. the ones containing at least one relevant path) with respect to all the available documents. Finally, the performances of the two systems are shown in the table: "Native" denotes the system based on the Native approach, whereas "Stratum" represents our previous prototype based on the Stratum approach.

Let us first focus on queries without personalized access. The Native approach shows a good efficiency in every context, providing a short response time (including query analysis, retrieval of the qualifying norm parts and reconstruction of the result) of approximately one or two seconds for most of the queries. Notice that the selectivity of the query predicates does not impair performances, even when large amounts of documents containing some (typically small) relevant portions have to be retrieved. In particular, due to the different ways the two systems work and store their data structures, their performances have different behaviors with respect to the involved kinds of selectivity. For instance, considering Q2, which only involves structural and textual constraints, we see that the Native system has to handle 7 times the data than with Q1 (path selectivity is 4.02% and 0.6%, respectively), while the Stratum one, storing entire documents, has to access a nearly 30 times larger amount of data (document selectivity is 3.2% and 0.12%, respectively). For these reasons, Stratum performances are far worse for Q2 than for Q1. From additional tests we effected, we found that a finer storage granularity would have partially helped the Stratum to achieve performances closer to the Native ones, but only for queries not involving the temporal constraint, such as Q1 and Q2. When the temporal constraint is present, as in Q3, Q4, and Q5, different granularity choices do not lead to significant improvements in the Stratum performance due to the many shortcomings of this approach. In particular:

- stratum-level constraints have to be evaluated in a second moment, so that, even if a granularity finer than the whole document is adopted, a large quantity of additional information has to be retrieved anyway for their evaluation;
- for the same reason, the Stratum is not able to optimize query execution with an access plan filtering the data always on the most selective constraints first;
- the structure of a document is analyzed twice: a first time in the XML engine when the structural constraint is resolved and a second time in the Stratum to correctly evaluate the other constraints.

On the other hand, the Native system is able to deliver a fast and reliable performance in all cases, since it practically avoids the retrieval of useless document parts and is not as demanding as the Stratum in terms of main memory space. Notice that this property is also very promising towards future extensions to cope with concurrent multi-user query processing, since memory requirements are not crucial for performance.

As far as applicability constraints are concerned, the time needed to answer the personalized access versions of the Q1–Q5 queries is approximately 0.5-1% higher than for the query versions without applicability constraints, in both approaches. Moreover, in the Native system, since the applicability annotations of each part of an XML document are stored as simple integers, the size of the tuples with semantic versioning is practically unchanged (only a 3-4% storage space overhead is required with respect to documents without semantic versioning), even with quite complex annotations involving several applicability extensions and restrictions.

In conclusion, the Native approach clearly outperforms the Stratum Approach in every test condition and, thus, represent our cutting-edge solution for personalized access to large repositories of multi-version eGov resources. Finally, we only report a comment about the performance of the Native prototype in querying the other two collections C2 and C3 and, therefore, concerning the scalability of the system. We ran the same queries of the previous tests on the larger collections and saw that the computing time always grew sub-linearly with the number of documents. For instance, query Q1 executed on the 10,000 documents of collection C2 (which is as double as C1) took 1,366 msec (i.e. the system was only

Table 1. Features of the test queries and query execution time (time in milliseconds, collection C1)

Query	Constraints				Selectivity		Performance (msec)	
	Tm	St	Tx	Ap	**Paths**	**Docs**	**Stratum**	**Native**
Q1	–	✓	✓	–	0.6%	0.12%	2891	1046
Q2	–	✓	✓	–	4.02%	3.2%	43240	2970
Q3	✓	✓	–	–	2.9%	2.66%	47638	6523
Q4	✓	✓	✓	–	0.68%	0.12%	2151	1051
Q5	✓	✓	✓	–	1.46%	0.12%	3130	2550
Q1-A	–	✓	✓	✓	0.23%	0.05%	3043	1095
Q2-A	–	✓	✓	✓	1.65%	1.31%	43729	3004
Q3-A	✓	✓	–	✓	1.3%	1.19%	49358	6760
Q4-A	✓	✓	✓	✓	0.31%	0.05%	2277	1020
Q5-A	✓	✓	✓	✓	0.77%	0.06%	3201	2602

30% slower); similarly, on the 20,000 documents of collection C3, the average response time was 1,741 msec (i.e. the system was less than 30% slower than with C2). Also in the presence of the other queries, the measured trend was the same, thus showing the good scalability of the system in every type of query context.

CONCLUSION

In this Chapter, we presented the results of a research we carried out in the framework of a national research project in order to support efficient and personalized access to multi-version resources in an eGov scenario. We defined a data model supporting ontology-based personalized access to XML resources, built a prototype system implementing the data model and evaluated its performance through some exploratory experiments. The results we obtained are very encouraging as to query response time, storage requirements and system scalability figures.

Ongoing research work and desiderata for the evolution of our approach are outlined in the Section which follows.

FUTURE RESEARCH DIRECTIONS

The framework we presented in this Chapter can be extended and completed in many directions.

First of all, with reference to the complete infrastructure that we discussed in Sec. 3 and which is needed to make our proposal self-contained and fully operational in a real eGov environment, the design and implementation of further components is still needed, including administration and maintenance facilities. In particular, the identification and classification services still need to be examined thoroughly. To this end, advanced retrieval and reasoning strategies should be devised in order to provide efficient and effective automatic identification and classification of citizens.

Further work should also consider the assessment of our prototype systems in a concrete working environment, with real users and in the presence of a large repository of real legal documents. Specifically, a civic ontology based on a corpus of real norms (concerning infancy schools) is currently under development. In this way, we also plan to complement our system-oriented evaluation approach with user-oriented evaluations, measuring end-user performance and satisfaction in using our framework and pointing out the benefits of exploiting our techniques. Moreover, other kind of measures relevant for content providers (e.g. effort required for maintaining the civic ontology, for annotating the XML resources, for managing the repository contents) should also be taken into account to complete the assessment picture. Moreover, some feedback from eGov-promoting Agencies and PAs willing to boost eGov services should be collected in order to rank the various metrics according to the desired priorities.

Additional future research directions include the ability to handle ontologies containing more complex citizen class hierarchies and the management of ontology evolution issues. As a matter of fact, we are currently working on extending our approach in order to fully support ontologies with generic class relationships, containing, for instance, multiple-inheritance IS-A hierarchies and equivalence relations between classes. To this aim, the XML documents annotation scheme and their storage organization must be enhanced. The solution we are currently working out is based on the transformation of multiple-inheritance hierarchies into a forest of tree-shaped hierarchies, obtained by splitting classes with multiple ancestors across multiple taxonomies (preserving one of their ancestors in each taxonomy) and then connecting the split results with equivalence relations. As to the annotation, this solution requires the pre-order numbering scheme to be extended with an additional number denoting the taxonomy in the forest. Finally, at the present stage of the research, temporal (versioned) ontologies are not needed and we only consider temporal versioning of XML resources. However, we believe that it would be also very challenging to consider ontology versioning (which would add a temporal perspective on applicability) in our framework and to analyze in depth how proposed ontology versioning models, like the one in (Klein & Fensel, 2001), and available tools, such as t-Protégé (t-Protégé, n.d.), an extension of Protégé supporting temporal aspects, could aid in this respect.

REFERENCES

Al-Khalifa, S., Jagadish H. V., Patel, J. M., Wu, Y., Koudas, N. & Srivastava, D. (2002). Structural Joins: A Primitive for Efficient XML Query Pattern Matching. In *Proceedings of the 18th International Conference on Data Engineering (ICDE)* (pp. 141–154). Los Alamitos, CA: IEEE Computer Society Press.

Baader, F., Hoorocks, I. & Sattler, U. (2002). Description Logics for the Semantic Web. *Künstliche Intelligenz, 16*(4), 57–59.

Benjamins, V. R., Casanovas, P., Breuker, J. & Gangemi, A. (Eds.) (2005). *Law and the Semantic Web - Legal Ontologies, Methodologies, Legal Information Retrieval, and Applications*, Lecture Notes in Computer Science: Vol. 3369. Heidelberg, Germany: Springer-Verlag.

Berners-Lee, T., Hendler, J., & Lassila, O. (2001). The Semantic Web, *Scientific American, 284*(5), 34–43.

Breuker, J., Tiscornia, D., Winkels, R. & Gangemi, A. (Eds.) (2004). *Journal of Artificial Intelligence and Law, 12*(4): Special issue on Ontologies for Law.

Callan, J., Smeaton, A., Beaulieu, M., Borlund, P., Brusilovsky, P., Chalmers, M., Lynch, C., Riedl, J., Smyth, B., Straccia, U. & Toms, E. (2003). *Personalization and recommender systems in digital libraries. Joint NSF-EU DELOS Working Group Report.* Sophia Antipolis, France: ERCIM. Retrieved January 15, 2008, from http://www.ercim.org/publication/ws-proceedings/Delos-NSF/Personalisation.pdf

Casanovas, P., Biasiotti, M. A., Francesconi, E. & Sagri, M.T. (2007). In *Proceedings of the Second ICAIL Legal Ontologies and Artificial Intelligence Techniques Workshop (LOAIT).* IAAIL Workshop Series. Oisterwijk, The Netherlands: Wolf Legal Publishers.

Cornelis, B. (2003). *Personalizing search in digital libraries*. Unpublished master's thesis, University of Maastricht, Maastricht, The Netherlands.

ECeGov (n.d.). The European Commission e-Government Home Page. Retrieved January 15, 2008, from http://europa.eu.int/information_society/eeurope/2005/all_about/egovernment/index_en.htm

ECeG Project (2003). The "Semantic web techniques for the management of digital identity and the access to norms" PRIN Project Home Page. Retrieved January 15, 2008, from http://www.cirsfid.unibo.it/eGov03/

Frias-Martinez, E., Magoulas, G., Chen, S. & Macredie, R. (2006). Automated user modeling for personalized digital libraries. *International Journal of Information Management, 26*(3), 234–248.

Gauch, S., Chaffee, J. & Pretschner, A. (2003). Ontology-Based User Profiles for Search and Browsing. *Web Intelligence and Agent Systems, 1*(3-4), 219–234.

Godoy, D. & Amandi, A. (2005). User Profiling for Web Page Filtering. *IEEE Internet Computing, 9*(4), 56–64.

Golemati, M., Katifori, A., Vassilakis, C., Lepouras, G. & Halatsis, C. (2007). Creating an Ontology for the User Profile: Method and Applications. In *Proceedings of the First IEEE International Conference on Research Challenges in Information Science (RCIS)* (pp. 407–412). Los Alamitos, CA: IEEE Computer Society Press.

Grandi, F., Mandreoli, F., Bergonzini, M. & Tiberio, P. (2003). A Temporal Data Model and Management System for Normative Texts in XML Format. In R. H. L. Chiang, A. H. F. Laender & E.-P. Lim (Eds.), *Proceedings of the Fifth ACM Intlernational Workshop on Web Information and Data Management (WIDM)* (pp. 29–36). New York, NY: ACM Press.

Grandi, F., Mandreoli, F., Scalas, M. R. & Tiberio, P. (2004). *Management of the Citizen's Digital Identity and Access to Multi-version Norm Texts on the Semantic Web*. Paper presented at the International Symposium on Challenges in the Internet and Interdisciplinary (IPSI), Pescara, Italy.

Grandi, F., Mandreoli, F., & Tiberio, P. (2005a). Temporal Modelling and Management of Normative Documents in XML Format. *Data & Knowledge Engineering, 54*(3), 327–354.

Grandi, F., Scalas, M. R., Mandreoli, F. & Martoglia, R. (2005b). Personalized Access to Multi-version Documents for E-Government Applications. In P. Isaías, P. Kommers & M. McPherson, *Proceedings of IADIS International Conference e-Society 2005* (pp. 553–558). Lisbon, Portugal: IADIS Press.

Grandi, F., Mandreoli, F., Martoglia, R., Ronchetti, E., Scalas, M. R. & Tiberio, P. (2006). An eGovernment System for Temporal- and Semantic-aware Access to Norms. In A. Abecker, A. Sheth, G. Mentzas & L. Stojanovic (Eds.), *Semantic Web meets eGovernment: Papers from the AAAI Spring Symposium (SWEG)* (pp. 80–86). Menlo Park, CA: AAAI Press.

Grust, T. (2002). Accelerating XPath Location Steps. In M. J. Franklin, B. Moon & A. Ailamaki, *Proceedings of the 2002 ACM SIGMOD International Conference on Management of Data* (pp. 109–120). New York, NY: ACM Press.

Guarino, N. (1998). *Formal Ontology in Information Systems*. Amsterdam, The Netherlands: IOS Press.

Horrocks, I. & Patel-Schneider, P. F. (2003). Reducing OWL Entailment to Description Logic Satisfiability. In D. Fensel, K. P. Sycara & J. Mylopoulos (Eds.), *The Semantic Web - ISWC 2003, Second International Semantic Web Conference* (pp. 17–29). Lecture Notes in Computer Science: Vol. 2870. Heidelberg, Germany: Springer-Verlag.

Klein, M. C. A. & Fensel, D. (2001). *Ontology versioning on the Semantic Web.* In I. F. Cruz, S. Decker, J. Euzenat & D. L. McGuinness (Eds.), *Proceedings of SWWS 2001, The first Semantic Web Working Symposium* (pp. 75–91). Amsterdam, The Netherlands: IOS Press.

Kobsa, A. (2001). Generic User Modeling Systems. *User Modeling and User-Adapted Interaction, 11*(1-2), 49–63.

Lehmann, J., Biasiotti, M. A., Francesconi, E. & Sagri, M. T. (Eds.) (2005). *Proceedings of the First ICAIL Legal Ontologies and Artificial Intelligence Techniques Workshop (LOAIT)*, IAAIL Workshop Series. Oisterwijk, The Netherlands: Wolf Legal Publishers.

LKIF-Core (n.d.). A core ontology of basic legal concepts. ESTRELLA Project. Retrieved January 15, 2008, from http://www.estrellaproject.org/lkif-core/

Mandreoli, F., Martoglia, R., & Ronchetti, E. (2006). Supporting Temporal Slicing in XML Databases. In Y. E. Ioannidis, M. H. Scholl, J. W. Schmidt, F. Matthes, M. Hatzopoulos, K. Böhm, A. Kemper, T. Grust & C. Böhm (Eds.), *Advances in Database Technology - EDBT 2006. 10th International Conference on Extending Database Technology* (pp. 295–312). Lecture Notes in Computer Science: Vol. 3896. Heidelberg, Germany: Springer-Verlag.

Mandreoli, F., Martoglia, R., Grandi, F., & Scalas, M. R. (2007). Efficient Management of Multiversion XML Documents for e-Government Applications. In J. Filipe, J. Cordeiro & V. Pedrosa (Eds.), *Web Information Systems and Technologies – International Conferences WEBIST 2005/2006. Revised Selected Papers* (pp. 283–294). Lecture Notes in Business Information Processing: Vol. 1. Heidelberg, Germany: Springer-Verlag.

Micarelli, A., Gasparetti, F., Sciarrone, F. & Gauch, S. (2007). Personalized Search on the World Wide Web. In P. Brusilovsky, A. Kobsa & W. Nejdl (Eds.), *The Adaptive Web - Methods and Strategies of Web Personalization* (pp. 195–230). Lecture Notes in Computer Science: Vol. 4321. Heidelberg, Germany: Springer-Verlag.

Middleton, S. E., Shadbolt, N. & De Roure, D. C. (2004). Ontological user profiling in recommender systems. *ACM Transactions on Information Systems, 22*(1), 54–88.

OWL (2004). The Web Ontology Language Home Page. W3C Consortium. Retrieved January 15, 2008, from http://www.w3.org/2004/OWL/

Palmirani, M., & Brighi, R. (2002). Normasystem: A legal document system for managing consolidated acts. In A. Hameurlain, R. Cicchetti & R. Traunmüller (Eds.), *Database and Expert Systems Applications: 13th International Conference, DEXA 2002* (pp. 310-320). Lecture Notes in Computer Science: Vol. 2453. Heidelberg, Germany: Springer-Verlag.

Perugini, S., Gonçalves, M. A., & Fox, E.A. (2004). Recommender Systems Research: A Connection-Centric Survey. *Journal of Intelligent Information Systems, 23*(2), 107-143.

Pretschner, A. (1998). *Ontology based personalized search.* Unpublished master's thesis, University of Kansas, Lawrence, Kan.

Protégé (n.d.). The Protégé Home Page. Stanford University. Retrieved January 15, 2008, from http://protege.stanford.edu/

Razmerita, L., Angehrn, A. & Maedche, A. (2003). Ontology-based User Modeling for Knowledge management Systems. In P. Brusilovsky, A. T. Corbett & F. de Rosis (Eds.), *User Modeling 2003, 9th International Conference, UM2003* (pp. 213–217). Lecture Notes in Computer Science: Vol. 2702. Heidelberg, Germany: Springer-Verlag.

Resnick, P. & Varian, H. R. (Eds.) (1997). *Communications of the ACM, 40*(3): Special issue on Recommender systems.

Rich, E. (1999). Users are individuals: individualizing user models. *International Journal on Human-Computer Studies, 51*(2), 323–338.

Riecken, D. (2000). Personalized views of personalization. *Communications of the ACM, 43*(8), 27–28.

Rodotà, S. (2001). Introduction to the "One world, one privacy" session. *Proceedings of 23rd Data Protection Commissioners Conf.*, Paris, France. Retrieved January 15, 2008, from http://www.paris-conference-2001.org/eng/contribution/rodota_contrib.pdf

Shen, X., Tan, B. & Zhai, CX. (2007). Privacy protection in personalized search, *ACM SIGIR Forum, 41*(1), 4–17.

SOAP/XMLP (2000). The XML Protocol Working Group Home Page. W3C Consortium. Retrieved January 15, 2008, from http://www.w3.org/2000/xp/Group/

t-Protégé (n.d.). The t-Protégé Project Home Page. University of Peloponnese. Retrieved January 15, 2008, from http://t-protege.uop.gr/

Trajkova, J. & Gauch, S. (2004). Improving ontology-based user profiles. In *RIAO 2004 Conference Proceedings* (pp 380–389). Paris, France: C.I.D. Retrieved January 15, 2008, from http://www3.riao.org/Proceedings-2004/papers/0290.pdf

USeGov (2006). The U.S. President's e-Government Initiatives Home Page. Retrieved January 15, 2008, from http://www.whitehouse.gov/omb/egov/

Visser, P. R. S & Bench-Capon, T. J. M. (1998). A Comparison of Four Ontologies for the Design of Legal Knowledge Systems. *Artificial Intelligence and Law, 6*(1), 27–57.

UDDI (n.d.). The Universal Description Discovery and Integration Specification, OASIS Organization. Retrieved January 15, 2008, from http://www.oasis-open.org/committees/tc_home.php?wg_abbrev=uddi-spec

XML (n.d.). The eXtensible Markup Language Home Page. W3C Consortium. Retrieved January 15, 2008, from http://www.w3.org/XML/

XPDL (n.d.). The XML Process Definition Language. WfMC Coalition. Retrieved January 15, 2008, from http://www.wfmc.org/standards/docs.htm

XSL/XSLT (n.d.). The eXtensible Stylesheet Language Family Home Page. W3C Consortium. Retrieved January 15, 2008, from http://www.w3.org/Style/XSL/

XQuery (n.d.). The XML Query Home Page.W3C Consortium. Retrieved January 15, 2008, from http://www.w3c.org/XML/Query

WS-BPEL (n.d.). The Web Services Business Process Execution Language, OASIS Organization. Retrieved January 15, 2008, from http://www.oasis-open.org/committees/tc_home.php?wg_abbrev=wsbpel

FURTHER READINGS

Abecker A., Sheth A., Mentzas G. & Stojanovic L. (Eds.) (2006). *Semantic Web Meets eGovernment - Papers from 2006 AAAI Spring Symposium.* Technical Report SS-06-06, Menlo Park, CA: AAAI Press.

Anttiroiko, A. V. & Malia, M. (Eds.) (2006). *Encyclopedia of Digital Government* (3 Volumes). Hershey, PA: IGI Global.

Bonett, M. (2001). Personalization of Web Services: Opportunities and Challenges. *Ariadne, 28*. Retrieved January 15, 2008, from http://www.ariadne.ac.uk/issue28/personalization/

Braynov, S. (2004). Personalization and Customization Technologies. In H. Bidgoli (Ed.), *The Internet Encyclopedia - Vol. 2* (pp. 51–62), Hoboken, NJ: John Wiley and Sons.

Brusilovsky, P., Kobsa, A. & Nejdl, W. (Eds.) (2007). *The Adaptive Web - Methods and Strategies of Web Personalization*. Lecture Notes in Computer Science: Vol. 4321. Heidelberg, Germany: Springer-Verlag.

Curtin, G. G., Sommer, M. H. & Vis-Sommer, V. (Eds.) (2003). *The World of E-Government*. Binghamton, NY: Haworth Press.

Davies, J., Fensel, D. & van Harmelen, F. (Eds.) (2002). *Towards the Semantic Web: Ontology-driven Knowledge Management*. Hoboken, NJ : John Wiley and Sons.

The European Union eGovernment Research & Development Portal (n.d.). Retrieved January 15, 2008, from http://ec.europa.eu/egovernment

Grandi, F. (2004). Introducing an Annotated Bibliography on Temporal and Evolution Aspects in the World Wide Web. *ACM SIGMOD Record, 33*(2), 84–86.

Pascual, P. J. (2003). *E-Government*. Bangkok, Thailand: UNDP-APDIP. Retrieved January 15, 2008, from http://en.wikibooks.org/wiki/E-government

Sharman, R., Kishore, R., & Ramesh, R. (Eds.) (2007). *Ontologies - A Handbook of Principles, Concepts and Applications in Information Systems*. Integrated Series In Information Systems: Vol. 14, Heidelberg, Germany: Springer-Verlag.

Staab, S. & Studer, R. (Eds.) (2004). *Handbook on Ontologies*. International Handbooks on Information Systems, Heidelberg, Germany: Springer-Verlag.

Website of the Workshop on an Open XML Interchange Format for Legal and Legislative Resources (n.d.). Retrieved January 15, 2008, from http://www.metalex.eu/

ENDNOTES

1. In order to avoid unauthorized accesses to protected information, we assume citizens can be uniquely and trustworthy recognized on the Web (e.g. through an electronic ID card or digital signature) so that they can be always granted the privileges to read all and only their data from the various PA information servers. In this way, the required portions of their digital identity can effectively be reconstructed on demand via the activation of the appropriate identification services.
2. The norms are translated in our multi-version XML data model through a semi-automated process involving a human expert by means of an "intelligent" interactive editor (Palmirani & Brighi, 2002), which can be used to easily annotate the norms with the required temporal and semantic attributes and to record the annotated new norms in a legal database.

Chapter IX
Context and Adaptivity-Driven Visualization Method Selection

Maria Golemati
University of Athens, Greece

Costas Vassilakis
University of Peloponnese, Greece

Akrivi Katifori
University of Athens, Greece

George Lepouras
University of Peloponnese, Greece

Constantin Halatsis
University of Athens, Greece

ABSTRACT

Novel and intelligent visualization methods are being developed in order to accommodate user searching and browsing tasks, including new and advanced functionalities. Besides, research in the field of user modeling is progressing in order to personalize these visualization systems, according to its users' individual profiles. However, employing a single visualization system, may not suit best any information seeking activity. In this paper we present a visualization environment, which is based on a visualization library, i.e. is a set of visualization methods, from which the most appropriate one is selected for presenting information to the user. This selection is performed combining information extracted from the context of the user, the system configuration and the data collection. A set of rules inputs such information and assigns a score to all candidate visualization methods. The presented environment additionally monitors user behavior and preferences to adapt the visualization method selection criteria.

INTRODUCTION

New visualization systems are continually equipped with advanced features in order to enhance search and browsing activities. However, regardless of a thorough visualization design, systems remain unable to satisfy any possible need and task. This is due to not only the huge volumes of information which exist in digital format and the diversity in digital collections' parameters, but also because users who rely on electronic media in order to forage the information they need, often come up with specific and complicated demands. As this new era in information approach is getting shaped, a number of extra factors emerge.

To effectively achieve an information retrieval goal, any individual user's characteristics play a decisive role as they present different behavior when solving different tasks or even the same task under different circumstances. Thus, recording these characteristics a system could be evaluated as suitable or not for a specific user or user group. On the other hand, the particularities of a searching task, as well as the corpus which hosts the possible results, provide key information for the effectiveness of a specific system in the completion of a specific task. Consequently, any individual visualization system is never enough for any possible need and task.

The development of user-adaptive systems is a promising approach to address this problem, as these systems are designed to be customized to the needs and desires of their specific users. Building and then exploiting user models, user-adaptive systems incorporate dynamic processes which allow humans to define their function according to the surrounding situation.

In this paper, the user characteristics, the data collection particularities and the system capabilities are matched with the visualization method properties in a context-based adaptive visualization environment to be used in the Historical Archive of the University of Athens, in order to support information seeking tasks. The presented work introduces new techniques for supporting the adaptation and personalization issues in the design and development of Intelligent User Interfaces, mainly by adapting services to user preferences and device characteristics of the user (display and input devices available), while system constraints and resource availability (memory size and processor speed) are also taken into account.

In the next section of this paper, background issues and related work in the field of user modeling and user adaptive systems is surveyed. In the following sections, we analyze the notion of context modeling in our system and describe the process of visualization method selection, which is also exemplified through a hypothetical user session with the proposed system. In the last two sections, future trends are discussed and conclusions are drawn.

BACKGROUND

The problem of context management constitutes a new approach to the design of context-aware systems. (Zimmermann A., Specht M. & Lorenz A., 2005) refers to this problem combining personalization and contextualization. It defines that an *adaptive system (contextualized and personalized or both) follows an adaptation strategy (e.g. pacing or leading) to achieve an adaptation goal (e.g. intuitive information access or easy use of a service). To achieve an adaptation goal, it considers relevant information about the user and the context and adapts relevant system components on the basis of this information*".

(Domik G. O. & Gutkauf B, 1994) claims that a visualization system needs to adapt to desires, abilities and disabilities of the user, interpretation aim, resources (hardware, software) available, and the form and content of the data to be visualized. It distinguishes four different models: user model, problem domain/task model, resource model and data model and gives the design of computer tests and games to test user abilities (color perception, colour memory, colour ranking, mental rotation and motor coordination). (Fischer G., Lemke A., Mastaglio T., & Morch A., 1991) suggests the following three kinds of user modeling:

- the explicit modeling, which involves asking the user straightforward questions. Such kind of information is usually collected in the beginning of the user's interaction with the system.
- the implicit modeling, according to which the system extracts information from the user's work and interaction with the system. For example, recording the keys pressed and functions used, or the choices a user makes.
- special tasks to solve, where the user is submitted in solving special predefined tasks, designed for the purpose of extracting certain abilities of a user.

Each type of model further individualizes and enriches the information of the previous one(s).

The IVEE (Ahlberg, C., & Wistrand, E., 1995) is a visualization system, which supports multiple views of the data collection together with a functionality to format a query in a dynamic way. According to the authors of the system, a successful visualization environment depends on a whole set of visualizations appropriate for various tasks and data types, as it can be customized in a variation of existing conditions. In IVEE this notion is applied, providing the user with a variety of visualizations and features to customize to different preferences, abilities and needs. The system is only implemented in the context of movie searching and does not support document properties such as hierarchical structure, hypertext structure etc.

In the Periscope system (Wiza W., K. Walczak & W. Cellary, 2004) a holistic, an analytical, a hybrid as well as a specialized interface model have been implemented both in 2 and 3 dimensions to give the user the opportunity to select a specific presentation method to focus on certain properties of the results obtained. The system allows the user to assign search result attributes to visualization dimensions and therefore modify the method of visualization to highlight important features of the search result. Furthermore, the system provides the possibility to make comparisons between results from two or more different queries in a single 3D scene.

The problem discussed in this work is a specific instance of the generic problem of expressing and evaluating user preferences, which has been discussed, among others, in (Agrawal, R. & Wimmers, E. L., 2000) and (Seunghwa, L. & Eunseok, L., 2007). In (Agrawal, R. & Wimmers, E. L., 2000), a generic scheme is proposed, which allows autonomy and combination of various preferences. The personal preference model used in this work follows these basic principles accommodating additionally the context parameters which held when some user preference was expressed. Under this enhanced scheme, when some preference is considered the context parameters recorded in the preference are compared to the ones currently effective and the result of this comparison indicates how strongly this preference should be taken into account.

Based on the above research and taking into consideration the added value of the user and other feature modeling we suggest an adaptive visualization environment which adapts to specific users, tasks and environments. The result is a novel context-sensitive information space, which adjusts its appearance and functionality to best serve the user in any given situation.

CONTEXT MODELING

Modeling the context of the Historical Archive consists not only of the user characteristics, preferences and needs, but also of the platform available to perform the task and moreover the properties of the document collection to be retrieved. Consequently, the concept of context modeling includes each of the following cases:

Explicit user context: this is the initial user information. For example, the gender, the age, the profession, the educational level, the cognitive abilities, the user's experience in using computers and so forth, may constitute the explicit user context. Such information can be extracted through interviewing the user the first time s/he accesses the Historical Archive and it is used to initially populate the specific user's *preferences database*. For example, for users with little computer experience a low preference score for visualization methods with complicated controls is recorded, whereas for users with elevated color perception, high preference scores towards methods using color coding are registered. Demographic data (e.g. gender and age) and personal information (e.g. profession) are used to classify the user into a *user stereotype*, which is also associated with a set of preferences; this classification eases the initial preference database population.

These preferences are extracted from the user's preferences database the next time the same user visits again the Historical Archive, and are taken into consideration in the process of selecting the set of candidate visualization methods for the task at hand. Note that these initially set preferences may be later modified if the users' behavior in the system suggests that the recorded preferences do not apply as registered.

Implicit user context: this is additional information extracted while the user is working with a single visualization method. For example, his/her preferences and/or likes/dislikes of the visualization methods, his/her difficulties in understanding a method in finding the information needed etc, constitute the implicit user context. This information is registered to enhance the user profile with additional data which will also be considered in any future selection of the appropriate visualization method for the specific user.

System context. This concerns information relative to the software/hardware available to perform the visualization. For example, the existence or not of VR equipment, the memory size and processor power are elements of the system context. The system context is exploited by the adaptation mechanism to determine the most appropriate visualization method to employ. For example, a 3D visualization method can be more efficiently displayed when 3D monitors and/or other VR equipment is available. Note that the absence of such hardware may not preclude the use of 3D visualization methods, and, inversely, their presence does not imply that only 3D methods will be used; system context is co-evaluated along with other parameters to finally select the most prominent visualization method.

Document collection context. This concerns information relative to the portion of corpus of the Historical Archive that will be visualized in a given situation. Such a corpus has many particularities. For example, it may contain documents in various formats (text or scanned images, while for some documents only their *metadata* may be available); The documents may be related or not according to some criterion; selected documents may be classified under a taxonomy or they may have been retrieved using a query; and so forth. The most special case of the Historical Archive data collection is the minutes from the various University meetings, since a single document of this class may span across different thematic categories, affect multiple departments, reference or be referenced by multiple other documents etc. Consequently, these documents require a different visualization method, depending both on the data characteristics and on the user's needs as well.

The above-mentioned contexts provide valuable knowledge to the process of the selection of the most appropriate visualization method to display the information. This knowledge is processed using a set of rules, assigning to each method a score – effectively a value indicating its perceived usefulness for the running case. The algorithm used to perform this assessment is described in the next section.

VISUALIZATION METHODS AND THEIR SELECTION

The process of selecting the most appropriate visualization method to display to the user needs an explicit model of the visualization methods' properties to express their specific features. This arrangement enables the process of matching the contexts against the visualization methods. A set of rules combines all these data and assigns a *totalscore* to each available visualization system. The property model and the selection method are described in the following paragraphs.

Visualization Method Properties

In designing a visualization system several issues are taken into account. The principal goal is to bridge the user with the information source. This is a complicated task, as many parameters have to be taken into account. Typically, the design of a visualization system has a specific focus which can be achieved using intelligent procedures. In this way, every one of the systems has its own properties, which make it unique in improving a specific aspect of the information foraging.

For example, there are visualization methods which try to display full text documents in the most effective way, using thumbnails, highlights, document size and type cues, color coding, showing relations between terms, etc. Other methods, concentrate on improving focus+context techniques, in order to give the user alternative views to the document collection, using zoom in and out functionalities, graph rotation, hyperbolic spaces etc. A very common issue in large document collections which are structured in hierarchical way is how to visualize this hierarchy in an effective and easy to explore way. Important solutions to this issue have been proposed by introducing the third dimension in the visualization design, using tree-like layouts, real world metaphors, nested items, transparency/solidity functionalities etc. One of the main concerns a Historical Archive has to deal with is the managing of temporal information, i.e. information that varies with time. To facilitate the user in retrieving such information, visualization methods employ time axes in a variety of ways: bar charts, time lines, spirals etc. Another important concern in designing a visualization method is the representation of the relation between documents. This issue is effectively addressed using links between related documents, or clustering techniques, which bring together the related documents, color coding to reveal existing relations, etc. In a similar way the problem of the representation of the relation between the query terms and the displayed results is addressed.

Finally, since a data collection is not restricted to text documents, many visualization methods focus on designing novel techniques to support users in retrieving and viewing picture, audio and/or video documents.

For the purposes of this work, visualization methods have been categorized using the classification scheme presented in (Katifori, A., Halatsis, C., Lepouras, G., Vassilakis, C., & Giannopoulou, E., 2007); according to this scheme, visualization methods are primarily classified according to the visualization type they employ, which may be one of the following:

1. Indented list,
2. Node–link and tree,
3. Zoomable,
4. Space-filling,
5. Focus + context or distortion,
6. 3D Information landscapes.

Each category is further divided in two subcategories, namely 2D and 3D, taking into account the number of display dimensions it employs. While this classification scheme is introduced in the context of ontology visualization, it is generic enough to accommodate all visualization types used in this work. Using this classification facilitated the assignment of "suitability scores" for the available visualization methods, since scores were assigned at category level and were subsequently fine-tuned for each distinct visualization method within every category. The work reported in (Katifori, A., et al., 2007) includes also discussions on functional and non-functional visualization method aspects (task support, 2d vs. 3d, navigation and interaction issues and scalability issues), which have been also taken into account.

A list of basic features of visualization systems is depicted in Table 1 (the list includes only the features currently considered by the system; incorporation of additional features is being considered for future extensions). The first column lists the visualization method property, while within the second column the possible values for this property are presented. Each value is followed by an indicative list of visualization methods for which the specific property/value combination applies. Note that some visualization methods may support multiple values for a specific property [e.g. the PLAO (Lecolinet, E., Likforman-Sulem, L., Roberrt, L., Role, F., & Lebrave, J-L, 1998) visualization method may operate both in 2 and 3 dimensions], in which case the method is repeated under all pertinent list elements. Note also that in some cases, either a feature is supported or not (e.g. color coding). In these cases, no value list is provided in the second column; a dash is used instead, followed by the list of methods supporting the feature. For the compilation of the properties list appearing in table 1, a number of bibliographic sources including (Shneiderman, B., 1996), (Card, S. K., Mackinlay J. D., & Shneiderman B., 1999) and (Chi, E. H, 2000) were consulted.

Visualization Method Selection

The visualization method selection procedure matches properties from the user, system and collection contexts against the visualization system properties. This matching is enabled through a rule database, containing rules of the following format:

(context-property, vis-method-property, score)

Table 1. Properties of visualization systems and respective property values

Number of dimensions	• 2 (PLAO, IVEE, …) • 2 ½ (Data Mountain, LookMark, …) • 3 (IVEE, Perspective Tunnel, Task Gallery, PLAO, …)
Metaphor	• Landscape (Information City, Vineta, …) • Book and Library (WebBook, virtual library, …) • Perspective Planes & Panels (Data Mountain, Lookmark, etc) • 3D Geometric Shapes (Inform. Pyramids, VizNet, …) • Trees and Graphs (Starwalker, Visible Threads, ….)
Interactive browsing supported for documents of type:	• Article (UVA, SPIRE, Doc Cube, …) • Publication (Bead, Vineta, Cat-A-Cone, UVA, …) • Hypertext (LookMark, WebBook, …) • Photograph/Video (Viz-Net, Dynamic Timelines, …)
Supports user-defined grouping for documents of type:	• Articles (-) • Books (WebBook, Web Forager, …) • Hypertext (WebBook, Web Forager, …) • Photographs/Video (-)
Color coding	• - (File System Navigator, Harmony Information Landscape, …)
Term frequency	• - (Tile bars, PRISE, Themescape, …)

where context-property is a property from the user, system or collection context, *vis-method-property* is a visualization system property and score is a numeric metric in the range [-10, 10] expressing how appropriate visualization methods having the specific *vis-method-property* are considered for contexts where the particular context-property holds. For example, the rule:

(sysctx-display-3D, vismeth-noDimensions-3, 6)

declares that visualization methods employing three dimensions are considered quite appropriate for system contexts with 3D displays, while the rule:

(colctx-origin-dynamic, vismeth-itemgroup-hierarchical, -4)

expresses the belief that a visualization method employing hierarchical item grouping is inappropriate for collections that have been formulated by means of submitting queries.

For compiling the rule database, and in particular for assigning scores to (*context-property, vis-method-property*) pairs, users and visualization system experts were interviewed. In these interviews, subjects were asked to state how helpful/hindering each context property was considered in their opinion for performing each type of visualization. The interview results along with published evaluation results of visualization systems [e.g. (Robertson G., Czerwinski M., Larson K., Robbins D., Thiel D. & van Dantzich M., 1998; Shneiderman, B., Feldman, D., Rose, A., & Ferre G., X., 2000; Robertson, G. G., Van Dantzich, M., Robbins, D., Czerwinski, M., Hinckley, K., Risden, K., Thiel, D. & Gorokhovsky, V., 2000; Modjeska, D., 2000)] were used as input for the population of the rule database.

When a collection needs to be visualized, the system firstly compiles the full set of context properties, which is denoted as *CP*. Subsequently, it traverses the list of available visualization methods, extracting for each method M the set of method properties *PM*, which is used to compute a total score for method M. The total score is given by adding the score field *s* of all rules $R = (cp, vp, s)$, for which $cp \in CP$ and $vp \in PM$. Finally, the visualization method with the highest total score is selected to perform the visualization. Effectively, this step examines whether the properties of the visualization method are considered appropriate for the current context parameters, as this is expressed in the rule base. Note that under this scheme, the absence of any rule correlating a context property *cp* with a visualization method property *vp* has the effect that *vp* is considered "neutral" for contexts having the property *cp*; thus, there is no need to use rules of the form *(cp, vp, 0)* to explicitly state property orthogonalities.

An issue that has been commented on by users in the scheme above is that it is extremely prone to selecting different methods for consecutive visualization requests, even though the gains (as quantified by the respective method scores) may be marginal. Since users have been found to prefer a more "stable" work environment, a provision has been added in the score calculation procedure, to increase the score for the currently used method by a value of 5. This adjustment effectively directs the algorithm to perform a visualization method switch only when considerable gains will be attained, favoring thus environment stability. The value of 5 is currently a "magic number", but in the future it is planned to incorporate it into the user context, in the sense that some users have a stronger preference towards stable environments (thus a higher "bonus" value could be used), while other users are more "adventurous", so small bonus values (or even no bonus at all) should be given to the current method, in order to pursue even marginal gains from visualization method switching.

Since for the computation of the method scores the full set of context properties *CP* is matched against the full rule set *RS*, the complexity of this operation is $O(|CP| * |RS|)$. Note that the number of visualization methods does not appear in this formula but is indirectly considered, since the introduction of new visualization methods increases the cardinality of the rule set. Inclusion of additional visualization methods also increases the space required for storing the final result, which is O(|VM|) [where VM denotes the set of available visualization methods].

Adaptive Features in Method Selection

The visualization method selection process described in section 4.2 does not take into account the dynamic profile of the user, as this is exhibited by the user's preferences and dislikes while working with the system. This dynamic portion of the user context is accommodated by complementing the rule list described in section 4.2 with a user-specific preferences database, which hosts information regarding:

- whether the user has considered a visualization method suitable/not suitable for a specific context.
- whether the user likes/dislikes a specific visualization method altogether.

This information is collected from the user, when the visualization task is completed (the respective window is closed) and when an alternate visualization method is requested. More specifically, the "close window" user interface widget unfolds a drop-down menu with the options "The visualization was satisfactory", "The visualization was not helpful for this data collection" and "The visualization was obscure/unusable", from which the user selects one. If the response to this drop-down is "The visualization was obscure/unusable", then the dynamic user profile is augmented with a record of the form:

(dislike, viz-method)

stating that the user has a negative stance against the specific visualization method in general. Note that this does not inhibit the use of the visualization method in a future case; in presence of such rules, the visualization method selection procedure reduces the total score for the method (as described below), the method however *could* be selected if it is found to score significantly higher than other methods a specific context. If the user selects one of the two first replies, then a record of the form:

(eval, system-context, collection-context, viz-method, score)

is added to the dynamic user profile, where *score* is "1" or "-1", depending on which response was selected. Note that when the user chooses one of the first two replies, the visualization method is considered helpful/not helpful *for the current context.*

The rules within the dynamic user profile are taken into account for selecting the most prominent visualization method in system context SC and collection context CC according to the following scheme:

- if a *(dislike, viz-method)* rule exists in the dynamic user profile, then the total score for the specific visualization method is decremented by 15.
- for the second form of rules, when the total score for a specific visualization method is computed the system retrieves all the rules R_{dc} = *(eval, sys-con, col-con, viz-meth, score)* pertaining to this method. Subsequently, a *similarity metric* between *(sys-con, col-con)* and *(SC, CC)* is computed, to determine which of the rules is associated with a context that best matches the current context. The value of the similarity metric falls in the range [-10, 10], with -10 meaning "totally different contexts" and 10 meaning "exactly matching" ones. The similarity

metric between *(sys-con, col-con)* and *(SC, CC)* is calculated as follows:

1. the set of all rule context facts RCF = sys-con ∪ col-con and the set of all current context facts CCF = SC ∪ CC are computed, and the similarity metric is initialized to 0.
2. ∀rcf∈RCF, it is checked if rcf∈CCF. If this condition is true, the similarity score is incremented by 1, otherwise the similarity score is decremented by 1. Note that each element of RCF (and CCF) fully represents all aspects of a context element, e.g. the elements *sysctx-display-3D* and *colctx-origin-dynamic* specify that a 3D display is used and that the collection has been formulated through a query, respectively. Therefore, if the element of RCF appears in CCF, the two contexts are identical regarding the particular context element; otherwise the contexts are different in the specific respect (and CCF would contain a different element, e.g. *sysctx-display-2D* or *colctx-origin-static*).
3. Finally, the computed similarity score ss_{val} is normalized in the range [-10, 10] by dividing by the cardinality of RCF and multiplying by 10.

Note that the context similarity computation procedure described above considers all context elements to be equally important, since any match (mismatch) contributes by 1 (-1) to the final result. Assigning different weights to context elements for the purposes of context similarity computation is an issue under investigation and will be incorporated in a future system release.

The rule with the highest positive similarity metric is finally selected, the similarity metric is multiplied by the "score" field of the rule (1 or -1, depending on whether the visualization was considered helpful or not in the specific context) and the result is added to the total score for the visualization method under consideration. If no rule has a positive similarity metric, the total score for the visualization method is not altered.

The rationale behind the computations performed using the second rule form is that if a visualization was found to be helpful/not helpful in some context, then it is "almost certain" this perception will hold for identical contexts; if, however, two contexts differ in a number of parameters, then the certainty level for this belief drops. This certainty level is reflected in the context similarity metric, while the multiplication by the "score" field simply renders the outcome positive for "helpful" visualizations and negative for "not helpful" ones.

Besides the "close window" widget, the user interface hosts the "Switch visualization" button, which provides the ability to visualize the same collection with an alternate method. In this case, the visualization methods are listed in descending order of their scores; a small sample of each visualization is presented, allowing the user to get a preview of the method before it is selected. A user may reach this decision because "An alternate view to the data is desired", "The visualization was not helpful for this data collection" and "The visualization was obscure/unusable", which are the options listed when the "Switch visualization" button is clicked. In all cases, the dynamic user profile is updated in the same way that was described for the "close window" widget.

Example

In this section we present a sample interaction of a user with the proposed system, to clarify the modeling of contexts and the score computation algorithm. In this session, the user's interaction with the system begins by submitting the free text query "Faculty of Science" to the system (the name of the faculty to which the department belongs), expecting to view tracks of the Department she is interested in, from its very beginning up to recently. The system evaluates the query against the contents of the knowledge base and determines that:

1. The query *exactly matches* a branch in the "Academic departments" taxonomy (the "Faculty of Science" branch), which is superimposed on the Historical Archive's document collection. Though this is not a document *per se*, it is an important part of the knowledge base and is thus considered in the search.
2. The query matches metadata associated with a number of documents within the knowledge base. In particular, 136 documents have an author matching "Faculty of Science" (e.g. "Dean of the Faculty of Science" and 203 documents have a recipient matching "Faculty of Science").
3. The query matches the full text of 484 documents of the knowledge base.

Subsequently, the system structures the result collection as a hierarchy, having the query as its root node, and the three subcategories identified above as its direct descendents. Each subcategory, in turn, contains the corresponding result items; the second subcategory, in particular, has an extra level of classification, separating documents whose author matched the query from documents whose recipient matched the query.

At this stage, the system has all contexts available (explicit user context, system context, implicit/dynamic user context and document collection context) and may proceed to select the most prominent visualization method. The following factors are considered (in the following, not all rules are expressly listed for brevity reasons):

1. the document collection has an hierarchical structure, so due to the rule *(colctx-structure-hierarchical, vismeth-itemgroup-hierarchical, +4)* the visualization methods that are able to intuitively present hierarchies [Cone Tree (Robertson, G., Mackinlay, J., & Card, S., 1991), the Information Pyramids (Keith A., 2000) and the Gopher VR and MoireGraphs (Jankun, T. J., & Kwan, L. M., 2003)] increment their score by 4.
2. The system has no 3D output hardware, so the rule (sysctx-display-2D, vismeth-noDimensions-3, -5) decrements the score of all 3D methods (including the Cone Tree, Information Pyramids and Gopher VR listed in the previous factor) by 5.
3. The number of direct descendents from the current root (query) is small (3), so the score of the Cone Tree is further decremented by 3 (because its the space exploitation advantage is lost in such collection contexts).
4. The score of the Cone Tree method is incremented by 4 because the user has found it useful in a situation having common elements with the current one (the recorded system and collection contexts in the respective dynamic user profile rule have some properties similar with the situation at hand) and the score of the Information Pyramids method is incremented by 2, because the contexts recorded in the respective dynamic user profile rule are less similar with the current situation.

By summing up the points added/subtracted to the score of each visualization method, the system finally determines that the MoireGraphs algorithm (figure 1) achieves the highest score at this stage so it is selected for performing the visualization. In the moiré graph the query is the current focus, while the three result categories are the direct context. The MoireGraphs visualization has been tuned to display two context levels, thus the direct descendents of result categories are also shown, in smaller sizes.

Now the user focuses on the Taxonomy node, since this was the query target. The new docu-

Figure 1. The Moire graph visualization

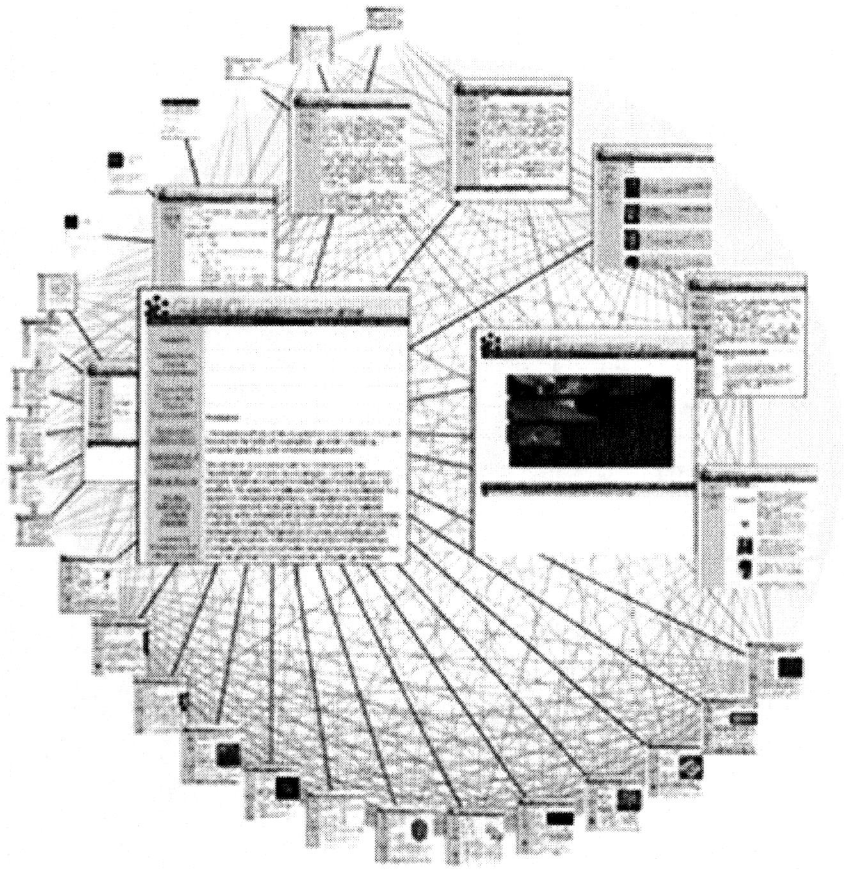

ment collection to be visualized (the taxonomy and the documents linked to each branch of it) has hierarchical structure too, but the number of direct descendents of the current root (Faculty of Science) is now considerably higher (12, which is the number of departments and administrative divisions directly subject to the faculty of science). In this respect item (3) of the factor list above does not apply, thus the Cone Tree visualization method accumulates the highest score and is selected for performing the visualization (Figure 2). In this snapshot, the Faculty of Science node is the central node in the second level, while the single node at the top level is the "University" entity. The user will locate the "Department of Informatics" node at the third level, set it as "current" and will then select "View related documents" to display all documents related with the Department of Informatics.

The document collection to be now presented has no hierarchical structure [property #1] and contains a considerable amount of individual documents (more than 3000) [property #2]. The first collection property adds gives an edge of 4points to the score of visualization methods not being based on hierarchies (Task Gallery, Data Mountain, Web Forager, Periscope-AVE, Virtual Library) against those who rely on hierarchical structure, due to the existence of the rule *(colctx-origin-dynamic, vismeth-itemgroup-hierarchical, -4)*. The first three of these methods are however inappropriate for large document collections (property #2), so their score is reduced; similarly, Virtual Library's score is decremented since it

Figure 2. Visualizing the taxonomy using cone trees

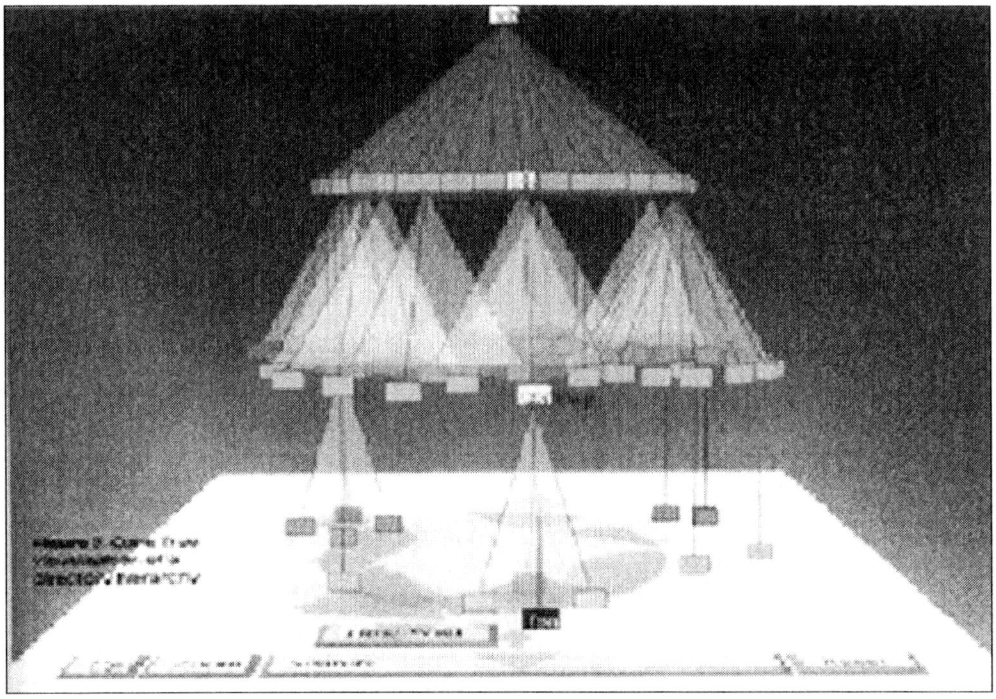

Figure 3. Periscope-AVE visualization

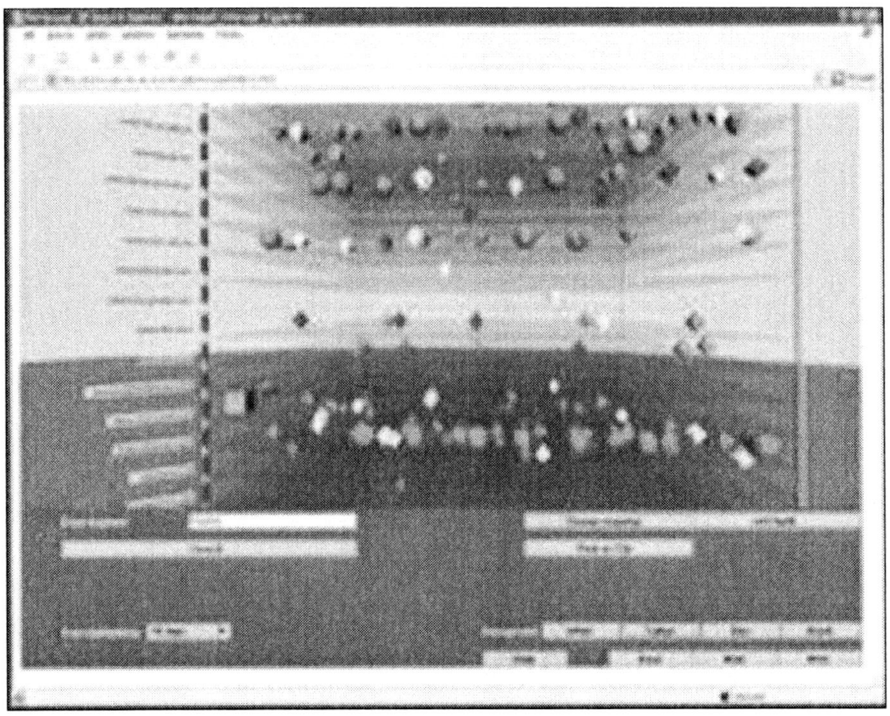

is more oriented to books rather than arbitrary document collections. After these computations, only the score of Periscope-AVE has not been decremented, and therefore this methods is selected for performing the visualization.

The user may finally select the desired categorization the documents (e.g. by purpose) and/or exploit the search mechanism of Periscope-AVE to locate the documents related to teaching in the Department of Informatics, which was the original goal.

FUTURE RESEARCH DIRECTIONS

The architectural approach described in this chapter although focused on the domain of historical archives is generic enough to be used as a basis for implementing systems in other application areas, such as digital libraries, legal databases and so forth. Naturally, in any such domain, the particularities of the specific document collection will have to be studied and expressed in the format required by the score computation algorithm. Additionally, in many application areas specialized visualization algorithms have been developed; the appropriateness of any such method, in relation with any individual context parameter must be assessed and recorded in the database.

Detailed studies on if and how each context parameter affects the effectiveness of visualization methods employing certain techniques, in order to provide a more elaborate population of the rule base, are also required. A thorough system evaluation, which will provide feedback both on the overall system effectiveness and for fine-tuning the rule database, and especially the "score" field, is also needed.

The adaptation scheme described in this chapter relies on explicit user input, either provided during the profile population stage or given at the end of each task (expression of satisfaction/dissatisfaction by the user). There exist however additional information elements that can be exploited to assess the suitability and/or usefulness of a particular visualization for a specific user in a given context: these information elements can be sourced from user activity and behavior monitoring, including metrics such as idle time, use of "reset visualization" functions, erroneous activities etc. This approach requires the use of additional architectural modules, similar to the "browser/user data sensing" and "data recorder" used in (Chittaro & Ranon, 2002), while the visualization algorithms themselves need to be extended with facilities that will detect and characterize "erroneous" user activities (e.g. clicking on non-functional areas of the visualization, using "undo" operations and so forth). Generalization and abstraction mechanisms may also be introduced to allow for speedier configuration of the rule database. These mechanisms will detect common features in visualization method assessments (either explicit or derived) and formulate generic rules which will affect all methods sharing these features. For instance, if a user is found to dislike WebBook and Virtual library, the system may derive that the specific user does not prefer visualizations employing the "Book and Library" metaphor and thus introduce a personalization rule for decrementing the score of these algorithms.

Finally, since the number of different visualization methods, rules and user preferences within the system is expected to increase, the efficiency of the algorithm selection method will need to be addressed. Research results from the area of *efficient top-k evaluation* algorithms [e.g. (Mamoulis, N., Yiu, M., L., Cheng K. H. & Cheung D. W., 2007) and (Marian, A., Amer-Yahia, S., Koudas, N., Srivastava, D., 2005)] can be considered to this end.

REFERENCES

Agrawal R. & Wimmers, E. L. (2000). A Framework for Expressing and Combining Preferences.. *Proceedings of ACM SIGMOD*, 297-306

Ahlberg, C., & Wistrand, E. (1995). IVEE: An Information Visualization & Exploration Environment. *Proceedings of IEEE Viz*

Card, S. K., Mackinlay J. D., & Shneiderman B. (1999). *Information Visualization: Using Vision to Think*. Morgan-Kaufmann, San Francisco, California.

Chi, E. H. (2000). A Taxonomy of Visualization Techniques using the Data State Reference Model. *Proceedings of the IEEE Symposium on Information Visualization 2000 (InfoVis'00)*, 69-75

Chittaro L. & Ranon R. (2002). Dynamic Generation of Dynamic VRML Content: a General Approach and its Application to 3D E-Commerce. Proceedings of Web3D Conference, pp. 145-154.

Domik G. O., & Gutkauf B (1994). User modeling for adaptive visualization systems. In R. Daniel Bergeron and Arie E. Kaufman, editors, *Proceedings of the IEEE Conference on Visualization.*

Fischer G., Lemke A., Mastaglio T., & Morch A. (1991). The role of Critiquing in Coorporative Problem Solving. *ACM Transactions on Information Systems* (9), 123 – 151

Jankun, T. J., & Kwan, L. M. (2003). Moire-Graphs: Radial Focus+Context Visualization and Interaction for Graphs with Visual Nodes, *IEEE Symposium on Information Visualization, Seattle, Washington*

Katifori, A., Halatsis, C., Lepouras, G., Vassilakis, C. & Giannopoulou, E. (2007). Ontology Visualization Methods-A Survey. *ACM Computing Surveys* (39) 4, 2007.

Lecolinet, E., Likforman-Sulem, L., Roberrt, L., Role, F., & Lebrave, J-L, (1998). An Integrated Reading and Editing Environment for Scholarly Research on Literary Works and their Handwritten Sources. *Proceedings of ACM Digital Libraries Conference.*

Mamoulis, N., Yiu, M., L., Cheng K. H. & Cheung D. W. (2007). Efficient top-k aggregation of ranked inputs. *ACM Transactions on Database Systems* (32) 3.

Marian, A., Amer-Yahia, S., Koudas, N., Srivastava, D. (2005). Adaptive Processing of Top-k Queries in XML. Proceedings of the 21st International Conference on Data Engineering, 162-173.

Modjeska, D. (2000). View vs. Overview: Hierarchical Data Visualization in Desktop Virtual Reality. *Proceedings of NordiCHI 2000.*

Robertson G., Czerwinski M., Larson K., Robbins D., Thiel D. & van Dantzich M. (1998). Data Mountain: Using Spatial Memory for Document Management, *Proceedings of ACM UIST '98 Symposium on User Interface Software& Technology*

Robertson, G. G., Van Dantzich, M., Robbins, D., Czerwinski, M., Hinckley, K., Risden, K., Thiel, D. & Gorokhovsky, V. (2000). The Task Gallery: A 3D Window Manager. *CHI Letters, 2(1),* 494-501.

Robertson, G., Mackinlay, J., & Card, S. (1991). Cone Trees: Animated 3D Visualizations of Hierarchical Information. *Proceedings of CHI '91*, 189-194.

Seunghwa, L. & Eunseok, L. (2007). A Collective User Preference Management System for U-Commerce. In *Managing Next Generation Networks and Services*, Springer Berlin / Heidelberg, 21-30.

Shneiderman, B. (1996). The eyes have it: a task by data type taxonomy for information visualization. *Proceedings of the IEEE Visual Languages.*

Shneiderman, B., Feldman, D., Rose, A., & Ferre G., X. (2000). Visualizing Digital Library Search Results with Categorical and Hierarchical Axes. *Proceedings of the 5th ACM International Conference on Digital Libraries*, 57-66.

Wiza W., K. Walczak & W. Cellary (2004). Periscope - A System for Adaptive 3D Visualization of Search Results, *Web3D 2004 Symposium - the 9th International Conference on 3D Web Technology, Monterey, California (USA), ACM SIGGRAPH*, 29-39.

Zimmermann A., Specht M. & Lorenz A. (2005). Personalization and Context Management. *User Modleing and User-Adapted Interaction*. 15, 275-302.

ADDITIONAL READING

Alimohideen, J., Renambot, L., Leigh, J., Johnson, A., Grossman, R. & Sabala, M. (2006). PAVIS – Pervasive Adaptive Visualization and Interaction Service. *CHI 06 Workshop on Information Visualization and Interaction Techniques for Collaboration Across Multiple Displays.*

Andrews, K. (2002). Visual Exploration of Large Hierarchies with Information Pyramids. *Proceedings of the Sixth International Conference on Information Visualization (IV'02)*, IEEE Computer Society Press, London, England, 793-798.

Benyon, D., Turner, P. & Turner, S. (2005). *Designing Interactive Systems: People, Activities, Contexts, Technologies*. Addison Wesley, ISBN: 978-0321116291.

Brodlie, K. W., Brooke, J., Chen, M., Chisnall, D., Hughes, C., John, N. W., Jones, M. W., Riding, M., Roard, N., Turner, M. J., & Wood, J. (2006) A Framework for Adaptive Visualization. *IEEE Visualization 2006.*

Brusilovsky, P. (2003), Adaptive navigation support in educational hypermedia: the role of student knowledge level and the case for meta-adaptation, *British Journal of Educational Technology*, Vol. 34 (4) pp 487-497.

Card, S. K., Mackinlay, J., Shneiderman, B. (1999). *Readings in Information Visualization: Using Vision to Think*. Morgan Kaufmann, ISBN: 978-1558605336.

Chen, H., Nunamaker J. Jr., Orwig R., & Titkova, O. (1998). Information Visualization for Collaborative Computing. *IEEE Computer*, Vol. 31, Issue 8, 75 – 82.

Cockburn, A., & Mckenzie D. (2002). Evaluating the Effectiveness of Spatial Memory in 2D and 3D Physical and Virtual Environments. *Proceedings of ACM Computer-Human Interaction Conf. Human Factors in Computing Systems*, ACM Press, 203-210.

Dumais, S. T., Cutrell, E., Cadiz, E., J. J., Jancke, G., Sarin R. & Robbins D. C. (2003). Stuff I've Seen: A system for personal information retrieval and re-use. *Proceedings of SIGIR 2003.*

Golemati, M., Halatsis, C., Vassilakis, C., Katifori, A. & Lepouras, G. (2006). A Context-Based Adaptive Visualization Environment. *Proceedings of the IV 06 Conference.*

Herman, I., Melançon, G., & Scott Marshall, M. (2000). Graph Visualization and Navigation in Information Visualization: a Survey, *IEEE Transactions on Visualization and Computer Graphics*, 24-43

Katifori, A., Torou, E., Halatsis, C., Vassilakis, C., & Lepouras G. (2006). A Comparative Study of Four Ontology Visualization Techniques in Protégé: Experiment Setup and Preliminary Results. *Proceedings of the 10th Information Visualization Conference*, London

Katifori, A., Vassilakis, C., Lepouras G., Daradimos, I., AND Halatsis, C. (2006). Visualizing a Temporally – Enhanced Ontology. *Proceedings of the AVI Conference*, Venice, Italy

Lepouras, G. (2004). Applying Clustering Algorithms to Web-based Adaptive Virtual Environments. To appear in Journal of Computational

Methods in Sciences and Engineering, http://pelopas.uop.gr/~gl/papers/JCMSE_algorithmsAdaptiveVE.pdf [Last accessed: November 2007]

Lepouras, G., & Vassilakis C. (2005). Adaptive Virtual Museums on the Web. Book chapter in book *Adaptable and Adaptive Hypermedia Systems*, Sherry Y. Chen & George Magoulas (eds), Idea Group Publishing.

Lepouras, G., & Vassilakis C. (2006). Adaptive Virtual Reality Shopping Malls. *Encyclopedia of E-Commerce, E-Government and Mobile Commerce*, Idea Group Publishing.

Löffler, J., Fellner, D. W. (2002). Adaptive visualization of distributed 3D documents using image streaming techniques. *Proceedings of the sixth Eurographics workshop on Multimedia*, 9-19.

Loke, S. (2006). *Context-Aware Pervasive Systems: Architectures for a New Breed of Applications*. Auerbach publications, ISBN: 978-0849372551

Marucci, L., Paternò F. (2002). Helping users through ubiquitous personalised, interactive support in a sightseeing visit. Proceedings ECCE11 - Eleventh European Conference on Cognitive Ergonomics, Catania, 2002, pp.245-250.

Not, E., Petrelli, D., Sarini, M., Stock, O., Strapparava, C., and Zancanaro, M. (1998). Hypernavigation in the physical space: adapting presentations to the user and to the situational context. The New Review of Hypermedia and Multimedia, Vol. 4, 1998 pp 33 – 46

Ringel, M., Cutrell, E., Dumais S. T., & Horvitz, E. (2003). Milestones in time: The value of landmarks in retrieving information from personal stores. *Proceedings of Interact 2003*.

Roussinov, D. (1999). Internet search using adaptive visualization. *Conference on Human Factors in Computing Systems*, 69-70.

Sarini, M. & Strapparava, C. (1998). Building a User Model for a Museum Exploration and Information-Providing Adaptive System. Proceedings of the 2nd Workshop on Adaptive Hypertext and Hypermedia, HYPERTEXT'98, Pittsburgh, USA, June 20-24, 1998.

Shneiderman, B. (1992). Tree visualization with Tree-maps. A 2-d space-filling approach. *ACM Transactions on Graphics*. Vol. 11, No. 1, September 92-99

Smallman, H., S., St. John, M., Oonk, H. M., & Cowen, M. B. (2001). Information Availability in 2D and 3D Displays, *IEEE Computer Graphics and Applications*, vol. 21, no. 5, 51-57.

Spence, R. (2001). *Information Visualization*. Addison-Wesley, ISBN: 978-0201596267.

Wu, J., & Storey, M.-A. (2000). A multi-perspective software visualization environment, *Proceedings of the 2000 conference of the Centre for Advanced Studies on Collaborative research*, ACM.

Section III
Adaptive Processing and Communication

Chapter X
Integrating Semantic Knowledge with Web Usage Mining for Personalization

Honghua Dai
DePaul University, USA

Bamshad Mobasher
DePaul University, USA

ABSTRACT

Web usage mining has been used effectively as an approach to automatic personalization and as a way to overcome deficiencies of traditional approaches such as collaborative filtering. Despite their success, such systems, as in more traditional ones, do not take into account the semantic knowledge about the underlying domain. Without such semantic knowledge, personalization systems cannot recommend different types of complex objects based on their underlying properties and attributes. Nor can these systems possess the ability to automatically explain or reason about the user models or user recommendations. The integration of semantic knowledge is, in fact, the primary challenge for the next generation of personalization systems. In this chapter we provide an overview of approaches for incorporating semantic knowledge into Web usage mining and personalization processes. In particular, we discuss the issues and requirements for successful integration of semantic knowledge from different sources, such as the content and the structure of Web sites for personalization. Finally, we present a general framework for fully integrating domain ontologies with Web usage mining and personalization processes at different stages, including the preprocessing and pattern discovery phases, as well as in the final stage where the discovered patterns are used for personalization.

INTRODUCTION

With the continued growth and proliferation of e-commerce, Web services, and Web-based information systems, personalization has emerged as a critical application that is essential to the success of a Website. It is now common for Web users to encounter sites that provide dynamic recommendations for products and services, targeted banner advertising, and individualized link selections. Indeed, nowhere is this phenomenon more apparent as in the business-to-consumer e-commerce arena. The reason is that, in today's highly competitive e-commerce environment, the success of a site often depends on the site's ability to retain visitors and turn casual browsers into potential customers. Automatic personalization and recommender system technologies have become critical tools, precisely because they help engage visitors at a deeper and more intimate level by tailoring the site's interaction with a visitor to her needs and interests.

Web personalization can be defined as any action that tailors the Web experience to a particular user, or a set of users (Mobasher, Cooley & Srivastava, 2000a). The experience can be something as casual as browsing a Website or as (economically) significant as trading stocks or purchasing a car. Principal elements of Web personalization include modeling of Web objects (pages, etc.) and subjects (users), categorization of objects and subjects, matching between and across objects and/or subjects, and determination of the set of actions to be recommended for personalization. The actions can range from simply making the presentation more pleasing to anticipating the needs of a user and providing customized information.

Traditional approaches to personalization have included both content-based and user-based techniques. Content-based techniques use personal profiles of users and recommend other items or pages based on their content similarity to the items or pages that are in the user's profile. The underlying mechanism in these systems is usually the comparison of sets of keywords representing pages or item descriptions. Examples of such systems include Letizia (Lieberman, 1995) and WebWatcher (Joachims, Freitag & Mitchell, 1997). While these systems perform well from the perspective of the end user who is searching the Web for information, they are less useful in e-commerce applications, partly due to the lack of server-side control by site owners, and partly because techniques based on content similarity alone may miss other types of semantic relationships among objects (for example, the associations among products or services that are semantically different, but are often used together).

User-based techniques for personalization, on the other hand, primarily focus on the similarities among users rather than item-based similarities. The most widely used technology user-based personalization is collaborative filtering (CF) (Herlocker, Konstan, Borchers & Riedl, 1999). Given a target user's record of activity or preferences, CF-based techniques compare that record with the historical records of other users in order to find the users with similar interests. This is the so-called *neighborhood* of the current user. The mapping of a visitor record to its neighborhood could be based on similarity in ratings of items, access to similar content or pages, or purchase of similar items. The identified neighborhood is then used to recommend items not already accessed or purchased by the active user. The advantage of this approach over purely content-based approaches that rely on content similarity in item-to-item comparisons is that it can capture "pragmatic" relationships among items based on their intended use or based on similar tastes of the users.

The CF-based techniques, however, suffer from some well-known limitations (Sarwar, Karypis, Konstan & Riedl, 2000). For the most part these limitations are related to the scalability and efficiency of the underlying algorithms, which requires real-time computation in both the neighborhood formation and the recommendation phases. The effectiveness and scalability of collaborative filtering can be dramatically enhanced by the application of Web usage mining techniques.

In general, *Web mining* can be characterized as the application of data mining to the content, structure, and usage of Web resources (Cooley, Mobasher & Srivastava, 1997; Srivastava, Cooley, Deshpande & Tan, 2000). The goal of Web mining is to automatically discover local as well as global models and patterns within and between Web pages or other Web resources. The goal of *Web usage mining,* in particular, is to capture and model Web user behavioral patterns. The discovery of such patterns from the enormous amount of data generated by Web and application servers has found a number of important applications. Among these applications are systems to evaluate the effectiveness of a site in meeting user expectations (Spiliopoulou, 2000), techniques for dynamic load balancing and optimization of Web servers for better and more efficient user access (Palpanas & Mendelzon, 1999; Pitkow & Pirolli, 1999), and applications for dynamically restructuring or customizing a site based on users' predicted needs and interests (Perkowitz & Etzioni, 1998).

More recently, Web usage mining techniques have been proposed as another user-based approach to personalization that alleviates some of the problems associated with collaborative filtering (Mobasher et al., 2000a). In particular, Web usage mining has been used to improve the scalability of personalization systems based on traditional CF-based techniques (Mobasher, Dai, Luo & Nakagawa, 2001, 2002).

However, the pure usage-based approach to personalization has an important drawback: the recommendation process relies on the existing user transaction data, and thus items or pages added to a site recently cannot be recommended. This is generally referred to as the "new item problem". A common approach to resolving this problem in collaborative filtering has been to integrate content characteristics of pages with the user ratings or judgments (Claypool et al., 1999; Pazzani, 1999). Generally, in these approaches, keywords are extracted from the content on the Website and are used to either index pages by content or classify pages into various content categories. In the context of personalization, this approach would allow the system to recommend pages to a user, not only based on similar users, but also (or alternatively) based on the content similarity of these pages to the pages the user has already visited.

Keyword-based approaches, however, are incapable of capturing more complex relationships among objects at a deeper semantic level based on the inherent properties associated with these objects. For example, potentially valuable relational structures among objects such as relationships between movies, directors, and actors, or between students, courses, and instructors, may be missed if one can only rely on the description of these entities using sets of keywords. To be able to recommend different types of complex objects using their underlying properties and attributes, the system must be able to rely on the characterization of user segments and objects, not just based on keywords, but at a deeper semantic level using the domain ontologies for the objects. For instance, a traditional personalization system on a university Website might recommend courses in Java to a student, simply because that student has previously taken or shown interest in Java courses. On the other hand, a system that has knowledge of the underlying domain ontology might recognize that the student should first satisfy the prerequisite requirements for a recommended course, or be able to recommend the best instructor for a Java course, and so on.

An *ontology* provides a set of well-founded constructs that define significant concepts and their semantic relationships. An example of an ontology is a relational schema for a database involving multiple tables and foreign keys semantically connecting these relations. Such constructs can be leveraged to build meaningful higher-level knowledge in a particular domain. Domain ontologies for a Website usually include concepts, subsumption relations between concepts (concept hierarchies), and other relations among concepts that exist in the domain that the Web site represents. For example, the domain ontologies of a movie Website usually include concepts such as "movie," "actor," "director," "theater," and so forth. The genre hierarchy can be used to represent different categories of movie concepts. Typical relations in this domain may include "Starring" (between actors and movies), "Directing," "Playing" (between theaters and movies), and so forth.

The ontology of a Website can be constructed by extracting relevant concepts and relations from the content and structure of the site, through machine learning and Web mining techniques. But, in addition to concepts and relations that can be acquired from Web content and structure information, we are also interested in usage-related concepts and relations in a Website. For instance, in an e-commerce Website, we may be interested in the relations between users and objects that define different types of online activity, such as browsing, searching, registering, buying, and bidding. The integration of such usage-based relations with ontological information representing the underlying concepts and attributes embedded in a site allows for more effective knowledge discovery, as well as better characterization and interpretation of the discovered patterns.

In the context of Web personalization and recommender systems, the use of semantic knowledge can lead to deeper interaction of the visitors or customers with the site. Integration of domain knowledge allows such systems to infer additional useful recommendations for users based on more fine grained characteristics of the objects being recommended, and provides the capability to explain and reason about user actions.

In this chapter we present an overview of the issues related to and requirements for successfully integrating semantic knowledge in the Web usage mining and personalization processes. We begin by providing some general background on the use of semantic knowledge and ontologies in Web mining, as well as an overview of personalization based on Web usage mining. We then discuss how the content and the structure of the site can be leveraged to transform raw usage data into semantically-enhanced transactions that can be used for semantic Web usage mining and personalization. Finally, we present a framework for more systematically integrating full-fledged domain ontologies in the personalization process.

BACKGROUND

Semantic Web Mining

Web mining is the process of discovering and extracting useful knowledge from the content, usage, and structure of one or more Web sites. Semantic Web mining (Berendt, Hotho & Stumme, 2002) involves the integration of domain knowledge into the Web mining process.

For the most part the research in semantic Web mining has been focused in application areas such as Web content and structure mining. In this section, we provide a brief overview and some examples of related work in this area. Few studies have focused on the use of domain knowledge in Web usage mining. Our goal in this chapter is to provide a road map for the integration of semantic and ontological knowledge into the process of Web usage mining, and particularly, in its application to Web personalization and recommender systems.

Domain knowledge can be integrated into the Web mining process in many ways. This includes leveraging explicit domain ontologies or implicit domain semantics extracted from the content or the structure of documents or Website. In general, however, this process may involve one or more of three critical activities: domain ontology acquisition, knowledge base construction, and knowledge-enhanced pattern discovery.

Domain Ontology Acquisition

The process of acquiring, maintaining and enriching the domain ontologies is referred to as "ontology engineering". For small Web sites with only static Web pages, it is feasible to construct a domain knowledge base manually or semi-manually. In Loh, Wives and de Oliveira (2000), a semi-manual approach is adopted for defining each domain concept as a vector of terms with the help of existing vocabulary and natural language processing tools.

However, manual construction and maintenance of domain ontologies requires a great deal of effort on the part of knowledge engineers, particularly for large-scale Websites or Websites with dynamically generated content. In dynamically generated Websites, page templates are usually populated based on structured queries performed against back-end databases. In such cases, the database schema can be used directly to acquire ontological information. Some Web servers send structured data files (e.g., XML files) to users and let client-side formatting mechanisms (e.g., CSS files) work out the final Web representation on client agents. In this case, it is generally possible to infer the schema from the structured data files.

When there is no direct source for acquiring domain ontologies, machine learning and text mining techniques must be employed to extract domain knowledge from the content or hyperlink structure of the Web pages. In Clerkin, Cunningham and Hayes (2001), a hierarchical clustering algorithm is applied to terms in order to create concept hierarchies. In Stumme, Taouil, Bastide, Pasquier and Lakhal (2000) a Formal Concept Analysis framework is proposed to derive a concept lattice (a variation of association rule algorithm). The approach proposed in Maedche and Staab (2000) learns generalized conceptual relations by applying association rule mining. All these efforts aim to *automatically* generate machine understandable ontologies for Website domains.

The outcome of this phase is a set of formally defined domain ontologies that precisely represent the Website. A good representation should provide machine understandability, the power of reasoning, and computation efficiency. The choice of ontology representation language has a direct effect on the flexibility of the data mining phase. Common representation approaches are vector-space model (Loh et al., 2000), descriptive logics (such as DAML+OIL) (Giugno & Lukasiewicz, 2002; Horrocks & Sattler, 2001), first order logic (Craven et al., 2000), relational models (Dai & Mobasher, 2002), probabilistic relational models (Getoor, Friedman, Koller & Taskar, 2001), and probabilistic Markov models (Anderson, Domingos & Weld, 2002).

Knowledge Base Construction

The first phase generates the formal representation of concepts and relations among them. The second phase, knowledge base construction, can be viewed as building mappings between concepts or relations on the one hand, and objects on the Web. The goal of this phase is to find the instances of the concepts and relations from the Website's domain, so that they can be exploited to perform further data mining tasks. Learning algorithms plays an important role in this phase.

In Ghani and Fano (2002), a text classifier is learned for each "semantic feature" (somewhat equivalent to the notion of a concept) based on a small manually labeled data set. First, Web pages are extracted from different Websites that belong to a similar domain, and then the semantic features are manually labeled. This small labeled data set is fed into a learning algorithm as the training data to learn the mappings between Web objects and the concept labels. In fact, this approach treats the process of assigning concept labels as filling "missing" data. Craven et al.

(2000) adopt a combined approach of statistical text classification and first order text classification in recognizing concept instances. In that study, learning process is based on both page content and linkage information.

Knowledge-Enhanced Web Data Mining

Domain knowledge enables analysts to perform more powerful Web data mining tasks. The applications include content mining, information retrieval and extraction, Web usage mining, and personalization. On the other hand, data mining tasks can also help to enhance the process of domain knowledge discovery.

Domain knowledge can improve the accuracy of document clustering and classification and induce more powerful content patterns. For example, in Horrocks (2002), domain ontologies are employed in selecting textual features. The selection is based on lexical analysis tools that map terms into concepts within the ontology. The approach also aggregates concepts by merging the concepts that have low support in the documents. After preprocessing, only necessary concepts are selected for the content clustering step. In McCallum, Rosenfeld, Mitchell and Ng (1998), a concept hierarchy is used to improve the accuracy and the scalability of text classification.

Traditional approaches to content mining and information retrieval treat every document as a set or a bag of terms. Without domain semantics, we would treat "human" and "mankind" as different terms, or, "brake" and "car" as unrelated terms. In Loh et al. (2000), a concept is defined as a group of terms that are semantically relevant, for example, as synonyms. With such concept definitions, concept distribution among documents is analyzed to find interesting concept patterns. For example, one can discover dominant themes in a document collection or in a single document; or find associations among concepts.

Ontologies and domain semantics have been applied extensively in the context of Web information retrieval and extraction. For example, the ARCH system (Parent, Mobasher & Lytinen, 2001) adopts concept hierarchies because they allow users to formulate more expressive and less ambiguous queries when compared to simple keyword-based queries. In ARCH, an initial user query is used to find matching concepts within a portion of concept hierarchy. The concept hierarchy is stored in an aggregated form with each node represented as a term vector. The user can select or unselect nodes in the presented portion of the hierarchy, and relevance feedback techniques are used to modify the initial query based on these nodes.

Similarly, domain-specific search and retrieval applications allow for a more focused and accurate search based on specific relations inherent in the underlying domain knowledge. The CiteSeer system (Bollacker, Lawrence & Giles, 1998) is a Web agent for finding interesting research publications, in which the relation "cited by" is the primary relation discovered among objects (i.e., among published papers). Thus, CiteSeer allows for comparison and retrieval of documents, not only based on similar content, but also based on inter-citation linkage structure among documents.

CiteSeer is an example of an approach for integrating semantic knowledge based on Web structure mining. In general, Web structure mining tasks take as input the hyperlink structure of Web pages (either belonging to a Website or relative to the whole Web), and output the underlying patterns (e.g., page authority values, linkage similarity, Web communities, etc.) that can be inferred from the hypertext co-citations. Another example of such an approach is the PageRank algorithm, which is the backbone of the Google search engine. PageRank uses the in-degree of indexed pages (i.e., number of pages referring to it) in order to rank pages based on quality or authoritativeness. Such algorithms that are based on the analysis of structural attributes can be further enhanced by integrating content semantics (Chakrabarti et al.,

1998). Web semantics can also enhance crawling algorithms by combining content or ontology with linkage information (Chakrabarti, van den Berg & Dom, 1999; Maedche, Ehrig, Handschuh, Volz & Stojanovic, 2002).

The use of domain knowledge can also provide tremendous advantages in Web usage mining and personalization. For example, semantic knowledge may help in interpreting, analyzing, and reasoning about usage patterns discovered in the mining phase. Furthermore, it can enhance collaborative filtering and personalization systems by providing concept-level recommendations (in contrast to item-based or user-based recommendations). Another advantage is that user demographic data, represented as part of a domain ontology, can be more systematically integrated into collaborative or usage-based recommendation engines. Several studies have considered various approaches to integrate content-based semantic knowledge into traditional collaborative filtering and personalization frameworks (Anderson et al., 2002; Claypool et al., 1999; Melville, Mooney & Nagarajan, 2002; Mobasher, Dai, Luo, Sun & Zhu, 2000b; Pazzani, 1999). Recently, we proposed a formal framework for integrating full domain ontologies with the personalization process based on Web usage mining (Dai & Mobasher, 2002).

WEB USAGE MINING AND PERSONALIZATION

The goal of personalization based on Web usage mining is to recommend a set of objects to the current (active) user, possibly consisting of links, ads, text, products, and so forth, tailored to the user's perceived preferences as determined by the matching usage patterns. This task is accomplished by matching the active user session (possibly in conjunction with previously stored profiles for that user) with the usage patterns discovered through Web usage mining. We call the usage patterns used in this context *aggregate usage profiles* since they provide an aggregate representation of the common activities or interests of groups of users. This process is performed by the recommendation engine which is the online component of the personalization system. If the data collection procedures in the system include the capability to track users across visits, then the recommendations can represent a longer term view of user's potential interests based on the user's activity history within the site. If, on the other hand, aggregate profiles are derived only from user sessions (single visits) contained in log files, then the recommendations provide a "short-term" view of user's navigational interests. These

Figure 1. General framework for Web personalization based on Web usage mining: The offline pattern discovery component

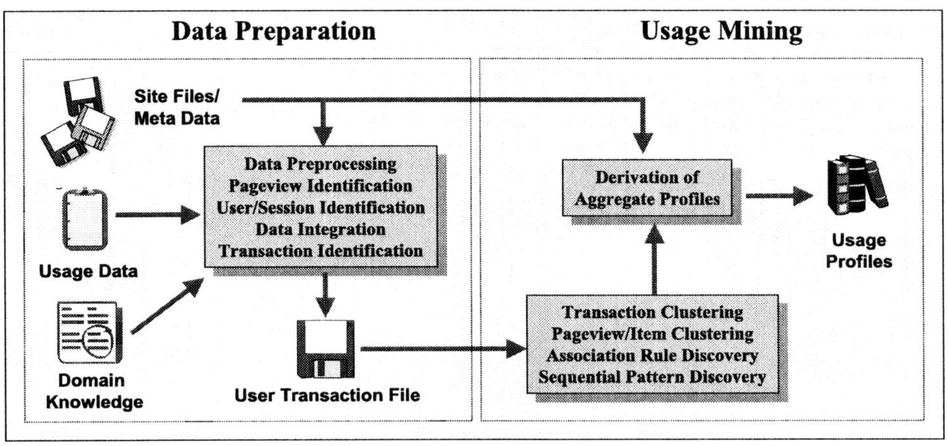

recommended objects are added to the last page in the active session accessed by the user before that page is sent to the browser.

The overall process of Web personalization based on Web usage mining consists of three phases: data preparation and transformation, pattern discovery, and recommendation. Of these, only the latter phase is performed in real-time. The data preparation phase transforms raw Web log files into transaction data that can be processed by data mining tasks. A variety of data mining techniques can be applied to this transaction data in the pattern discovery phase, such as clustering, association rule mining, and sequential pattern discovery. The results of the mining phase are transformed into aggregate usage profiles, suitable for use in the recommendation phase. The recommendation engine considers the active user session in conjunction with the discovered patterns to provide personalized content.

The primary data sources used in Web usage mining are the server log files, which include Web server access logs and application server logs. Additional data sources that are also essential for both data preparation and pattern discovery include the site files (HTML, XML, etc.) and meta-data, operational databases, and domain knowledge. Generally speaking, the data obtained through these sources can be categorized into four groups (see also Cooley, Mobasher, & Srivastava, 1999; Srivastava et al., 2000).

- **Usage data:** The log data collected automatically by the Web and application servers represents the fine-grained navigational behavior of visitors. Depending on the goals of the analysis, this data needs to be transformed and aggregated at different levels of abstraction. In Web usage mining, the most basic level of data abstraction is that of a *pageview*. Physically, a pageview is an aggregate representation of a collection of Web objects contributing to the display on a user's browser resulting from a single user action (such as a clickthrough). These Web objects may include multiple pages (such as in a frame-based site), images, embedded components, or script and database queries that populate portions of the displayed page (in dynamically generated sites). Conceptu-

Figure 2. General framework for Web personalization based on Web usage mining: The online personalization component

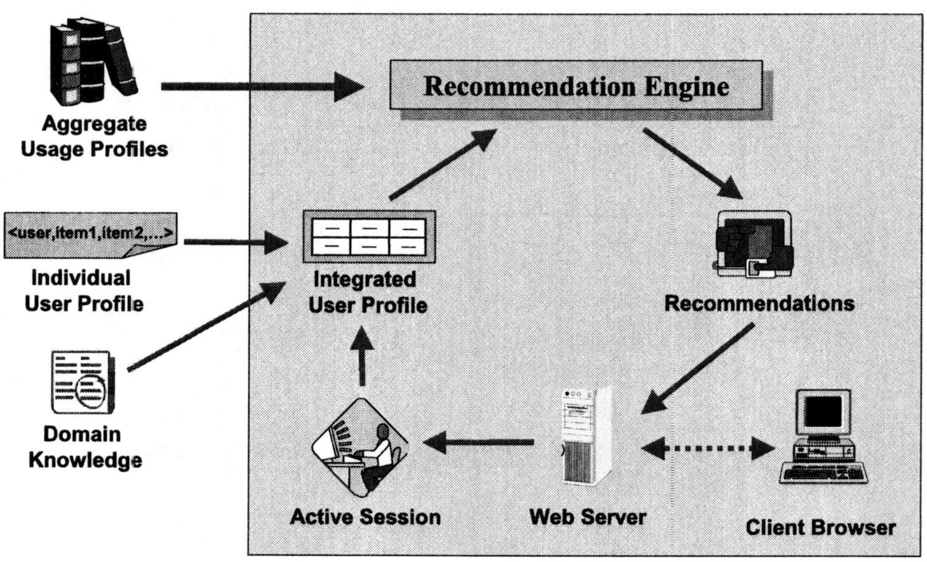

ally, each pageview represents a specific "type" of user activity on the site, e.g., reading a news article, browsing the results of a search query, viewing a product page, adding a product to the shopping cart, and so on. On the other hand, at the user level, the most basic level of behavioral abstraction is that of a *server session* (or simply a *session*). A session (also commonly referred to as a "visit") is a sequence of pageviews by a single user during a single visit. The notion of a session can be further abstracted by selecting a subset of pageviews in the session that are significant or relevant for the analysis tasks at hand. We shall refer to such a semantically meaningful subset of pageviews as a *transaction*. It is important to note that a transaction does not refer simply to product purchases, but it can include a variety of types of user actions as captured by different pageviews in a session.

- **Content data:** The content data in a site is the collection of objects and relationships that are conveyed to the user. For the most part, this data is comprised of combinations of textual material and images. The data sources used to deliver or generate this data include static HTML/XML pages, image, video, and sound files, dynamically generated page segments from scripts or other applications, and collections of records from the operational database(s). The site content data also includes semantic or structural meta-data embedded within the site or individual pages, such as descriptive keywords, document attributes, semantic tags, or HTTP variables. Finally, the underlying domain ontology for the site is also considered part of content data. The domain ontology may be captured implicitly within the site, or it may exist in some explicit form. The explicit representation of domain ontologies may include conceptual hierarchies over page contents, such as product categories, structural hierarchies represented by the underlying file and directory structure in which the site content is stored, explicit representation of semantic content and relationships via an ontology language such as RDF, or a database schema over the data contained in the operational databases.
- **Structure data:** The structure data represents the designer's view of the content organization within the site. This organization is captured via the inter-page linkage structure among pages, as reflected through hyperlinks. The structure data also includes the intra-page structure of the content represented in the arrangement of HTML or XML tags within a page. For example, both HTML and XML documents can be represented as tree structures over the space of tags in the page. The structure data for a site is normally captured by an automatically generated "site map" which represents the hyperlink structure of the site. A site mapping tool must have the capability to capture and represent the inter- and intra-pageview relationships. This necessity becomes most evident in a frame-based site where portions of distinct pageviews may represent the same physical page. For dynamically generated pages, the site mapping tools must either incorporate intrinsic knowledge of the underlying applications and scripts, or must have the ability to generate content segments using a sampling of parameters passed to such applications or scripts.
- **User data:** The operational database(s) for the site may include additional user profile information. Such data may include demographic or other identifying information on registered users, user ratings on various objects such as pages, products, or movies, past purchase or visit histories of users, as well as other explicit or implicit representation of users' interests. Obviously, capturing such data would require explicit interactions

with the users of the site. Some of this data can be captured anonymously, without any identifying user information, so long as there is the ability to distinguish among different users. For example, anonymous information contained in client-side cookies can be considered a part of the user's profile information, and can be used to identify repeat visitors to a site. Many personalization applications require the storage of prior user profile information. For example, collaborative filtering applications, generally, store prior ratings of objects by users, though, such information can be obtained anonymously, as well.

For a detailed discussion of preprocessing issues related to Web usage mining see Cooley et al. (1999). Usage preprocessing results in a set of n pageviews, $P = \{p_1, p_2, \cdots, p_n\}$, and a set of m user transactions, $T = \{t_1, t_2, \cdots, t_m\}$, where each t_i in T is a subset of P. *Pageviews* are semantically meaningful entities to which mining tasks are applied (such as pages or products). Conceptually, we view each transaction t as an l-length sequence of ordered pairs:

$$t = \left\langle (p_1^t, w(p_1^t)\ (p_2^t, w(p_2^t)\ \cdots, (p_l^t, w(p_l^t)) \right\rangle,$$

where each $p_i^t = p_j$ for some j in $\{1, \cdots, n\}$, and $w(p_i^t)$ is the weight associated with pageview p_i^t in transaction t, representing its significance (usually, but not exclusively, based on time duration).

For many data mining tasks, such as clustering and association rule discovery, as well as collaborative filtering based on the kNN technique, we can represent each user transaction as a vector over the n-dimensional space of pageviews. Given the transaction t above, the transaction vector $\vec{t}$ is given by: $t = \left\langle w_{p_1}^t, w_{p_2}^t, \cdots, w_{p_n}^t \right\rangle$, where each $w_{p_i}^t = w(p_j^t)$, for some j in $\{1, \cdots, n\}$, if p_j appears in the transaction t, and $w_{p_i}^t = 0$, otherwise. Thus, conceptually, the set of all user transactions can be viewed as an $m \times n$ transaction-pageview matrix, denoted by TP.

Given a set of transactions as described above, a variety of unsupervised knowledge discovery techniques can be applied to obtain patterns. These techniques such as clustering of transactions (or sessions) can lead to the discovery of important user or visitor segments. Other techniques such as item (e.g., pageview) clustering and association or sequential pattern discovery can be used to find important relationships among items based on the navigational patterns of users in the site. In each case, the discovered patterns can be used in conjunction with the active user session to provide personalized content. This task is performed by a recommendation engine.

REQUIREMENTS FOR SEMANTIC WEB USAGE MINING

In this section, we present and discuss the essential requirements in the integration of domain knowledge with Web usage data for pattern discovery. Our focus is on the critical tasks that particularly play an important role when the discovered patterns are to be used for Web personalization. As a concrete example, in the last part of this section we discuss an approach for integrating semantic features extracted from the content of Web sites with Web usage data, and how this integrated data can be used in conjunction with clustering to perform personalization. In the next section, we go beyond keyword-based semantics and present a more formal framework for integrating full ontologies with the Web usage mining and personalization processes.

Representation of Domain Knowledge

Representing Domain Knowledge as Content Features

One direct source of semantic knowledge that can be integrated into mining and personalization processes is the textual content of Web site pages. The semantics of a Web site are, in part, represented by the content features associated with items or objects on the Web site. These features include keywords, phrases, category names, or other textual content embedded as meta-information. Content preprocessing involves the extraction of relevant features from text and meta-data.

During the preprocessing, usually different weights are associated with features. For features extracted from meta-data, feature weights are usually provided as part of the domain knowledge specified by the analyst. Such weights may reflect the relative importance of certain concepts. For features extracted from text, weights can normally be derived automatically, for example as a function of the term frequency and inverse document frequency (tf.idf) which is commonly used in information retrieval.

Further preprocessing on content features can be performed by applying text mining techniques. This would provide the ability to filter the input to, or the output from, other mining algorithms. For example, classification of content features based on a concept hierarchy can be used to limit the discovered patterns from Web usage mining to those containing pageviews about a certain subject or class of products. Similarly, performing learning algorithms such as, clustering, formal concept analysis, or association rule mining on the feature space can lead to composite features representing concept categories or hierarchies (Clerkin, Cunningham, & Hayes, 2001; Stumme et al., 2000).

The integration of content features with usage-based personalization is desirable when we are dealing with sites where text descriptions are dominant and other structural relationships in the data are not easy to obtain, e.g., news sites or online help systems, etc. This approach, however, is incapable of capturing more complex relations among objects at a deeper semantic level based on the inherent properties associated with these objects. To be able to recommend different types of complex objects using their underlying properties and attributes, the system must be able to rely on the characterization of user segments and objects, not just based on keywords, but at a deeper semantic level using the domain ontologies for the objects. We will discuss some examples of how integrated content features and usage data can be used for personalization later in this Section.

Representing Domain Knowledge as Structured Data

In Web usage mining, we are interested in the semantics underlying a Web transaction or a user profile which is usually composed of a group of pageview names and query strings (extracted from Web server logs). Such features, in isolation, do not convey the semantics associated with the underlying application. Thus, it is important to create a mapping between these features and the objects, concepts, or events they represent.

Many e-commerce sites generate Web pages by querying operational databases or semi-structured data (e.g., XML and DTDs), from which semantic information can be easily derived. For Web sites in which such structured data cannot be easily acquired, we can adopt machine learning techniques to extract semantic information. Furthermore, the domain knowledge acquired should be machine understandable in order to allow for further processing or reasoning. Therefore, the extracted knowledge should be represented in some standard knowledge representation language.

DAML+OIL (Horrocks & Sattler, 2001) is an example of an ontology language that combines the Web standards from XML and RDF, with the reasoning capabilities from a description logic *SHIP(DL)*. The combinations of relational models and probabilistic models is another common approach to enhance Web personalization with domain knowledge and reasoning mechanism. Several approaches to personalization have used Relational Models such as Relational Markov Model (Anderson et al., 2002). Both of these approaches provide the ability to represent knowledge at different levels of abstraction, and the ability to reason about concepts, including about such relations as subsumption and membership.

In Dai & Mobasher (2002), we adopted the syntax and semantics of another ontology representation framework, *SHOQ(D),* to represent domain ontologies. In *SHOQ(D),* the notion of *concrete datatype* is used to specify literal values and *individuals* which represent real objects in the domain ontology. Moreover, *concepts* can be viewed as sets of individuals, and *roles* are binary relations between a pair of concepts or between concepts and data types. The detailed formal definitions for concepts and roles are given in Horrocks & Sattler (2001) and Giugno & Lukasiewicz (2002). Because our current work does not focus on reasoning tasks such as deciding subsumption and membership, we do not focus our discussion on these operations. The reasoning apparatus in *SHOQ(D)* can be used to provide more intelligent data mining services.

Building "Mappings" Between Usage-Level and Domain-Level Instances

During usage data preprocessing or post processing, we may want to assign domain semantics to user navigational patterns by mapping the pageview names or URLs (or queries) to the instances in the knowledge base. To be more specific, instead of describing a user's navigational path as: "a_1, a_2, ..., a_n" (where a_i is a URL pointing to a Web resource), we need to represent it using the instances from the knowledge base, such as: "movie(name=Matrix), movie(name=Spiderman), …, movie(name=Xman)." With the help of a pre-acquired concept hierarchy, we may, for example, be able to infer that the current user's interest is in the category of "Action&Sci-Fi." We refer to this "semantic" form of usage data as "Semantic User Profiles." These profiles, in turn, can be used for semantic pattern discovery and online recommendations. In the context of personalization applications, domain-level (semantic) instances may also need to be mapped back to Web resources or pages. For example, a recommendation engine using semantic user profiles may result in recommendations in the form of a movie genre. This concept must be mapped back into specific pages, URLs, or sections of the site relating to this genre before recommendations can be relayed to the user.

Using Content and Structural Characteristics

Classification algorithms utilizing content and structural features from pages are well-suited for creating mappings from usage data to domain-level instances. For example, in Craven et al. (2000) and Ghani & Fano (2002) classifiers are trained that exploit content or structural features (such as terms, linkage information, and term proximity) of the pageviews. From the pageview names or URLs we can obtain the corresponding Web content such as meta-data or keywords. With help from text classification algorithms, it is possible to efficiently map from keywords to attribute instances (Ghani & Fano, 2002).

Another good heuristics used in creating semantic mappings is based on the anchor text associated with hyperlinks. If we can build the complete user navigational path, we would be able to acquire the anchor text for each URL or pageview name. We can include the anchor text as part of the content features extracted from the body of documents or in isolation. However, whereas the text features in a document represent the semantics of the document, itself, the anchor text represents the semantics of the document to which the associated hyperlink points.

Using Query Strings

So far, we have overlooked the enormous amount of information stored in databases or semi-structured documents associated with a site. Large information servers often serve content integrated from **multiple** underlying servers and databases (Berendt, & Spiliopoulou, 2000). The dynamically generated pages on such servers are based on queries with multiple parameters attached to the URL corresponding to the underlying scripts or applications. Using the Web server query string recorded in the server log files it is possible to reconstruct the response pages. For example, the following are query strings from a hypothetical online bookseller Web site:

http://www.xyz.com/app.cgi?action=viewitem&item=1234567&category=1234
http://www.xyz.com/app.cgi?action=search&searchtype=title&searchstring= web+mining

http://www.xyz.com/app.cgi?action=order&item=1234567&category=1234& couponid=3456

If the background database or semi-structured documents are available, then we can access the content of the instances in the response pages via the name-value pairs from the query strings. This enriches our knowledge base of user interest. In the above bookseller Web site example, if we were able to access background database, we would be able to get the content of item "1234567" in category "1234". In this case, we could have the book name, price, author information of this item. We could recommend other books in the same content category or written by the same author. More generally, in well-designed sites, there is usually an explicitly available semantic mapping between query parameters and objects (such as products and categories), which would obviate the need to reconstruct the content of dynamic pages.

Levels of Abstraction

Capturing semantic knowledge at different levels of abstraction provides more flexibility both in the mining phase and in the recommendation phase. For example, focusing on higher-level concepts in a concept hierarchy would allow certain patterns to emerge which otherwise may be missed due to low support. On the other hand, the ability to drill-down into the discovered patterns based on finer-grained subconcepts would provide the ability to give more focused and useful recommendations.

Domain knowledge with attributes and relations requires the management of a great deal more data than is necessary in traditional approaches to Web usage mining. Thus, it becomes essential to prune unnecessary attributes or relations. For example, it may be possible to examine the number of distinct values of each attribute and generalize the attributes if there is a concept hierarchy over the attribute values. In Han & Fu (1995) a multiple-level association rule mining algorithm is proposed that utilizes concept hierarchies. For example, the usage data in our hypothetical movie site may not provide enough support for an association rule: "Spiderman, Xmen → Xmen2", but mining at a higher level may result in obtaining a rule: "Sci-Fi&Action, Xmen → Xmen2". In Anderson et al. (2002) relational Markov models are built by performing shrinkage (McCallum et al., 1998) between the estimates of parameters at all levels of abstractions relative to a concept hierarchy. If a pre-specified concept hierarchy does not exist, it is possible to automatically create such hierarchies through a variety of machine learning techniques, such as hierarchical agglomerative clustering (Stumme et al., 2000).

Integration of Semantics at Different Stages of Knowledge Discovery

The semantic information stored in the knowledge base can be leveraged at various steps in the knowledge discovery process, namely in the preprocessing phase, in the pattern discovery phase, or during the post-processing of the discovered patterns.

Preprocessing Phase

The main task of data preprocessing is to prune noisy and irrelevant data, and to reduce data volume for the pattern discovery phase. In Mobasher, Dai, Luo, & Nakagawa (2002), it was shown that applying appropriate data preprocessing techniques on usage data could improve the effectiveness of Web personalization. The concept level mappings from the pageview-level data to concepts can also be performed in this phase. This results in a transformed transaction data to which various data mining algorithms can be applied. Specifically, the transaction vector t given previously can be transformed into a vector $t' = \langle w^t_{o_1}, w^t_{o_2}, \cdots, w^t_{o_k} \rangle$, where each o_j is a semantic object appearing in one of the pageviews contained in the transaction, and $w^t_{o_j}$ is a weight associated with that object in the transaction. These semantic objects may be concepts appearing in the concept hierarchy or finer-grained objects representing instances of these concepts.

Pattern Discovery Phase

Successful utilization of domain knowledge in this phase requires extending basic data mining algorithms to deal with relational data to concept hierarchies. As an example, consider a distance-based data mining technique such as clustering. The clustering of flat single-relation data (such as Web user transactions) involves the computation of similarities or distance among transaction vectors. In such cases, normally simple vector-based operations are used. However, in the presence of integrated domain knowledge represented as concept hierarchies or ontologies, the clustering algorithms will have to perform much more complex similarity computations across dimensions and attributes. For example, even if the two user transactions have no pageviews in common, they may still be considered similar provided that the items occurring in both transactions are themselves "similar" based on some of their attributes or properties. The integration of domain knowledge will generate "semantic" usage patterns, introducing great flexibility as well as challenges. The flexibility lies in the pattern discovery being independent of item identities. The challenge is in the development of scalable and efficient algorithms to perform the underlying computational tasks such as similarity computations. We discuss this issue further below.

Post-Processing Phase

Exploiting domain knowledge in this phase can be used to further explain usage patterns or to filter out irrelevant patterns. One possibility is to first perform traditional usage mining tasks on the item-level usage data obtained in the preprocessing phase, and then use domain knowledge to interpret or transform the item level user profiles into "domain-level usage profiles" (Mobasher & Dai, 2002) involving concepts and relations in the ontology. The advantage of this approach is that we can avoid the scalability issues that can be endemic in the pattern discovery phase. The disadvantage is that some important structural relationships may not be used during the mining phase resulting in lower quality patterns.

Aggregation Methods for Complex Objects

To characterize patterns discovered through data mining techniques, it is usually necessary to derive aggregate representation of the patterns. An example of this situation is clustering applications. In the context of Web user transactions, clustering may result in a group of sessions or visitors that are considered similar because of their common navigational patterns. The vector representation of these transactions facilitates the aggregation tasks: the centroid (mean vector) of the transaction cluster acts as a representative of all of the transactions in that cluster. However, in the case of semantically enhanced transactions, the aggregation may have to be performed independently for each of the attributes associated with the objects contained in the cluster.

For example, clustering may result in a group of users who have all visited pages related to several movies. To be able to characterize this group of users at a deeper semantic level, it would be necessary to create an aggregate representation of the collection of movies in which they are interested. This task would require aggregation along each dimension corresponding to the attributes of "movie" instances, such as "genre", "actors", "directors", etc. Since each of these attributes require a different type of aggregation function depending on the data type and the domain, it may be necessary to associate various aggregation functions with the specification of the domain ontology, itself. In the next section we present one approach for solving this problem.

Measuring Semantic Similarities

Measuring similarities (alternatively, distances) among objects is a central task in many data mining algorithms. In the context of Web usage mining this may involve computing similarity measures among pageviews, among user transactions, or among users. This also becomes a critical task in personalization: a current user's profile must be matched with similar aggregate profiles representing the discovered user patterns or segments. As in the case of the aggregation problem discussed above, when dealing with semantically enhanced transactions, measuring similarities poses additional challenges. This is because the similarity of two transactions depends on the similarities of the semantic objects contained within the transactions.

Let us again consider the *static* vector model for representing a Web transaction t (or a user profile): $t = \langle w^t_{p1}, w^t_{p2}, \ldots, w^t_{pn} \rangle$. Computing similarity between two such vectors is straightforward and can be performed using measures such as cosine similarity, Euclidean distance, Pearson correlation (e.g., in case the weights represent user ratings).

When such vectors are transformed according to the underlying semantics, however, the computation of similarities will involve the computation of semantic similarities among the concepts or objects, possibly using different domain-specific similarity measures. Let A and B be two transformed transactions, each represented as a set of semantic objects in a site:

$$A = \{a_1, a_2, \cdots, a_m\} \text{ and } B = \{b_1, b_2, \cdots, b_l\}.$$

The computation of vector similarity between A and B, $Sim(A,B)$, is dependent on the semantic similarities among the component objects, $SemSim(a_i,b_j)$. For instance, one approach might be to compute the weighted sum or average of the similarities among object pairs. such as in:

$$Sim(A,B) = \frac{\sum_{a \in A} \sum_{b \in B} SemSim(a,b)}{|A| \cdot |B|}$$

In general, computing the semantic similarity, $SemSim(a,b)$, is domain dependent and requires knowledge of the underlying structure of among objects. If both objects can be represented using the same vector model (e.g., pages or documents represented as bags of words), we can compute their similarity using standard vector operations. On the other hand, if their representation includes attributes and relations specified in the domain ontology, we need to first make sure that the objects can be classified under a common ontological schema and then measure similarities along the different dimensions corresponding to each attribute. The notion of semantic matching among objects and classes has been a subject of considerable study recently (Rodriguez & Egenhofer, 2003; Palopoli, Sacca, Terracina, & Ursino, 2003; Ganesan, Garcia-Molina, & Widom, 2003).

For example, such an approach was used in Jin & Mobasher (2003) in the context of collaborative filtering with movies. In this work, association analysis was first performed on the "genre" attribute to define a genre hierarchy. Furthermore, the "year" attribute was discretized into intervals, while other attributes, such as "cast", were treated as a bag of words. These preprocessing steps allowed for the definition of appropriate similarity measures for each attribute. Finally, the semantic similarity between two movies, i and j, was defined as a linear combination of attribute-level similarities:

$$SemSim(i,j) = \alpha_1 * CastSim(i,j) + \alpha_2 * DirectorSim(i,j) + \alpha_3 * GenreSim(i,j) + ...,$$

where, α_i are predefined weights for the corresponding attributes.

Example: Using Content Features for Semantic Web Usage Mining

As an example of integrating semantic knowledge with the Web usage mining process, let us consider the especial case of using textual features from the content of Web pages to represent the underlying semantics for the site. As noted earlier, each pageview p can be represented as a k-dimensional feature vector, where k is the total number of extracted features (words or concepts) from the site in a global dictionary. This vector can be given by:

$$p = \langle fw(p,f_1), fw(p,f_2), \cdots, fw(p,f_k) \rangle$$

where $fw(p, f_j)$ is the weight of the jth feature in pageview p, for $1 \leq j \leq k$. For the whole collection of pageviews in the site, we then have an $n \times k$ pageview-feature matrix $PF = \{p_1, p_2, \cdots, p_n\}$.

There are now at least two basic choices as to when content features can be integrated into the usage-based personalization process: pre-mining integration or post-mining integration.

The pre-mining integration involves the transformation of user transactions, as described earlier, into "content-enhanced" transactions containing the semantic features of the pageviews. While, in practice, there are several ways to accomplish this transformation, the most direct approach involves mapping each pageview in a transaction to one or more content features. The range of this mapping can be the full feature space, or feature sets (composite features) which in turn may represent concepts and concept categories. Conceptually, the transformation can be viewed as the multiplication of the transaction-pageview matrix TP, defined earlier, with the pageview-feature matrix PF. The result is a new matrix $TF = \{t_1, t_2, \cdots, t_n\}$, where each t_i is a k-dimensional vector over the feature space. Thus, a user transaction can be represented as a content feature vector, reflecting that user's interests in particular concepts or topics.

Various data mining tasks can now be performed on the content-enhanced transaction data. For instance, if we apply association rule mining to such data, then we can get a group of association rules on content features. As an example, consider a site containing information about movies. This site may contain pages related to the movies themselves, actors appearing in the movies, directors, and genres. Association rule mining process could generate a rule such as: {"British", "Romance", "Comedy" $\Rightarrow$ "Hugh Grant"}, suggesting that users who are interested in British romantic comedies may also like the actor Hugh Grant (with a certain degree of confidence). During the online recommendation phase, the user's active session (which is also transformed into a feature vector) is compared with the discovered rules. Before recommendations are made, the matching patterns must be mapped back into Web pages or Web objects. In the above example, if the active session matches the left hand side of the association rule, the recommendation engine could recommend other Web pages that contain the feature "Hugh Grant".

The post-mining integration of semantic features involves combining the results of mining (performed independently on usage and content data) during the online recommendation phase. An example of this approach was presented in Mobasher et al. (2000b), where clustering algorithms were applied to both the transaction matrix *TP* and the transpose of the feature matrix *PF.* Since both matrices have pageviews as dimensions, the centroids of the resulting clusters in both cases can be represented as sets of pageview-weight pairs where the weights signify the frequency of the pageview occurrence in the corresponding cluster. We call the patterns generated from content data "content profiles", while the patterns derived from usage data are called "usage profiles". Though they share the same representation, they have different semantics: usage profiles represent a set of transactions with similar navigational behavior, while content profiles contain groups of Web pages with (partly) similar content.

Specifically, given a transaction cluster (respectively, a feature cluster) *cl,* we can construct the usage (respectively, content) profile pr_{cl} as a set of pageview-weight pairs by computing the centroid of *cl:*

$$pr_{cl} = \{\langle p, weight(p, pr_{cl})\rangle \mid weight(p, pr_{cl}) \geq \mu\},$$

where:

- the significance weight, $weight(p, pr_{cl})$, of the page p within the usage (respectively, content) profile pr_{cl} s given by:
$$weight(p, pr_{cl}) = \frac{1}{|cl|} \cdot \sum_{s \in cl} w(p,s)$$
- $w(p,s)$ is the weight of page p in transaction (respectively, feature) vector s in the cluster *cl;* and
- the threshold μ is used to focus only on those pages in the cluster that appear in a sufficient number of vectors in that cluster.

Each such profile, in turn, can be represented as a vector in the original n-dimensional space of pageviews. This aggregate representation can be used directly in the recommendation phase: given a new user, u who has accessed a set of pages, P_u, so far, we can measure the similarity of P_u to the discovered profiles, and recommend to the user those pages in matching profiles which have not yet been accessed by the user. Note that this approach does not distinguish between recommendations emanating from the matching content and usage profiles. Also note that there are many other ways of combining usage profiles and content profiles during the online recommendation phase. For example, we can use content profiles as the last resort in the situation where usage profiles can not provide sufficient number of recommendations.

A FRAMEWORK FOR ONTOLOGY-BASED PERSONALIZATION

At a conceptual level, there may be many different kinds of objects within a given site that are accessible to users. At the physical level, these objects may be represented by one or more Web pages. For example, our hypothetical movie site may contain pages related to the movies, actors, directors, and studios. Conceptually, each of these entities represents a different type of semantic object. During a visit to this site, a user may implicitly access several of these objects together during a session by navigating to various pages containing them. In contrast to content features, ontological representation of domain knowledge contained in the site makes it possible to have a uniform architecture to model such objects, their properties, and their relationships. Furthermore, such a representation would allow for a more natural mapping between the relational schema for the backend databases driving Web applications and the navigational behavior of users.

In this section we will present a general framework for utilizing domain ontologies in Web usage mining and personalization. Figure 3 lays out a

Figure 3. A General framework for personalization based on domain ontologies

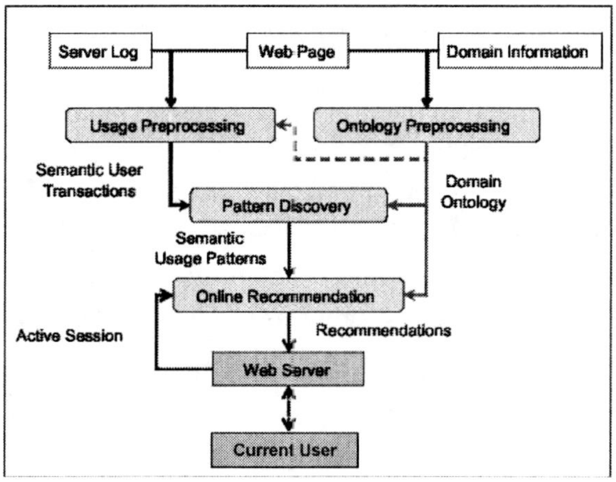

general process for such an integrated approach. In keeping with our earlier discussion, it is composed of three main phases: preprocessing, pattern discovery and online recommendation. Each of these phases must take into account the object properties and their relationships as specified in a domain ontology.

We assume that the site ontology is already available (either specified manually, or extracted automatically using ontology learning techniques). The goal of the preprocessing phase is to transform users' navigational transactions into "semantic transaction" by mapping accessed pages and resource to concepts and objects of the specified ontology. The goal of the pattern discovery phase is to create aggregate representation of groups of semantic objects that are implicitly accessed by similar users, thus providing a semantic characterization of user segments with common behavior or interests. Finally, in the recommendation phase, the discovered semantic patterns are utilized in conjunction with an ongoing record of a current user's activity (including, possibly the user's stored profile) to recommend new resources, pages, or objects to that user.

Knowledge Representation

General ontology representation languages such as DAML+OIL (Horrocks, 2002) provide formal syntax and semantics for representing and reasoning with various elements of an ontology. These elements include "individuals" (or objects), "concepts" (which represent sets of individuals), and "roles" (which specify object properties). In DAML+OIL, the notion of a concept is quite general and may encompass a heterogeneous set of objects with different properties (roles) and structures. We, on the other hand, are mainly interested in the aggregate representations for groups of objects that have a homogenous concept structure (i.e., have similar properties and data types). For example, we may be interested in a group of movie objects, each of which has specific values for properties such as "year", "genre", and "actors." We call such a group of objects a *class*. Thus, in our framework, the notion of a class represents a restriction of the notion of a concept in DAML+OIL. It should be noted, however, that the users of a Web site, in general, access a variety of objects belonging to different classes. Thus, this homogeneity assumption would imply that semantic objects within user transactions must first be classified into homogenous classes as a preprocessing step.

More specifically, we define a *class* C as a set of objects together with a set of *attributes*. These attributes together define the internal properties of the objects in C or relationships with other concepts that involve the objects in C. Thus attributes of a class correspond to a subset of the set of roles in the domain ontology. We denote the domain of values of an attribute r as D_r. Furthermore, because we are specifically interested in aggregating objects at the attribute level, we extend the notion of a role to include a domain-specific combination function and an ordering relation.

More formally, a class C is characterized by a finite set of attributes AC, where each attribute a in AC is defined as follows.

Definition: Let C be a class in the domain ontology. An *attribute a AC* is a 4-tuple, where $a = \langle T_a, D_a, \prec_a, \psi_a \rangle$
- T_a is the *type* for the values for the attribute a.
- D_a is the domain of the values for a;
- $\prec_a$ is an ordering relation among the values in D_a; and
- ψ_a is a *combination function* for the attribute a.

The "type" of an attribute in the above definition may be a concrete datatype (such as "string" or "integer") or it may be a set of objects (individuals) belonging to another class.

In the context of data mining, comparing and aggregating values are essential tasks. Therefore, ordering relations among values are necessary properties for attributes. We associate an ordering relation $\prec_a$ with elements in D_a for each attribute a. The ordering relation $\prec_a$ can be null (if no ordering is specified in the domain of values), or it can define a partial or a total order among the domain values. For standard types such as values from a continuous range, we assume the usual ordering. In cases when an attribute a represents a concept hierarchy, the domain values of a are a set of labels, and $\prec_a$ is a partial order representing the "is-a" relation.

Furthermore, we associate a data mining operator, called the *combination function*, ψ_a, with each attribute a. This combination function defines an aggregation operation among the corresponding attribute values of a set of objects belonging to the same class. This function is essentially a generalization of the "mean" or "average" function applied to corresponding dimension values of a set of vectors when computing the centroid vector. In this context, we assume that the combination function is specified as part of the domain ontology for each attribute of a class. An interesting extension would be to automatically learn the combination function for each attribute based on a set of positive and negative examples.

Classes in the ontology define the structural and semantic properties of objects in the domain which are "instances" of that class. Specifically, each object o in the domain is also characterized by a set of attributes A_o corresponding to the attributes of a class in the ontology. In order to more precisely define the notion of an object as an instance of a class, we first define the notion of an instance of an attribute.

Definition: Given an attribute $a = \langle T_a, D_a, \prec_a, \psi_a \rangle$ and an attribute $b = \langle T_b, D_b, \prec_b, \psi_b \rangle$, b is an *instance* of a, if $D_b \subseteq D_a$, $T_b = T_a$, $\psi_b = \psi_a$, and $\prec_b$ is a restriction of $\prec_a$ to D_b. The attribute b is a *null instance* of a, if Db is empty.

Definition: Given a class C with attribute set $A_C = \{a_1^C, a_2^C, \cdots, a_n^C\}$, we say that an object o is *an instance of* C, if o has attributes $A_o = \{a_1^o, a_2^o, \cdots, a_n^o\}$ such that each is a, possibly null, instance of a_1^C.

Based on the definitions of attribute and object instances, we can now provide a more formal representation of the combination function ψ_a. Let C be a class and $\{o_1, o_2, \cdots, o_m\}$ a set of object instances of C. Let $a \in A_C$ be an attribute of class C. The combination function ψ_a can be represented by:

$$\psi_a\left(\left\{\langle a_{o_1}, w_1\rangle, \langle a_{o_2}, w_2\rangle, \cdots, \langle a_{o_m}, w_m\rangle\right\}\right) = \langle a_{agg}, w_{agg}\rangle$$

where each belonging to object o_i is an instance of the attribute a, and each w_i is a weight associated with that attribute instance (representing the significance of that attribute relative to the other instances). Furthermore, a_{agg} is a *pseudo instance* of a meaning that it is an instance of a which does not belong to a real object in the underlying domain. The weight w_{agg} of a_{agg} is a function of $w_1, w_2, ..., w_n$.

Given a set of object instances, of a class *C*, a *domain-level aggregate profile* for these instances is obtained by applying the combination function for each attribute in *C* to all of the corresponding attribute instances across all objects $o_1, o_2, ..., o_n$.

Ontology Preprocessing

The ontology preprocessing phase takes as input domain information (such as database schema and metadata, if any) as well as Web pages, and generates the site ontology. For simple Web sites, ontologies can be easily designed manually or derived semi-automatically from the site content. However, it is more desirable to have automatic ontology acquisition methods for a large Web site, especially in Web sites with dynamically generated Web pages. E-commerce Web sites, for instance, usually have well-structured Web content, including predefined metadata or database schema. Therefore it is easier to build automatic ontology extraction mechanisms that are site-specific.

There have been a number of efforts dealing with the ontology learning problem (Clerkin et al., 2001; Craven et al., 2000; Maedche & Staab, 2000). A wide range of information, such as thesauri, content features, and database schema can help to identify ontologies. Many of these approaches have focused on extracting ontological information from the Web, in general. In Berendt et al. (2002) the notion of "Semantic Web Mining" was introduced, including a framework for the extraction of a concept hierarchy and the application of data mining techniques to find frequently occurring combinations of concepts.

An Example

As an example, let us revisit our hypothetical movie Web site. The Web site includes collections of pages containing information about movies, actors, directors, etc. A collection of pages describing a specific movie might include information such as the movie title, genre, starring actors, director, etc. An actor or director's information may include name, filmography (a set of movies), gender, nationality, etc. The portion of domain ontology for this site, as described, contains the classes **Movie, Actor** and **Director** (Figure 4). The collection of Web pages in the site represents a group of embedded objects that are the instances of these classes.

In our example, the class **Movie** has attributes such as *Year, Actor* (representing the relation "acted by"), *Genre,* and *Director*. The *Actor* and *Director* attributes have values that are other objects in the ontology, specifically, object instances of classes **Actor** and **Director,** respectively. The attribute *Year* is an example of an attribute whose datatype is positive integers with the usual ordering. The attribute *Genre* has a concrete datatype whose domain values in D_{Genre} are a set of labels (e.g., "Romance" and "Comedy"). The ordering relation $\prec_{Genre}$ defines a partial order based on the "is-a" relation among subsets of these labels (resulting in a concept hierarchy of Genres, a portion of which is shown in Figure 4).

Figure 5 shows a **Movie** instance "About a Boy" and its related attributes and relations extracted from a Web page. The schema of the class **Movie** is shown at the bottom left portion

Figure 4. Ontology for a movie Web site

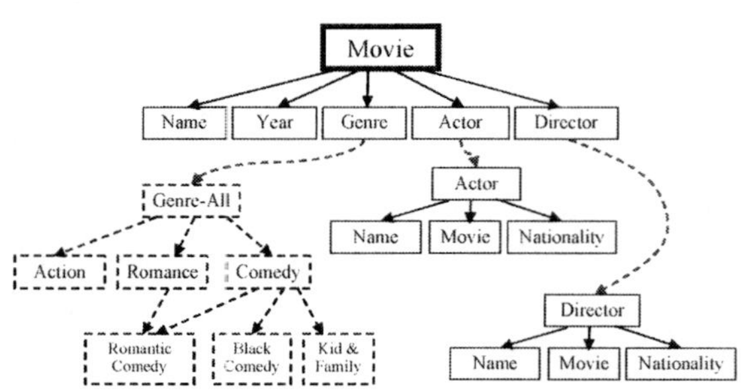

Figure 5. Example of ontology preprocessing

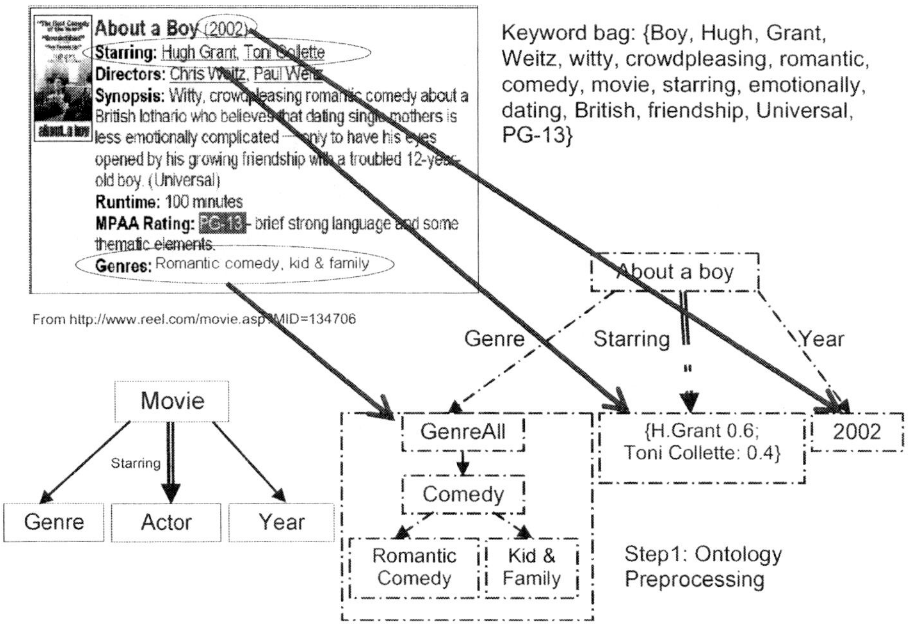

of the figure. Here we treat the classes **Genre** and **Year** as attributes of the class **Movie**. The instances of the ontology are shown at the bottom right of the figure. The *Genre* attribute contains a partial order among labels representing a concept hierarchy of movie genres. We use a restriction of this partial order to represent the genre to which the **Movie** instance belongs. The diagram also shows a keyword bag containing the important keywords in that page.

An attribute a of an object o has a domain D_a. In cases when the attribute has unique a value for an object, D_a is a singleton. For example, consider an object instance of class **Movie,** "About a Boy" (see Figure 5). The attribute *Actor* contains two objects "H. Grant" and "T. Collette" that are instances of the class **Actor** (for the sake of presentation we use the actors' names to stand for the object instances of **Actor**). Therefore, D_{Actor} = {"H. Grant", "T. Collette"}. Also, a real object may have values for only some of the attributes. In this case the other attributes have empty domains. For instance, the attribute *Director* in the example has an empty domain and is thus not depicted in the figure. We may, optionally, associate a weight with each value in the attribute domain D_a (usually in the range [0,1]). This may be useful in capturing the relative importance of each attribute value.

For example, in a given movie the main actors should have higher weights than other actors in the cast. In our example, the object "H. Grant" has weight 0.6 and the object "Toni Collette" has weight 0.4. Unless otherwise specified, we assume that the weight associated with each attribute value is 1. In the object o shown in Figure 5, the domain for the attribute *Genre* is the set of labels {Genre-All, Action, Romance, Comedy, Romantic Comedy, Black Comedy, Kids & Family}. The ordering relation $\prec^{o}_{Genre}$ is a restriction of $\prec_{Genre}$ to the subset {Genre-All, Comedy, Romantic Comedy, Kids & Family}.

Pattern Discovery

As depicted in Figure 3 domain ontologies can be incorporated into usage preprocessing to generate semantic user transactions, or they can be integrated into pattern discovery phase to generate semantic usage patterns. In the following example, we will focus on the latter approach.

Given a discovered usage profile (for example, a set of pageview-weight pairs obtained by clustering user transactions), we can transform it into a domain-level aggregate representation of the underlying objects (Dai & Mobasher, 2002). To distinguish between the representations we call the original discovered pattern an "item-level" usage profile, and we call the new profile based on the domain ontology a "domain-level" aggregate profile. The item-level profile is first represented as a weighted set of objects: $pr = \{\langle o_1, w_1\rangle, \langle o_2, w_2\rangle, \cdots, \langle o_n, w_n\rangle$ in which each o_i is an object in the underlying domain ontology and w_i represents o_i's significance in the profile *pr*. Here we assume that, either using manual rules, or through supervised learning methods, we can extract various object instances represented by the pages in the original page- or item-level usage profile. The transformed profile represents a set of objects accessed together frequently by a group of users (as determined through Web usage mining). Objects, in the usage profile, that belong to the same class are combined to form an aggregated pseudo object belonging to that class. An important benefit of aggregation is that the pattern volume is significantly reduced, thus relieving the computation burden for the recommendation engine. Our goal is to create an aggregate representation of this weighted set of objects to characterize the common interests of the user segment captured by the usage profile at the domain level.

Given the representation of a profile *pr* as a weighted set of objects, the objects in *pr* may be instances of different classes $C_1, C_2, ..., C_k$ in the ontology. The process of creating a domain-level aggregate profile begins by partitioning *pr* into collections of objects with each collection containing all objects that are instances of a specified class (in other words, the process of classifying the object instances in *pr)*. Let G_i denote the elements of *pr* that are instances of the class C_i.

Having partitioned *pr* into *k* groups of homogeneous objects, $G_1, ..., G_k$, the problem is reduced to creating aggregate representation of each partition G_i. This task is accomplished with the help of the combination functions for each of the attributes of C_i some of whose object instances are contained in G_i. Once the representatives for every partition of objects are created, we assign a significance weight to each representative to mark the importance of this group of objects in the profile. In our current approach the significance weight for each representative is computed as the weighted sum of all the object weights in the partition. However, significance weight can be computed using other numeric aggregation functions.

Examples Continued: Generating Domain-Level Aggregate Profiles

To illustrate the semantic aggregation process, let us return to our movie site example. The aggregation process requires that a "combination function" be defined for each attribute of an object in the domain ontology. Figure 6 and 8 show an example of such process. Each movie object has attribute "Name", "Actor", "Genre" and "Year". For the attribute *Name,* we are interested in all the movie names appearing in the instances. Thus we can define ψ_{Name} to be the union operation performed on all the singleton *Name* attributes of all movie objects. On the other hand, the attribute *Actor* contains a weighted set of objects belonging to class **Actor**. In fact, it represents the relation "Starring" between the actor objects and the movie object. In such cases we can use a vector-based weighted mean operation as the combination function. For example, we will determine the aggregate weight of an actor object *o* by:

Figure 6. Creating an aggregate representation of a set of movie objects

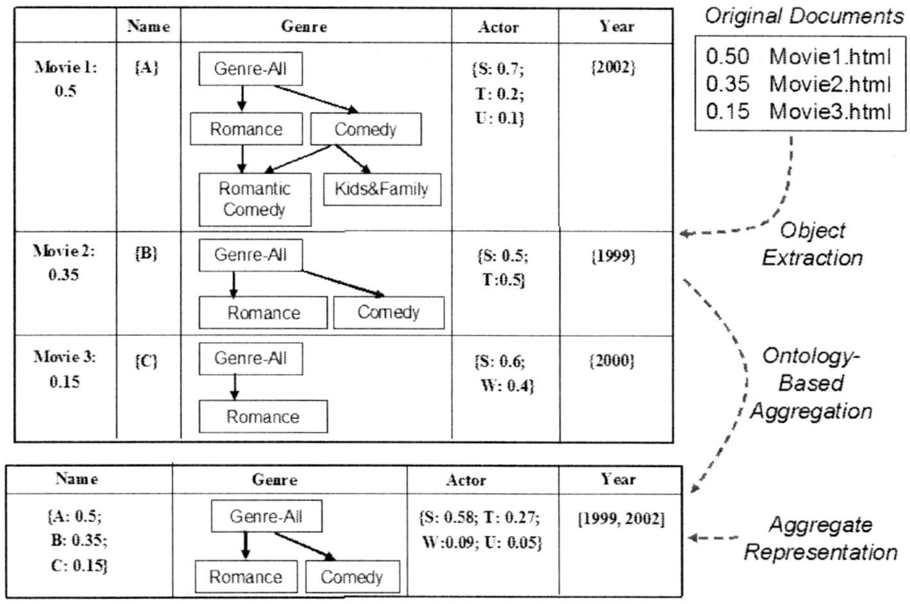

$$w'_o = \left(\sum_i w_i \cdot w_o\right) / \sum_i w_i .$$

Applying ψ_{Actor} in our example will result in the aggregate actor object {⟨*S*, 0.58⟩, ⟨*T*, 0.27⟩, ⟨*U*, 0.09⟩}. As for the attribute *Year,* the combination function may create a range of all the *Year* values appearing in the objects. Another possible solution is to discretize the full *Year* range into decades and find the most common decades that are in the domains of the attribute. In our example, using the range option, this may result in an aggregate instance [1999, 2002] for the *Year* attribute.

The attribute *Genre* of **Movie** contains a partial order representing a concept hierarchy among different *Genre* values. The combination function, in this case, can perform tree (or graph) matching to extract the common parts of the conceptual hierarchies among all instances. Extracting the common nodes from this hierarchy may also depend on the weights associated with the original objects leading to different weights on the graph edges. For example, given that the higher weight Movies 1 and 2 have "Romance" in common, this node may be selected for the aggregate instance, even though it is not present in Movie 3. However, the weight of "Romance" may be less than that of "Comedy" which is present in all three movies.

Figure 6 shows the item-level usage profile and its representation as a weighted set of objects, as well as the resulting domain-level aggregate profile. Note that the original item-level profile gives us little information about the reasons why these objects were commonly accessed together. However, after we characterize this profile at the domain-level, we find some interesting patterns: they all belong to *Genre* "Comedy" (and to a lesser degree "Romance), and the actor *S* has a high score compared with other actors.

Online Recommendation Phase

In contrast to transaction-based usage profiles, semantic usage profiles capture the underlying common properties and relations among those objects. This fine-grained domain knowledge, captured in aggregate form enables more powerful approaches to personalization. As before, we consider the browsing history of the current user, i.e., active session, to be a weighted set of Web pages that the user has visited. The same transformation described in the last subsection can be used to create a semantic representation of the user's active session. We call this representation the *current user profile*.

Figure 7 presents the basic procedure for generating recommendations based on semantic profiles. The recommendation engine matches the current user profile against the discovered domain-level aggregate profiles. The usage profiles with matching score greater than some pre-specified threshold are considered to represent this user's potential interests. A successful match implies that the current user shares common interests with the group of users represented by the profile. The matching process results in an *extended user profile* which is obtained by applying the aggregation process described above to the domain-level profiles and the original user profile.

Figure 7. Online recommendation enhanced by domain ontologies

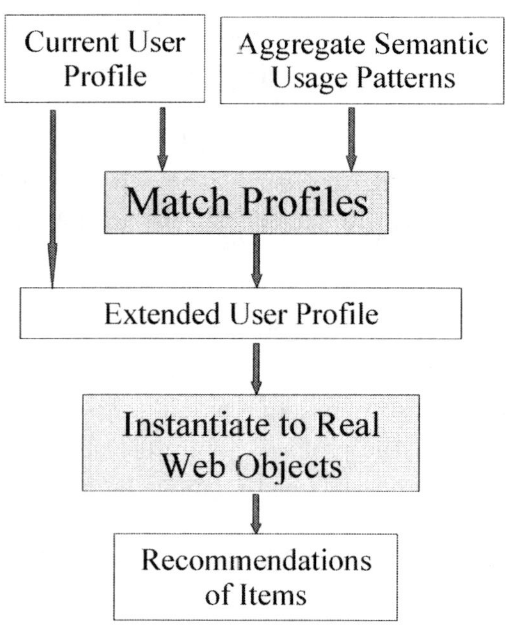

The recommendation engine then instantiates the user's extended profile to real Web objects and will recommend them to the user. We can also exploit structural relationships among classes during the recommendation process. For example, if a concept hierarchy exists among objects, and the recommendation engine can not find a good match for a user profile at a certain concept level, then it can generalize to a more abstract level (e.g., from "romantic comedy" to "romance").

This approach has several advantages over traditional usage-based personalization. First, it retains the user-to-user relationships that can be captured by the discovered usage profiles. Secondly, in contrast to standard collaborative filtering, it provides more flexibility in matching aggregate usage profiles with the current user's activity because the matching process involves comparison of features and relationships, not exact item identities. Thirdly, the items do not have to appear in any usage profiles in order to be recommended, since fine-grained domain relationships are considered during the instantiation process. The previous example shows that this approach can also be used to solve the "new item" problem. Furthermore, it can alleviate the notorious "sparsity" problem in collaborative filtering systems by allowing for "fuzzy" comparisons between two user profiles (or ratings). The basis for matching profiles does not have to be similar ratings on the same items. The comparison can be based on showing interest in different objects with similar properties (for example, purchasing items that have same brand). Therefore, even if the raw transaction or rating data is sparse, the semantic attributes of items or users can be used to indirectly infer potential interest in other items.

CONCLUSION

We have explored various approaches, requirements, and issues for integrating semantic knowledge into the personalization process based on Web usage mining. We have considered approaches based on the extraction of semantic features from the textual content contained in a site and their integration with Web usage mining tasks and personalization both in the pre-mining and the post-mining phases of the process. We have also presented a framework for Web personalization based on full integration of domain ontologies and usage patterns. The examples provided throughout this chapter reveal how such a framework can provide insightful patterns and smarter personalization services.

We leave some interesting research problems for open discussion and future work. Most important among these are techniques for computing similarity between domain objects and aggregate domain-level patterns, as well as learning techniques to automatically determine appropriate combination functions used in the aggregation process.

More generally, the challenges lie in the successful integration of ontological knowledge at every stage of the knowledge discovery process. In the preprocessing phase, the challenges are in automatic methods for the extraction and learning of the ontologies and in the mapping of users' activities at the clickstream level to more abstracts concepts and classes. For the data mining phase, the primary goal is to develop new approaches that take into account complex semantic relationships such as those present in relational databases with multiple relations. Indeed, in recent years, there has been more focus on techniques such as those based relational data mining. Finally in the personalization stage, the challenge is in developing techniques that can successfully and efficiently measure semantic similarities among complex objects (possibly from different ontologies).

In this chapter we have only provided an overview of the relevant issues and suggested a road map for further research and development in this area. We believe that the successful integration of semantic knowledge with Web usage mining is likely to lead to the next generation of personalization tools which are more intelligent and more useful for Web users.

REFERENCES

Anderson, C., Domingos, P., & Weld, D. (2002). Relational markov models and their application to adaptive Web navigation. *Proceedings of the Eighth ACM SIGKDD International Conference on Knowledge Discovery and Data Mining* (KDD-2002), Edmonton, Alberta, Canada.

Berendt, B., & Spiliopoulou, M. (2000). Analysing navigation behaviour in Websites integrating multiple information systems. *VLDB Journal, Special Issue on Databases and the Web, 9*(1), 56-75.

Berendt, B., Hotho, A., & Stumme, G. (2002). Towards semantic Web mining. *Proceedings of the First International Semantic Web Conference* (ISWC02), Sardinia, Italy.

Bollacker, K., Lawrence, S., & Giles, C.L. (1998). Citeseer: An autonomous Web agent for automatic retrieval and identification of interesting publications. *Proceedings of the Second International Conference on Autonomous Agents*, Minneapolis, Minnesota.

Chakrabarti, S., Dom, B., Gibson, D., Kleinberg, J., Raghavan, P., & Rajagopalan, S. (1998). Automatic resource list compilation by analyzing hyperlink structure and associated text. *Proceedings of the 7th International World Wide Web Conference*, Brisbane, Australia.

Chakrabarti, S., van den Berg, M., & Dom, B. (1999). Focused crawling: A new approach to topic-specific Web resource discovery. *Proceedings of the 3rd World Wide Web Conference*, Toronto.

Claypool, M., Gokhale, A., Miranda, T., Murnikov, P., Netes, D., & Sartin, M. (1999). Combining content-based and collaborative filters in an online newspaper. *Proceedings of the ACM SIGIR '99 Workshop on Recommender Systems: Algorithms and Evaluation*, Berkeley, California.

Clerkin, P., Cunningham, P., & Hayes, C. (2001). Ontology discovery for the semantic Web using hierarchical clustering. *Semantic Web Mining Workshop at ECML/PKDD-2001*, Freiburg, Germany.

Cooley, R., Mobasher, B., & Srivastava, J. (1997). Web mining: Information and pattern discovery on the World Wide Web. *Proceedings of the International Conference on Tools with Artificial Intelligence*, 558-567, Newport Beach. IEEE Press.

Cooley, R., Mobasher, B., & Srivastava, J. (1999). Data preparation for mining World Wide Web browsing patterns. *Journal of Knowledge and Information Systems, 1*(1), 5-32.

Craven, M., DiPasquo, D., Freitag, D., McCallum, A., Mitchell, T., Nigam, K., & Slattery, S. (2000). Learning to construct knowledge bases from the World Wide Web. *Artificial Intelligence, 118*(1-2), 69-113.

Dai, H., & Mobasher, B. (2002). Using ontologies to discover domain-level Web usage profiles. *Proceedings of the 2nd Semantic Web Mining Workshop at ECML/PKDD 2002*, Helsinki, Finland.

Ganesan, P., Garcia-Molina, H., & Widom, J. (2003). Exploiting hierarchical domain structure to compute similarity. *ACM Transactions on Information Systems, 21*(1), 63-94.

Getoor, L., Friedman, N., Koller, D., & Taskar, B. (2001). Learning probabilistic models of relational structure. *Proceedings of the 18th International Conference on Machine Learning.*

Ghani, R., & Fano, A. (2002). Building recommender systems using a knowledge base of product semantics. *Proceedings of the Workshop on Recommendation and Personalization in E-Commerce*, 2nd International Conference on Adaptive Hypermedia and Adaptive Web Based Systems, Malaga, Spain.

Giugno, R., & Lukasiewicz, T. (2002). P-SHOQ(D): A probabilistic extension of SHOQ(D) for probabilistic ontologies in the semantic Web. *Proceedings of the 8th European Conference on Logics in Artificial Intelligence*, Cosenza, Italy.

Han, J., & Fu, Y. (1995). Discovery of multiple-level association rules from large databases. *Proceedings of the 1995 International Conference on Very Large Data Bases* (VLDB95), Zurich, Switzerland.

Herlocker, J., Konstan, J., Borchers, A., & Riedl, J. (1999). An algorithmic framework for performing collaborative filtering. *Proceedings of the 22nd ACM Conference on Research and Development in Information Retrieval* (SIGIR'99), Berkeley, CA.

Horrocks, I. (2002). DAML+OIL: A description logic for the semantic Web. *IEEE Data Engineering Bulletin, 25*(1), 4-9.

Horrocks, I., & Sattler, U. (2001). Ontology reasoning in the SHOQ(D) description logic. *Proceedings of the 17th International Joint Conference on Artificial Intelligence*, Seattle, WA.

Hotho, A., Maedche, A., & Staab, S. (2001). Ontology-based text clustering. *Proceedings of the IJCAI-2001 Workshop Text Learning: Beyond Supervision*, Seattle, WA.

Jin, X., & Mobasher, B. (2003). Using semantic similarity to enhance item-based collaborative filtering. *Proceedings of The 2nd IASTED International Conference on Information and Knowledge Sharing*, Scottsdale, Arizona.

Joachims, T., Freitag, D., & Mitchell, T. (1997). Webwatcher: A tour guide for the World Wide Web. *Proceedings of the 15th International Conference on Artificial Intelligence*, Nagoya, Japan.

Lieberman, H. (1995). Letizia: An agent that assists Web browsing. *Proceedings of the 1995 International Joint Conference on Artificial Intelligence*, Montreal, Canada.

Loh, S., Wives, L.K., & de Oliveira, J.P. (2000). Concept-based knowledge discovery in texts extracted from the Web. *SIGKDD Explorations, 2*(1), 29-39.

Maedche, A., & Staab, S. (2000). Discovering conceptual relations from text. *Proceedings of the European Conference on Artificial Intelligence* (ECAI00), Berlin.

Maedche, A., Ehrig, M., Handschuh, S., Volz, R., & Stojanovic, L. (2002). Ontology-focused crawling of documents and relational metadata. *Proceedings of the 11th International World Wide Web Conference* (WWW02), Honolulu, Hawaii.

McCallum, A., Rosenfeld, R., Mitchell, T., & Ng, A. (1998). Improving text classification by shrinkage in a hierarchy of classes. *Proceedings of the 15th International Conference on Machine Learning*, Madison, Wisconsin.

Melville, P., Mooney, R.J., & Nagarajan, R. (2002). Content-boosted collaborative filtering for improved recommendations. *Proceedings of the 18th National Conference on Artificial Intelligence* (AAAI02), Edmonton, Alberta, Canada.

Mobasher, B., Cooley, R., & Srivastava, J. (2000a). Automatic personalization based on Web usage mining. *Communications of the ACM, 43*(8), 142-151.

Mobasher, B., Dai, H., Luo, T., & Nakagawa, M. (2001). Effective personalization based on association rule discovery from Web usage data. *Proceedings of the 3rd ACM Workshop on Web Information and Data Management* (WIDM01), Atlanta, Georgia.

Mobasher, B., Dai, H., Luo, T., & Nakagawa, M. (2002). Discovery and evaluation of aggregate usage profiles for Web personalization. *Data Mining and Knowledge Discovery, 6,* 61-82.

Mobasher, B., Dai, H., Luo, T., Sun, Y., & Zhu, J. (2000b). Integrating Web usage and content mining for more effective personalization. *E-Commerce and Web Technologies: Proceedings of the EC-WEB 2000 Conference*, Lecture Notes in Computer Science (LNCS) 1875, 165-176. Springer.

Palopoli, L., Sacca, D., Terracina, G., & Ursino, D. (2003). Uniform techniques for deriving similarities of objects and subschemes in heterogeneous databases. *IEEE Transactions on Knowledge and Data Engineering, 15*(1), 271-294.

Palpanas, T., & Mendelzon, A. (1999). Web prefetching using partial match prediction. *Proceedings of the 4th International Web Caching Workshop* (WCW99), San Diego, CA.

Parent, S., Mobasher, B., & Lytinen, S. (2001). An adaptive agent for Web exploration based on concept hierarchies. *Proceedings of the International Conference on Human Computer Interaction*, New Orleans, LA.

Pazzani, M. (1999). A framework for collaborative, content-based and demographic filtering. *Artificial Intelligence Review, 13*(5-6), 393-408.

Perkowitz, M., & Etzioni, O. (1998). Adaptive Websites: Automatically synthesizing Web pages. *Proceedings of the 15th National Conference on Artificial Intelligence*, Madison, WI.

Pitkow, J., & Pirolli, P. (1999). Mining longest repeating subsequences to predict WWW surfing. *Proceedings of the 2nd USENIX Symposium on Internet Technologies and Systems*, Boulder, Colorado.

Rodriguez, M.A., & Egenhofer, M.J. (2003). Determining semantic similarity among entity classes from different ontologies. *IEEE Transactions on Knowledge and Data Engineering, 15*(2), 442-456.

Sarwar, B.M., Karypis, G., Konstan, J., & Riedl, J. (2000). Analysis of recommender algorithms for e-commerce. *Proceedings of the 2nd ACM E-Commerce Conference* (EC'00), Minneapolis, MN.

Srivastava, J., Cooley, R., Deshpande, M., & Tan, P. (2000). Web usage mining: Discovery and applications of usage patterns from Web data. *SIGKDD Explorations, 1*(2), 12-23.

Spiliopoulou, M. (2000). Web usage mining for Web site evaluation. *Communications of ACM, 43*(8), 127-134.

Stumme, G., Taouil, R., Bastide, Y., Pasquier, N., & Lakhal, L. (2000). Fast computation of concept lattices using data mining techniques. *Proceedings of the Knowledge Representation Meets Databases Conference* (KRDB00), Berlin.

Chapter XI
Adaptive Presentation and Scheduling of Media Streams on Parallel Storage Servers

Constantinos Mourlas
National & Kapodistrian University of Athens, Greece

ABSTRACT

One way to implement adaptive software is to allocate resources dynamically during run-time rather than statically at design time. Design of adaptive software and adaptive execution of processes are key factors that improve versatility of software and decrease maintenance costs. In this chapter we study the development of adaptive software focusing on a design strategy for the implementation of parallel media servers with an adaptable behaviour. This strategy makes the timing properties and the quality of presentation of a set of media streams predictable. The proposed adaptive scheduling approach exploits the performance of parallel environments and seems a promising method that brings the advantages of parallel computation in media servers. The proposed mechanism provides deterministic service for both Constant Bit Rate (CBR) and Variable Bit Rate (VBR) streams. We present an efficient placement strategy for data frames as well as an adaptability strategy that allows appropriate frames to be dropped without sacrificing the ability to present multimedia applications predictably in time.

INTRODUCTION

One property of most User Interfaces is the presentation of multiple streaming media (video and audio) that must be presented within a predefined range of acceptable levels of quality, i.e. satisfying a set of Quality of Service (QoS) constraints. The network servers which serve such interfaces differ enough from traditional storage servers since they store and manipulate continuous media data (video and audio) which consist of of media quanta (video frames and audio samples) that must be presented using the same timing sequence with which they were captured. For example, throughput must be maintained continuously for acceptable video playouts, and jitter must be kept within strict bounds of the order of 10ms for digital audio to be intelligible to humans.

Adaptive Systems Programming is a new direction for programming such complex systems which need to adapt their execution at run time according to new system requirements and requests that arrive from a dynamic and complex runtime environment where other processes coexist and share the same resources. Research results have been applied on system programming and implementations of advanced and evolving environments like multimedia servers, streaming media presentations, ubiquitous computing, soft real-time systems, agent computing and Grid computing applications. Adaptive Scheduling which is a special case of adaptive systems programming, and resource allocation strategies must be provided by the Continuous media (CM) server such that the required CM data will be available for the time they are needed. Hence, media servers need to ensure that the retrieval and storage of such CM streams proceed at their pre-specified real-time rates.

The proposed work is focused on the design and implementation of a predictable parallel media server with an adaptive behaviour. We focus mainly on resource management of the parallel server in order to provide on-demand support for a large number of concurrent continuous media objects in a predictable manner. With the ability to manage parallel data retrievals on media servers that satisfy the real-time requirements of each stream we could be able to concurrently support more predictable continuous media applications than on traditional single processing servers.

In a subsequent step, we extend our resource management strategy to provide *adaptability*. Instead of rejecting requests, adaptability allows more requests to be served by a suitable choice of frame dropping. The proposed adaptability management provides this feature without sacrificing the ability to present multimedia applications predictably in time. Our resource and adaptability management strategies have been especially designed for parallel media servers and support both CBR and VBR encoded media streams (video and audio) in a predictable manner.

THE ARCHITECTURE OF THE PARALLEL MEDIA SERVER

One common server architecture is the single processing model. However, this single processor server model has its limitations like performance, scalability, low transfer rate and low capacity. Recently, much research has been made on the topic of parallel systems in the community of parallel computing. In order to design a general purpose architecture which can be adapted to the current user requirements, a scalable parallel multimedia server shall be designed.

We will use the traditional model for a parallel media server previously described in (Wu & Shu, 1996; Jadav et al., 1997b). In that architecture there exist three kinds of nodes: storage nodes, delivery nodes and one control node (see Figure 1). The three kinds of nodes are explained in greater detail below:

Storage nodes are responsible for storing video and audio clips, retrieving requested data blocks and sending them to delivery nodes within a time limit. In addition, partitioned media blocks are wide striped among storage nodes in a round-robin fashion to balance the workload.

Delivery nodes are responsible for serving stream requests that have been previously accepted for service. Their main function is to request the striped data from the storage nodes through the internal interconnection network, re-sequence the packets received if necessary and then send the packets over the wide area network to the clients.

Figure 1. The logical model of the parallel media server

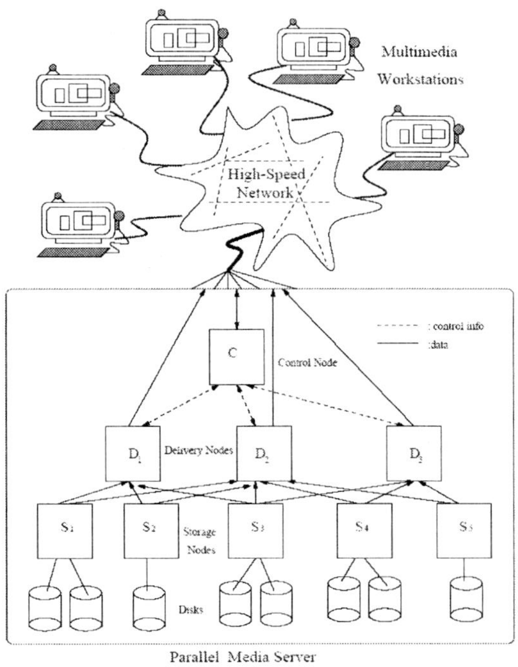

The logical storage and delivery nodes can be mapped to different as well as to the same physical node. The model where a node can be both a storage node and a delivery node is called "flat" architecture and it is more suitable to be implemented on a cluster of workstations interconnected by high-speed links. In this paper, we are focused on "flat" architectures.

Due to the fact that many parallel tasks share the server resources (storage and delivery nodes) and execute periodic reads for data retrieval to satisfy the stream's real-time constraints, it happens for one task to wait till some resources of the media server become available by other tasks. Since tasks are inter-dependent and share both storage and delivery nodes our main problem is the scheduling of the incoming requests to improve performance and high level of system utilization. The required real-time scheduling algorithm needs to prevent under-utilization of the resources and ensure load balancing. These problems are addressed in the following section.

THE PROPOSED SCHEDULING ALGORITHM

It is well understood that scheduling policies are critical to performance of continuous media servers. Without scheduling and resource management, streams may conflict each other. Therefore may be delayed and the quality of a multimedia presentation cannot be guaranteed. Furthermore, buffers are used for a smooth delivery of data to the clients through the storage and delivery nodes. Continuous media streams that are not well scheduled may require large buffer space. The work we present here on scheduling of a parallel media server is focused on deterministic guarantees, so that the application can maintain the requested QoS level without encountering unpredictable delay and jitter while reproducing the video display and audio sound. The proposed scheduling algorithm guarantees the QoS of every (accepted) stream, efficiently utilizes server resources, reduces the required buffer size, increases system throughput and finally provides adaptability.

As mentioned earlier, the data is compressed and striped across all storage nodes in a round-robin fashion. Although data blocks are wide striped, without properly scheduling of data retrievals, resource conflicts may be occurred such as port contention where two storage nodes are transmitting to a single delivery node at the same time. Another resource conflict that may also happen is disk contention where more than one request retrieves blocks from the same storage node at the same time instance.

The work described in this chapter, is concentrated on the special case of conflict-free scheduling that provides deterministic guarantees for both CBR and VBR stream requests. It is well understood that providing deterministic service for CBR streams is easier due to the fact that a CBR stream requests the same amount of data in every interval. For presentational purposes, the initial version of our scheduling algorithm that schedules CBR requests is presented first. In a following subsection we extend our scheduling algorithm to include VBR streams taking into account the fluctuations in the bit rates of multiple requests that may overload throughput capacity of the storage nodes.

Deterministic Guarantees for CBR Streams Encoded at Different Playback Rates

We will describe how requests for media streams can be modeled as a set of periodic tasks and we give a formal evaluation of some components such as the period and the data retrieval section of each task. Time is divided into time frames (or rounds) where the length of every time frame T_i equals to T which is a constant value. R_i is the required playback rate for stream s_i that has been pre-determined during the compression phase of that stream. Note that, for a CBR stream s_i, the value R_i is constant during the length of the stream. Different CBR streams stored in a media server usually have been encoded in different playback rates for different qualities of audio and video objects. Due to the fact that the data transfer rate of a single disk or a disk array can be much higher than the playback rate of a stream, multiple media streams can be served by a storage server in every T time units while the individual playback rate R_i is still preserved. Our aim in the design of a parallel media server is to supply the stream with enough data to ensure that the playback processes do not starve.

Therefore, every stream s_i is represented by a periodic task τ_i where in every period (i.e. in every time frame) T needs to retrieve $F_i = T * R_i$ amount of data to guarantee that the stream s_i will meet its real-time requirements. The above equation determines the stripe fragment size F_i of stream s_i which is different in general for every stream according to its playback rate R_i. Every media stream s_i is striped across all nodes in a round-robin fashion where the stripe fragment size of s_i equals to F_i. The average time to retrieve F_i bytes from the storage node and transmit them to a delivery node is given by equation

$$t^i_s = t_{avg\text{-}seek} + t_{avg\text{-}rot} + t_{r\text{-}Fi} + t_{nw\text{-}Fi} \quad (1)$$

where $t_{avg\text{-}seek}$ and $t_{avg\text{-}rot}$ are the average seek and rotational latencies for the disks being used, $t_{r\text{-}Fi}$ is the disk data transfer time for F_i bytes and $t_{nw\text{-}Fi}$ is the internal network latency to transport F_i bytes from a storage node to a delivery node. Thus, t^i_s is the length of the data retrieval section of the periodic task τ_i. Note that the equation (1) uses average seek and rotational latencies for disk accesses. Since these latencies are variable, there will be boundary conditions when the time to retrieve F_i bytes is much more (less) than the average value. If some clients require strict performance guarantees, then one can categorize users into those requiring hard and soft deadlines and use the maximum values of the disk overheads for admitting such users.

Since the stripe fragments of a continuous media are consecutively distributed in all N storage nodes, if a task τ_i at time frame m retrieves data from node k, it will retrieve data from node $(k+1)$ $mod\,N$ at time frame $(m+1)$. A complete schedule is represented by a schedule table consisting of N consecutive time frames. Let u_i be the set of tasks allocated to the delivery node i for service. We define as the utilization factor U_i of a delivery node i, the sum given by the formula:

$$U_i = \sum_{\tau_j \in u_i} \frac{t^j_S}{T}, \quad 0 \le i \le N-1 \quad (2)$$

The value U_i of a delivery node i changes only when a new request is allocated to the delivery node i by the control node, or when an existing request completed its execution and quits. U_i represents the load of the delivery node i and its value can never be greater than one. Note that, the utilization factor of a storage node varies from one time frame to the other. More precisely, the load of one storage node in the frame T_i moves to the next storage node in frame T_{i+1} and returns in frame T_{i+N}.

This work is concentrated on the special case of scheduling called conflict-free scheduling (Wu & Shu, 1996). It is an extension of the work presented in (Lin & Wu, 1999) and (Reddy, 1995) based on a conflict-free stream scheduling algorithm that eliminates contentions so that high system performance and stream throughput can be achieved. The algorithm guarantees that once the first round has a conflict-free scheduling, the following time frames will not have conflict. Our first extension of that scheduling scheme is described in the following paragraphs and provides better flexibility and better performance for large-scale parallel media servers. Based on the extended scheduling scheme we will be able to provide streams of different playback rates and make maximum utilization of resources which are not possible in the original version of the algorithm described in (Lin & Wu, 1999) and (Reddy, 1995). In the next subsection, we extend further our scheduling strategy to accommodate VBR stream requests.

A conflict-free schedule is a schedule that in every time instance the following scenario will never occur: two media streams request data from the same storage server or two storage servers transmit data to the same delivery node. In order to construct such a schedule we implement every frame (or round) in such a way that only one storage node transmits data to one delivery node. Note that, a starting sequence which designates the transmission order between storage nodes and delivery nodes needs to be assigned at the first basic time frame T_0. Different but equivalent basic time frames exist each one with a different starting sequence and any of that frames can be selected as the basic frame T_0. Since the blocks of the media streams are consecutively distributed in all N storage nodes, when delivery node 0 schedules a request that retrieves a block from storage node 1 the same request retrieves blocks from storage nodes 2,3,...,-1,0 in the next N-1 frames (see Figure 2).

Figure 2. Equivalent schedule tables starting from a different basic time frame T0

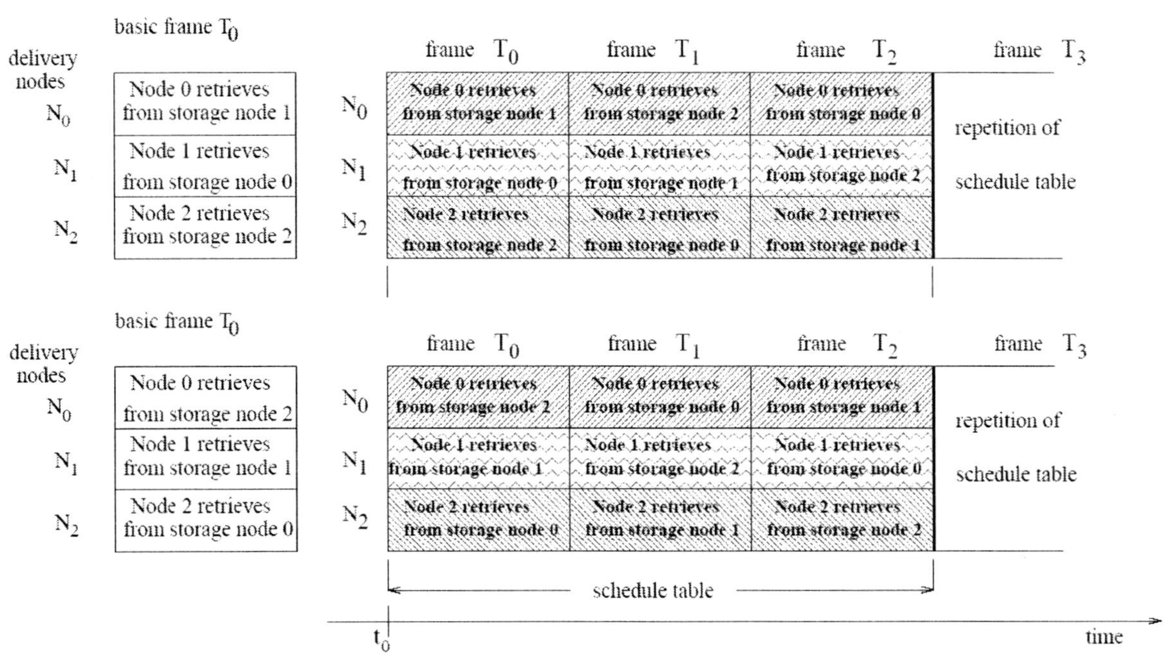

The proposed algorithm schedules the stream requests as follows: When a new request r_k for a media object arrives where its starting block is stored in node *j*, the first step is to test schedulability of the new request. The control node checks the loads of the delivery nodes and finds the node *i*, $(0 \leq i \leq N-1)$ with the minimum load U_i. Then, it checks if the condition $(U_i + t^k_s / T \leq 1)$ is satisfied for that node. If the condition is satisfied then the node *i* is declared as the delivery node of the stream s_k and it will serve together with the previous streams the new one during its lifetime. The new request r_k starts receiving data when delivery node *i* is connected with storage node *j* for first time after the receipt of request r_k and the schedule table is updated accordingly. Notice the possibility to delay the beginning of service for a request till delivery node is connected for the first time after the receipt of the request with the corresponding storage node. In case that the above condition cannot be satisfied the request is rejected or postponed for later service. An important property of the proposed algorithm is that when the control node finds a delivery node *i* to serve the request r_k and the condition $(U_i + t^k_s / T \leq 1)$can be satisfied, immediately it is guaranteed that the new load U_i', $(U_i' = U_i + t^k_s / T \leq 1)$ can be accommodated also by the storage nodes.

The proposed conflict-free scheduling algorithm can be illustrated by a single example. Suppose that a parallel media server with a "flat" architecture supports 3 nodes (N=3). The stream parameters of the example are presented in Table 1. Suppose that an empty basic frame T_0 is given and all the media requests arrive in sequence during the time interval $[t_0-T, t_0)$. An entry in a time frame (i.e. a shaded area) shows the data retrieval section of the request and the storage node number from where the stripe fragment is retrieved (see Figure 3). The retrieval of the stripe fragments of a single stream are separated by one time frame. In our example, delivery node 0 schedules the first request r_0 that retrieves a stripe fragment from storage node 2 in time frame T_0. The same request retrieves blocks from storage nodes 0 and 1 in the next two frames. A complete schedule is represented by a schedule table consisting of 3 time frames (see Figure 3). Notice also that request r_4 is delayed for T time units before it is served.

Table 1. The stream parameters used in the example

Stream Parameters			
Request	Type	Playback Rate	Starting Storage Node
r_0	video	1.5 Mbits/sec	2
r_1	audio	0.6 Mbits/sec	1
r_2	audio	0.4 Mbits/sec	0
r_3	video	1.2 Mbits/sec	0
r_4	video	2.2 Mbits/sec	1

Deterministic Guarantees for VBR Streams

The problem of providing deterministic guarantees for VBR streams is harder due to the following two reasons:

1. the load of a stream on the storage units varies from one round to the other, and
2. scheduling the first block of a VBR stream does not mean that the rest blocks of the stream can be scheduled.

One approach for the solution of the problem is to compute the peak rate of the stream and reserve enough bandwidth on storage nodes to satisfy the peak requirements of the stream. This pessimistic approach results to the underutilization of resources since the peak demand is observed only for short durations compared to the whole duration of the stream. When many streams are served on the parallel server, it is very possible that the peak demands of the streams do not overlap with each other. Thus, it is true that we can actually serve more streams than it is allowed by the peak-rate allocation, without reducing the quality

Figure 3. The basic frame T_0, the arrival order of the requests and the complete schedule of the example

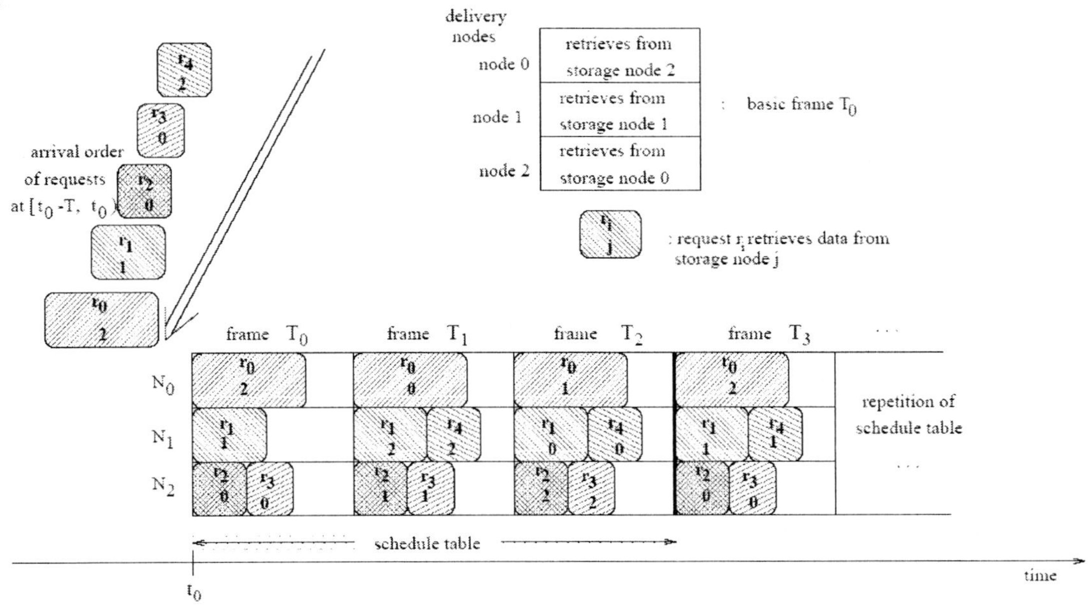

provided by the server. We propose an extension of the previous scheduling algorithm for CBR streams that allows the system to increase the number of accepted requests for streams while providing deterministic service.

In the previous subsection, every CBR stream s_i is represented by a periodic task τ_i where in every time frame T needs to retrieve a constant data length block F_i determined by the equation $F_i = T * R_i$. R_i is the required playback rate for stream which is a constant value for every different CBR stream. Using VBR streams, the bit rate R_i is variable which means that the stripe fragment size for VBR streams is also variable and thus the workload for the storage devices changes from one frame to the other.

Our approach considers the variations in loads and provides guarantees for VBR streams as follows: Time is divided as described above into time frames of equal size T. We introduce the parameter FR_i which denotes the frame rate of real-time playback (frames per second) for a video stream s_i (or samples per second for audio stream) determined when the media was captured. Thus, the number of frames included in every stripe fragment of the media stream s_i is given by the number $FR_i * T$. Our new requirement that we set here is that the result of the product $FR_i * T$ must always be an integer value for all the streams stored in our parallel server. The stripe fragment size $F_i[k]$ on round k is given by the expression: $F_i[k] = sizeof(FR_i * T \text{ frames on round } k)$. We therefore store and read the data in units of $F_i[k]$ which is of variable length on every different round. Every VBR stream s_i is striped across all nodes in a round-robin fashion where the stripe fragment size for round k equals to $F_i[k]$. Notice that just as with CBR streams, data required during a round is located on a single storage node. The time duration $t^i_s[k]$ to retrieve $F_i[k]$ bytes from the storage node and transmit them to delivery node during the k_{th} round is given by equation 1 described in the previous section.

In our approach, a presentation requiring service for a VBR stream supplies the media server with a *load vector* for that stream according to its demands. More precisely, the load vector $LV_i[k]$, $0 \leq k < dur(s_i)$ describes th time required for a storage node to retrieve and transmit $F_i[k]$ data units to a delivery node on each round k. The term $dur(s_i)$ defines the length of the stream s_i in rounds. The load vector $LV_i[]$ for stream s_i can be stored on the Control Node in a form of a special file. We can easily conclude that compared to the size of the video or audio file, the size of the load vector file is not significant.

The Control Node keeps track also of the utilization of every delivery node i of the server in the form of a utilization vector $U_i[]$. The utilization vector $U_i[]$ for delivery node i stores the actual utilization of that node in each round over sufficient period of time. Let u_i be the set of tasks allocated to the delivery node i for service. We define as the utilization $U_i[k]$ of a delivery node i during the round k, the sum given by the formula:

$$U_i[k] = \sum_{\tau_j \in u_i} \frac{t_S^j[k]}{T}, \quad 0 \leq i \leq N-1 \qquad (3)$$

The values of the $U_i[]$ vector of a delivery node i are modified when a new request is allocated to the delivery node i by the control node, or when an existing request completed its execution and quits. In addition, the utilization of a delivery node changes from one time frame to the other due to the variable bit rate of the streams. $U_i[k]$ represents the load of the delivery node i on round k and its value can never be greater than one. The utilization vector $U_i[]$ of a delivery node i stores the current as well as the future utilization values for that delivery node. Before a stream is accepted by the control node, its load vector is combined with the utilization vector of every delivery node to check if there exists a delivery node where its new load never exceeds its capacity (i.e. its utilization is always lower than or equal to one during the length of the candidate stream). Let $U_i[j]$ denote the utilization of delivery node i in round j when a new request for stream s_r arrived at the server. Let the starting block of the stream s_r be on a storage node where delivery node i will be connected to that node after k time frames ($0 \leq k \leq N-1$, where N is the total number of storage nodes). Then, the stream can be admitted if there exists a delivery node i that all the following m conditions:

$$U_i[j+k+m] = \frac{LV_r[m]}{T} \leq 1, \ 0 \leq k < dur(s_r) \ where$$

$$U_i[j+k+m] = \sum_{\tau_j \in u_i} \frac{t_S^j[j+k+m]}{T}, \text{ and } LV_r[m] = t_s^r[m] \qquad (4)$$

can be satisfied. The term k denotes the startup latency for that stream. In case that multiple delivery nodes satisfy the above conditions, the delivery node with the minimum value of k can be selected to provide the minimum startup latency. If the request is accepted then the utilization vector of the selected delivery node is updated accordingly. Let $dur(s_r)$ be the length of the stream s_r measured in time frames. The control node requires at most $N * dur(s_r)$ additions to determine if a stream can be accepted or not for service, where N is the number of delivery nodes of the parallel server.

ADAPTABILITY MANAGEMENT

A request of a media stream for service can be accepted or not following the aforementioned admission control policy. When a request is rejected it means that at least one of the m conditions given by (4) cannot be satisfied. In other words, if we accept such a request then there will be a future time instance lying between the time of acceptance and the duration of that stream when a storage node will be overloaded. Due to the fact that media presentations have not to be considered as hard real-time applications, we need a media server that enables us to drop the frame rate of a candidate stream to smaller values rather than rejecting that request.

Thus, we need to extend our approach on deterministic scheduling of media streams in order to support adaptability of media flows without sacrificing the ability to present multimedia applications predictably in time. Suppose that a request to serve a specific stream includes quality of service (QoS) specifications which are expressed with temporal and spatial resolutions. The temporal resolution can be expressed by the number of frames per second or sample rate and the spatial resolution can by expressed by data size or number of bits per pixel. For example, in one simple digital video application, the user may choose 22 frames per second for its temporal resolution and a spatial resolution of 160 by 120 pixels wide with an 8-bit color resolution. The video quality requirements can be specified using the following attributes:

- **[fps]:** The value of *fps* defines the temporal resolution of a video presentation by giving the number of frames per second. The value of this attribute can be any positive integer or a range of positive integers. For example giving *fps=14-18* as attribute to a video object, it means that the accepted values for this video presentation can be any rate between 14 and 18 frames per second.
- **[spatial-res]:** The *spatial-res* definition of a video presentation specifies the spatial resolution in pixels required for displaying the video object. If an ordered list of resolutions is given (e.g. *spatial-res=[180130, 12070]*) then the video object will be presented with the highest possible spatial resolution according to the availability of system resources and can be altered at run time.
- **[color-res]:** This attribute specifies the color resolution in bits required for displaying the video object. The value must be greater than 0. Typical values are 2, 8, 24,.. . If an ordered list of integer values is given (e.g. *color-res=[8,2]*) then the video object will be presented with a color resolution that is equal with one of the values of the list. During object presentation the highest color resolution is tried to be used first and this has to be decided at run time according to the availability of system resources.

The audio quality requirements can be specified using the attributes:

- **[sample-rate]:** The value of *sample-rate* defines in kHz the rate that the analog signal is sampled. If we need, for example, telephone quality the analog signal should be sampled 8000 times per second (i.e. *sample-rate = 8*).
- **[sample-size]:** This attribute specifies the sample size in bits of each sample. If an ordered list of integer values is given (e.g. *sample-size=[16,8]*) then each sample will be represented with a number of bits equal with one of the values given. For telephone quality, each sample of the signal is coded with 8 bits whereas for CD quality it is coded with 16 bits. The highest value that can be used for every sample has to be decided at run time according to the availability of the resources.

The above attributes form a complete set for QoS definition of every distinct continuous media that participate in a multimedia presentation. Using the above list of attributes and supporting an adaptability management module in our parallel media server we will be able to satisfy more requests by gracefully degrading their bit rates, instead of rejecting them. In this chapter, we consider only temporal adaptability achieved by frame dropping. Thus, when a video request with attribute *fps=6-8* asks for service from the

the parallel server, then the runtime system of the server will try to provide the best value in the range and it will be also authorized to modify this value at run-time towards the upper (8 fps) or the lower bound (6 fps) value according to the availability of the resources. The recommended strategy follows:

As we have already described, the number of frames included in every stripe fragment of a media stream s_i is constant given by the number $FR_i * T$. We store and read the data in units of $F_i[k]$ which are in general of variable length for every different round. Notice that data required during a round is located on a single storage node. In our adaptability strategy all the frames that are used for the lowest-rate reconstruction are grouped at the beginning of the data unit. Assume that a VBR stream has been compressed with $FR = 8$ *fps* and a request for that stream arrived at the control node of the server with quality attribute *fps=6-8*. Assume also that the length of every time frame T_i equals to 1 *sec*. The original frame pattern of that stream is $F_1F_2F_3F_4F_5F_6F_7F_8$.

By grouping the frames for each rate starting from 1 *fps* to 8 *fps*, our storage pattern becomes $F_1F_5F_7F_3F_4F_6F_2F_8$. Using this ordering, the system can degrade the request from 1 *fps* to the maximum possible frame rate 8 *fps*. For frame rate 1 *fps* only the first frame F_1 is retrieved, for frame rate 2 *fps* the frames F_1F_5 are retrieved, for frame rate 3 *fps* the frames $F_1F_5F_7$ are retrieved, for frame rate 4 *fps* the frames $F_1F_5F_7F_3$ and so on. Delivery nodes re-sequence the retrieved frames and then send them to the clients. Notice that the frames are evenly spaced throughout the round and causes less jitter than would be caused by dropping the last frames of the original ordering. As shown above, we group all of the frames of each rate together in each read unit. In addition, all of the frames that are used for the lowest-rate reconstruction are grouped at the beginning of the data unit. In our example, where *fps=6-8* the runtime system is authorized to retrieve six ($F_1F_5F_7F_3F_4F_6$), seven ($F_1F_5F_7F_3F_4F_6F_2$) or eight ($F_1F_5F_7F_3F_4F_6F_2F_8$) frames per second according to the availability of the resources.

The load vector of a stream becomes now a two-dimensional array $LV_i[j][k]$, $1 \leq j \leq max\_frames_i$, $0 \leq k < dur(si)$. The values in the first dimension $LV_i[1][k]$ specify the time required in every round k for a storage node to retrieve and transmit only one frame from the set of frames included in the stripe fragment $F_i[k]$. The values in $LV_i[2][k]$ specify the time to retrieve and transmit 2 frames and so on, until $LV_i[max\_frames_i][k]$ that specify the time required to retrieve and transmit all the frames in every stripe fragment $F_i[k]$. The size of the load vector $LV_i[][]$ is n times larger than the size of the previous one-dimensional vector $LV_i[]$, where n is the length of the first dimension of the vector $LV_i[][]$. If a small range of different frame rates for different qualities is supported then the size of every different load vector $LV_i[][]$ remains in acceptable levels.

Without adaptability, the load of a candidate stream is combined with the utilization vector of every delivery node to check if there exists a node where its new load never exceeds its capacity. If such a node exists the request is accepted, otherwise it is rejected. Using a frame placement strategy similar to the one described above and using the two-dimensional *load vector* $LV_i[][]$ for each stream s_i the admission control policy can be improved providing different levels of adaptability. Suppose that a request specifies the expected quality of service from the server by giving the lower and the upper bound for the expected frame rate (e.g. $fps = 18 - 22$). Let *min_fps* and *max_fps* to indicate the lower and the upper bound of the expected quality for a video presentation. The admission control mechanism is authorized to select any value in the range [*min_fps, max_fps*] when it is trying to find a delivery node where its new load never exceeds its capacity. Formally, a new set of conditions have to be satisfied similar to the ones described in (4). Let $U_i[j]$ denote the utilization of delivery node i in round j when a new request for stream

s_r arrived at the server. Let the starting block of the stream s_r be on a storage node where delivery node i will be connected to that node after k time frames ($0 \leq k \leq N-1$, where N is the total number of storage nodes). Let $LV_r[n][k]$ be the load vector of stream s_r which includes the time required in every round k for a storage node to retrieve and transmit n frames grouped at the beginning of the stripe fragment $F_r[k]$. Then, the stream can be admitted if there exists a delivery node i that the following conditions are satisfied:

$$\forall m \; \exists n : U_i[j+k+m] = \frac{LV_r[n][m]}{T} \leq 1, \quad where$$
$$0 \leq m < dur(s_r), \; \min\_fps_r \leq n \leq \max\_fps_r \tag{5}$$

More advanced admission control strategies can be easily implemented using the proposed data structures and the frame placement policy. Such strategies will give the possibility for a stream to increase or decrease dynamically its frame rate during its presentation, towards the lower or the upper bound according to the availability of resources. These more sophisticated adaptive mechanisms are required in interactive environments where the user can suspend the presentation of a continuous media stream with no prior notification.

RELATED WORK

Much interesting work has been done in this field for single processor servers, trying to provide media servers with schemes for effectively scheduling the available disk bandwidth and storage capacity so that high levels of concurrency and system utilization can be sustained [Cho & Shin, 1998; Gemmell et al., 1995]. Additional research has been focused on the design of parallel on-demand media servers (Jadav et al., 1997a, Cho & Shin, 1998; Rottmann et al., 1997). A great part of the current research community effort has been also focused on new data layout schemes (Rottmann et al., 1996), striping mechanisms, admission control and disk scheduling (Rottmann et al., 1997) for storage device arrays of parallel (Lee, 1998) and clustered multimedia servers (Khaleel & Reddy, 1999). The problem of providing deterministic service for VBR streams in a single processor system has been studied in (Wijayaratne & Reddy, 2000) where the notion of the *demand trace* of every VBR stream was introduced.

However, the stream scheduling problem has not been formally addressed. The system resources cannot be fully utilized without a sophisticated scheduling strategy (Hicks et al., 2003). A very interesting approach described in (Lin & Wu, 1999) and (Reddy, 1995) provides accurate scheduling of video streams, maximizes system throughput and minimizes the usage of buffers. The main limitation of the method described in (Lin & Wu, 1999; Reddy, 1995) is that schedules only CBR video streams with the restrictive assumption that all the streams have been encoded using a unique base stream rate R. The presented work is an extension of that scheduling strategy and supports both CBR and VBR media streams (s_is) video and audio encoded using different playback rates (R_is), which is an interesting feature not supported in the original version of the algorithm.

CONCLUSION

This chpater is focused on the adaptability and the resource management problems of parallel media servers. A conflict-free scheduling scheme was presented that provides on-demand support for a large number of concurrent continuous media objects in a predictable manner. The proposed algorithm supports both CBR and VBR encoded media streams video and audio at different playback rates. Using that algorithm, we are able to achieve optimal scheduling in distributed memory parallel architectures. More precisely, the proposed real-time scheduling algorithm guarantees the QoS level of every accepted stream, efficiently utilizes server resources, reduces the required buffer size and increases system throughput.

The most interesting feature of the scheduling algorithm is the adaptive behaviour, able to support different quality levels for every connection. The server is able at runtime to allow appropriate media frames to be dropped in a predictable manner without fully suspending service to any one user.

FUTURE RESEARCH DIRECTIONS

While our work is a promising first step, many interesting directions remain. To understand the scalability of the architecture, we plan to explore a prototype implementation and simulations experiments that prove the efficiency and adaptive behaviour of the proposed scheduling strategy. In addition, we intend to examine the effect of bandwidth variations of the network during the transmission of the media data from the server to the clients giving the possibility for a stream to increase or decrease dynamically its frame rate during its presentation, towards the lower or the upper bound according to the bandwidth availability.

On possible application of adaptive scheduling that we would like to study in the near future will be the execution environment of Grids which offer a dramatic increase in the number of available processing and storing resources that can be delivered to applications. However, efficient job submission and management continue being far from accessible to ordinary scientists and engineers due to their dynamic and complex nature. Application of adaptive scheduling strategies for job execution will allow an easier and more efficient execution of jobs. The adaptive behaviour of job execution in large Grids can be achieved using a scheduling strategy that takes into account job migration, performance degradation, better resource discovery, requirement change, owner decision or remote resource failure (Huedo et al., 2004).

REFERENCES

Cho J. and Shin H. (1997). Scheduling video streams in a large-scale video-on-demand server. Parallel Computing - Special Issue on parallel processing and multimedia, 23(12):1743{1756, December.

Garofalakis, M. N., Ozden B. Ä, and Silberschatz A. (1998). On Periodic Resource Scheduling for Continuous Media Databases, *In Proceedings of the 8th International Workshop on Research Issues in Data Engineering*, February.

Gemmell D.J., Vin H.M., Kandlur D.D., Rangan P.V., and Rowe L.A. (1995). Multimedia Storage Servers: *A Tutorial. IEEE Computer*, 28(5):40{49, May.

Hicks M., Nagarjan A., and Renesse R.. User-specified Adaptive Scheduling in a Streaming Media Network. OpenARCH'03. San Francisco, CA. April 2003.

Huedo E. , Montero R. , Llorente I., A framework for adaptive execution in grids, In Software: Practice and Experience, Vol. 34, No 7, pp. 631 - 651, 2004, John Wiley & Sons.

Jadav D., Srinilta C., and Choudhary A. (1997a). Batching and dynamic allocation techniques for increasing the stream capacity of an on-demand media server. *Parallel Computing - Special Issue on parallel processing and multimedia*, 23(12):1727{1742, December.

Jadav D., Srinilta C., Choudhary A., and Berra Bruce P.(1997b). An evaluation of design tradeo®s in a high performance media-on-demand server. *Multimedia Systems*, 5(1):53{68, 1997b 17.

Khaleel A. and Reddy A. (1999). Evaluation of data and request distribution policies in clustered servers, *In Proceedings of the High Performance Computing*, 1999.

Lee B.Y.J. (1998). Parallel video servers: A tutorial. IEEE Multimedia, 5(2):20{28, 1998.

Lin C-S, Shu W., and Wu Y. M. (1999). Performance study of synchronization schemes on parallel cbr video servers, *In Proceedings of the Seventh ACM International Multimedia Conference*, November.

Rottmann V., Berenbrink P., and Luling R. (1996). A comparison of data layout schemes for multimedia servers, *In European Conference on Multimedia Applications, Services, and Techniques* (ECMAST'96), pages 345{364, 1996.

Reddy N.L.A. (1995). Scheduling and data distribution in a multiprocessor video server, *In Proceedings of the 2nd IEEE Int'l Conference on Multimedia Computing and Systems*, pp. 256{263, 1995.

Rottmann V., Berenbrink P., and Lauling I.R. (1997). A simple distributed scheduling policy for parallel interactive continuous media servers. *Parallel Computing - Special Issue on parallel processing and multimedia*, 23(12):1757{1776, December.

Wijayaratne R., and Reddy N.L.A. (2000). Providing QOS guarantees for disk I/O. *Multimedia Systems*, 8(1):57{68.

Wu Y.M. and Shu W. (1996). Scheduling for large-scale parallel video servers, *In Proceedings of the Sixth Symposium on the Frontiers of Massively Parallel Computation*, pp. 126{133, October.

ADDITIONAL READING

Ramanujan R. and Thurber K. (1998). An active network-based design of a QoS adaptive video multicast service," in Proceedings of the Workshop on Network and Operating System Support for Digital Audio and Video, July.

Fu X., Shi W., Akkerman A., and Karamcheti V. (2001). CANS: Composable, adaptive network services infrastructure, *In Proceedings of the USENIX Symposium on Internet Technologies and Systems* (USITS), March.

Atkin B. and Birman P.K. (2003). Evaluation of an adaptive transport protocol, *In Proceedings of the IEEE INFOCOM Conference*, April.

Li B. and Nahrstedt K. (1999). Dynamic reconfiguration for complex multimedia applications, *In Proceedings of the IEEE International Conference on Multimedia Computing and Systems*, June, pp. 165–170.

Noble B. and Satyanarayanan M. (1999). Experience with adaptive mobile applications in Odyssey. *Mobile Networks and Applications*, Vol. 4.

Rejaie R., Handley M., and Estrin D. (1999). Quality adaptation for congestion controlled video playback over the internet, *In Proceedings of the ACM SIGCOMM Conference*.

Bjørndalen M.J., Anshus J.O., Larsen T., Bongo L., and Vinter B. (2002), Scalable processing and communication performance in a multi-media related context, *In Proceedings of the IEEE EUROMICRO Conference*, September.

Doerr S.B, Venturella T., Jha R., Gill D. C., and Schmidt C.D. (1999). Adaptive Scheduling for Real-time, Embedded Information Systems, *In Proceedings of the 18th IEEE/AIAA Digital Avionics Systems Conference* (DASC), St. Louis, Missouri, October 24-29.

Section IV
Innovative Applications with Adaptive Behaviour

Chapter XII
Impact of Cognitive Style on User Perception of Dynamic Video Content

Gheorghita Ghinea
Brunel University, UK

Sherry Y. Chen
Brunel University, UK

ABSTRACT

This study investigated two dimensions of cognitive style, including Verbalizer/Imager and Field Dependent/Field Independent and their influence on user perceived quality of multimedia video. Perceived user quality was characterised using the Quality of Perception (QoP) metric, which captures the infotainment duality of multimedia presentations. Results indicate that, generally, clip dynamism impacts on user QoP; in particular, it is worthwhile to remark that in the clips with strong and medium dynamism, Field Dependent users performed worse than the other two groups, while Field Dependent users had a (slightly) better performance than Field Independent users in clips with weak dynamism.

INTRODUCTION

Notions of quality are of paramount importance in distributed multimedia systems – simply stated, a user will not invest time, money or, indeed, other resources if (s)he does not believe that (s)he is getting quality commensurate with expectations. Whilst efforts to characterize distributed multimedia quality have been forthcoming along the years (Apteker et al., 1995; Cranley et al., 2003; Steinmetz, 1996; Wilson and Sasse, 2001), the proliferation of multimedia applications, display devices and – last but certainly not least – users, have led researchers to investigate novel ways of exploiting perceptual quality measures to transmit bandwidth-intensive multimedia content over fixed size pipes to an increasing numbers of users.

Information transfer constitutes, in most cases, an important side of multimedia applications. Nonetheless, a dimension that is often overlooked in such cases, particularly in respect of quality considerations is the one of *cognitive style* (an individual's characteristic and consistent approach to organising and processing information (Weller et al., 1994)), especially since it affects the ways through which people organize and perceive information. Accordingly, in this chapter, we propose to explore the impact of cognitive style on a user's perception of quality for dynamic multimedia content. In particular, we will focus on two dimensions of cognitive style: the *Verbalizer/Imager* and *Field Dependent/Field Independent*, because the former refers to information representation, while the latter relates to information organization.

USER COGNITIVE STYLES

Cognitive style refers to a user's information processing habits, representing an individual user's typical mode of perceiving, thinking, remembering, and problem solving (Messick 1976). Jonassen and Grabowski (1993) defined cognitive style as inbuilt and relatively consistent preferences in organising and representing information. It is notable that there is a number of dimensions of cognitive styles, such as Holism/Serialism (Pask, 1976), Divergent/Convergent (Hudson, 1966), Field Dependence/Independence (Witkin et al., 1977), and Verbalizer/Imager (Riding, 1991). Among these, Field Dependence/Independence and Verbalizer/Imager are related to perceptual multimedia. The former concerns how users process and organize information, whereas the latter emphasises how users perceive the presentation of information.

Field Dependence/Independence is related to the degree to which a user's perception or comprehension of information is influenced by the context (Jonassen and Grabowski, 1993). The key issue of Field Dependence lies within the differences between Field Dependent and Field Independent learners, which are presented below:

- **Field Dependence:** the individuals are considered to have a more social orientation than Field Independent persons since they are more likely to make use of externally developed social frameworks. They tend to seek out external referents for processing and structuring their information, are better at learning material with human content, are more readily influenced by the opinions of others, and are affected by the approval or disapproval of authority figures.
- **Field Independence:** the individuals tend to exhibit more individualistic behaviors since they are not in need of external referents to aide in the processing of information. They are more capable of developing their own internal referents and restructuring their knowledge, are better at learning impersonal abstract material, are not easily influenced by others, and are not overly affected by the approval or disapproval of superiors (Witkin et al. 1977).

The Imagers/Verbalizer dimension describes the tendency for individuals to represent information being processed in the form of text or in the form of images (Riding and Cheema, 1991). Their different characteristics are:

- **Imagers:** Imagers tend to be internal and passive. Imagers perform better if the environment presents text and also pictorial material such as pictures, diagrams, charts, and graphs. Imagersprefer to process information by seeing and they will learn most easily through visual and verbal presentations, rather than through an exclusively verbal medium.
- **Verbalisers:** Verbalisers tend to be external and stimulating. Verbaliser individuals perform better if the environment presents only information in the form of text. Verbalizers prefer to process information through words and find they learn most easily by listening and talking (Laing, 2001).

These two dimensions of cognitive styles have been investigated by previous work in respect of the user computing experience. For example, a study by Chuang (1999) produced four-courseware versions: animation+text, animation+voice, animation+text+voice, and free choice. The result showed that Field Independent subjects in the animation+text+voice group or in the free choice group scored significantly higher than those did in the animation+text group or in the animation+voice group. No significant presentation effect was found for the Field Dependent subjects, however. Furthermore, Riding and Douglas (1993), with a sample of 15-16-year-old students, found that the computer-presentation of material on motorcar braking systems in a text+picture format facilitated the learning process of Imagerscompared to the situation where the same content was presented in a text+text version. They further found that in the recall task in the text+picture condition, 50% of the Imagersused illustrations as part of their answers, compared to only 12% of the Verbalisers. Thus, generally, Imagerslearn best from pictorial presentations, while Verbalisers learn best from verbal presentations.

There is, however, a paucity of studies investigating the relationship between the use pattern of these two dimensions of cognitive styles in multimedia systems in general, and specifically in distributed multimedia systems, where quality fluctuations can and do occur owing to dynamically varying network conditions. As the QoP metric is one which has an integrated view of user-perceived multimedia quality in such distributed systems, it is of particular interest to investigate the impact of cognitive styles on QoS-mediated QoP, as it will help in achieving a better understanding of the factors involved in such environments (distance learning and CSCW, to name but two) and ultimately help in the elaboration of robust user models which could be used to develop applications that meet with individual needs.

MULTIMEDIA LEARNING: A PERCEPTUAL EXPERIENCE?

Multimedia has been identified as a potential method of improving the learning process. Its use encourages user interaction, thus ensuring that users cannot become a passive participant of the learning experience (Neo and Neo, 2004). Previous research has also found that the use of rich multimedia in learning tools not only increases interaction, but increases interest, motivation and retention of information (Demetriadis et al, 2003). It was also found that students sometimes preferred the use of multimedia for teaching to the standard teacher-student paradigm as it is more user-centred (Zwyno, 2003).

Multimedia Perceptual Quality

Some research groups, having recognised that user perception should be the driving force in networking and operating systems research, have researched the link between differing QoS parameters and the user's satisfaction level associated with the multimedia presentation. Accordingly, previous research on user perception of multimedia presentations has investigated media synchronisation perception and the bounds within which media components can drift in and out of sync without being detectable or perceived as annoying by users (Blakowski and Steinmetyz, 1996). Lip synchronisation is a special case of synchronisation between the video and audio streams of a presentation in which the focus is on ensuring that words being spoken by, for example, a newscaster are synchronised with the movement of his/her lips. Given the importance of lip synchronisation in distributed multimedia applications such as teleconferencing, Steinmetz (1996) looked at the acceptable delay and jitter bounds for lip synchronisation, while Kouvelas *et al.* (2001) studied strategies for maintaining lip synchronisation over the Internet. On the other hand, user perception of pointer synchronisation, namely the synchronisation between audio and an object being pointed at, is important in Computer Supported Co-operative Work environments, and has been looked at in Blakowski and Steinmetz, 1996).

Related, non-synchronisation, work on user perceptual impact of multimedia displayed with different technical parameters includes research by Apteker *et al* (1995), which showed that there is a non-linear dependency between varying frame rates and user satisfaction with a multimedia presentation. This result leads to an interesting trade-off raising the possibility of sacrificing a small amount of user perceptual satisfaction in return for the release of a much larger relative amount of bandwidth, which could then be potentially used by future multimedia sessions. Similar work by Fukuda *et al* (1997) investigated the relationship between spatial resolution, Signal to Noise Ratio, number of frames per second (fps) and user satisfaction, while Anderson and Blockland (1997) investigated the intelligibility of speech when low frame rate multimedia video is employed. Both Watson and Sasse (1998) and Wijesekera *et al* (1996) have reported how users perceive or notice media losses. On the other hand, research has also been done measuring users' attitudes towards multimedia and automated telephone interfaces. Key service attributes such as ease of use, reliability, perceived efficiency and friendliness are being focused on. All this research (including ones dealing with synchronisation perception) have only investigated a part of the user perceptual experience, namely that of the user satisfaction component of a multimedia presentation, and have completely ignored the fundamental and essential aspect of user understanding and assimilation of the same presentation.

Multimedia: The Challenges

However, the potential of multimedia has to date, not been fully realised. Users perceive, process and organise information in individualistic ways, yet current multimedia CAL applications fail to take this into consideration (Stash et al, 2004). Allowing users to choose their preferred method of multimedia presentation, will let them learn more in a shorter period of time as they will be more receptive to the content (Carver et al, 1999). However, more research must be performed in this area before the potential is realised (Stash et al, 2004).

Previous research has shown that different cognitive style groups perform better with certain multimedia presentation methods. Chuang (1999) found that Field Independent students performed significantly better than Field Dependent students when using a rich multimedia interface. However, no significant preferences were found for Field Dependent students. Conversely, research performed by Marisson and Frick (1994) found that Field Dependent individuals would show improved learning with the use of audio. As a result of these findings, it is clear that more research must be performed in order to clearly identify what multimedia presentation methods are preferred by different cognitive style groups.

Ford et al. (1994) suggest that students with different cognitive styles utilise different strategies to seek and process information and that these strategies will have different levels of effectiveness for students in different contexts. Norcio and Stanley (1989) also state that students' requirements of multimedia interfaces are likely to change as they become more knowledgeable in the subject content being delivered. These statements suggest that students may prefer different multimedia presentation methods in different contexts. For example, students may prefer one method of presentation when they are a novice in a subject and may prefer another method of presentation when they are an expert in that same subject. However this remains to be conclusively proved.

Although the use of multimedia in teaching has its benefits, careful consideration must be given to how it is implemented, as ineffective use of multimedia can lead to high cognitive load, frustration and reduced interest (Zhang et al, 2004). Plass and Homer (2002) found that students that were allowed a choice of presentation methods learnt content effectively, whereas students who were assigned a particular presentation method performed poorly as the presentation method did not suit their cognitive style.

A particular challenge of employing multimedia for learning is the integration of new multimedia technologies into the classroom. Several important factors such as availability of relevant hardware, equipping educators with the relevant skills to use the tools and user acceptance must be considered when utilising multimedia (Neo and Neo, 2004).

Measuring the Perceptual Multimedia Experience

The focus of our research has been the enhancement of the traditional view of multimedia with a user-level defined *Quality of Perception* (QoP). This is a measure which encompasses not only a user's satisfaction with multimedia clips, but also his/her ability to perceive, synthesise and analyse the informational content of such presentations, thus providing a more complete characterisation of the communication goals of multimedia. With it users are asked to indicate, on a scale of 1-6, how much they enjoyed the multimedia presentation (with scores of 1 and 6 respectively representing "no" and, "absolute" user satisfaction), while their knowledge of the informational component is examined via a series of questions, and expressed as a percentage measure reflecting the proportion of correct answers received (Ghinea and Thomas, 1998). The former component is denoted by QoP-LOE (Level of Enjoyment), whilst the latter is QoP-IA (Information Assimilation).QoP thus represents, to the best of our knowledge, the only metric for perceptual quality evaluation which takes into account multimedia's *infotainment* characteristic, and in this chapter we study the effect of individual differences, as given by a user's cognitive style, on QoP, when multimedia is affected by dynamic variation of content.

PROCEDURE

Participants

The study reported in this paper was conducted at Brunel University's School of Information Systems, Computing and Mathematics. 126 participants took part in the study. Participants' cognitive styles were categorised according to Riding's Cognitive Style Analysis in which the two dimensions of cognitive styles considered are: Field Dependent/Field Independent and Verbalizer/Visualiser. Participants' breakdown according to cognitive styles is given in Figure 1. All participating users were inexperienced in the content domain of the multimedia video clips visualized as part of our experiments, which will be described next.

Material

A total of 12 video clips were used in our study. The multimedia clips were visualized under a Microsoft Internet Explorer browser with a Microsoft Media player plug-in, with users subsequently filling in a Web-based questionnaire to evaluate

Figure 1. The cognitive styles of the participants

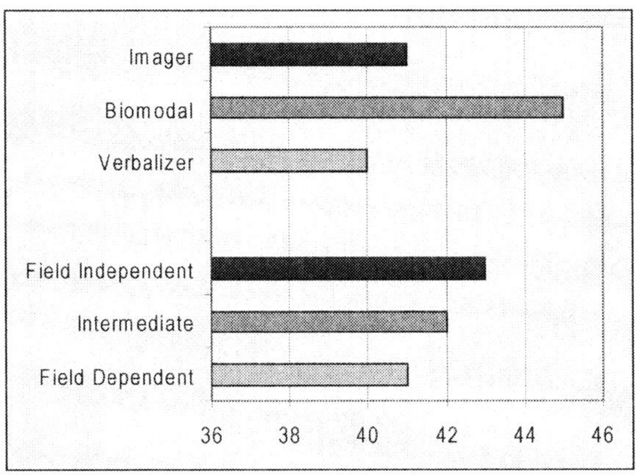

QoP for each clip. All multimedia clips used in our study were visualised a frame rate of 25 fps and with full colour 24-bit quality, parameters which represent optimal playback conditions in distributed multimedia systems.

These 12 clips had been used in previous QoP experiments (Ghinea and Thomas, 1998), and were between 30-44 seconds long and digitised in MPEG-1 format. The subject matter they portrayed was varied and taken from selected television programmes, thereby reflecting informational and entertainment sources that average users might encounter in their everyday lives. Also varied was the dynamism of the clips (i.e., the rate of change between the frames of the clip), which ranged from a relatively static news clip to a highly dynamic space action movie (Table 1).

Cognitive Style Analysis

The cognitive style dimensions investigated in this study include Field Dependence/Independence and Verbalizer/Visualiser. A number of instruments have been developed to measure these two dimensions. Riding's (1991) Cognitive Style Analysis (CSA) was applied to identify each participant's cognitive styles in this study, because the CSA offers computerised administration and scoring. In addition, the CSA can offer various English versions, including Australasian, North American and UK contexts.

The CSA uses two sub-tests to identify Field Dependence/Independence. The first presents items containing pairs of complex geometrical figures that the individual is required to judge as either the same or different. The second presents items each comprising a simple geometrical shape, such as a square or a triangle, and a complex geometrical figure, as in the GEFT, and the individual is asked to indicate whether or not the simple shape is contained in a complex one by pressing one of two marked response keys (Riding and Grimley, 1999).. The first sub-test is a task requiring Field Dependent capacity. Conversely, the second sub-test requires the disembedding capacity associated with Field Independence.

The CSA uses two types of statement to measure the Verbal-Imagery dimension and asks participants to judge whether the statements are true or false. The first type of statement contains information about conceptual categories while the second describes the appearance of items. There are 48 statements in total covering both types of statement. Each type of statement has an equal number of true statements and false statements. It is assumed that Imagersrespond more quickly to the appearance statements, because the objects can be readily represented as mental pictures and the information for the comparison can be obtained directly and rapidly from these images. In the case of the conceptual category items, it is assumed that Verbalisers have a shorter response time because the semantic conceptual category membership is verbally abstract in nature and cannot be represented in visual form. The computer records the response time to each statement and calculates the Verbal-ImagerRatio. A low ratio corresponds to a Verbaliser and a high ratio to a Visualizer, with the intermediate position being described as Bimodal.

Table 1. Multimedia video content

VIDEO CATEGORY	Dynamism		
	Low	Medium	High
1. Action Movie			X
2. Animated Clip		X	
3. Band Clip		X	
4. Chorus Clip	X		
5. Commercial/Ad Clip		X	
6. Cooking Clip	X		
7. Documentary Clip		X	
8. News Clip	X		
9. Pop Music Clip		X	
10. Rugby Clip			X
11. Snooker Clip	X		
12. Weather Forecast Clip	X		

This study followed Riding's recommendation for the measurements of Field Dependence/Independence and Verbalizer/Visualizer. In terms of Field Dependence/Independence, Riding's (1991) recommendations are that scores below 1.03 denote Field Dependent individuals; scores of 1.36 and above denote Field Independent individuals; students scoring between 1.03 and 1.35 are classed as Intermediate. Regarding the measurement of Verbalizer/Visualizer, the recommendations are that scores below 0.98 denote Verbalizers; scores of 1.09 and above denote Visualizers; students scoring between 0.98 and 1.09 are classed as Bimodal.

Procedure

The experiment consisted of several steps. Initially, the CSA was used to classify users' cognitive styles as Field Dependent/Intermediate/Field Independent and Verbalizer/ Bimodal/Imager. Subjects then viewed the 7 multimedia video clips. In order to counteract any order effects, the order in which clips were visualised was varied randomly for each participant. After the users had seen each clip once, the window was closed, and they had to answer a number of questions about the video clip they had just seen. The actual number of such questions depended on the video clip, and varied between 10 and 12. After the user had answered the set of questions pertaining to a particular video clip and the responses had been duly recorded, (s)he was asked to rate the enjoyment quality of the clip that had just been seen on a Likert scale of 1–6 (with scores of 1 and 6 representing the worst and, respectively, best perceived qualities possible). The user then went on and watched the next clip.

Users were instructed not to let personal bias towards the subject matter in the clip or production-related preferences (for instance the way in which movie cuts had been made) influence their enjoyment quality rating of a clip. Instead, they were asked to judge a clip's enjoyment quality by the degree to which they, the users, felt that they would be satisfied with a general purpose multimedia service of such quality. Users were told that factors which should influence their quality rating of a clip included clarity and acceptability of audio signals, lip synchronisation during speech, and the general relationship between visual and auditory message components.

Data Analyses

In this study, the independent variables include the participants' cognitive styles, as well as clip categories and their degree of dynamism. The dependent variables were the two components of Quality of Perception: the level of understanding (QoP-IA, expressed as a percentage measure describing the proportion of questions that the user had correctly answered for each clip) as well as the level of enjoyment (QoP-LOE, expressed on a 6-point Likert scale).

All QoP-IA questions used definite answers. For example, from the Rugby video clip used in our experiments, "What teams are playing?" was asked. This question has an unambiguous answer (England and New Zealand), which is presented in the clip, and it was therefore possible to determine if a participant had answered this question correctly or not. Since, in our experiments, questions can only be answered if certain information is assimilated from specific information sources (for example, the words of a song can only be gained from the audio stream), it is possible to determine the percentage of correctly answered questions that relate to the different information sources within specific multimedia video clip. For each feedback question, the source of the answer was determined as having been assimilated from one of the following information sources:

- V: Information relating specifically to the video window, for example, pertaining to the activity of lions in a documentary clip.
- A: Information which is presented in the audio stream.

T: Textual information contained in the video window, for example: information contained in a caption (for example: the newscaster's name).

Thus, by calculating the percentage of correctly absorbed information from different information sources, it was possible to determine from which information sources participants absorbed the most information. Using this data it is possible to determine and compare, over a range of different multimedia content, potential differences that might exist in QoP-IA

Data were analysed with the Statistical Package for the Social Sciences (SPSS) for Windows version (release 9.0). An ANalysis Of VAriance (ANOVA), suitable to test the significant differences of three or more categories, and t-test, suitable to identify the differences between two categories (Stephen and Hornby, 1997), were applied to analyse the participants' responses. A significance level of $p < 0.05$ was adopted for the study.

RESULTS AND DISCUSSION

Dynamism Impact: Field Dependent vs. Field Independent

Multimedia clip dynamism was found to significantly impact upon participants' level of understanding in our study (Figure 2). The level of significance was found to be p=.000 for Field Dependent users and p=.001 for Intermediate and Field Dependent users. All users performed worst in the clips with strong dynamism. In particular, Field Dependent users do not perform as well as Field Independent and Intermediate users. As suggested by previous works (Chen and Macredie, 2002; Chen, 2002), Field Dependent users' performance was hindered in situations where they need to extract cues by themselves. Thus, in multimedia clips with strong dynamism that provided too many cues, Field Dependent users might find it difficult to select relevant cues.

The dynamism of the visualized clips also influenced the level of enjoyment experienced

Figure 2. Impact of dynamism on QoP-IA (Field Dependent vs. Field Independent)

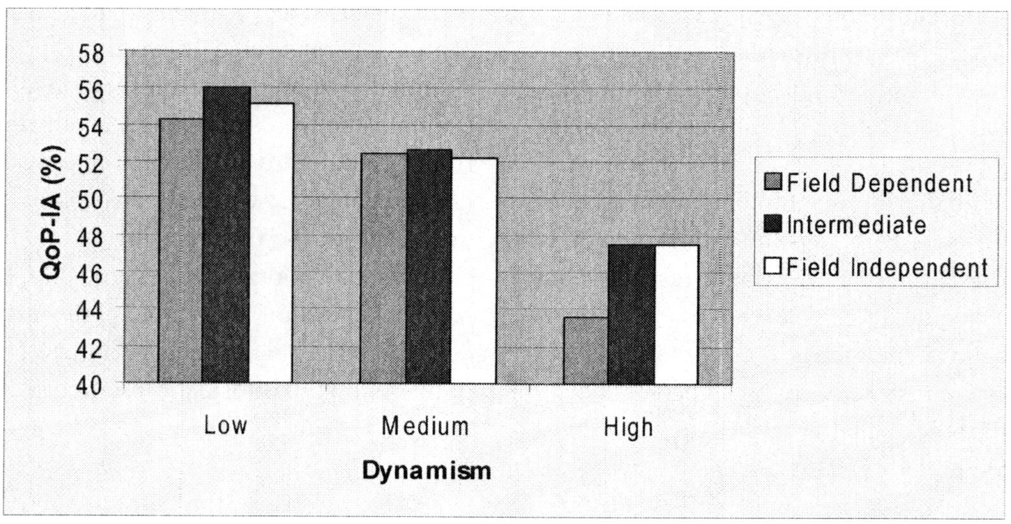

by participants (p=.000). If a per-cognitive style analysis is pursued, we find that the level of enjoyment is influenced by the dynamism of the multimedia clip for both Field Independent (p=.004) and Field Dependent (p=.000) users. As shown in Figure 3, both Field Independent and Field Dependent users experienced higher levels of enjoyment from the clips with medium dynamism, while strongly dynamic clips were liked least of all. However, dynamism does not seem to be a factor influencing multimedia clip enjoyment of Intermediate users. One possible interpretation is that individuals possessing an Intermediate cognitive style employ a more versatile repertoire of information seeking strategies. Versatile users, who have acquired the skill to move back and forth between different information seeking strategies, are more capable of adapting themselves to suit the subject content presented by the multimedia video clips. This finding is consistent with the views of previous work, namely that a versatile strategy can be better equipped for multimedia learning technology (Chen and Ford, 1998; Paterson, 1996).

Dynamism Impact: Imager vs. Verbaliser

Analysis of the results obtained from the experiment shows that the degree of clip dynamism significantly impacts upon the QoP-IA component of QoP, irrespective of the user's cognitive style (Verbalizers: F=6.359; df-within = 549; p=.002; Visualizers: F=9.368; df-within = 645; p<.001; Bimodals: F=8.217; df-within = 381; p<.001). The analysis has highlighted, moreover, the fact that the highest QoP-IA scores are obtained for clips which have a low degree of dynamism. Conversely, multimedia clips which have a high degree of dynamism have a negative impact on the user assimilation of the informational content being conveyed by the respective clips (Figure 4). Thus, clips which have relatively small interframe variability will facilitate higher QoP-IA scores: an object which might appear for only 0.5 seconds in a highly dynamic clip is less easily remembered than when it appears for one second in a clip which is less dynamic.

As far as the QoP-LOE component is concerned (Figure 3), analysis of our results

Figure 3. Impact of Dynamism on QoP-LOE (Field Dependent vs. Field Independent)

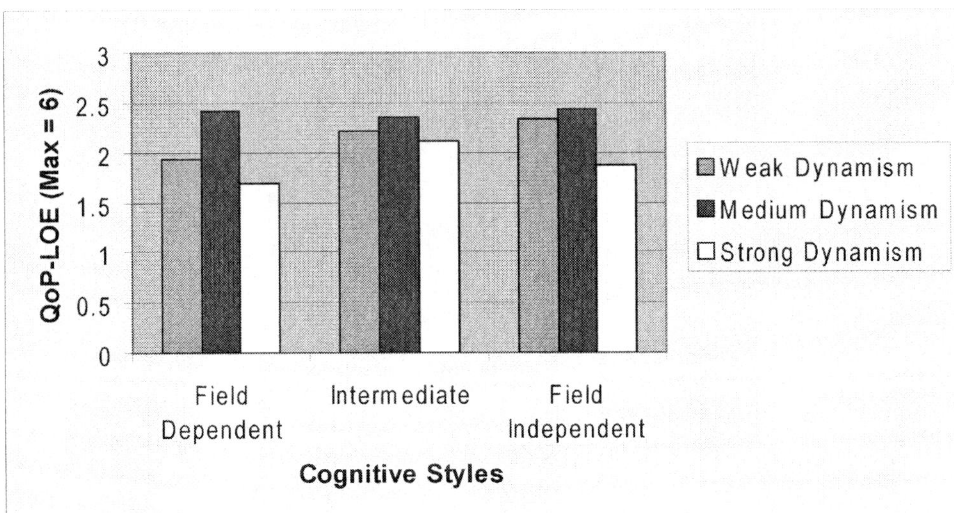

Figure 4. Impact of dynamism on QoP-IA (Verbalisers vs. Imagers)

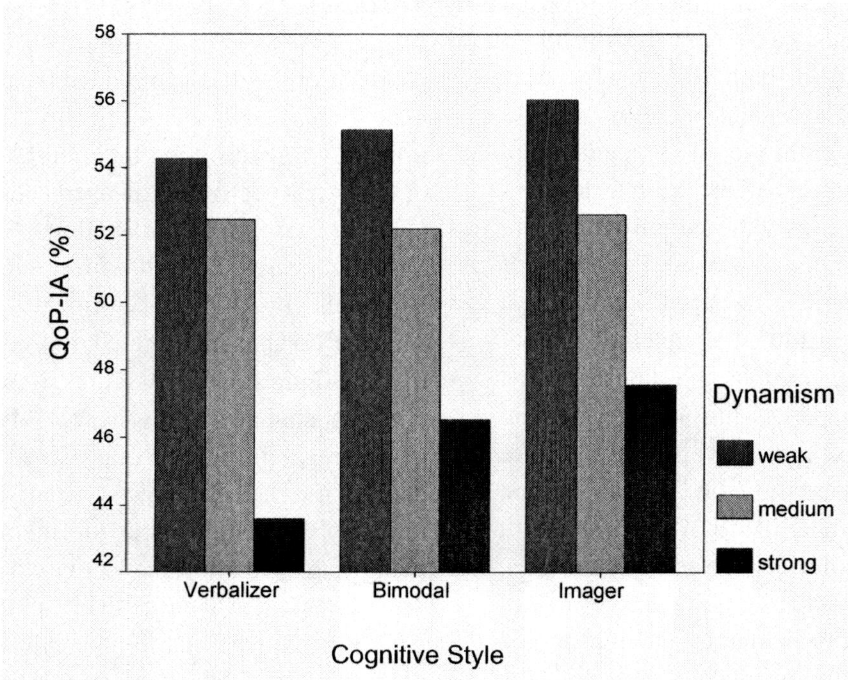

Figure 5. Impact of dynamism on QoP-LOE (Verbalisers vs. Imagers)

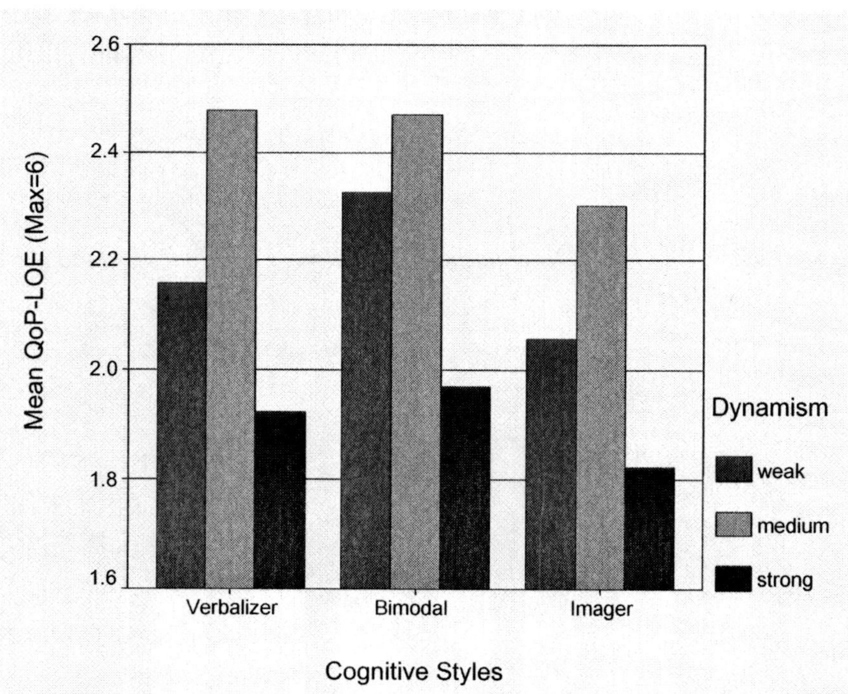

reveals that whilst dynamism is a significant factor in the case of Verbalizers ($F=8.009$; df-within = 549; $p<.001$) and Imagers ($F=4.691$; df-within = 645; $p=.009$), this is not true for Bimodals ($F=2.824$; df-within = 381; $p=.061$), although there is a trend toward significance for this cognitive style category as well. As suggested by previous research (Riding and Rayner, 1998), Bimodals can tailor learning strategies to the specific learning environments so the features of learning environments have no significant effects on their enjoyment. For Verbalizers and Imagers, however, it was found that clips of medium dynamism had the highest levels of QoP-LOE, which suggests that such users do not find enjoyable clips which are static (or, conversely, highly dynamic). Whilst the user may feel somewhat overwhelmed by a fast-paced clip, (s)he might possibly feel uninterested by a static clip with (almost) repetitive frame displays; it should come as no surprise, then, that such users prefer clips of medium dynamism, where they do not feel overwhelmed, but neither are they bored by the presentation of the subject matter concerned.

CONCLUSION

In concluding, we remark that our results show that clip dynamism, has, for all users, a significant effect on information assimilation– irrespective of a particular user's cognitive style. Accordingly, the highest Information assimilationscores were obtained for clips with medium dynamism, for all categories of users. At the other end of the spectrum, highly dynamic clips were shown to have a detrimental impact on information assimilation, with users obtaining low information assimilation scores for clips in this particular class. Whilst we believe that the explanation behind these results might lie in the fact that the rapid temporal changes of dynamic clips make it difficult for the user to focus on their informational content, the observation that users do not obtain the highest Information assimilationscores for static clips might be explained by their failure to capture and focus user attention. Lastly, it is worthwhile to remark that in the clips with strong and medium dynamism, Field Dependent users performed worse than the other two groups while Field Dependent users had a (slightly) better performance than Field Independent users in the clips with weak dynamism. This may be due to the fact that weak dynamism clips provide less confusion and may thus be suitable for Field Dependent users who have difficulties in dealing with complexity.

FUTURE RESEARCH DIRECTIONS

This study is a small step towards understanding the interplay between cognitive styles and the two main quality facets, subjective and technical, of distributed multimedia applications. However, cognitive styles are only one aspect of personal characteristics that impact perceptions of work [Stewart and Barrick, 2003]. In the future, other human factors - such as gender differences, prior knowledge, or alternative construction of cognitive styles - could be examined in this context, as could a wider variety of multimedia content (for example, games, with a higher degree of interactivity). It would also be interesting to explore what effect content presented in different languages have on learner's strategies for acquiring information, and whether these change with cultural or linguistic dimensions. These are all important considerations for personalisation.

Traditional statistics were used to analyse data in this study, but the limitations of using traditional statistics to analyse data is that there is a need to have assumptions. Such assumptions may have limitations for the findings that we discovered. On the other hand, data mining can be used to analyse data without any assumptions. In other words, we can discover findings from data themselves. By doing so, some hidden relationships can be discovered. Thus, a direction for future research is to conduct data analyses with data mining.

In light of our findings, it would also be worthwhile to explore how perceptual quality is affected by users having to pay for the content that they are accessing, or how, indeed, expectations are affected by this – would a user who has paid for bronze access to content still expects high quality (or how would he rate a low quality clip)? Conversely, would a user who has paid for gold access penalise more harshly low quality clips? Or, because s/he now has higher expectations (having paid for gold access), would s/he be even more strict in rating what are even high quality clips?

In addition, 'what users prefer' may be different from 'what is appropriate to users', so further research is needed to examine their differences in terms of cognitive styles. Such work can help to develop a better understanding of individual strategies used by different cognitive style groups so that designers can exploit the full potential of the QoP-QoS interplay and provide multimedia presentations with an enhanced QoP. The ultimate goal of such an understanding is to build robust user models for the development of personalised distributed multimedia environments and to integrate users' individual differences into truly end-to-end communication architectures.

REFERENCES

Anderson A. and Blockland A. Intelligibility of Speech Mediated by Low Frame-Rate Video, in C. Benoit (ed.) *Proceedings of the Audio-Visual Speech Processing Conference*, Rhodes, Greece 1997.

Apteker R.T., Fisher J.A., Kisimov V.S., and Neishlos H. Video Acceptability and Frame Rate, *IEEE Multimedia*, 2(3), pp. 32-40, 1995.

Blakowski, G. and Steinmetz R. A Media Synchronisation Survey: Reference Model, Specification, and Case Studies, *IEEE Journal on Selected Areas in Communications,* 14(1), pp. 5–35, 1996.

Chen, S. Y. A Cognitive Model for Non-linear Learning in Hypermedia Programmes. *British Journal of Educational Technology* 33 (4) 453-464, 2002

Chen, S. Y. and Ford, N. J. Modelling User Navigation Behaviours in a Hypermedia-Based Learning System: An Individual Differences Approach. *International Journal of Knowledge Organization* 25 (3) 67-78, 1998.

Chen, S. Y. and Macredie, R. D. Cognitive Styles and Hypermedia Navigation: Development of A Learning Model. *Journal of the American Society for Information Science and Technology* 53 (1) 3-15, 2002.

Chuang, Y-R. Teaching in a Multimedia Computer Environment: A study of effects of learning style, gender, and math achievement, 1999. Available: http://imej.wfu.edu./articles/1999/1/10/index/asp [21/12/2001]

Cranley, N., Murphy, L. and Perry, P. User-perceived quality-aware adaptive delivery of MPEG-4 content, *Proceedings of the 13th international workshop on Network and operating systems support for digital audio and video*, 42-49, Monterey, CA, 2003.

Demetriadis, S., Triantafilou, E., and Pombortis, A. A Phenomenographic Study of Students' Attitudes Toward the Use of Multiple Media for Learning, *ACM SIGCSE Bulletin, Proceedings of the 8th annual conference on Innovation and technology in computer science education*, June 30 – July 2 2003, Thessaloniki, Greece, pp 183 – 187, 2003.

Ford, N.,Wood, F.,Walsh, C. Cognitive styles and searching. Online CD-ROM Rev. 18(2), 79–86, 1994.

Fukuda, K., Wakamiya, N., Murata, M., and Miyahara, H., QoS Mapping between User's Preference and Bandwidth Control for Video Transport, in *Proceedings of the 5th International Workshop on QoS*, Paris, France, pp. 291-301, 1997.

Ghinea, G and Thomas, J P., QoS Impact on User Perception and Understanding of Multimedia Video Clips, in *Proceedings of ACM Multimedia '98*, Bristol, United Kingdom, pp. 49-54, 1998.

Hudson, L. Contrary Imaginations, Penguin, Harmondsworth, 1966.

Jonassen, D. H. and Grabowski, B. Individual Differences and Instruction. New York: Allen & Bacon, 1993.

Kouvelas, I., Hardman, V., and Watson, A., Lip Synchronisation for use over the Internet: Analysis and Implementation, in *Proceedings of IEEE Globecom '96*, London, United Kingdom, retrieved from the World Wide Web: http://www-mice.cs.ucl.ac.uk/multimedia/publications.

Laing, M. Teaching Learning and Learning Teaching: An Introduction to Learning Styles. *New Frontiers in Education* 31(4), 463-475, 2001.

Marrison, D. L. and Frick, M. J. The Effect of Agricultural Students' Learning Styles on Academic Achievement and Their Perceptions of Two Methods of Instruction. *Journal of Agricultural Education*, 35 (1) 26-30, 1994.

Messick, S. (1984) The nature of cognitive style: problems and promise in educational practice, *Educational Psychologist* 19, 59–74.

Neo, T. and Neo, M. Classroom innovation: engaging students in interactive multimedia learning, *Campus-Wide Information Systems*, 21(3), pp 118 – 124, 2004.

Pask, G. Styles and strategies of learning, British Journal of Educational Psychology 46, pp. 128–148, 1976.

Paterson P. The influence of learning strategy in a computer mediated learning environment Paper presented at ALT-Conference '96, 1996. Available: http://www.warwick.ac.uk/alt-/alt-96/papers.html [19/11/1997]

Riding, R.J, and Cheema, I.. Cognitive styles: An overview and integration. *Educational Psychology*, 11(3 & 4), 193-215, 1991.

Riding R.J. and Douglas, G.. The effect of cognitive style and mode of presentation on learning performance, *British Journal of Educational Psychology*, 63, 297-307, 1993.

Riding, R. J. *Cognitive Styles Analysis*, Birmingham: Learning and Training Technology, 1991.

Riding, R.J. and Grimley, M. Cognitive style and learning from multimedia materials in 11 year old children. *British Journal of Educational Technology* 30 (2) 43-56, 1999..

Riding, R.J. and Rayner, S.G. Cognitive Styles and Learning Strategies, London: David Fulton Publisher, 1998.

Steinmetz, R. Human Perception of Jitter and Media Synchronisation, *IEEE Journal on Selected Areas in Communications*, 14(1), pp. 61 –72, 1996.

Watson A and Sasse, M.A. Measuring Perceived Quality of Speech and Video in Multimedia Conferencing Applications, in *Proceedings of ACM Multimedia '98*, Bristol, United Kingdom, pp. 55-60, 1998.

Wijesekera, D. and Srivastava, J. Quality of Service (QoS) Metrics for Continuous Media, *Multimedia Tools and Applications*, 3(1), pp. 127-166, 1996.

Witkin, H. A., Moore, C. A., Goodenough, D. R., and Cox., P. W. Field-dependent and field independent cognitive styles and their educational implications. *Review of Educational Research*, 47, 1-64, 1977.

Zwyno, M. S. Student Learning Styles, Web Use Patterns and Attitudes Towards Hypermedia-Enhanced Instruction, *Proceedings of the 33rd ASEE/IEEE Frontiers in Education Conference*, Colorado, USA, pp 1-6, 2003.

ADDITIONAL READING

Blakowski, G., and Steinmetz R., A Media Synchronisation Survey: Reference Model, Specification, and Case Studies, IEEE Journal on Selected Areas in Communications, 14(1), 5 - 35, January 1996

Bouch, A., Kuchinsky, A., and Bhatti, N., Quality is in the eye of the beholder. *Proc. of the CHI 2000 Conference on Human Factors in Computing Systems*, The Hague, The Netherlands, pp. 297-304, 2000.

Bouch, A., Sasse, M.A., and DeMeer, H., Of Packets and People: A User-Centred Approach to Quality of Service. *Proc. of IWQoS 2000*, Pittsburgh, PA, pp. 189-197, 2000.

Calcaterra, A., Antonietti, A., and Underwood, J. Cognitive style, hypermedia navigation and learning. Computers & Education. 44(4), 441-457, 2005.

Chen, S. Y., Ghinea, G. and Macredie, R. D. A Cognitive Approach to User Perception of Multimedia Quality: An Empirical Investigation. International Journal of Human-Computer Studies. 64(12), 1200-1213, 2006.

Chilton, M. A., Hardgrave, B. C., Armstrong, D. J. Person - Job Cognitive Style Fit For Software Developers. Journal of Management Information Systems, 22(2), 193-226, 2005.

Claypool, M., and Tanner, J., The Effects of Jitter on the Perceptual Quality of Video, *ACM Multimedia'99 (Part 2),* Orlando, FL, pp. 115-118, 1999.

Dogan, S., Eminsoy, S., Sadka, A. H., and Kondoz, A. M., Personalised multimedia services for real-time video over 3G mobile networks. *Third International Conference on 3G Mobile Communication Technologies, 2002. (Conf. Publ. No. 489)*, pp. 366–370, 2002.

Falmagne, J.C., *Handbook of Perception and Human Performance",* Vol. 1, Chapter 1, Psychophysical Measurement and Theory, John Wiley, 1986

Faraday, P. and Sutcliffe, A., An Empirical Study of Attending and Comprehending Multimedia Presentations. In *Proc. of ACM Multimedia '99,* Boston, Massachusetts, USA, pp. 265-275, 1999.

Frias-Martinez, E., Chen, S. Y., and Liu, X. Automatic Cognitive Style Identification of Digital Library Users for Personalization. Journal of the American Society for Information Science and Technology. 58(2), 237-251, 2007.

Ghinea, G. and Angelides, M.C. Quality of Perception in m-Commerce, Mobile Commerce Applications, N.S. Shi (ed.), pp. 284-302, Idea Group Publishing, 2004

Ghinea, G. and Chen, S. Digital Multimedia Perception and Design, Idea Group Publishing, 2006

Ghinea, G. and Chen, S. Y. Perceived Quality of Multimedia Educational Content: A Cognitive Style Approach. ACM Multimedia Systems Journal. 11(3), 271-279, 2006.

Ghinea, G. and Chen, S. Y. The Impact of Cognitive Styles on Perceptual Distributed Multimedia Quality. British Journal of Educational Technology. 34(4), 393-406, 2003.

Ghinea, G. and Thomas, J.P. Quality of Perception: User Quality of Service in Multimedia Presentations, IEEE Transactions on Multimedia, 7(4), 786-789, 2005.

Goodenough, D. The role of individual differences in field dependence as a factor in learning and memory. Psychological Bulletin. 83, 675-694, 1976.

Graff, M. Learning from Web-based Instructional Systems and Cognitive Style. British Journal of Educational Technology 34(4), 407-418, 2003.

Gulliver S.R. and Ghinea, G. Stars in their Eyes: What Eye-Tracking Reveals about Multimedia Perceptual Quality, IEEE Transactions on Systems, Man and Cybernetics, Part A, 34(4), 472-482, 2004.

Gulliver, S.R., Serif T. and Ghinea, G. Pervasive and Standalone Computing: the Perceptual Effects of Variable Multimedia Quality, International Journal of Human Computer Studies, 60, 640-665, 2004.

Hardman, V., Sasse, M. A., and Kouvelas, I., Successful multi-party audio communications over the Internet. Communication of the ACM, 41 (5), 74-80, 1998.

Just, M. A. and Carpenter, P. A., Eye Fixations and Cognitive Processes. Cognitive Psychology, 8, 441-480, 1976.

Kim, K. and Allen, B. Cognitive and Task Influences on Web Searching Behavior. Journal of the American Society for Information Science and Technology. 53(2), 109-199, 2002.

Lee, C. H., Cheng, Y. W., Rai, S., and Depickere, A. What affect student cognitive style in the development of hypermedia learning system. Computers & Education. 45(1), 1-19, 2005.

Liegle, J. O. and Janicki, T. N. The effect of learning styles on the navigation needs of Web-based learners. Computers in Human Behavior. 22 (5), 885-898, 2006.

Miller, L. E. and Escolme, K. M. (1990) Cognitive Style of International and Domestic Graduate Students in Agricultural Education and Agricultural Economics. 34, 52-56.

Parkinson, A., Redmond, J. A., and Walsh, C. Accommodating field-dependence: a cross-over study. *Proceedings of the 9th annual SIGCSE conference on Innovation and technology in computer science education*. pp 72-76, 2004.

van den Branden Lambrecht, C.J., and Verscheure, O., Perceptual Quality Measure using a Spatio-Temporal Model of the Human Visual System, *Proceedings of the SPIE*, Vol. 2668, pp. 450 - 461, San Jose, CA, January 28 - February 2 1996,

Verscheure, O. and Hubaux, J. Perceptual Video Quality and Activity Metrics: Optimisation of Video Services based on MPEG-2 encoding", *Proceedings of COST-237 Workshop,* Barcelona, Spain, November 1996

Watson, A. and Sasse, M.A., Evaluating Audio and Video Quality in Low-Cost Multimedia Conferencing Systems, *Interacting with Computers*, 8(3), 255-275, 1996

Webster, A.A., Jones, T.C., Pinson, M.H., Voran, S.D., and Wolf, S., An objective video quality assessment system based on human perception, *SPIE Human Vision, Visual Processing, and Digital Display IV,* Vol. 1913, pp. 15 - 26, San Jose, CA, February 1993

Zywno, M. Hypermedia Instruction and Learning Outcomes at Different Levels of Bloom's Taxonomy of Cognitive Domain. Global Journal of Engineering Education. 7(1), 59-70, 2003.

Chapter XIII
Building Digital Memories for Augmented Cognition and Situated Support

Mathias Bauer
mineway GmbH, Germany

Alexander Kröner
German Research Center for Artificial Intelligence (DFKI GmbH), Germany

Michael Schneider
German Research Center for Artificial Intelligence (DFKI GmbH), Germany

Nathalie Basselin
German Research Center for Artificial Intelligence (DFKI GmbH), Germany

ABSTRACT

Limitation of the human memory is a well-known issue that anybody has experienced. This chapter discusses typical components and processes involved in the building and the exploitation of augmented memories. SPECTER, an adaptive, self-learning system supports the user in everyday activities by interpreting sensor information captured in the environment and deriving adequate suggestions for actions to be taken in the current situation. A particular form of introspection allows the user to reflect on the digital memory's contents and the system behavior, thus leaving the user in control. An empirical study in a shopping scenario evaluates the benefits and limitations of the approach taken.

INTRODUCTION

Limitation of the human memory is a well-known issue that anybody has experienced. Do you remember how the colleague you just met was dressed, how much you paid for your television, what you prepared this year for dinner to your various guests, which books you looked at the last time you visited a bookstore, and, by the way, when exactly was it again? Human sensory, short-term and long-term memories appear to have limitations or problems which disable us to store and retrieve all data.

Human sensory memory consists of a buffer in which items perceived are stored. There exists one per perception channel (e.g. view, touch). The storage time usually lasts 200 to 500 ms after the perception of an item. George Sperling conducted several studies and reported that sensory memory could store a maximum of 12 perceived items, but, because of the fast degradation of this memory, only a few could actually be memorized and reported by the subjects (Sperling, 1960).

While limitations of the short-term human memory are still controversial, views argue that short-term memory would have capacity- and / or time-limitations. According to Miller (Miller, 1956) this memory would have limitations regarding enumerations of more than seven items plus or minus two or, according to more recent research (Henderson, 1972), the upper capacity limit would rather be between 3 and 5 chunks. In addition, memory has various biases such as for instance the one to remember rather the first or last items of an enumeration than the ones in between. Diverse strategies therefore allow for dealing with these issues. While the storable number of chunks would be limited, the easiest way to remember a long number or list of letters is, according to Herbert Simon, to divide them into chunks of three letters or numbers. Phone numbers are indeed usually divided into chunks of three or two numbers. To cope with the time limitation of the short-term memory, rehearsal of chunks is an efficient way to store them longer into the short-term memory.

Long-term memory problems have also been studied and categorized into "seven sins" by Schacter (2001). Three of the seven sins involve forgetting: "transience", i.e. the decreasing ability to access memory over time, "absent-mindedness", i.e. lapses of attention and forgetting to do things, and "blocking", i.e. temporary inaccessibility of some data. Three other sins involve distortion problems: "misattribution", i.e. a right memory is associated with a wrong source or one believes to have seen or heard something while this is not the case, "suggestibility", i.e. implanting of misinformation via leading questions for instance, and "bias", i.e. distortion of past memories by current knowledge. The seventh sin is of less interest for the purpose of this chapter since it consists of "persistence", i.e. pathological inability to forget, which can happen after a traumatic-stress. In order to cope with the usual memory problems, people often resort to memory aids such as sticky notes and mnemonics.

Some of the previously mentioned limitations of the human memory can be addressed by exploiting one of the strengths of computers: the ability to store huge amounts of information for an unlimited time without loss of precision. And actually, state-of-the-art mobile devices in general provide features for creating reminders, linking notes to time and dates, and for managing time.

However, these techniques require the user to capture this data manually, and thus the quality of such memories greatly depends on her cognition and carefulness (please note that throughout this chapter we will refer to the user of our system in the female form.). These issues can be addressed by capturing and recording the desired data *automatically* within an intelligent environment. Such records can then be used not only to augment the user's memory, but also to enable new types of user support, such as contextual reminders or reflection on missed opportunities. This chapter provides a discussion of various challenges related to building and exploiting such augmented personal memories in everyday's life. We concentrate on a number of crucial aspects: the importance of abstraction processes for building this memory and the design of a user interface for supporting interaction between user and memory. We illustrate our approach with examples of processing and exploiting information about the user's location in the shopping assistant SPECTER (System for Perception of and Empathetic Communication Toward Environmental Resources). This research was supported by the German Federal Ministry of Education and Research respectively under grant 524-40001-01 IW C03 (project SPECTER) and 01 IW F03 (project SharedLife).

BACKGROUND

While digital memories can be created manually by the user—for instance, Gemmell et al. (2002) reported on benefits of a manually-created document-centered memory—, an automated capturing and recording process is not only more convenient for the user, but also allows a system to record information that the user herself may have missed, thus virtually extending her perception.

The automated construction of digital memories by means of an intelligent environment brings about some specific challenges related to capturing, storing, and processing sensor data. For instance, with a long-term application in mind, it will usually be impossible to judge if a perception made by a machine will be of value for future decisions. This suggests to capture as much data as possible and to be restrictive when dismissing information—which imposes strong constraints regarding efficiency and flexibility on storage and retrieval mechanisms.

For the exploitation of such digital memories, it is crucial to support the user in her interaction with the voluminous records of fine-grained, unstructured, and—depending on the number of applied sensor devices—manifold perceptions provided by an intelligent environment. Such support can be achieved in two ways: by an abstraction process translating sensor data into symbolic information that can be understood by the user, and by a user interface supporting the user in performing typical memory-related tasks.

Abstraction of Perceptions

With the ultimate goal of assisting the human with valuable information from past events, the extraction of meaningful information from a stream of system-made perceptions has been investigated in various scenarios. For instance, Clarkson (2002) illustrates how records of raw data automatically captured by wearable sensors could be mined in order to identify re-occurring situations. Horvitz et al. (2004) analyze a log of a user's desktop actions (e.g., "created a document") together with her calendar entries in order to identify clusters of related actions, which can then be exploited to support the user with a diary-like organization of her recent computer work. Pollack et al. (2003) illustrates how these ideas can be transferred to a user's everyday. AI planning technology and machine learning are employed to detect deviations from normal activity patterns and to provide adaptive, personalized reminders. Similarly, Patterson et al. (2004) analyze records of motion data in order to detect route errors of individuals with mild cognitive disabilities using transportation services.

Despite the great difference in the quality of data used in these examples, abstraction turns out to be indispensable in order to provide the user with an appropriate view on a digital memory. However, for the realization of user support based on sensor data, the abstraction process should not be limited to a particular data layer, since raw sensor data may form the input of such a memory as well as user actions of varying complexity. As depicted in Figure 5, a permanent stream of incoming low-level measurement data represents the world as being perceived by the system's various sensors such as GPS, RFID readers etc. To make these ephemeral snapshots of the environment accessible to the system's internal reasoning processes, these data are stored in a structure that constitutes an *extensional* representation of relations representing SPECTER's limited view of its context.

Using background knowledge—encoded in the form of rules, theories, or pattern libraries—these data are subject to interpretation processes that transform them into symbolical, abstract concepts, thus allowing an *intensional* representation of the essentials hidden in the incoming stream of measurements. Iterating this process eventually leads to a multi-layered representation of SPECTER's view of the world at various levels of abstraction. This multitude of abstraction levels is used to both support reasoning processes by providing input at the right level of "preprocessing" and improve communication with the user by presenting information at the appropriate granularity. See (Saitta & Zucker, 1998) and (Mustiere et al., 2000) for a thorough discussion of knowledge representation and abstraction frameworks in the context of learning applications.

From a technical—machine learning—point of view, data abstraction amounts to deriving additional attributes from a given data set, thus enhancing the representation of observed cases with more elaborate feature vectors. For propositional learning algorithms this is the most straightforward way to make use of background knowledge in the attempt to detect useful patterns in the training data. See e.g. (Atzmueller, 2006) for a discussion of this aspect.

In anticipation of the sample scenario to be described below, let's have a look at the way SPECTER deals with the user's motion in space as recorded using GPS receivers and similar localization technology. After cleaning the data in a preprocessing step by removing obvious measurement errors, the user's current path—represented by geographical coordinates and time stamps—can be classified using prototypical trajectories extracted from previous observations. The result of this classification is enriched by additional attributes representing properties of the user's movement and locations visited. Here background knowledge comes in the form of functions to extract concepts such as average speed, number of stops, length of loops etc. and annotations of places such as restaurant, department store etc. The feature vectors so created are used to determine a user's motion profile which—in the next stage of abstraction—forms part of the input of a plan recognition engine and finally a general situation classifier. Depending on her expertise and preferences, the appropriate level of abstraction can be selected by the system for effective communication with the user.

Interaction with Digital Memories

While a sophisticated abstraction process is crucial for the value of a digital memory, the user additionally requires a user interface supporting her interaction with the memory in order to actually benefit from captured and derived data. The retrieval methods provided to the user play a crucial role. Previous research addressed this issue in a variety of ways. For instance, information may be visually aligned and clustered in order to support the user while browsing a digital memory (see, e.g., (Dumais et al., 2003)). For explicit retrieval, Lamming et al. (1994) emphasize the special value of context for retrieval, while van den Hoven (2004) explores an object-centered approach to recollection. We contribute an approach which integrates these ideas with results from a study about how users actually apply such records in an everyday setting—a question widely neglected by previous research.

Besides such manual retrieval, augmented memories are also of particular value for proactive user support. For instance, Lee et al. (2006) describe how memories related to some previously retrieved real-world event may be displayed in order to assist the user in discovering relationships. Holz et al. (2005) discuss a variation of this idea based on a task model: Here, a knowledge worker is supported with documents automatically retrieved from a corporate memory in order to augment the user's perception of documents relevant to the current task. Other example scenarios include preventing nursing accidents by means of contextual reminders of instructions (Kuwahara et al., 2003) and social matching based on shared experiences (Sumi et al., 2002). However, even a sophisticated abstraction cannot guarantee a perfect match between the user's and the system's perception of a certain situation. Therefore, *transparency* of all system aspects becomes a key issue which means that the user has to be provided with tools to both inspect and manipulate not only the recorded information, but also the system's interpretation of this data and the implications derived. This holds true especially with respect to another application of digital memories: a user might want to review memories not only in order to learn about the system's processes, but also about herself (for an example of such interest for statistics, see the public annual reports of Nicholas Feltron's life at http://www.feltron.com/). Therefore, a user interface to digital memories should support such an *introspection* approach—a "...process of inward attention or reflection, so as to examine the contents of the mind..." (Sharples et al., 1989), an issue rarely addressed so far.

BUILDING AUGMENTED MEMORIES

The process of building an augmented memory described in the following mainly relies on automated mechanisms while simultaneously allowing (but not requiring) perfect control by the user—a crucial prerequisite to meet the transparency requirements. Its outcome is an event-based memory of user experiences. Here, we think of an "experience" as a piece of information composed from a user action, its context (e.g., location, time), and some rating associated with these data. The latter ones may be assigned explicitly by the user, or be computed by the system.

Scenario

The automatic collection of personal experiences relies on environments instrumented with various sensors. Retail stores can be expected to constitute the first group of instrumented environments to make an impact in everyday's life (Walmart, Tesco and METRO Group are early RFID adopters). Furthermore, smart homes (e.g., Siemens and Samsung's smart kitchens and homes), but also any kind of public places such as hospitals and offices are obvious candidates for increasing instrumentation.

In order to learn about the use of memories in these environments, we conducted a contextual inquiry where 5 subjects were observed in their preparation to go shopping and while shopping in non-instrumented environments. They were observed at home, in public transportation, downtown, visiting specialized, generalist, or grocery stores. Some had a shopping list, some not, the lists were either written on paper or stored on their PDAs. One subject was shopping without the help of a PDA, while the 4 others who were PDA owners shopped with the help of the "Tasks" application of the Pocket PC or with shopping dedicated applications: VOShoppingList (http://www.voscorp.com/) or HandyShopper (http://www.ggaub.com/hs/). The reason for selecting preferably subjects regularly using PDAs for shopping was to observe the purpose they use it for (which information do they store, for which tasks do they use it) and how the interaction with the PDA and the real world takes place.

The details of this study would have exceeded the scope of this chapter; therefore, we focus on selected results. It has been observed that shopping involves intensive gathering and processing of information from the environment, which in turn substantially involves memory: while shopping for groceries, people recall their past experiences with products to choose which ones to buy. They also try to remember which products are missing or will soon be missing at home. Product comparison and price comparison is also an important task in shopping, especially when the products to compare are complex or expensive (digital cameras, for instance). Subjects tried to remember the prices, the product features as well as the different models available in the various stores they visited and tried to optimize their moves in the city and in huge supermarkets or department stores. Subjects also tried to estimate the total cost of their purchases before going to the cashier. This results in a relatively high cognitive load.

The observation showed that the subjects sometimes tried to achieve conflicting goals and optimize the costs of various shopping aspects: people try to make the best purchase at the best price, to minimize the shopping time and thus the walking time, but also to minimize their fatigue due to walking distances, reflection, and memorization. However, investing in memorization and reflection allows for optimizing store visits, save time and purchase at the best price. A mobile memory assistant could support the shopping task using ubiquitous features to support the human memory by noticing surrounding artifacts (for instance the content of the fridge), storing past experiences, as well as the products for which the user showed interest in a store by storing the product reference, description, price and store where it has been seen.

We set up various instrumented shopping environments (cell phones, digital cameras, audio CDs) and linked these to the shopping assistant SPECTER, which supports its user in the previously mentioned tasks by means of an automatically built digital memory. Thus the system memorizes on the user's behalf the places she visited, the products she looked at and their different properties (see the middle part of Figure 1). The user can consult these records at any time; in addition, the system supports the user's natural memory by reminding her of past experiences related to her current situation: for instance, if the user takes two products from a shelf, then

Figure 1. Exploiting a digital memory for user support in a camera-shopping scenario. The screenshot in the middle shows an excerpt of experiences recorded by SPECTER. The screen on the right-hand side presents a feature comparison of two cameras.

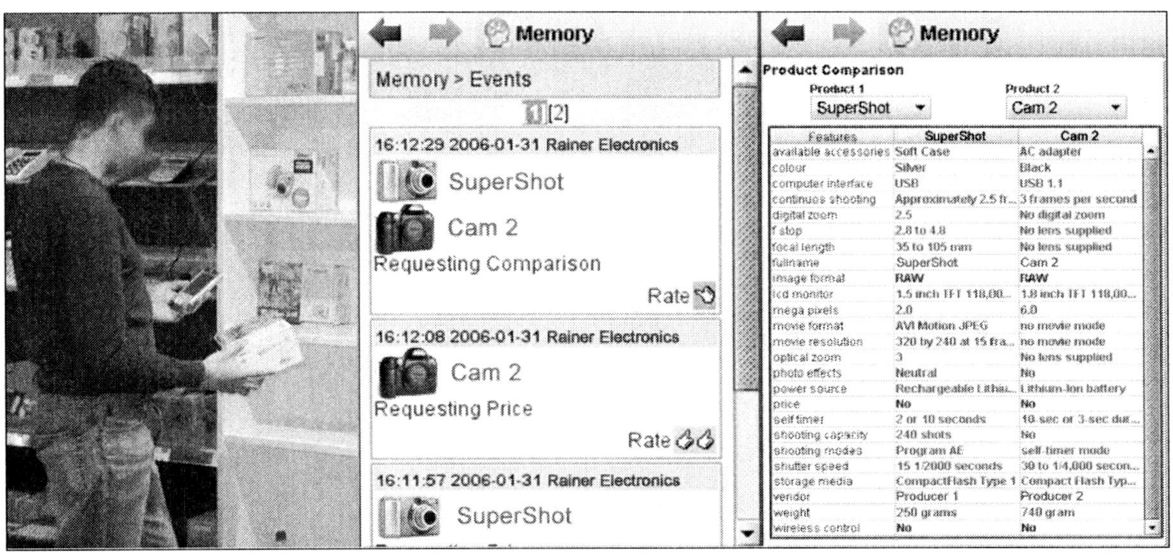

the system displays a comparison of both products' features (see the right-hand side of Figure 1). In the following, we will describe processes involved in the building and the exploitation of such a memory in more detail.

Capturing and Recording

Situated in an open, potentially complex environment, a memory-based system like SPECTER has to deal with a broad range of diverse information items. These items might be provided by a heterogeneous set of information sources like sensors and devices worn by the user herself, applications and sensors run by the environment, or virtual information sources like web services or background information provided by some world or domain model. Accordingly, a flexible and extendable mechanism for the representation and handling of relevant knowledge is required. In the following we will first describe how information is created and distributed in the environment in a general way. We will then see how information about a user's context and her behavior is represented in the environment and the augmented memory.

As mentioned above, information that is used as input to the augmented memory might originate from a variety of different sources, where each source is likely to observe just a small fraction of the environment. Instead of building and maintaining a single huge context model, each information source is responsible for constructing a partial model describing the environment's aspects it can provide information for. Whenever some knowledge source discovers a change in state, it constructs a minimal model that describes the new state of the affected property and publishes this model on the web under a unique URL.

A model shared by a temperature sensor for instance could contain the only statement that the temperature in room C0.03 was 21 degree Celsius on June 5th, 2007 at 11 o'clock. Each model contains a timestamp that states when the information was discovered. Already at this level domain-dependant abstraction processes may be applied to the information, especially if the information without such an abstraction process would generally not be understandable. An example would be the removal of a physical item from the field of a radio frequency identification (RFID) antenna. According to the situational context this event could have many different interpretations, ranging from the intended removal of a product from a shelf in the shop to the borrowing of a book in the library.

If a more complete picture of the current situation is required, an augmented-memory system may merge multiple individual knowledge models representing different aspects of the environment into a single, larger model. In the case of overlapping and contradicting partial models, such a system will have to resolve conflicts according to its trust into the respective reliability of the knowledge sources involved. Resolving conflicts on the application level has the big advantage to allow different instances of an augmented memory (possibly owned by different users) to apply their individual models of trust independently. Figure 2 illustrates how partial models (black bars) provided by different sources may be merged into a more complex model of the current situation (dashed contour). Although the proposed framework does not impose restrictions on the granularity of shared

Figure 2. Merging of partial knowledge models (black bars) to construct the current world state.

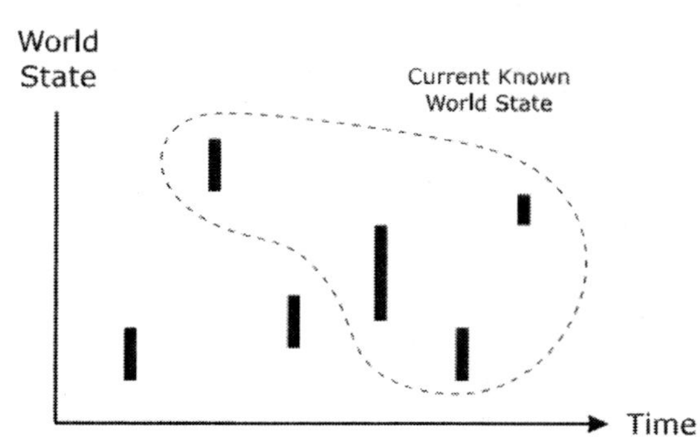

models, it is reasonable to separate independent statements into individual models. On the one hand, this minimizes the processing overhead (bandwidth, parsing, memory, and processing) for systems that are only interested in parts of the shared knowledge, and on the other hand reduces the danger of conflicts between models from different sources that describe similar properties of the environment.

So far, the described framework is independent of any concrete knowledge representation. It is even possible for each knowledge source to use its own representation framework, as long as the augmented memory application is able to merge knowledge models from different sources. Nevertheless, for practical reasons knowledge sources and the augmented memory system should agree on a shared knowledge representation, which is then used throughout the whole system. We will later see how we used RDF and an OWL ontology to represent knowledge models.

Simply providing knowledge models under some URL is not sufficient to build an augmented memory. The memory system additionally needs a way to locate relevant knowledge models and to get notified about updates. For this reason we introduced the concept of so-called RDF:Stores (cf. (Schneider, 2006)). An RDF:Store serves as a yellow-page service for RDF-based knowledge models. Whenever a knowledge source publishes a new model, it posts the model URL to the current RDF:Store. The RDF:Store then downloads the contents of advertised model and creates an index about the concepts and instances used. Memory-based systems can later look up the URLs of models containing information about a certain item instance or describing a certain property via a query interface. Additionally, a trigger can be defined which proactively notifies the memory system whenever a new model matching a configurable filter is added to the RDF:Store.

Information provided by the environment and stored in an augmented memory needs to be represented in a way that is understandable and interpretable by both the human user of the memory and the automated reasoning processes of the memory implementation. A common solution in such cases is the use of an ontology which defines a shared vocabulary for the exchange of semantically rich information. The ontology used in the SPECTER implementation is expressed in the Web Ontology Language (OWL, see http://www.w3.org/TR/owl-ref/) and is based on the Suggested Upper Merged Ontology and Mid-Level Ontology (SUMO and MILO, see http://ontology.teknowledge.com/). Domain-specific extensions were added for individual application scenarios where necessary.

When representing the content of an augmented memory it is reasonable to distinguish between two different kinds of information: General information about the user's actual context (like the current state of the environment), and information about dynamic processes like the user's concrete behavior and actions. While contextual information is represented in a straightforward manner by asserting properties to object instances, the representation of dynamic processes is somewhat more complex.

Observations of higher-level user actions are represented as instances of SUMO processes. Figure 3 shows an excerpt of the SUMO process hierarchy. As an example, the "Comparing" pro-

Figure 3. Excerpt of the SUMO process hierarchy

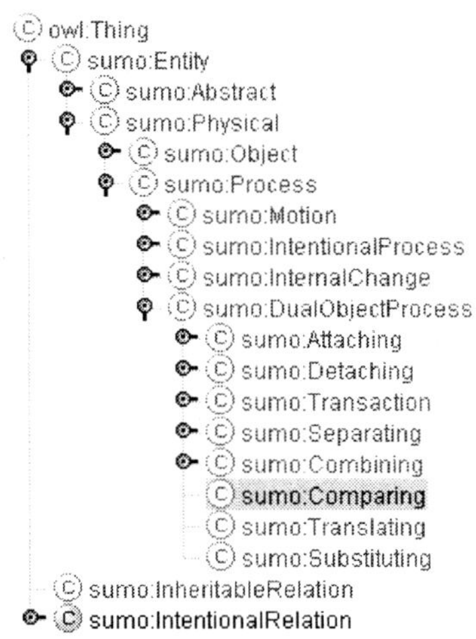

cess is highlighted, which is used in the digital camera shopping example mentioned above to model the act of comparing two or more camera against each others. Although all associated properties of the process class might be used for a detailed description of the observed action, a few properties are of special interest in the context of augmented memories and are specified whenever possible:

- **agent:** The agent (or person) that performed the shared interaction. In most cases this will be the user of the augmented memory itself, but the agent could also be some proactive application that initiates an interaction with the user.
- **patient:** The physical or virtual items that are involved in the described process.
- **whenFn:** The time interval during which the process was performed.
- **partlyLocated:** The location where the observed process took place (if applicable).
- **subProcess:** A more fine-grained description of the observed process (if applicable).

In order to represent information about the source of the observed information, the process instance that describes the observed action itself is wrapped into a "Perception" instance. Here, the property "agent" refers to the information source, and the "patient" property refers to the actual interaction Process.

Figure 4 shows the ontological representation of the camera comparison action that the user performed in the digital camera shopping scenario described above. The shaded boxes represent individuals of the denoted classes. The arrows represent relationships between these individuals through the denoted properties. Due to space restrictions and reasons of clarity we have omitted the representation of the Comparison process's sub processes as well as all properties used for the annotation of the individuals in a human readable format (textual description, pictograms, etc.).

Besides the ontological representation of the user's context and behavior the systems benefits from a semantic representation of the objects involved in our memory entries. In our shopping scenarios we could greatly simplify the task of modeling the offered goods by reusing product information that is available free-of-charge from Amazon's e-commerce web service (http://www.amazon.com/gp/aws/landing.html). The information provided by this service includes product names, short and long descriptions, pictures, prices, category information, technical proper-

Figure 4. Exemplary representation of a camera comparison with instances (grey boxes) and used properties (white boxes)

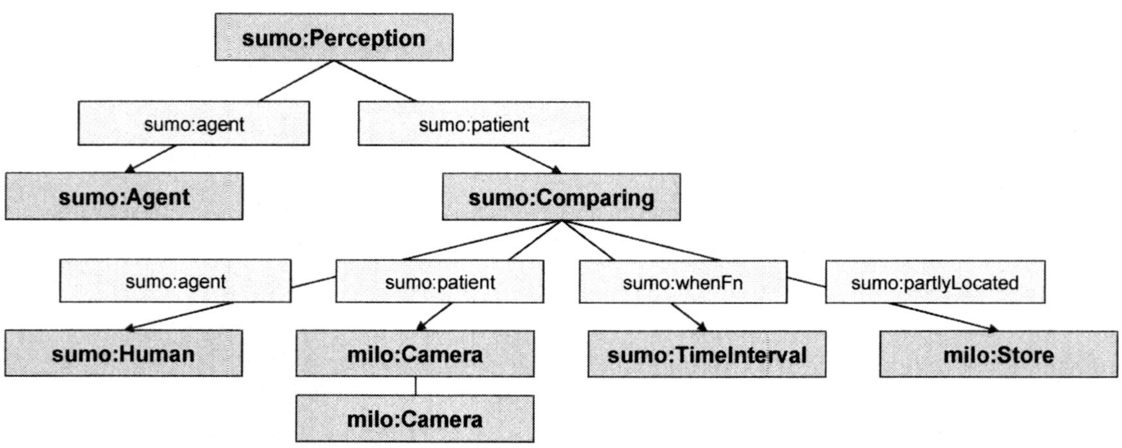

Figure 5. The abstraction process in SPECTER

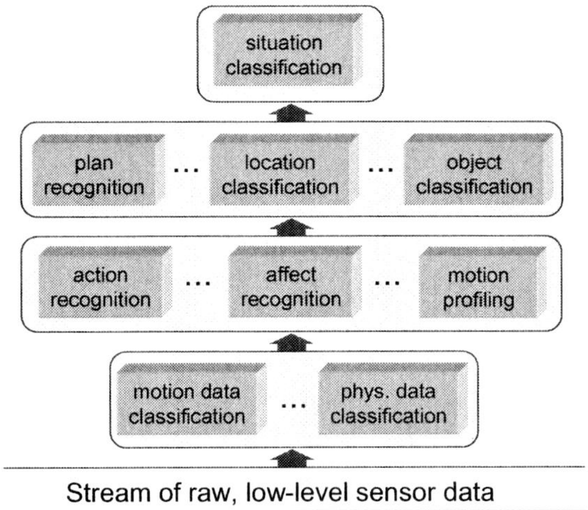

Figure 6. Components and processes applied for building augmented memories

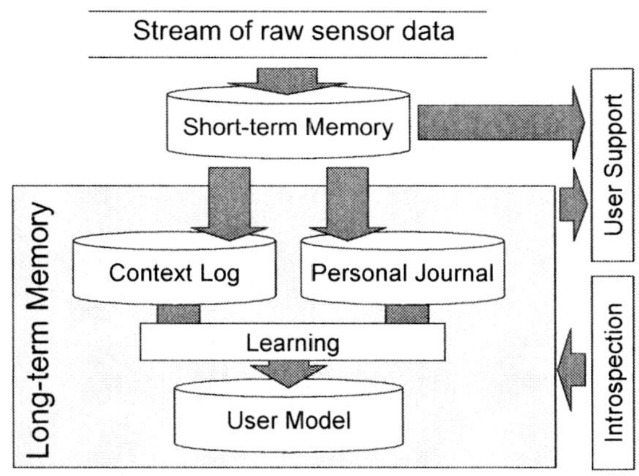

ties, etc. and is available for all products that are listed on Amazon.com. A script on our server allows fetching a model for each product under a unique URL which encodes the Amazon Standard Identification Number (ASIN) of the desired product. The script decodes the requested ASIN from the URL and invokes Amazon's web service to retrieve the according product description. As the returned result is given in a proprietary XML format, the script finally generates a valid OWL model of the requested product information. Thus, we are able to automatically generate a detailed model describing any product available at Amazon.com on the fly.

Processing Perceptions

The system's observations have to undergo further processing steps before they can be exploited for user support. Components of SPECTER involved in this processing are depicted in Figure 6; there, analogies to notions known from biology and psychology are used to describe processes related to building augmented memories. In this model, incoming perceptions are stored in a *short-term memory* which serves two main purposes. First, it is of special relevance for the recognition of situations and thus situated user support. Facts stored in the short-term memory describe the user's current context. This context is matched against patterns of service bindings specified in the user model (see next section). The second major purpose of the short-term memory is the identification of related perceptions, which can be combined to complex events and episodes. This leads to our two-fold approach to a *long-term memory* for intelligent environments. First of all, perceptions are stored without modification in a context log. This log works primarily as the system's memory. It is linked to the *personal journal* whose entries represent episodes created from one or more perceptions. These entries are annotated with contextual information (e.g., location, time, kind of motion) extracted from the referred perceptions; their creation is controlled by rules expressing commonsense knowledge and domain knowledge. Thus, the personal journal offers the user the right level of granularity when accessing the augmented memory. In the course of introspection, the user may interact with journal entries in various ways, e.g., by assigning ratings in order to express a personal impression related to a situation, or by applying them in order to customize automated user support. From the system's point of view, both context log and personal journal provide input to the processes performed in the short-term memory. In addition, they are exploited for building and refining the user model.

All of these components depend on—or are actively involved in—an abstraction process which starts on the level of perceptions and leads to statements in the user model. We will illustrate this idea in the following by discussing the processing of the user's motion data. As pointed out by Bogdanovych et al. (2007), this data is of special value for estimating the user's *current* shopping mood. Thus, the interpretation of this data is not only valuable for user support, but also to create contextual information for the creation of journal entries.

Motion Profiles

When discussing the abstraction process we already briefly mentioned the use of location and motion data to interpret the user's observed behavior. Now let's have a look at this line of reasoning in the context of the abovementioned short-term/long-term memory framework.

SPECTER computes a two-part motion profile from low-level position data as provided e.g. by the increasingly widespread GPS receivers or any other positioning method based on WLAN, infrared beacons or similar (Zeimpekis et al., 2003).

The low-level input to the system consists of a permanent stream $S = \langle p_1, ..., p_n, ...\rangle$ of positions passed by the user where $p_i = \langle x_i, y_i, z_i, t_i\rangle$. In the case of GPS data, x_i and y_i correspond to latitude and longitude values, respectively, z_i measures the current elevation, t_i is a time stamp. In a first step, these data are cleaned from obvious measurement errors that may occur in the initialization phase. They can be easily recognized by looking at the distances covered during the last timestamp.

A motion profile MP(S) = $\langle mod_p(S), mod_m(S)\rangle$ based on S consists of two components. $mod_p(S)$ encodes properties of the various positions contained in S while $mod_m(S)$ represents essential aspects of the user's movements in terms of abstract features immediately determined from S such as average speed, number and duration of stays, loops etc.

The contents of $mod_p(S)$ plays a role both in short-term and long-term memory. Immediate, situation-dependent user support relies on the short-term memory. Depending on the background knowledge available, the *x/y/z*-positions recorded in S are enhanced with identifiers for the associated places (e.g. "university library" or "Paolo e Tonio") and possibly additional tags representing classifications such as "restaurant" taken from a domain ontology. This information about the places visited by the user so far is used by the system to make predictions and recommendations regarding locations to be visited in the near future. Similar information collected about other system users is used to identify typical combinations in the form of association rules such as:

"If the user has visited 'Kulturcafe' and (then) 'Sport Scheck', then she will also visit 'H&M'."

or

"If the user has visited a shoe shop and a department store, then she will also visit a restaurant."

Note that such rules come with confidence and support values indicating the reliability of such a rule. Comparing the left-hand side of such rules with the user's immediate past enables the system to e.g. proactively check for availability of a restaurant according to the user's food taste—stored in another facet of the system's long-term memory.

In addition to these annotated sequences of places, modp(S) still contains the user's trajectory as a sequence of GPS locations. (Bauer & Deru, 2005) presents a method to identify prototypical patterns within collections of such trajectories (see

Figure 7. Trajectories recorded in a downtown area (left) and prototypical paths derived (right)

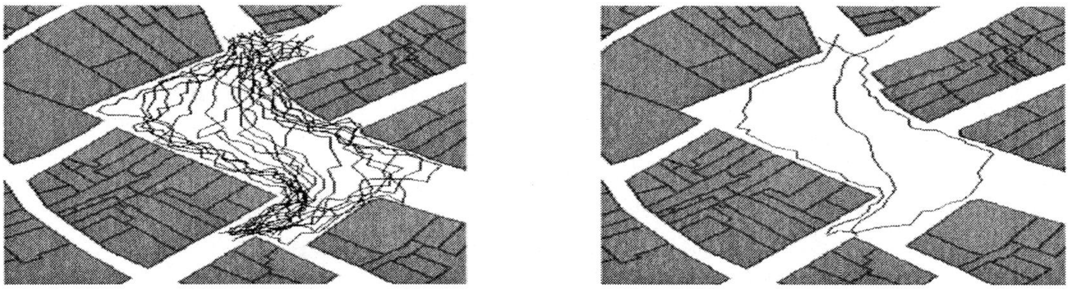

Figure 7). Again, comparing the data gathered for the current user to the prototypical patterns derived from observing other users, the future movements—and thus, the user's most likely path in the immediate future—can be predicted with a certain degree of confidence. For all this reasoning the system falls back on the short-term memory.

Combined with the user's reactions to these suggestions—i.e. her actual subsequent behavior—the location-dependent part of the motion profile enters the long-term memory where it serves as a basis to adjust the reliability values for prediction and classification rules and derive individual preference information for this user, thus updating her overall user model.

As already mentioned, the second part of the motion profile, $mod_m(S)$, deals with the user's motion itself. The feature vector computed characterizes the way the user is moving. A classifier in the form of a decision tree derived from the observed behaviors of all system users is applied to this vector to estimate the user's current mood and receptiveness for new information to be presented by the system. If, for example, the user seems to be in a hurry, it might be no good idea for the system to bother her with (currently) irrelevant details about a restaurant close by. So, the hypothesis of the user's current state—as estimated from the classification of her current motions—forms the basis for the filtering of information to be presented and the way this presentation will actually take place. An obviously confused user who has lost her way might need much more elaborate navigation hints than somebody just strolling through a pedestrian area. This situated reasoning takes place using the system's short-term memory.

Just as the other part of the motion profile, $mod_m(S)$ enters the system's long-term memory to be combined with the user's reaction to the system's behavior and the eventual update of her preferences regarding both presentations and information to be presented.

USER SUPPORT THROUGH AUGMENTED MEMORIES

A user's past experiences can be exploited for user support in quite diverse ways. We will in the following focus on an application well suited to illustrate the potential benefits of such services: decision support based on augmented memories. Here, the straightforward idea is that for a situation, experiences made by the user in similar situations might contain information worth to consider for upcoming decisions.

This suggests realizing a mobile assistant which grants the user access to her augmented memory at any time. However, depending on the diversity of situations experienced by the user, her information needs might differ widely: for instance, while exploring a store, a user might require information allowing her to judge an object at hand quickly. Here, a compilation of previous experiences might be more helpful than a rich description of previous encounters. However, when reviewing her user profile, the user might require such a rich description in order to understand the previously seen compilation. Such different applications impose strong requirements on the flexibility of retrieval and display methods employed for the design of a user interface to augmented memories.

Quan et al. (2003) experienced a similar need for a flexible presentation of RDF-encoded records describing a user's desktop communication. They addressed this issue by means of "views", which allow for presenting a given data set in various ways. Transferred to augmented memories, a view provides specific retrieval and visualization techniques for memories, and adapts to situational constraints. Following this approach, we realized several special-purpose views as well as some general-purpose views. The firmer views implement domain-specific visualizations, such as a feature comparison within a shopping scenario, which aligns the features of a given product with all other products of that category the user saw so far. The latter views address the domain-independent tasks mentioned before.

Figure 8 illustrates some of them within an "audio CD shopping" scenario. On the left-hand side, a function-oriented view presents functions applicable to an object. This view is applicable to each content element from the augmented memory, which includes events as well as their respective contents. The functions activate services provided by the system ("memory functions" such as "Similar CDs in memory") or by the user's current environment ("environment functions" such as "Similar CDs in <current store>"). In the middle, another view displays a list of objects extracted from the memory. Here, contextual information is suppressed—in contrast to the event-based view on the right-hand side, which displays actions and involved objects within their context (e.g., time, location).

These views can be replaced at any time by user or system in order to obtain a different perspective on the augmented memory. However, with respect

Figure 8. Supporting the user's interaction with her augmented memory by means of varying views on augmented memories in an audio CD shopping scenario. From the left to the right: functions, objects, events.

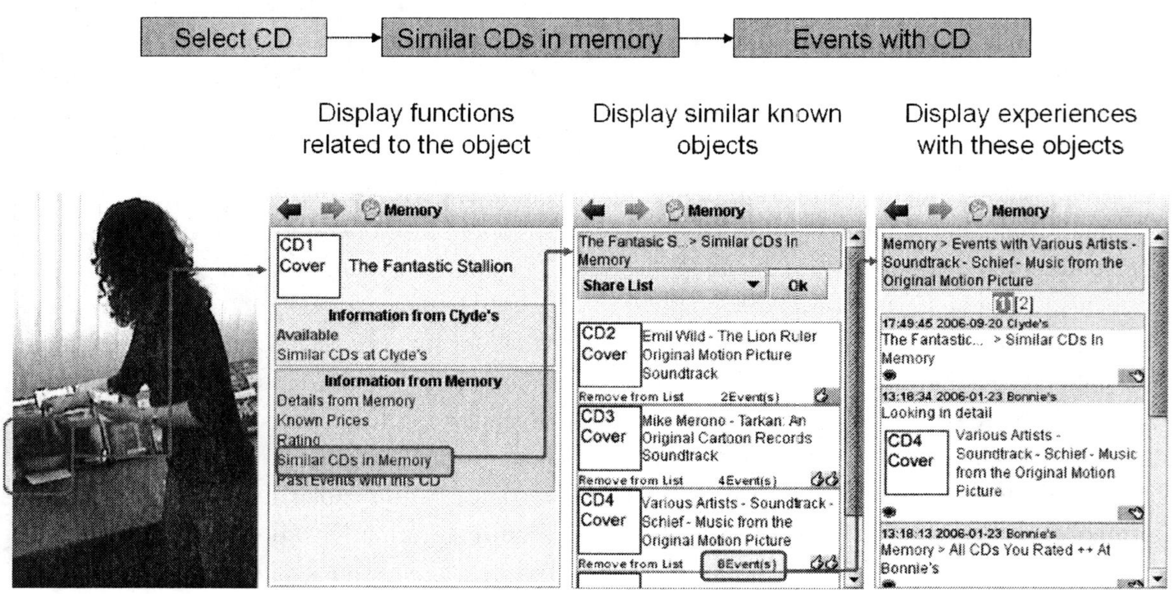

to the envisioned domain-independent application of augmented memories, this mechanism has to deal with a broad range of diverse memory contents—whose display has to be adapted to the surrounding view. Thus, again a mechanism is needed which allows for displaying the different pieces content in various ways. And again, the view paradigm provides a solution for this task. Since all memories are encoded by means of RDF, their respective contents can be mapped to RDF classes defined in the underlying content ontology. Kröner et al. (2006) explained how these classes can be associated with visualization templates, which can be selected by the display engine with respect to the current view and other situational constraints. The selection of these templates can be steered based on the ontology's class hierarchy, which enables the realization of a default visualization based on inheritance of templates.

The various views are interconnected by hyperlinks, which guide the user to related information, and which frequently involve a change in the view on the memory and thus support the user in retrieving and reviewing augmented memories. The hyperlinks have been optimized with respect to interaction patterns we observed in an empirical study. For instance, in Figure 8 the interaction begins with the user inspecting a music CD in one of the stores. This action automatically triggers a function-oriented view on the user's PDA. There, the user may ask for "Similar CDs in Memory" in order to learn about the offer. In response, she receives an object view on CDs she encountered earlier. Each object is connected to events involving it which allows the user to learn about contexts making reference to this CD.

While this approach supports the user in reflecting on memories, it still requires her initiative to begin such a process. However, it is easy to imagine occasions where the user won't take such initiative—for instance, because she isn't aware of the availability of memories relevant for her current situation. Thus, one should take into account for the design of such a memory-based system the option to augment the user's cognition with relevant memories. This requires that the system is equipped with a mechanism which allows it to initiate a reflection depending on the current situation. Within SPECTER's architecture, such services can be realized by applying perceptions stored in the short-term memory in order to retrieve corresponding memories from the long-term memory, which can then be exploited for triggering various supporting services.

We coined the notion "recomindation" in order to describe the (situated) reminding of the user on past events with the goal to express a recommendation regarding the user's next actions (Plate et al., 2006);. We implemented examples of such support within the previously mentioned "audio CD shopping" scenario. There, we defined events which triggered the automated choice of a view with information matching the event's nature—for instance, if a user removes a CD from the shelf, a view is displayed which provides various functions which allow to retrieve additional information from memory and environment (see left-hand side of Figure 8). The user is not actually required to use or confirm the presented information. Thus, there is a certain risk that the user misses relevant information despite the system's activity. However, the impact of such behavior can be reduced by means of the augmented memory: the system keeps a history of displayed views on the one hand side and a precise record of all initiated services within the memory on the other side. Thus, the user may benefit from previously ignored services during a later opportunity.

The participants of empirical studies within that setting appreciated the flexibility and the unobtrusiveness of this approach. Nevertheless, one shouldn't expect that such automated behavior is always in line with the individual user's preferences. Therefore, we will proceed with a discussion of further means of reflection, which enable the user to critique the system's behavior.

Reflection and Introspection

Up to this point we focused on supporting a user during her actions by means of augmented memories. However, humans frequently apply their memories outside of such situational constrained settings: for instance, humans use memories in preparation of future actions or review them in order to learn about themselves. Since augmented memories can be exploited in a similar fashion, their user interface should assist the user in this task as well. The need for such support is further emphasized by the personal nature of services grounded on augmented memories. Here, reflection on system behavior provides not only a way of making system behavior transparent, but also to resolve deviations between the user's expectations and actual system behavior.

In order to address these issues, we realized an "introspection environment", which aims at supporting the user in reflecting on the content of her augmented memory (see Figure 9). It embeds the previously discussed mobile interface in a desktop interface; the additional space is used to display detailed views on contents selected from the memory. The component can be controlled by the mobile interface or alternatively by a domain-specific menu. The latter one allows the user to evoke various functions related to an introspection process (e.g., summaries) or to the objects currently in the focus of the user's attention. Alternatively, the user may hand over initiative to the system by requesting for a guided introspection. Such a request evokes the BDI planner JAM (Huber, 1999), which employs the introspection environment's features to generate

Figure 9. A screenshot of SPECTER's user interface for computer-supported reflection on past experiences. The right-hand side shows an information piece retrieved from the memory, the middle related material (here: applicable functions), and the left-hand side a virtual character who guides the process.

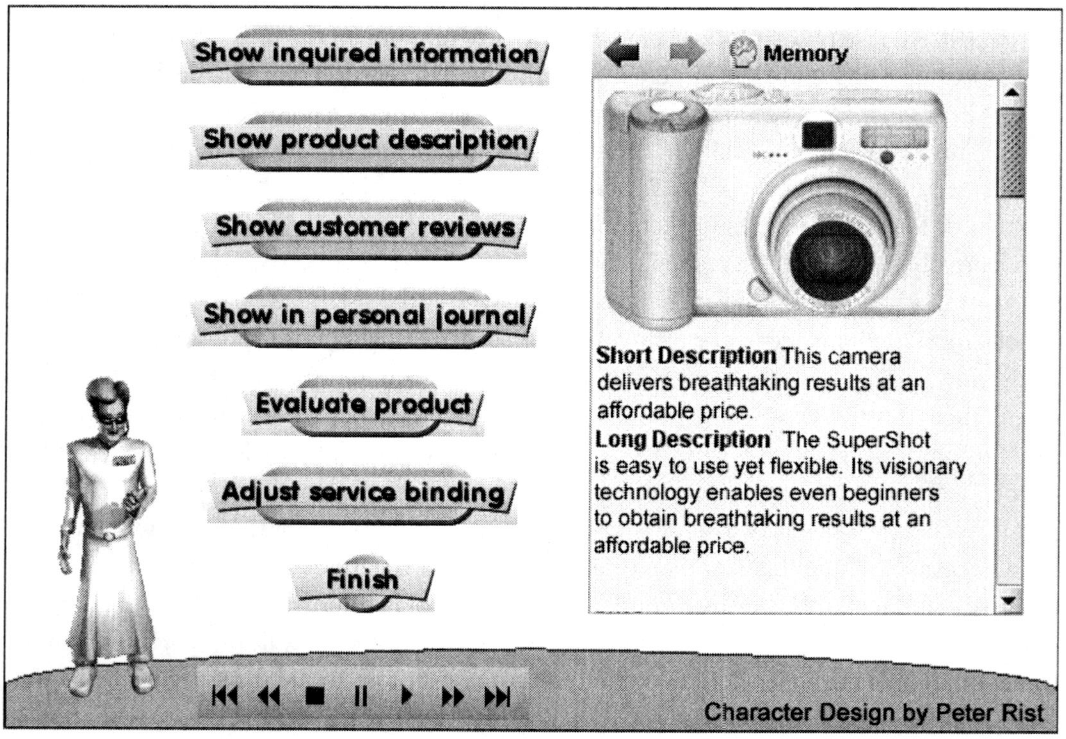

a presentation of events recently observed by the system. The presentation is conducted by a virtual character, which comments on the user's actions in the second person. In addition, the character serves as the system's "voice", which invites the user for introspection-related actions. This addresses in the very first place another important purpose of introspection: the communication of personal preferences to the system. Here, the user may actively provide explicit feedback about events, which is then applied in order to

personalize the system behavior. Ratings attached to user experiences are exploited to build a preference model, which affects indirectly the behavior of the system, e.g., of retrieval methods provided by the mobile interface. In contrast, ratings attached to system actions may have a direct impact on the course of the introspection process: During introspection, the system examines its own recent actions, with a special focus on actions rated negatively by the user. If such actions are found, then the planner embeds in the user's introspection process a system request to the user, whose subject is a negotiation of the respective system method's behavior between user and system.

We tested this component within the "audio CD shopping" scenario. The concept of introspection and reflection on past events was appreciated well. Participants found it useful to remember their past experiences to bring back certain facts into their "natural" memory and thus to prepare themselves for their next steps. Similarly, they appreciated to get an overview of their preferences and adjust ratings in order before their shopping trip.

Collaborative Critiquing of Situated User Support

General acceptance of a powerful system such as SPECTER can only be expected if it provides the user with means to:

- effectively *inspect* the current contents of her user model (UM); this includes a clear identification of the information sources and inference processes involved (e.g. was a particular fact explicitly entered by the user or indirectly inferred using some reasoning mechanisms?);
- easily *correct or modify* the contents of the UM whenever she feels incorrectly assessed or deliberately chooses to alter its contents to influence the system behavior (optimally, this includes enabling the user to estimate in advance the consequences of actively interfering with the user model);
- actively *survey, direct, or bias* processes drawing inferences from the UM contents, thus producing additional entries explicitly represented in the UM or deriving "intermediary" facts for internal use by the system.

A system that implements all of these aspects is called a *transparent user-modeling system* and the class of UMs so generated *transparent user models*. For a thorough discussion of this aspect, the reader is referred to (Bauer, 2004). For describing a very similar concept, Judy Kay coined the notion of "scrutable" UMs, see e.g. (Kay et al., 2001).

SPECTER provides a mechanism for collaborative critiquing that empowers even non-expert users to actively influence the system's behavior in case of dissatisfactory suggestions or service offers caused by incorrect associations between situations and actions (see the discussion of *triggers* in the CD shopping scenario). The rationale behind this mechanism is the assumption that an incorrect system reaction results from the erroneous classification of the user's current situation. As this classification is built upon models automatically derived from observations, this means the user needs a means to guide a machine-learning component towards the "right" classifier—in the sense of matching the user's intended semantics. With conventional machine-learning (ML) approaches, this is only possible for designated experts in this area.

The basic idea of our approach is to divide the work to be done between system and user according to their respective capabilities. While the system definitely "knows" how to exploit quantitative properties of the training data to select (statistically) relevant features and generate a classification model, the user can be expected to have sufficient background knowledge about the application domain and her own decision making.

Given a certain task at hand, the system first generates a decision tree using the features available in the training data. All of these features are explicitly represented as concepts of a domain ontology (Fensel, 2001). The domain ontology is a representation of (semantic) concepts of the application domain as well as relationships between them and an enumeration of individuals that can instantiate a concept.

Using a very simple interface (see Figure 10), the user can check which concepts were used to create the decision tree and criticize the system's choice by indicating which features should be ignored and which ones should be replaced by alternatives. Features marked as irrelevant are simply removed from the training set. Whenever the user indicates that some feature X should be replaced by another one, the system allows the user to interactively explore the semantic neighborhood of the feature under consideration. To this end, it determines the set of all domain concepts in the immediate neighborhood of the domain concept associated with X and presents them to the user. If the user does not find the desired concept among the system's suggestions, she can go on exploring the set of concepts until a suitable one is found.

The rationale behind this is the observation that a user—even if she is completely ignorant about ML—certainly has some idea of which factors influence her own behavior and which ones are (semantically) irrelevant. In the shopping episode classification example mentioned above, it is quite easy for the user to find out that e.g. the current temperature does not influence her shopping behavior (even if the statistical properties of the training data happen to tell something else) whereas the type of store (discounter, department store, etc.) certainly does.

Figure 10. Interaction with the learning component of SPECTER

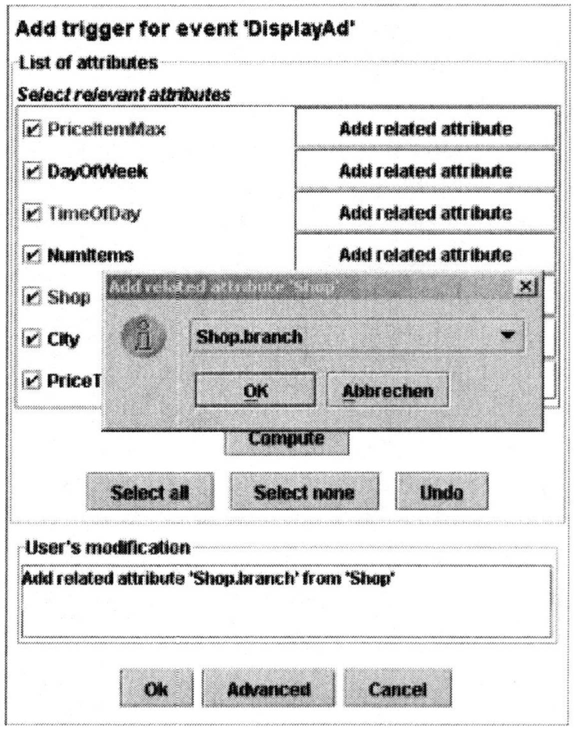

While the semantic correctness of a classification model obviously depends on the choice of the correct concepts to be included in the data representation, both accuracy and complexity of the models are strongly influenced by the way that information is actually captured and represented as features.

Assume the user decided to make the system take a particular ontology concept C into account. The system then derives a set of candidate features $F(C)$ for data representation using a number of heuristics which produce variants of the same information. If C can assume numerical values, the system derives both numerical variants representing the numerical values as contained in the training data such as to guarantee certain statistical properties (e.g. by applying sigmoid transformations to achieve uniform distributions) as well as categorical features (e.g. by partitioning the training data into equally sized bins). If C can assume categorical values $v_1, ..., v_n$, $F(C)$ contains e.g. Boolean features that represent whether or not the actual value of a data entry is or is not an element of some subset $V \subseteq \{ v_1, ..., v_n \}$.

Note that these—often very technical and hard to interpret—features are not meant to be presented to the user. All she sees are the more abstract semantic categories (concepts) used to represent the data and generate the classification model. (One exception are easily understandable Boolean features derived from categorical concepts.) The system then tries to generate a new model, this time using the features derived from the concepts picked by the user. Those features that are actually being used in the decision tree are incorporated into the ontology, using obvious naming conventions on the basis of the original concept name and the heuristics applied to derive that feature.

The light-shaded ovals in Figure 11 represent semantic concepts, the dark ones concepts representing heuristically derived features. The rectangles correspond to the individuals that may instantiate a particular ontology concept. Assume a shopping event is to be classified w.r.t. to whether or not the user is likely to spend too much money. The training data contain temporal information in the form of the respective *Day*, *Month*, and *Year* at which a certain shopping episode occurred. According to the training data, the *Day* is an appropriate feature for discriminating between critical (user spends too much) and non-critical shopping episodes.

The user—knowing there are certain days during a week when she tends to spend more money than usual—wants to provide this background knowledge to the system and thus criticizes

Figure 11. Part of an ontology dealing with temporal information

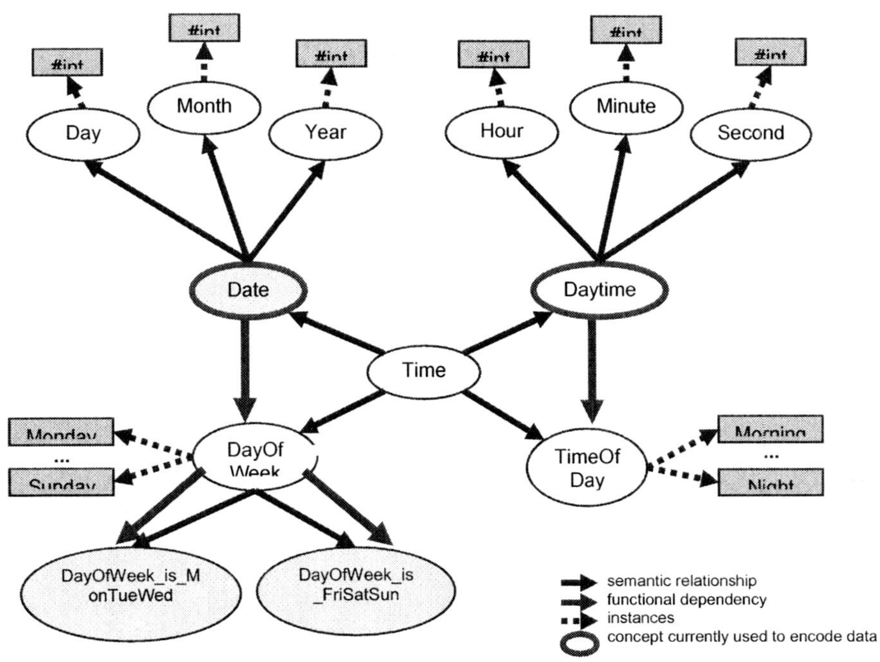

the system's use of the feature *Day*. Passing the abstract concept *Time* from which no immediate features can be derived (*Time* possesses no individuals that could instantiate it), the system arrives at the closest semantic neighbors *DayOfWeek*, *Daytime*, and *TimeOfDay*, all of which can be easily understood by the user. The system acknowledges the user's request to replace *Day* by *DayOfWeek* and generates a new model using a set of features derived from this concept. It turns out extensive shopping seems to occur most often towards the end of the week. As a consequence the intuitively understandable (Boolean) feature *DayOfWeek_is_Friday_or_Saturday* is used in the decision tree and added to the ontology.

That way, not only the current problem with the system performance in a particular class of situations can be remedied, but the system' s knowledge base is extended such as to provide a richer set of formalized semantic knowledge to be used for future reasoning

Evaluating Functions of Augmented Memories

We conducted a series of studies in order to learn about the possible uses of augmented memories. These studies aimed at identifying and evaluating functions of user support based on augmented memories. The studies were performed in a soundtrack CDs shopping scenario, which allowed the user to record and exploit experiences in various contexts (see Figure 12). A detailed analysis of these studies' outcome is provided by Plate et al. (2006); in the following, we will summarize some of their results.

In order to obtain initial content for their augmented memories, the 20 study participants were first asked to report on real past experiences with movies and the corresponding soundtrack CDs by means of an authoring interface. Later, they had to browse the soundtrack section of Amazon.com. Their interaction with the Web site was stored in their augmented memory. They then performed a system-guided introspection and reflection process in order to review and annotate the captured events.

Afterwards, they explored two mock-up CD stores (each one equipped with 250 CDs) located in an experiment room at our research institute in order to select 6 CDs for a duration of 30 minutes. From this selection, they obtained a subset of a fixed value as reward for their participation. The participants' interactions with the stores (e.g., "entered store", "looked at CD") were automatically captured by means of RFID technology, and were added to their respective augmented memory. By means of a mobile device, participants could consult the augmented memory at any time. Its user interface combined the template-based engine described above with features known from regular Web browsers (e.g., a navigation history). To make

Figure 12. A user study on functions of augmented personal memories in four phases

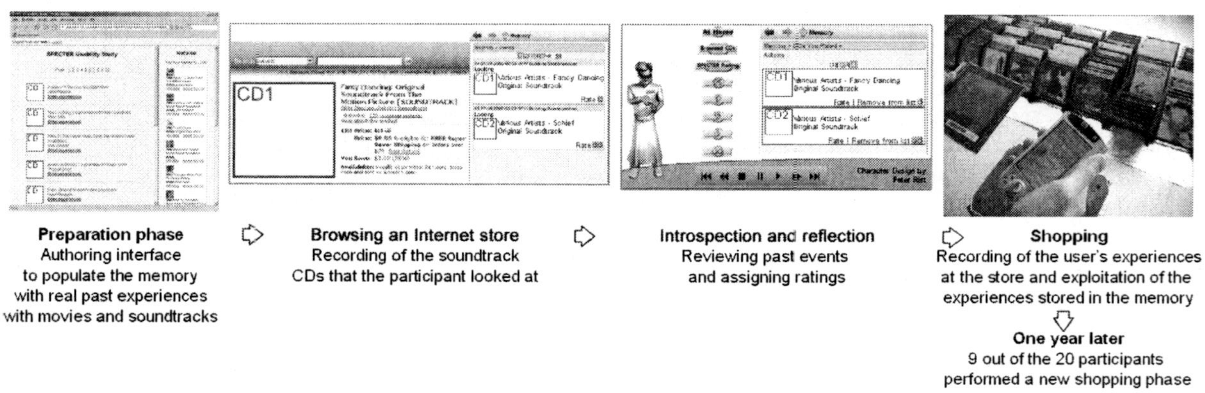

the scenario more realistic, we introduced a penalty for switching between the stores: when they wished to visit the other store, they had to leave the experiment room and to bring back a specific ticket from a pile of tickets in order to simulate the distance between the two stores, make them lose time and get their attention focused on a task independent to their primary goal. This obstacle aimed to enforce participants to make the best use of their visit in the current store, and to use their real and electronic memories before deciding to leave the store and return to the other one.

Furthermore, some situational triggers were specified in the participants' user models. These displayed automatically on the mobile device services related to the user's actions (in particular, entering a store or looking at a CD). This offer consisted of a set of links, which allowed to issue requests to the environment (e.g., after picking a CD, "Similar CDs in the store") as well as to the augmented memory (e.g., after entering a store, "CDs you saw in this store"). Using the mobile device, participants could consult the augmented memory at any time.

In addition to the records represented by the augmented memory, the participants' interaction with the user interface was logged and the participants also had to fill in a questionnaire.

A challenging aspect of a study concerning the use of a digital memory is the amazing performance of the human memory despite its limitations described in the introduction: one hypothesis was that participants would not use the digital memory if the desired information is readily available in their natural memory. We tried to test this hypothesis and evaluate the added value of augmented memories using a complex setting, but nevertheless had concerns due to the short duration between gathering and exploiting memories, which might affect the outcome of such a study as well. Therefore, one year later, 9 out of the 20 initial participants accepted to shop again in the mock-up stores in order to study the impact of this longer time span on the interaction with the digital memory. Here, we did not observe any significant change in the use of the system.

According to free text answers to the questionnaire, the purpose of the phase of introspection has been well understood by the participants: it has been perceived as a way to review past experiences and to annotate them, e.g. with ratings (45% of the free answers). Furthermore, introspecting has been perceived as a way to learn about oneself, in particular, about personal preferences (20% of the answers). 35% of the participants declared that the overview of their personal preferences helped them memorize relevant information and prepare the shopping phase. They further expressed that the time and effort invested in the reflection on past events was rewarded by a gain of time and a more precise support provided by the system during shopping. However, some participants mentioned that such support should also be provided by the mobile user interface in order to enable introspection during idle times (e.g., a bus ride).

The results of the studies show that in the shopping phase of the CD shopping scenario, the augmented memory in itself (a succession of events) had no direct use: indeed, the list of events in the augmented memories, filters on those events and the past events with a CD represent in total and in average 1.7 uses per participant during the shopping phase of 30 min during which in average, participants made 83.1 uses of functions. On the contrary, functions making use of the content of the augmented memory were very successful: 35.8% of the function uses were uses of functions remembering prices or listing, filtering or recominding CDs stored in the augmented memory. As expected in such a scenario involving many items of the same type due to the limitation of the natural memory to enumerate long and comprehensive item lists, functions listing CDs seen in the past were among the most often used memory-related functions: CDs rated "Excellent" by the participant, all CDs seen in the past, but also queries on the memory returning CD lists

(CDs with a positive rating seen in the past in the current store or another location and possibly with a price inferior to a certain amount). A notable and expected successful function is also the prices noticed in the past in different stores for a given product (9.5% of function uses).

The questionnaire administrated at the end of the long-term study highlighted that the recomindation function "CDs from memory similar to the one(s) considered" was not only used to recommend similar CDs that the user may have forgotten and which may be worth being bought. This function has also sometimes been used to recommend or discourage the purchase of the CD the user is considering: It provides more information about the considered CD with which the user may not be familiar and supports the purchase decision by informing the user that it is similar to certain CDs well known by the user. On the whole, it turned also out from the questionnaire that these recomindation functions were particularly popular.

The ubiquity of the system was also an important element of the success of the system in general and of some memory-related functions in particular. Here, the participants especially appreciated the system's recomindations after entering a store: here, the system proactively offered links to retrieve CDs available in the store seen in the past (used 53.2% of the times they entered a store), rated "Excellent" (6.5%) or similar to the ones rated "Excellent" (4.8%). In the contrary to what one might have been expected, this proactive service offer was in average not considered as obtrusive by the participants. One possible reason for this result might be that the user could just ignore this offer or return to their previous activity with a single click. One other probable reason might be that the service offer explicitly tailored to the limited set of user actions and goals in this setting—in fact, there was only a small risk of interrupting an ongoing interaction between user and augmented memory.

CONCLUSION

Dense records of perceptions made by an intelligent environment can be exploited to take a user's past experiences into account for user support. Thus, these records allow extending the user's perception in several ways: on the one hand side, the user may reflect on missed opportunities, and on the other side, her perception can be extended with past experiences. In this section, we used the implementation of the shopping assistant SPECTER in order to discuss two aspects which are especially crucial for the added value of such a memory for the user: the automated building of augmented memories, and interaction support with augmented memories.

Regarding the former aspect, we proposed the use of a lightweight yet flexible structure for storing RDF-encoded perceptions made by sensors. We used this approach as the basis for the implementation of components and processes which exploit the system's perceptions for building a user model on the one side and a diary-like structure on the other side—both components, which are required for the realization of user support from augmented memories. Here we argue that one of the key aspects in making an augmented memory accessible to the user is the abstraction of sensor data. In order to illustrate this idea, we showed how motion data are processed in SPECTER to motion profiles, which can be exploited for situation recognition as well as for annotation of entries in the user's personal journal with contextual information.

In the following, we employed this framework for realizing memory-based user support in an intelligent environment. We used an audio CD shopping scenario in order to illustrate how a user interface can support the user's interaction with her augmented memory. With respect to the diversity of memory contents and potential applications, we emphasized the need to provide the user with a flexible system of views, thus allowing her to change perspective on memories based on her current needs. Then, we used the implementation of such an interface in order to illustrate how an augmented memory can be exploited to realize situated reminders on past experiences. Here, we emphasized the need for making such support transparent to the user: the situation mapping as well as the memory contents have to be under control of the user. Therefore, we discussed in the following the implementation of a component for reflection and introspection support. In order to assist the user in dealing with the complexity of this task, we embedded a collaborative approach to the specification of situational triggers in the reflection process. The system applies machine-learning techniques to extract from the mass of data stored in the augmented memory feature candidates, which can then be critiqued by user based on semantic relationships—a process which aims at optimizing the skills of system and user.

FUTURE RESEARCH DIRECTIONS

In this chapter, we limited the discussion of issues related to building and exploiting of augmented memories to a specific setting: the application of augmented memories for user support in a shopping scenario. However, related research illustrates well that this concept is applicable to manifold domains. For instance, with respect to the aging society (see, for instance, the 2006 revision of the United Nations Dept. of Economic & Social Affairs / Population Division's report on World Population Prospects at http://www.un.org/esa/population/unpop.htm), augmented personal memories might provide a means to support elder people in their daily life with contextual reminders. Other promising applications arise from the exchange of augmented memories between users. Such sharing might help to establish an additional means of communication, and thus contribute to the building and strengthening of social relationships. Here, the proposed RDF basis for representing memories allows to link such shared memories easily with another rapidly growing field of applications—the Web 2.0. Thus, it is not surprising that issues related to sharing memories are already subject of remarkable research activities.

An instance of such research efforts is the project SharedLife, which builds on technology introduced in this chapter (Wahlster et al., 2006). The latter project provides also the background for an application of memory-like structures interesting for industry and home users as well: the digital product memory (Wahlster, 2007). Here, the objective is to record a product's "experiences" (e.g., temperature and humidity the product was exposed to) in a digital memory. This data can then be exploited for commercial purposes such as stock keeping or quality control. Furthermore, by transferring it to memories (such as the augmented personal memory) owned by the customers of such smart products, these can be linked to services provided by smart homes, e.g., a smart kitchen, which continues to monitor the quality of the product in the user's home.

Techniques for generating models of everyday's life (e.g. regarding motions, regular behaviors etc.) are likely to play a crucial role within the context of *Ambient Assisted Living* (cf. http://www.aal169.org/). This new paradigm aims at supporting elderly or persons suffering from dementia in their daily lives such as to allow them to lead a most normal life in their usual environment. Modeling their normal behaviors can be used to survey their health and activity states and activate emergency services in case of significant deviations from the expected behavior.

REFERENCES

Atzmueller, M. (2006). *Knowledge-Intensive Subgroup Mining - Techniques for Automatic and Interactive Discovery.* Dissertation, Department of Computer Science, University of Würzburg, Germany.

Bauer, M., & Baldes, S. (2005). An Ontology-Based Interface for Machine Learning. In: J. Riedl, A. Jameson, D. Billsus, and T. Lau (Eds.), *Proceedings of the 2005 International Conference on Intelligent User Interfaces* (pp. 314–316). New York, NY: ACM Press.

Bauer, M. and Deru, M. (2005) Motion-Based Adaptation of Information Services for Mobile Users. In L. Ardissono, P. Brna, and T. Mitrovic (Eds.), *LNAI 3538: Proceedings of the 10th International Conference on User Modeling (UM05)* (pp. 271–276). Berlin, Heidelberg: Springer.

Bogdanovych, A. & Bauer, M. (2007). *Using Trajectories of Avatars to Predict the Shopping Mood.* (paper submitted).

Clarkson, B. (2002). *Life Patterns: structure from wearable sensors.* PhD thesis, School of Architecture and Planning, Massachusetts Institute of Technology, Cambridge, MA, USA.

Dumais, S., Cutrell, E., Cadiz, J.J., Jancke, G., Sarin, R., & Robbins, D.C. (2003). Stuff I've seen: a system for personal information retrieval and reuse. In *SIGIR '03: Proceedings of the 26th annual international ACM SIGIR conference on Research and development in information retrieval* (pp. 72–79). New York, NY: ACM Press.

Fensel, D. (2001): Ontologies: a silver bullet for knowledge management and electronic commerce. Springer, Berlin.

Gemmell, J., Bell, G., Lueder, R., Drucker, S., & Wong, C. (2002). MyLifeBits: Fulfilling the Memex Vision. In *Proceedings of ACM Multimedia '02* (pp. 235–238), Juan-les-Pins, France.

Henderson, L. (1972). Spatial and verbal codes and the capacity of STM. *Quarterly Journal of Experimental Psychology*, 24, (pp. 485-495).

Holz, H., Maus, H., Bernardi, A., & Rostanin, O. (2005). A lightweight approach for proactive, task-specific information delivery. In *Proceedings of I-KNOW 2005 – Special Track on Business Process Oriented Knowledge Infrastructures BPOKI.*

Horvitz, E., Dumais, S., & Koch, P. (2004). Learning predictive models of memory landmarks. In *Proceedings of the CogSci 2004: 26th Annual Meeting of the Cognitive Science Society.* Chicago, USA.

Huber, M. J. (1999). JAM: A BDI-theoretic mobile agent architecture. In *Proceedings of the 3rd Conference on Autonomous Agents* (pp. 236–243). New York, NY: ACM Press.

Kröner, A., & Basselin, N. (2006). Situated Views on Augmented Memories. In P. Isaias, M.B. Nunes, I.J. Martinez (Eds.), *Proceedings of the IADIS International Conference WWW/Internet 2006* (vol. 2, pp. 272–277), Murcia, Spain.

Kuwahara, N., Noma, H., Kogure, K., Hagita, N., Tetsutani, N., & Iseki, H. (2003). Wearable autoevent-recording of medical nursing. In *Proceedings of the Ninth IFIP TC13 International Conference on Human-Computer Interaction (INTERACT 2003).*

Lamming, M., & Flynn, M. (1994). Forget-Me-Not: Intimate computing in support of human memory. In *Proceedings of FRIEND21, the 1994 International Symposium on Next Generation Human Interface*, Meguro Gajoen, Japan.

Lee, B., Klemmer, S. R., & Brafman, R. (2006). *Adaptive interfaces for declarative presentation of heterogeneous content.* Technical Report CSTR 2006-10 09/29/06, Stanford University, HCI Group, Stanford, CA, USA.

Miller, G. A. (1956). The magical number seven, plus or minus two: Some limits on our capacity for processing information. *Psychological Review, 63* (pp. 81–97).

Mustière, S., Zucker, J.-D., & Saitta, L. (2000). *An Abstraction-based Machine Learning approach to Cartographic Generalization*. Paper presented at the 9th International Symposium on Spatial Data Handling (SDH 2000), Beijing, China.

Patterson, D. J., Liao, L., Gajos, K., Collier, M., Livic, N., Olson, K., Wang, S., Fox, D. & Kautz, H. A. (2004). Opportunity Knocks: A System to Provide Cognitive Assistance with Transportation Services. In N. Davies, E. D. Mynatt, I. Siio (Eds.), *LNCS 3205: UbiComp 2004: Ubiquitous Computing: 6th International Conference* (pp. 433–450). Berlin, Heidelberg: Springer.

Plate, C., Basselin, N., Kröner, A., Schneider, M., Baldes, S., Dimitrova, V., & Jameson, A. (2006). Recomindation: New functions for augmented memories. In V. Wade, H. Ashman (Eds.), *LNCS 4018: Adaptive hypermedia and adaptive web-based systems – Proceedings of AH 2006* (pp. 141–150). Berlin, Heidelberg: Springer.

Pollack, M. E., Brown, L., Colbry, D., McCarthy, C. E., Orosz, C., Peintner, B.,Ramakrishnan, S., & Tsamardinos, I.. (2003). Autominder: An intelligent cognitive orthotic system for people with memory impairment. *Robotics and Autonomous Systems*, 44 (pp. 273–282).

Quan, D., Huynh, D., & Karger, D.R. (2003). Haystack: A platform for authoring end user semantic web applications. In *Proceedings of the 2nd International Semantic Web Conference (ISWC 2003)* (pp. 738–753). Florida, USA.

Schacter, D. L. (2001). *The seven sins of memory: how the mind forgets and remembers*. Boston, Houghton Mifflin.

Schneider, M. (2006). RDF:Stores – A Lightweight Approach on Managing Shared Knowledge. In *Proceedings of the 3rd International Conference on Ubiquitous Intelligence and Computing (UIC)*, Wuhan, China.

Sharples, M., Hogg, D., Hutchison, C., & Torrance, S. (1989). *Computers and Thought: A Practical Introduction to Artificial Intelligence*. Bradford Book.

Sperling, G. (1960). The information available in brief visual presentations. *Psychology Monographs, 74*(11) (pp. 1–29).

Sumi, Y., & Mase, K. (2002). Supporting awareness of shared interests and experiences in community. *International Journal of Human-Computer Studies*, 14(6) (pp. 127–146).

Van den Hoven, E. (2004). *Exploring graspable cues for everyday recollecting*. Paper presented at the PERVASIVE 2004 Workshop on "Memory and Sharing of Experience", Vienna, Austria.

Wahlster, W. (2007). Digital Product Memory: Embedded Systems Keep a Diary. In D. Harting, *tec.News 15* (pp. 6–9). Retrieved June 4, 2007, from http://www.harting.com/.

Wahlster, W., Kröner, A., & Heckmann, D. (2006). SharedLife: Towards Selective Sharing of Augmented Personal Memories. In O. Stock, M. Schaerf (Eds.), *Reasoning, Action and Interaction in AI Theories and Systems. Essays Dedicated to Luigia Carlucci Aiello*, LNAI 4155 (pp. 327–342). Berlin, Heidelberg: Springer.

Zeimpekis, V., Giaglis, G.M., & Lekakos, G. (2003). A Taxonomy of Indoor and Outdoor PositioningTechniques for Mobile Location Services. In *ACM SIGecom Exchanges*, 3(4) (pp. 19–27).

ADDITIONAL READING

Akinori, A., Ohsawa, Y. (Eds.). (2005). *International Series on Natural and Artificial Intelligence 3: Readings in Chance Discovery*. Magill (Adelaide): Advanced Knowledge International.

Abowd, G.D.; Mynatt, E.D.; Rodden, T. (2002). The human experience. *IEEE Pervasive Computing, 1*(1) (pp.48–57).

Atkinson, R.C., & Shiffrin, R.M. (1968). Human memory: A proposed system and its control processes. In K.W. Spence and J.T. Spence (Eds.), *The psychology of learning and motivation, 8*. London: Academic Press.

Bush, V. (1945): As we may think. *Atlantic Monthly, 176*(1) (pp. 101–108).

Clarkson, B., Mase, K., & Pentland, A. (2001). The Familiar: a living diary and companion. In *Proceedings of Computer-Human Interaction 2001* (pp. 271–272). New York, NY, USA: ACM.

Cutrell, R. Jeffries, & Gary M. Olson (Eds.), *Proceedings of the 2006 Conference on Human Factors in Computing Systems, CHI 2006* (pp. 571–580). New York, NY, USA: ACM.

Czerwinski, M., Gage, D. W., Gemmell, J., Marshall, C. C., Pérez-Quiñones, M. A., Skeels, M. M., & Catarci, T. (2006). Digital memories in an era of ubiquitous computing and abundant storage. *Communications of the ACM, 49*(1)*: Personal Information Management* (pp. 44–50). New York, NY, USA: ACM.

Fitzgibbon, A., & Reiter, E. (2003). *Memories for life – managing information over a human lifetime*. Cambridge, UK: Computer Laboratory, University of Cambridge.

Gama, J. and Gaber, M. M. (2007): Learning from Data Streams: Processing Techniques in Sensor Networks. Springer, Berlin.

Heckmann, D. (2006). *Ubiquitous User Modeling*. Berlin: Akademische Verlagsgesellschaft Aka GmbH, ISBN 3-89838-297-4 and ISBN 1-58603-608-4.

Kapoor, A., & Horvitz, E. (2007). Principles of Lifelong Learning for Predictive User Modeling. In C. Conati, K. F. McCoy, & G. Paliouras (Eds.), *LNCS 4511: User Modeling 2007, 11th International Conference* (pp. 37–46). Berlin, Heidelberg: Springer.

Mase, K., Sumi, Y., Fels, S. (Eds.). (2007). *Journal of Personal and Ubiquitous Computing, 11*(4)*: Memory and Sharing of Experiences*. London: Springer.

Mitchell, T. M. (1997): Machine Learning. Mcgraw-Hill Professional.

O'Hara K., Morris, R., Shadbolt, N., Hitch, G. J., Hall, W., & Beagrie N (2006). Memories for life: a review of the science and technology. *Journal of the Royal Society Interface 3*(8) (pp. 351–365). ISSN 1742-5689.

Prante, T., Meyers, B., Fitzpatrick, G., & Harvel, L.D. (Eds.). (2005). *Proceedings of the 1st International Workshop on Exploiting Context Histories in Smart Environments.*

Ronnie, L., Johansson, M., & Xiong, N. (2003). Perception management: an emerging concept for information fusion. *Information Fusion, 4*(3) (pp. 231–234).

Schneider, M., Kröner, A., & Wasinger, R. (2006). Augmenting interaction in intelligent environments through open personal memories. *Intelligent Environments, 2nd International Conference* (pp. 407–416).

Squire, L. R. (2004). Memory systems of the brain: A brief history and current perspective. *Neurobiology of Learning and Memory* 82 (pp. 171–177). Elsevier.

Tulving, E. (1985). How many memory systems are there? *American Psychologist 40* (pp. 385–398).

Vurgun, S., Philipose, M., & Pavel, M. (2007). A Statistical Reasoning System for Medication Prompting. In J. Krumm, G.D. Abowd, A. Seneviratne, & Th. Strang (Eds.), *LNCS 4717: UbiComp 2007: Ubiquitous Computing* (pp. 1–18). Berlin, Heidelberg: Springer.

Witten, I. H. and Frank, E. (2005): Data Mining. Practical Machine Learning Tools and Techniques. Morgan Kaufmann.

Yeh, R. B., Liao, C., Klemmer, S. R., Guimbretière, F., Lee, B., Kakaradov, B., Stamberger, J. A., & Paepcke, A. (2006). ButterflyNet: a mobile capture and access system for field biology research. In R. E. Grinter, T. Rodden, P. M. Aoki, E.

Chapter XIV
Open Learner Modelling as the Keystone of the Next Generation of Adaptive Learning Environments

Rafael Morales
Universidad de Guadalajara, Mexico

Nicolas Van Labeke
University of London, UK

Paul Brna
University of Edinburgh UK

María Elena Chan
Universidad de Guadalajara, Mexico

ABSTRACT

It is believed that, with the help of suitable technology, learners and systems can cooperate in building a sufficiently accurate learner model they can use to promote learner reflection through discussion of their knowledge, preferences and motivational dispositions (among other learner characteristics). Open learner modelling is a technology that can help set up this discussion by giving the learners a representation of aspects of the learner as "believed" by the system. In this way/role, open learner modelling can perform a critical role in a new breed of intelligent learning environments driven by the aim to support the development of self-management, signification, participation and creativity in learners. In this chapter we provide an analysis of the migration of open learner modelling technology to common e-learning settings, the implications for modern e-learning systems in terms of adaptations to support the open learner modelling process, and the expected functionality of a new generation of intelligent learning environments.

INTRODUCTION

The history of the use of computers for training and education started soon after the introduction of the first commercial computers. For some time, research and development in this area have been under the influence of two main visions: one which sees information and communication technologies as useful *tools* for improving people's access to learning resources and enhancing their teaching and learning experiences, and another one which sees computers as intelligent *agents* playing a proactive role in the educational context, much as students, teachers and tutors do. Practitioners strongly influenced by the first view have been mainly concerned with developing systems that can make the ever-evolving information and communication technologies more useful for training and education. In contrast, practitioners strongly influenced by the second view have been mostly interested in enhancing the learning experience by making computers as flexible and supportive of learning as human tutors are capable of being (ADL, 2001; Gibbons & Fairweather, 2000).

Widespread implementations of the first approach, current e-learning systems such as learning management systems based on content, metadata and web technologies, are mostly designed to make information and learning materials easily available to a broader audience, while providing a set of tools for supporting, and hopefully enhancing, human-to-human communication. Their way of supporting learning, however, usually combines two simple models: provision of a rigid and predefined path through educational and informational materials, and allowing free content browsing and choosing. The danger of this approach, of course, is to replicate the traditional and ineffective educational approaches of *one serves all* and unsupported *consumer freedom* on a massive scale. On the contrary, intelligent tutoring systems (Polson & Richardson, 1988; Wenger, 1987), as products from the second approach, have always cared for their learners as individuals and they have used adaptation and personalisation as essential mechanisms for achieving their purpose of promoting better learning by their users (Self, 1999). Nevertheless, intelligent tutoring systems have mostly stayed in their designers' laboratories, due to the difficulty of scaling them to more realistic settings and integrating them with other educational systems (Picard, Kort, & Reilly, 2007).

Learner models, understood as digital representations of learners, have been at the core of intelligent tutoring systems from their original inception (Carbonell, 1970). Learner models facilitate the knowledge about the learner necessary for achieving any personalisation through adaptation, while most intelligent tutoring systems have been designed to support the learning modelling process: a win-win strategy that have produced many successful systems in terms of their efficacy to improve learning. Learner modelling is a *necessary process* to achieve the adaptability, personalisation and efficacy of intelligent tutoring systems. Consequently, we need to introduce this same process into modern e-learning environments, and adapt it to its new working conditions, if we want an equivalent functionality in these systems (Brooks, Greer, Melis, & Ullrich, 2006; Brooks, Winter, Greer, & McCalla, 2004; Brusilovsky, 2004; Devedzic, 2003). Furthermore, a variation of learner modelling in which the learner plays an active role in the modelling process, known as *open learner modelling* (Morales, Pain, Bull, & Kay, 1999), sets the context for system and learners (and even other actors in the learning process, such as teachers) to discuss through suitable user interfaces the knowledge, preferences, motivational dispositions and other aspects of the learner as "believed" by the system. Beliefs can be inspected and negotiated (Bull, Brna, & Pain, 1995), leading to a better picture of the learner—or, at least, to a learner model which is known by the learner and the learner agrees more with. Learner reflection and awareness of their own conditions are promoted through this process, leading to a better informed learner that can make better decisions on what do to next (Cook & Kay, 1994), and preparing the path for the system to make suggestions based on its inspected, justified and negotiated beliefs.

In this chapter we provide an analysis of the migration of open learner modelling technology to common e-learning settings, the implications for modern e-learning systems in terms of adaptations to support the open learner modelling process, and the expected functionality of a new generation of intelligent learning environments. This analysis is grounded on the authors' recent experience on an e-learning environment called LeActiveMath, the main product of a European-funded research project aimed at developing a web-based learning environment for Mathematics in the state of the art.

The second section of this chapter sets the context of our work with a description of the general characteristics of the educational model of e-learning, which is followed by the proposal of a new educational model for next-generation intelligent learning environments with integrated open learner modelling technology. The third section is devoted to a brief presentation of the salient characteristics of the LeActiveMath system as representative of a general class of modern e-learning systems. The fourth section focuses on learner modelling in LeActiveMath. It includes a presentation of the motivations and issues addressed in the project, the inspection/challenge aspects of its open learner modelling, its scope and limitations. In the fifth section we explore the generalisation of the open learner modelling approach followed in LeActiveMath to the broader class of systems LeActiveMath represents. The sixth section contains a brief report of recent approaches to learner modelling and evaluation results. The chapter ends drawing some conclusions on the state of the art and sketching future research directions.

THE E-LEARNING EDUCATIONAL MODEL

There are at least five educational traditions that converge into common e-learning systems nowadays: expositive teaching, programmed instruction, distance and continuous education, administration and multimedia-based didactics.

Expositive teaching is certainly the most entrenched tradition in education. It gives the teacher the task of presenting information and carrying out demonstrations to a learner whose function is reduced to capture the information and transcribe it, only to give it back through exercises and assessment. In e-learning this means that educational materials have an expositive nature, with a minimum level of interaction, and the e-learning environment is an information container. Criticism to expositive teaching is widespread. Other approaches, such as discovery learning, the constructivist models, as well as the perspective of education communication have been developed mostly in opposition to frontal, expositive teaching. Influential authors that have lead movements against expositive teaching are, among others, Ausubel (1995), with significant and discovery learning, and Freire (1999) with his notion of "banking education" as an analogy to the informational deposit in expositive teaching.

Programmed instruction is an educational method based on educational materials with detailed step by step instructions for learner actions. Questions are provided as well to assess learner progress in acquiring the information from the materials. Regarding instructional design, it is the teacher who sets the materials and their sequencing, defines assignments, evaluates and generally dictates to the learner what to do. The e-learning environment acts as a space for delivering instruction and the assessment of information transfer. Programmed instruction was the first use of computers for teaching in the 70s, and it is the antecedent to closed instructional design based on structured content and previously defined closed questions and answers (Gibbons & Fairweather, 2000).

E-learning has also been developed using instructional models from traditional distance education, based on detailed description of the sequence of activities to be carried out by the learner and carefully designed characterisations of their products, under the assumption that there would be little support from teachers for the learning process—given that communication between learners and teachers in traditional distance education was mostly by post. E-learning that has evolved from traditional distance education settings towards the use of learning management systems (LMS) has maintained its pedagogical emphasis on the careful disposition of directions for activities to be carried out *outside* of the learning management system, considering the latter only as a medium to deliver instruction, not as an environment for teaching and learning (Bates, 2005).

From the management view of education e-learning imports its emphasis on organisational tools and spaces, such as agendas, programmes, content repositories and drop boxes for assignments and feedback (Chan Núñez, 2004). Information and communication technologies become the new raw materials for building organisational tools and very little else. On the other hand, a focus on the rich expressiveness of the new media as a tool for delivering information through all learner senses can be observed among the more significant didactical applications of new technologies. Learners are seen as a free explorer of educational materials in the context provided by the organisational tools.

Together, the five traditions outlined above exert their influence on the conception of e-learning environments as containers of educational materials to be browsed by, or detailed instructions to be executed along predefined paths by a preconceived hypothetical learner.

Interactivity and Self-Management

There are two concepts that have been reduced in their meaning as qualities of learning in virtual environments: interactivity and self-management. The execution of tasks by the learner, following the predefined path set in a learner management system, has been understood as self-managed because the learner makes decisions limited to the amount of time assigned to each one of them, behaving in a more or less disciplined way along the course. The learner decides on these behaviours, but not on the trajectories and contents. In this approach, the concept of self-management is reduced actually to the development of study habits, the discipline to fulfil tasks, and the responsibility to undertake each activity indicated. Self-management is therefore executed in a frame of provisions, decided by educators, which do not necessarily respond to the interests, necessities or capacities of the learner. So, what is it that the learner really manages?

Another term that is applied indiscriminately in e-learning is the one of *interactivity*. From a computational and informational perspective, a system exhibits interactivity if it allows for information flow in both directions with its user. However, from a perspective of meaning, we should distinguish between interactivity and *interaction*, the latter requiring not only information exchange but also a mutual influence between the subjects in the communication process. In courses with a design that guides the actions of the learner we can observe reactions of the learner as responses to predefined and anticipated situations, but their actions have no effect on the planning of the course.

In e-learning we have got to consider the systematic design of courses as a precious quality, but then e-learning ends up as a collection of closed systems. There is little space or time for the learner's perception of their own learning, or the recognition of what they have achieved, let alone their necessities and interests.

Towards a New Educational Model for E-Learning

In contrast to the "traditional" e-learning model depicted above, we would like to propose a new model based on the principles of self-management, creativity, signification and participation (UDG Virtual, 2004). That is to say at least three things: (1) all four principles should be identifiable as characteristics of learners in e-learning environments, especially after some time of being exposed to the model, (2) the design of the environment should be guided by them, and (3) teachers/tutors should undertake their tasks caring for the same principles.

Learner's self-management is understood here as their achievement of security and self-confidence, as their capacity to make decisions and be the driver of their own learning process, and as their commitment towards their own being and the tasks that fall under their responsibility. Creativity is understood as the capacity of a person to identify problems, to generate alternative ideas about the problems, to find alternative solutions, to express themselves and to innovate. Signification articulates itself with creativity as far as it assumes involvement with problems and their solutions, grounding of concepts on experience and capacity to generalise the acquired knowledge and transfer it to new situations. Finally, participation is understood here as cooperation, collaboration, and team work.

The principles of self-management, creativity, signification and participation are supported mainly by two theoretical approaches to learning: cognitivism and social constructivism (Ausubel, 1995; Vygotsky, 1996). These positions coincide with premises about competency-based learning (Gonczi & Athanasou, 1996), among others: learning by doing, learning by getting involved in tasks with a meaning for the (social) learner, role playing in a team carrying out collective tasks and project-based learning (Reigeluth, 1999).

We believe that open learner modelling can perform a critical role in the development of self-management, signification, participation and even creativity in learners; that its place is the centre of the e-learning environment, as its main access and meeting point. Through it, learners would be able to inspect their learning process and their achievements, to engage with them through challenging and negotiating the system view of it (in a general sense, including the views of others such as teachers and peer learners), to gain in security and self-confidence through visualising and reflecting on their progress. Through open learner modelling, learners would get support from the environment on their learning in a justified manner (e.g. "you can see I believe, for good reasons, that you are very close to mastery of this competency, so I recommend you to practice it a bit longer and then reflect on what you have done and achieved"), so they can make informed decisions on their learning process.

Open learner modelling needs to evolve in order to meet this challenge, and our work on the LeActiveMath project can be seen as a move in this direction.

THE LeAvtiveMath PROJECT AND SYSTEM

The LeActiveMath project was born from a desire to improve the support given to learn mathematics by ActiveMath, a "generic and adaptive web-based learning environment" (Melis et al., 2001) which used a book metaphor to present educational content for learners to choose from on the basis of their profile (e.g. educational level and field of studies), learning goals and scenarios (e.g. learning a topic for the first time, revising it or preparing for an assessment). The system used an XML-based knowledge representation for encoding mathematical documents and was clever enough to use it to choose the content that fit the learner's profile and request, and to present it in a variety of formats, achieving in this way a primitive sense of personalisation. The LeActiveMath project (LeActiveMath Consortium, 2007) aimed to transform ActiveMath into a next generation intelligent learning environment, in which the learner could take the initiative in their active and exploratory learning of Mathematics while the system supported them through a variety of mechanisms for adaptation and personalisation, from intelligent feedback and tutorial dialogue, through content suggestions to open learner modelling.

The new system, called LeActiveMath, fits the description given by the Advanced Distributed Learning Initiative (ADL, 2004b) for a second-generation e-learning system that combines a modern content-based approach from computer assisted instruction with adaptive educational strategies from intelligent tutoring systems. This mixture of approaches produced tensions during the design of the system in general, but particularly during the design of its learner modelling subsystem since this has to support a wide range of adaptive educational strategies, from coarse-grain book construction to tailored natural language dialogue, but with a general lack of something traditionally afforded in intelligent tutoring systems: painfully designed and dynamically constructed learning activities capable of providing large amounts of detailed information about learner behaviour. A learner model working in these conditions has to deliver more with less. It has to be able to answer questions about the learner on the basis of sparse information without pursuing blind over-generalisation.

Content-Based E-Learning

As in many other e-learning systems, LeActiveMath makes heavy use of pre-authored educational *content* to support learning, aiming to capitalise in this way from the efforts and expertise of a variety of authors at producing standardised educational materials. However, a big disadvantage of this approach is that educational content is for the most part opaque to learner modelling, in the absence of a domain expert subsystem to query about what is inside the content. The information available is hence reduced to the one explicitly provided by authors in the form of *metadata*, which is not ideal for reasons explained below. This configuration is common in content-oriented systems such as popular commercial and open source learning management systems, yet it is a bit paradoxical in the case of LeActiveMath, given the fact that its educational content is encoded in a language designed to represent the semantics of statements (Kohlhase, 2005), which is nevertheless used at large for providing links to other pieces of content (e.g. reference content) and for supporting multiple presentation formats (like HTML, MathML, PDF and SVG).

Content in e-learning systems tends to come in relatively big chunks with little flexibility, as compared to finer grained and highly flexible "content" traditionally found in intelligent tutoring systems. An advantage of the former approach is that the system is provided with a small number of big components, instead of a big number of small ones, to put together in a coherent way. As with jigsaw puzzles, the task in the first case is generally easier than in the second case. On the other hand, and from a learner modelling point of view, most pieces of content are hardly adaptable to suit the dynamic needs of the ongoing modelling task, while information about learner behaviour and performance tends to come, if at all, in big summary chunks at the end of the learner's interaction with each piece of content.

Metadata

As mentioned above, the absence of a domain expert inside an e-learning system such as LeActiveMath forces a learner modelling component to work on the basis of content metadata. There are at least three problems in this way of proceeding that need to be addressed. First, metadata is a heavy burden on authors since it amounts to doing the work twice: to say the thing and to say what has been said. The more detailed and accurate the metadata, the more extra work has to be done. Automatic production or verification of metadata would be very helpful, but it amounts to introducing some expensive domain expertise into the system or authoring tool.

Secondly, metadata tends to be subjective. Although there could be a lot of commonality in two experts view of their subject domain, there are also differences which sometimes are serious. Hence two authors could easily provide different metadata for equivalent pieces of content. The more flexible is the addition of new content and metadata to the system, the higher the diversity in criteria for defining metadata. A learner modelling component in these conditions must be tolerant of diversity.

Thirdly, metadata lacks details. A book's record in a library catalogue is never the same as the book itself, and this applies to metadata of electronic content as well. What matters to include as metadata is defined beforehand, whilst filling gaps later can be very expensive. A well-intentioned driver towards standardisation of metadata gets thwarted (from a modelling point of view) given the shallowness of current metadata standards such as LOM (IEEE, 2002).

Navigation Freedom

Guidance to learners through educational content in LeActiveMath, as well as many other e-learning systems, jumps between two extremes: predefined paths and content browsing. LeActiveMath contains a handful of predefined "books" on different areas of mathematics to be followed by learners, and learners can define new books according to their own goals. Once a book is defined, it can change only by the addition of new content recommended by the system from time to time. The learner has two choices: either to follow the books in the recommended order or to browse their content at will, with no further guidance other than a table of contents with indications of progress.

From a learner modelling perspective, both situations are for the most part equivalent, since neither of them accommodates the presentation of new content materials to the modelling needs. Whereas in intelligent tutoring systems, learner modelling can be used to lead the learner's progress through the subject domain, in e-learning it has to be *opportunistic*: taking advantage of whatever information is available at any time.

THE EXTENDED LEARNER MODEL

Along the LeActiveMath project we developed a learner modelling engine to support the new adaptive features of the LeActiveMath system, as well as to explore the possibilities of open learner modelling in this new context. We called it the Extended Learner Model (xLM) for reasons that will be apparent later. It was designed to deal with and benefit from the features of its host system but, nevertheless, it was expected to be easily detachable from it to serve similar e-learning systems, either as an embedded component or by offering its services on the Web.

Figure 1 illustrates the process by which xLM gets information concerning learner interaction with educational content. In essence, content encoded in LeActiveMath's mathematical content representation language OMDoc (Kohlhase, 2006) is transformed in a presentation language (HTML, MathML or PDF) using style-sheets and related technologies. Some of the content items and their presentations allow learners to interact with them in a way that the interaction can be captured by LeActiveMath and reported to xLM in the form of *event messages* containing data such as learner identifier, content item identifier, type of event reported and additional information such as (for some events) a measure of learner performance.

Figure 1. The process by which content is transformed into information about learners to feed learner models in xLM. Thick arrows represent information flow whereas thin arrows represent relationships between elements.

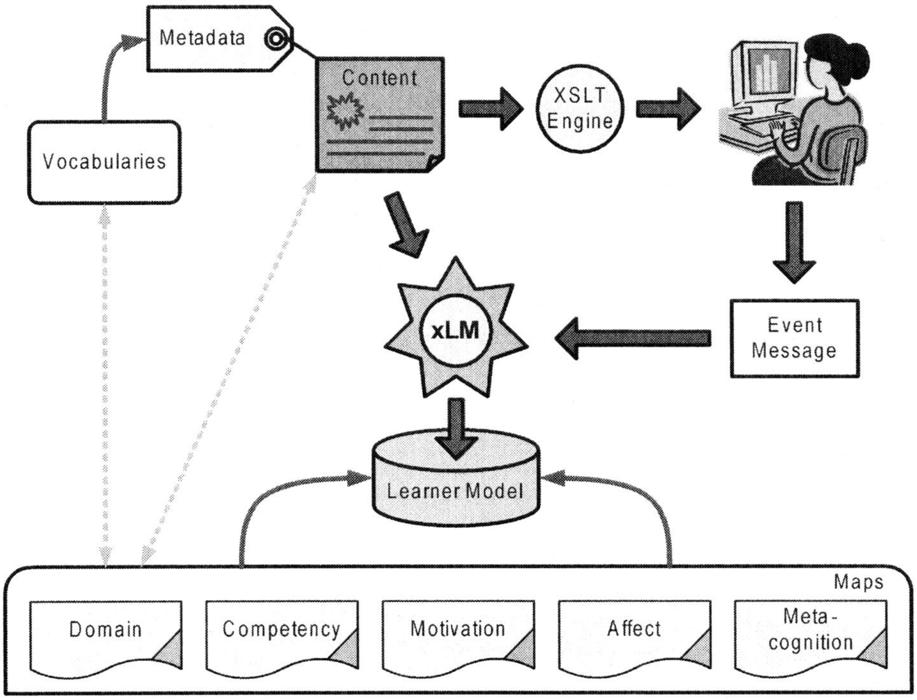

A variation of this scheme consists in the introduction of additional components acting as *diagnosers* of learner behaviour, which evaluate what happens during the interaction of learners with content and produce judgements on learners' states and dispositions. Examples of such additional diagnosers include an assessment tool that produces judgements on learners' levels of competency, a self-report tool through which learners provide judgements on their own affective states, and a situational model that produces judgements on learners' motivational state. A further variation of the scheme consists in learners interacting with their learner models instead of interacting with educational content. The models are made available through an xLM component called the extended Open Learner Model (xOLM) which provides learners with a graphical user interface to their models. It includes facilities for inspecting and challenging *beliefs* held in the models and the evidence supporting them. xOLM acts also as a diagnoser, producing judgements on learners' levels of metacognition.

Once xLM receives an event message, it proceeds to interpret it using the *event handler* that corresponds to the type of event reported in the message (Figure 2). The event handler uses the identifier of the content item, as reported in the message, to recover the item metadata that sets the context for interpreting the rest of the message. In particular, metadata provides information to identify the domain topics and competencies related to the event, while additional data in the event message helps to identify related affective and motivational factors, if any. Armed with all this information, the event handler produces *evidence* to update a selection of beliefs in a learner model, as identified by their *belief descriptor*: a juxtaposition of six identifiers, one for each of the learner dimensions modelled by xLM,

⟨*domain topic, misconception, competency, affective disposition, motivational disposition, metacognition*⟩.

Each element in a belief descriptor must either be empty or appear in the *concept map* that specifies the internal structure of the corresponding dimension in the learner models (see bottom of Figure 1). It is the composition of these maps, in the predefined way illustrated in Figure 3, what rules the composition of belief descriptors and defines the overall structure of learner models in xLM. The structure of the maps is used by *propagators* to spread the evidence produced by event handlers through the network of beliefs, producing in the end a relatively large collection of indirect evidence for a broader selection of beliefs than the ones directly addressed by the event. The final step in the process of learner modelling is updating the beliefs in the learner model in the light of the new evidence accumulated.

Learner Modelling Example

To illustrate what has been explained above, let us consider the case of a learner that is studying Differential Calculus and has finished the exercise on differentiation of linear functions shown in Figure 4. xLM receives an event message reporting that the learner has just finished successfully the exercise identified as:

mbase://LeAM_calculus/exercisesDerivs/mcq_const_lin_derivs

Then xLM requests the exercise metadata and receives the following information, among other:

- Exercise is for content items ex_diff_const. and ex_diff_lin, which are examples for differentiating a constant function and differentiating a learner function, respectively.
- Difficulty: very easy.

Figure 2. The process of interpreting events for producing evidence for beliefs in a learner model. Arrows represent information flow

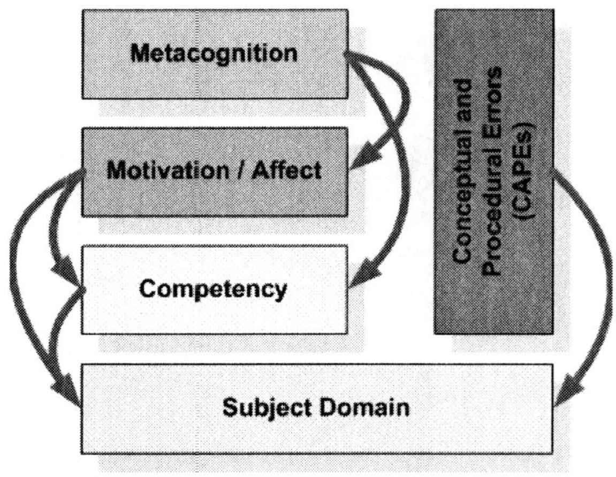

Figure 3. The layered structure of learner models determines the possible combinations of dimensions (the application of upper layers to lower layers) in learner model beliefs

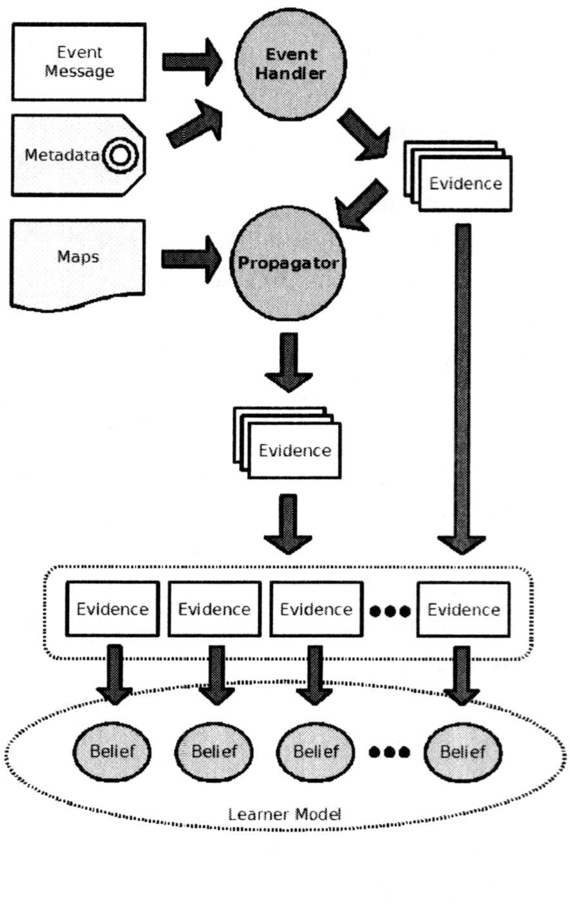

Figure 4. Example of the exercise and self-report tool in LeActiveMath

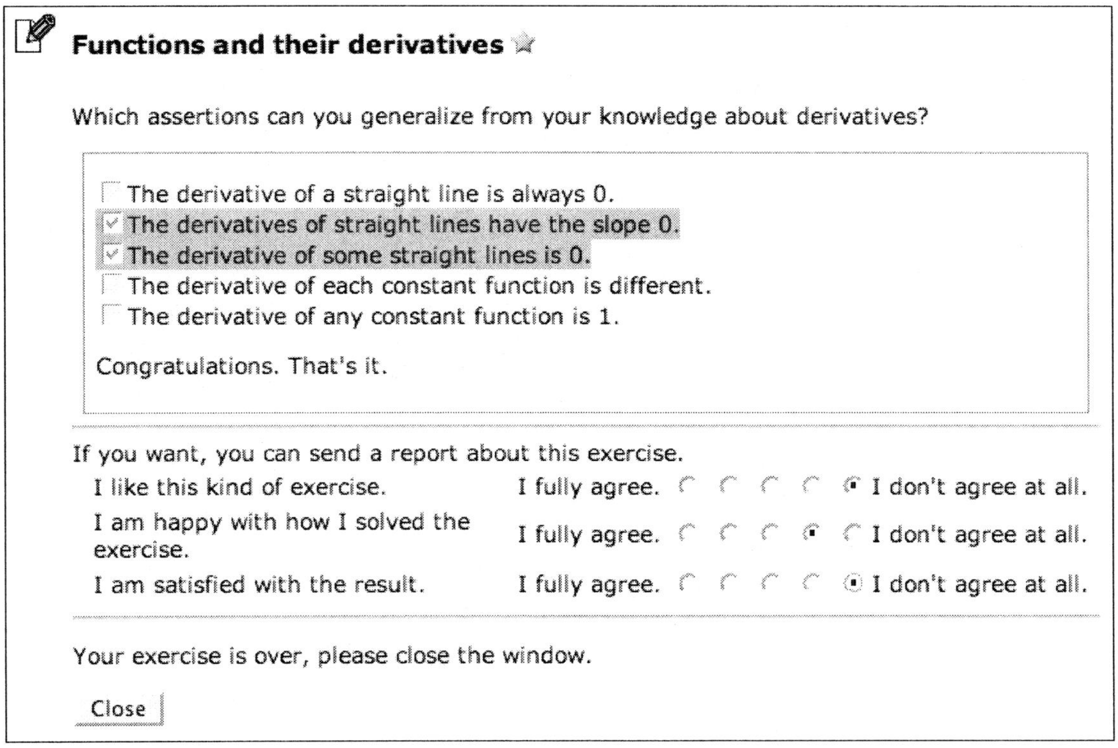

- Competency: think mathematically.
- Competency level: simple conceptual.

Subsequently, xLM goes from the exercise to the pair of examples of differentiation, to definitions of the corresponding differentiation rules, and so on up to the nodes diff_quotient, deriv_pt and derivative in the map of the subject domain, which stand for the domain topics of difference quotient, derivative at a point and derivative, respectively. With this information, xLM can now construct the descriptors for the beliefs the exercise provides new evidence for:

⟨diff_quotient,_,think,_,_,_⟩,
⟨deriv_pt,_,think,_,_,_⟩ and
⟨derivative,_,think,_,_,_⟩.

The beliefs corresponding to these belief descriptors are all on the competency level of the learner to think mathematically on/with the topics trained or tested by the exercise. Information on the difficulty and competency level of the exercise and the success rate achieved by the learner is used to calculate probabilities for the learner being at any of four possible competency levels. These probabilities are then transformed into a *belief function* (Shafer, 1976), a numeric formalism for representing beliefs that generalises probabilities and allows for a better representation of ignorance (lack of evidence) and conflict (conflicting evidence). Belief functions are the formalism used by xLM to represent its beliefs and their supporting evidence (Morales, Van Labeke, & Brna, 2006).

The initial set of direct evidence (three pieces, one for each belief) is sent as input to propagators, which produce new pieces of indirect evidence for beliefs with descriptors such as ⟨differentiation,_,think,_,_,_⟩, propagating on the domain map, and ⟨derivative,_,judge,_,_,_⟩, propagating on the competency map.

The learner's self-report of their affective state (bottom of Figure 4) would be delivered to xLM in another event message and then used to infer new evidence for beliefs on the affective dispositions of the learner towards domain topics and mathematical competencies, with descriptors such as

⟨*diff_quotient,_,_,liking,_,_*⟩

and

⟨*differentiation,_,think,affect,_,_*⟩.

Learner Model Inspection and Challenge

xLM provides LeActiveMath users with facilities for inspecting their learner models and for challenging beliefs hold in them. This has been accomplished via a dedicated graphical user interface (Figure 5) that allows learners to navigate through the web of beliefs and evidence built by xOLM over the user's interaction with LeActiveMath, as described in the previous section.

Toulmin Argumentation Pattern

The complexity of such a modelling process requires a mechanism to control the delivery of all this information in a way that maintains its significance. In xOLM, this mechanism is inspired by the Toulmin Argumentation Pattern (Toulmin, 1959) which, besides its (superficial) simplicity, does provides us with the possibility for managing both the exploration of the Learner Model and the challenge of its judgements. It also quite nicely supports a dynamic reorganisation of the evidence that helps to establish and clarify the justifications presented to the learner.

In xOLM, the mapping between each element of Toulmin's pattern (see Figure 6) and elements of xLM's internal representations is as follow:

Figure 5. xOLM graphical user interface to learner models

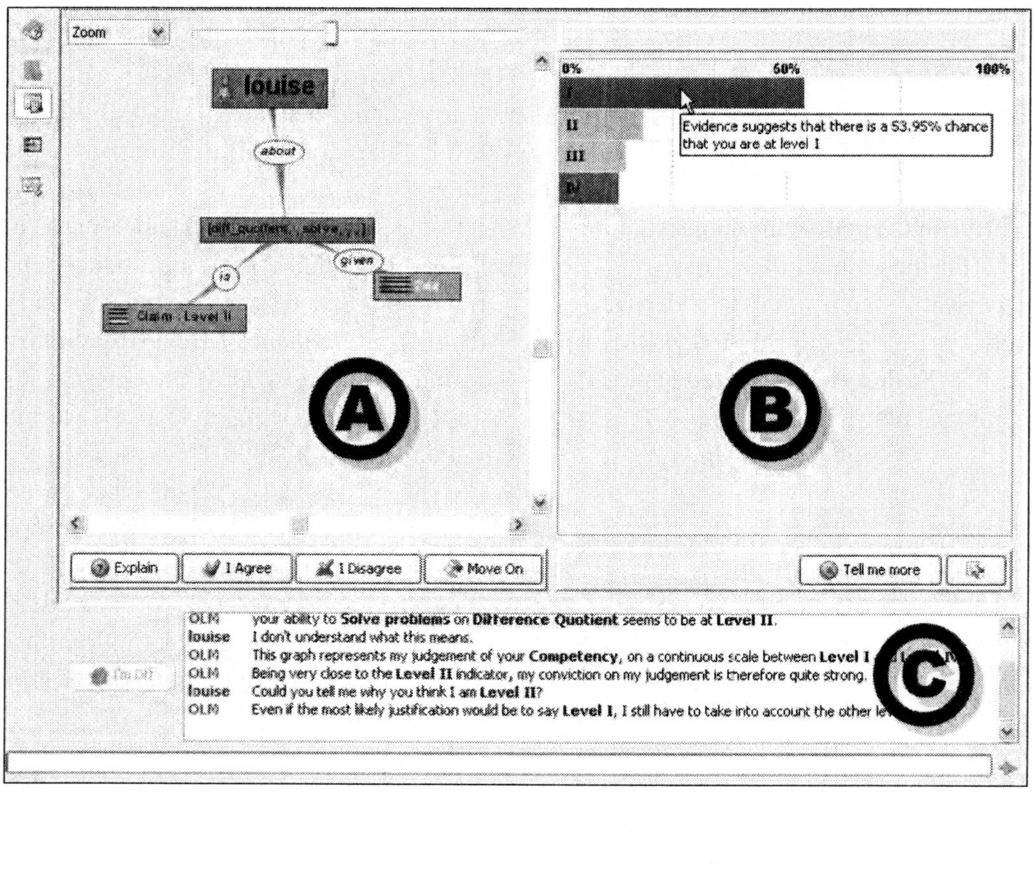

Figure 6. Toulmin's argumentation pattern

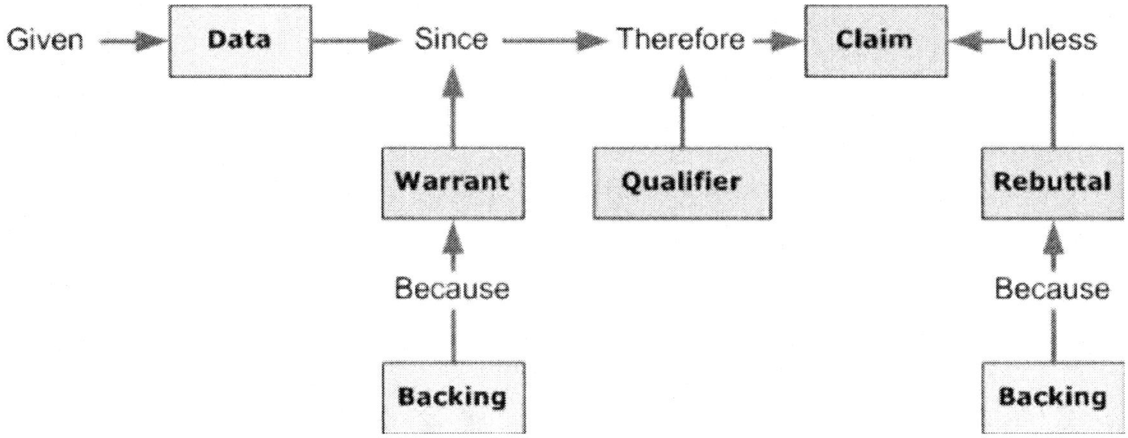

- The *Claim* is associated with a summary belief; that is a short, straightforward judgement about the learner's ability, or other disposition, on a given topic (i.e. "I think you are Level II on mathematical thinking on derivatives").
- The *Data* (or *Grounds*) is associated with a full belief, represented both by its pignistic probability function, its simplest internal encoding, and its mass function, its full internal encoding (Morales et al., 2006).
- *Warrants* are associated with the evidence supporting the belief, represented by mass functions. There will be one warrant for every piece of evidence used by xLM to build its current belief.
- *Backings* are associated with the attributes, both qualitative and quantitative, of the events whose interpretation has produced the evidence supporting the belief. Backings and warrants come in pairs for a single belief, although the same backing may be associated with distinct beliefs.

It has to be noted that xOLM does not consider any evidence gathered by xLM as *Rebuttal*, since any evidence in a learner model is supporting its corresponding belief. Rebuttal in xOLM exists only momentarily, as an explicit challenge from the learner to a belief held in the learner model, expressed through the graphical interface. However, once incorporated into the adjusted belief in the learner model, even the learner's challenge is evidence for the new belief and hence becomes a warrant.

Inspection and Challenge in the User Interface

The presentation of a belief—and its ultimate justification step-by-step—is controlled by the dual view, as seen in Figure 5: the Argument view (labelled A) and the Component view (labelled B). A verbalisation of the interaction between the learners and xOLM (labelled C) also acts as a complementary source of information and support.

The purpose of the Argument view is twofold: to provide the user both with a representation of the logic of the justification of the judgement made by xOLM and with an interface to navigate between the various external representations associated with each component of the justification. It is a direct reification of Toulmin's pattern, represented under the appearance of a dynamic and interactive graph. Each of the nodes of the graph is associated with one of the component of the argumentation pattern: the claim node associated with the summary belief, the data node associated with the belief itself, the warrant and backing nodes associated with individual evidence, etc. The shapes, colours, labels and icons of the nodes are appropriately designed in order to provide a quick and unambiguous identification of the corresponding element.

The Toulmin nodes are reactive to learners' interaction, acting as a trigger for the next step of the exploration. Upon selection, two actions are taking place: first, the appropriate external representation is immediately displayed in the right-hand side Component view; second, the Toulmin's pattern in the left-hand side is expanded to provide learners access to the next layer of the argumentation. Note that some intermediary nodes, not reactive to learner's interaction, have been added to introduce meaningful associations between the important parts of the graph (e.g. "about", "given", etc.); they are mostly linguistic add-ons for improving both the readability and the layout of the graph.

A mock interaction between a learner and xOLM is shown in Figure 7. It represents steps in the inspection-justification of a belief. Every step of the discussion is made manifest as a result of the learner requesting explanations as to why the xOLM made its judgement. At the interface level, the expansion of the Toulmin's pattern, combined with an external representation of the current component of the argumentation (see Figure 8), gives the learners the possibility to inspect—and ultimately challenge—several aspects of the xLM. A more detailed description of the interface can be found in (Van Labeke et al., 2007).

Design and Implementation Issues

Many things need to work together for the process described in the previous section to run smoothly. There are many decision points where trade-offs have been made between efficiency, generality, flexibility and availability of resources within the project.

Knowledge vs. Content

From the beginning of the project there were divergences regarding the nature of the material developed for the project in OMDoc. From one viewpoint, it can be seen as close to mathematical *knowledge*, given OMDoc's focus on mathematical meaning, rather than on visual presentation. From another viewpoint, the semantic nature of OMDoc is mediated by the nature of the documents it encodes and the processing capabilities of the interpreters. Formal mathematical documents encoded in OMDoc should be written with consistency and completeness in mind, since their purpose is to represent knowledge that can be verified, proved and otherwise interpreted and used by computers. On the other hand, educational mathematical documents are written pedagogically, their purpose being to provoke learning experiences. Educational documents can be rather inconsistent, repetitive and incomplete, even on purpose if that is believed to improve their pedagogical effect.

The issue got acute when it came to decide the shape for the subject domain map in xLM. One possibility was to build the maps from content items, so that content items (e.g. OMDoc concepts and symbols) were subjects of beliefs. On the one hand, the approach is quick and simple, and it is the one used by ActiveMath's old learner model. Authoring of new content would automatically update the map and every author could define topics for xLM to model learners on. Nevertheless, it is an approach prone to inconsistencies, repetitions and incompleteness in terms of learner models, very much as content could be. Another possibility was to develop an *explicit* ontological/conceptual map of the subject domain, as a more stable framework for xLM to ground beliefs on (Kay & Lum, 2004). Given the lack of a domain expert embedded in the LeActiveMath system, able to interpret content and answer questions about it, a map of the domain would deliver part of the hidden, implicit content semantics. A map

Figure 7. Belief inspection and justification in xOLM

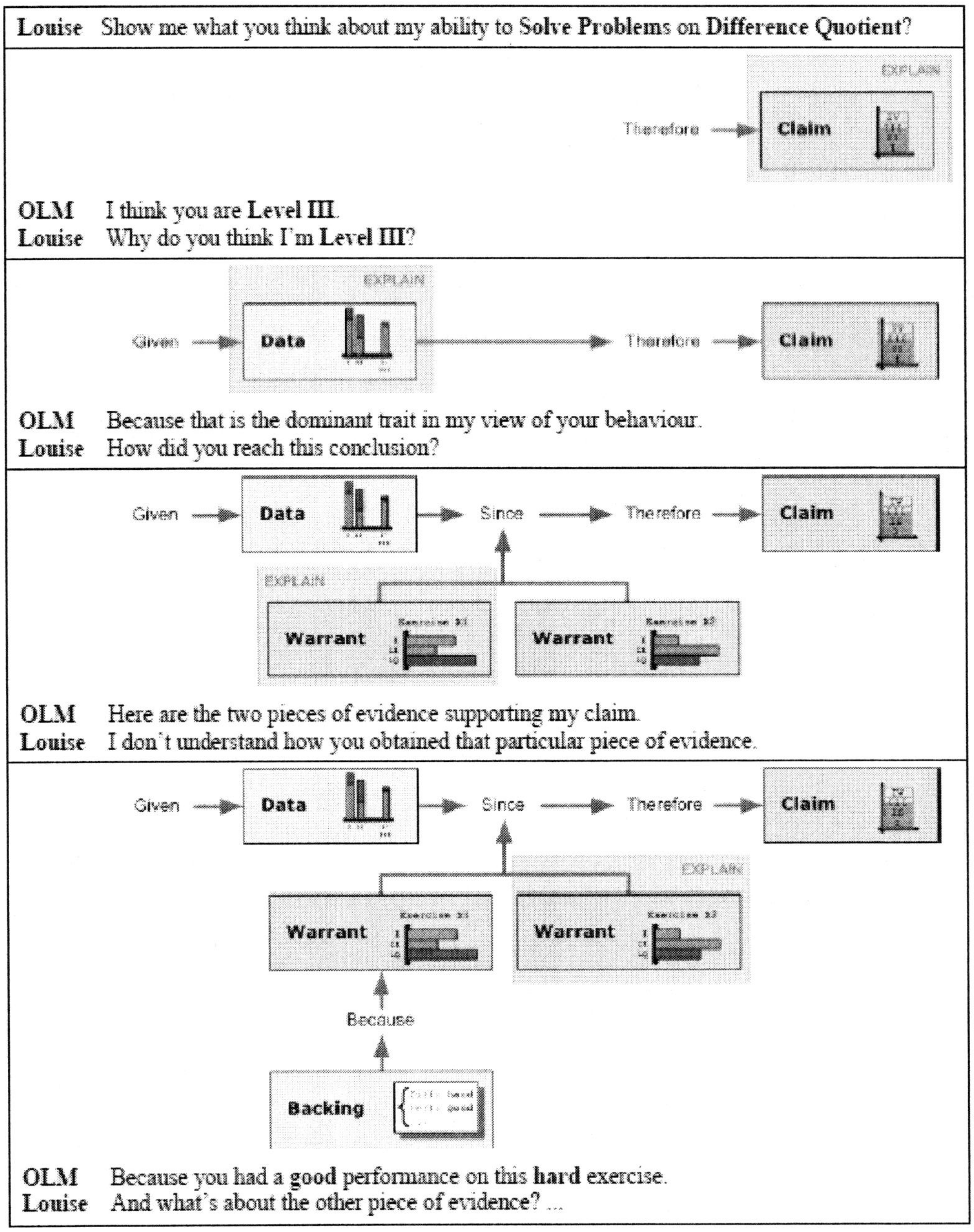

of the domain could help authors to better describe their content by making explicit references to the relevant parts of the map. On the other hand, since any subject domain can be described from many viewpoints, there can be many different, even conflicting maps of just about anything. A third option was to use a collection of content dictionaries written in OpenMath (Buswell, Caprotti, Carlisle, Dewar, & Kohlhase, 2004)—the formal, XML-based mathematical language on which OMDoc is based. However, this option was discarded because the content dictionaries

Figure 8. An expanded Toulmin's Argumentation Pattern, side-by-side with a dedicated external representation of the Warrant/Backing component

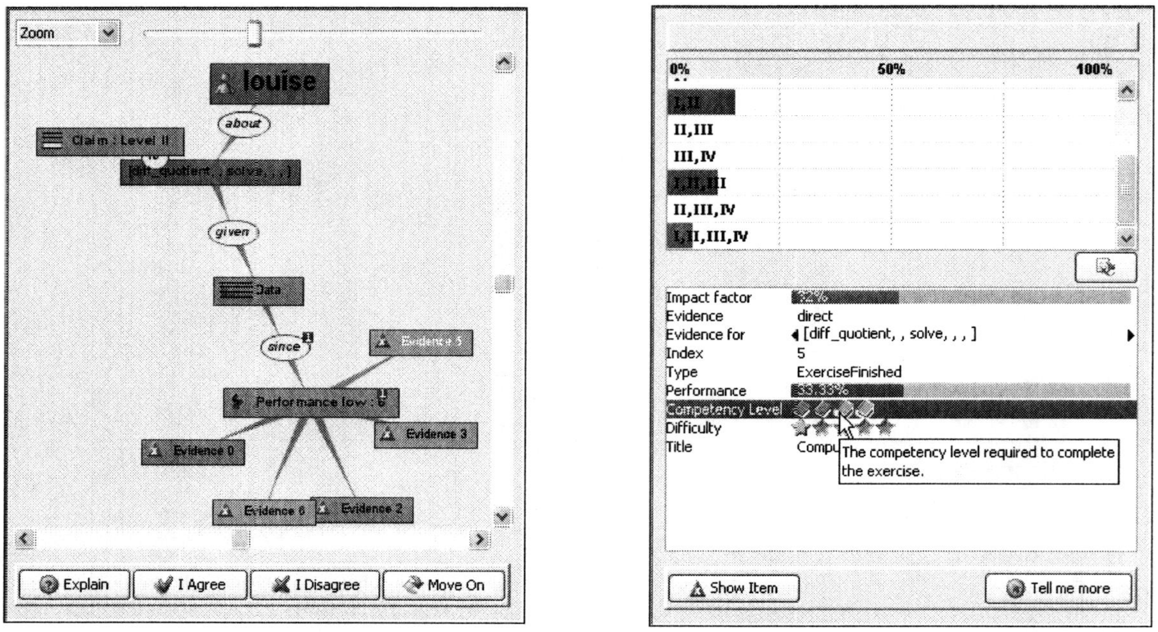

were found inadequate, both in terms of the topics covered and the relationships between them. Consequently, a separate concept map for the subject domain was the implementation decision of choice for xLM, and so a hand-crafted domain map was implemented as part of xLM which covers a subset of Differential Calculus—the main subject domain of LeActiveMath—and includes a mapping from content items to the relevant concepts, if available. It provides a solid ground for learner modelling which is less sensitive to changes in content.

Maps and Vocabularies

There is a weak relationship in between the map for competencies used by xLM and the vocabularies used for specifying the relevant competencies in content metadata. Certainly they are based on the same framework (OECD, 2003) and care has been taken to coincide, but this coincidence does not derive from any explicit link between them.

The mapping from content to topics is currently hardwired into the implementation of the handcrafted domain map, or generated dynamically at start up. In either case, it is hidden from content authors. In the same way, knowledge about vocabularies for metadata such as difficulty and competency level is hardwired into the code of xLM, particularly in event handlers and diagnosers such as the Situational Model and the Open Learner Model. There is no explicit link between this knowledge and the definition of the vocabularies.

Metadata and Its Usage

A core but limited subset of the available content metadata is actually taken into account while interpreting events. It is quite possible that making use of more metadata may provide knowledge of additional important features of content; features that can be the reasons behind apparently contradictory evidence. Nonetheless, since most metadata for the current LeActiveMath content has been produced based on the subjective appreciation of their authors, rather than on empirical evaluation of content, it may in reality provide very little extra information (coming from the same, biased source) and could be misleading.

Propagation Algorithm

A learner model in xLM is a large belief network constructed by composition of the maps that define the distinct dimensions of learners to be modelled (Figure 3). Every belief and evidence in this network is represented as a belief function. Propagators, that make use of the internal structure of the maps to propagate evidence, require the definition of a conditional belief function per association between elements in the maps. In the current implementation of xLM, however, a single conditional belief function is used for all associations in all maps, despite their many different types.

A careful analysis of the maps and the propagation algorithm is necessary to determine suitable adjustments. On the same line, there are a few parameters that can be fine tuned to optimise xLM performance in terms of accuracy, reliability and efficiency. Of particular interest is the issue of performance with larger maps.

Dynamic vs. Static Learner Models

Most of xOLM external representations provide the learners with an overview of the current state of the learner model (belief by belief) but not of its evolution across time. Although some attempts to give access to the dynamics of learner models have been tried, it became evident that they raised more issues than they solved; among them, the question of consistency across external representations (e.g. how to represent the dynamics of complex information such as that encoded in the pignistic function, the mass distribution, etc.); the question of controlling the dynamic representation (e.g. replaying, going backward, stopping, etc.); the question of integrating representations of dynamic and static aspects of learner models (e.g. selecting a step of a process to access the related evidence).

As with most learner models, an assumption underlying the implementation of xOLM is that the interest of the learners will be on the actual state of the beliefs rather than on their trajectories. This assumption needs to be carefully challenged in the future, by introducing dynamic aspects of xLM wherever they are likely to provide different information and support different (and improved) reflection by learners.

Support for Inspection of Learner Models

Inspecting a learner model is a complex task, so finding an adequate paradigm for this activity and producing a supportive interface is an important issue to address. Such an interface should allow learners to easily search for and localize beliefs in learner models. In fact, it should proactively suggest some beliefs to start with, based on what is stored in the learner model. It should present them in context, connected to the rest of the beliefs in the model, at least to be consistent with use of propagation of evidence in learner models, but most importantly for supporting learner metacognition (Flavell, 1979).

The current implementation of xLM includes a simple mechanism for identifying beliefs by their descriptors, plus minimal facilities to see beliefs in context (using a representation of the belief network as a sort of hyperbolic graph), but they should be seen more as proofs of concept than user-friendly facilities of xOLM graphical user interface.

To Show or Not to Show, Because it is Complex

xOLM was designed with the goal of given learners full access to what is held in learner models, from simple summaries of beliefs to their full representation in a knowledge representation formalism, from the interpretation of the events supporting a belief to the details of such events. A two-fold motivation sustained the goal through the design and implementation process: that the learner has got the right to know, and that having full access to the information in learner models would help learners to understand them better, answering their questions by going deeper into their models. We believed that hiding information from learners and presenting partial information in a simplified way only could have a detrimental effect on learners understanding their models, blurring the rationale behind the (summarised) beliefs. It would make it harder for learners to challenge a learner model they did not understand.

There seems to be trade-off between inspectability and readability, which has had an impact on the xOLM interface. It seems to be the case also that the difficulties for learners to understand their models are severe at both extremes (i.e. a heavy bias towards either inspectability or readability). The best solution seems to lie somewhere around the middle, yet such a solution has yet to be found.

Adaptive Open Learner Modelling

The same rationale that makes us believe that personalisation through proactive adaptation is a necessary ingredient of any system that aims to provide the best learning environment for each individual learner applies to the case of open learner modelling. That is to say, a learner interacting with their learner model will need personalised settings in order to take full advantage of the experience. There are, of course, many aspects of the interaction that can be adapted to the learner, among them the content of the model that is accessible to the learner at a given time, the amount of it that is presented at once, the media, modality and general organisation of its presentation, the navigation support and the stubbornness with which the system defends its beliefs. We are not aware of any research carried out in this direction.

GENERIC OPEN LEARNER MODELLING

We have envisioned a future for xLM in which it can be easily embedded into other educational systems or even deployed as a learner modelling server. There have been a few attempts to do this in the history of research in intelligent tutoring systems (Brooks et al., 2004; Kobsa & Pohl, 1995; Paiva & Self, 1995; Zapata-Rivera & Greer, 2004) with some level of success among the research community but no widespread usage outside of it, yet. Besides the obvious moves of making xLM appealing through its core functionality as an open learner modelling engine, and improving its use of Semantic Web technologies and standards, a proper parameterisation of its components would help xLM to better serve other educational systems. We can examine these issues from the perspective of the open learner modelling process described in the previous section.

To start with, the number of dimensions used by xLM, the way they are combined to set the framework for learner models (Figure 3) and the maps that give each dimension its structure and, combined as dictated by the framework, produce the network of beliefs held in learner models, need to be flexible. The maps should be encoded using a standardised language, such as XTM—XML for Topic Maps (TopicMaps.org, 2001)—and supplied to xLM as parameters. An explicit and strong connection between the maps and vocabularies for metadata would be beneficial too.

Knowledge of the content, structure and semantic of event messages recognisable by xLM (Figure 1) needs to be made explicit and accessible to xLM users (researchers and developers). It amounts to specifying a *data model*, as in SCORM (ADL, 2004c), plus its intelligent processing. For example, the current implementation of xLM supports event messages reporting log-ins and log-outs, starting and finishing exercises (including a measure of success rate), self-reports of affective states, diagnosis of motivational states and metacognitive skills, but all knowledge of which event messages are supported and how to interpret them is hardwired in the code of the xLM event handlers.

Propagation of evidence in learner models would greatly benefit from specialised conditionals attached to the associations in the concept maps. Consequently, finding an easy way to do this is an important problem. We are exploring a possible solution to it by defining a conditional per association type (Dichev & Dicheva, 2005) and adjusting it case by case, for each individual association on the maps, by taking into account the number of nodes each association connects—the more nodes connected, the conditional gets weaker.

For xOLM, the visible face of xLM, every event, map, metadata and vocabulary has to be provided with (internationalised) descriptions of their various constitutive elements, to be used in the graphical user interface to learner models. These descriptions are needed at various levels, as can be seen in Figure 5). Parameterising the evidence presentation view, particularly of the events whose interpretation delivers the evidence, means that important attributes have to be identified, their names and values to be described, as well as the (graphical) rendering used to display them properly. Parameterising the dialogue view (zone C in Figure 5, a verbalisation of the exchange between the learner and the xOLM) means that a verbal description of xOLM events has to be defined, including the templates to use and their arguments. The description of each argument needs to indicate how it should be formatted in the template. All references to belief elements need to be defined for their externalisation: descriptor, ability levels, and so on. For example, the belief descriptor ⟨deriv_pt,_,think,_,_,_⟩ needs to be transcribed according to the descriptions in the relevant topic maps (deriv_pt referring to the topic "derivative at a point" in the domain map and think referring to the competency of "mathematical thinking" in the competency map) and abstract ability levels currently used need to be mapped to the relevant vocabularies (e.g. for the case of a competency level, Level II could be transcribed as "medium").

We have presented xLM, the open learner modelling subsystem of a Web-based educational system for mathematics called LeActiveMath. We have described xLM functionality, particularly in relation to its use of technologies related to the Semantic Web, and discussed important design and implementation issues. Due to the fact that we aim at decoupling xLM from the LeActiveMath system so that it can serve a variety of educational systems, we have discussed a minimum set of requirements to accomplish our goal, emphasising the need to parameterise xLM and improve its usage of Semantic Web standards and technologies. Striving to generality has been, together with open learner modelling, a "salutary principle" for xLM (Self, 1988), yet the road ahead is full of challenges.

EVALUATION OF OPEN LEARNER MODELLING

Inspecting an open learner model cannot guarantee improved learning. In the worst case, the learner might be trapped in a cycle of introspection from which they find it hard to escape. In the best case, the learner not only learns the material that they are supposed to learn but also becomes a "better learner". Evaluation studies can help us map out the ways in which learners with different profiles/characters/background knowledge can benefit from different aspects of open learner models. Following Bull and Kay (2007), we might expect to find evaluations that are focused on one or more of "accuracy; reflection; planning and monitoring; collaboration and competition; navigation; right of access and control as well as issues of improving trust; and assessment". The methods used need to be varied, experiments with controlled conditions only go so far in terms of revealing the benefits and drawbacks of open learner modelling. Many of the studies focus on aspects of learners that are motivational or attitudinal, hence most studies rely to some extent on self report.

The evaluations of open learner models in use—either through small scale studies or larger ones—are broadly favourable. Bull, Quigley and Mabbott (2006) provide an example of a field evaluation of the deployment of their *OLMlets,* which have been designed by instructors. The system was used in five university courses in Electronic, Electrical and Computer Engineering. Mitrovic and Martin (2007) provide evidence that a fairly simple open learner model could lead to increased motivation for more able students and with less able students improving their performance.

Given that ultimately open learner models need to be deployed together with systems that are used widely with real students and in real institutional contexts, evaluations must necessarily go beyond small scale controlled studies. Simpler open learner models have begun to appear in real life settings. However, there are a number of research-based open learner models which have demonstrated promise in small scale studies. Three such systems can be found in a recent special issue of the International Journal of Artificial Intelligence in Education: Tchetagni, Nkambou and Bourdeau (2007) outline a system that seeks to encourage reflection; Van Labeke, Brna and Morales (2007) provide a more detailed exposition of the xOLM system described in this chapter, and Zapata-Rivera et al. (2007) provide an approach to open learner modelling for a range of stakeholders which is strongly focused on issues connected with evidence-based argumentation.

For the xOLM, this has now been subjected to a detailed evaluation which indicated a relationship between confidence and growth in knowledge for learners who had used the xOLM within the LeActiveMath environment, suggesting that open learner modelling, in this case, facilitates the learner's metacognitive skill (this is reported within Deliverable 44 of the LeActiveMath project by the evaluation team.). There is indeed room for further evaluation studies, but the evidence so far is encouraging.

FUTURE RESEARCH DIRECTIONS

We have argued in this chapter that open learner modelling can perform a critical role in a new breed of intelligent learning environments driven by the aim to support the development of self-management, signification, participation and creativity in learners. We believe that its place in such environments is at the centre, as a main access door and meeting point.

Open learner modelling needs to evolve in order to meet this challenge, and our work on the LeActiveMath project can be seen as an initial move in this direction. We have put open learner modelling as an important tool in a web-based, content+metadata system, and have shown how it can take advantage of Semantic Web technologies and sophisticated knowledge representation techniques, well suited for managing knowledge and uncertainty in e-learning environments.

In the previous section we outlined a set of outstanding issues that need to be addressed before we can accomplish our goal of pushing open learner modelling into e-learning. They are exclusive neither to our specific open learner modelling engine nor to the system hosting it. We have also sketched some moves towards making the Extended Learner Model a generic open learner modelling engine for e-learning systems based on standards and international reference models such as SCORM (ADL, 2004a). The road ahead looks bright and full of questions to answer.

REFERENCES

ADL. (2001). *Sharable Content Object Reference Model Version 1.2: The SCORM Overview*. Retrieved Nov 25, 2007, from http://adlnet.gov/downloads/AuthNoReqd.aspx?FileName=SCORM_1_2_pdf.zip&ID=240.

ADL. (2004a). *Sharable Content Object Reference Model (SCORM)*. Retrieved Nov 25, 2007, from http://www.adlnet.gov/dowloads/AuthNotReqd.aspx?FileName=SCORM.2004.3ED.DocSuit.zip&ID=237

ADL. (2004b). *Sharable Content Object Reference Model (SCORM) Overview*. Retrieved Nov 25, 2007, from http://www.adlnet.gov/donloads/AuthNotReqd.aspx?FileName=SCORM.2004 .3ED.DocSuite.zip&ID=237

ADL. (2004c). *Sharable Content Object Reference Model (SCORM) Run Time Environment*. Retrieved Nov 25, 2007, from http://www.adlnet.gov /dowloads/AuthNotReqd.aspx?FileName=SCORM.2004.3ED.DocSuite.zip&ID=237

Ausubel, D. P. (1995). *Educational Psychology: A Cognitive View*. London: Routledge.

Bates, T. (2005). *Technology, e learning and distance education*. London: Routledge.

Brooks, C., Greer, J., Melis, E., & Ullrich, C. (2006). Combining ITS and e-learning technologies: opportunities and challenges. In M. Ikeda, K. Ashley & T-W. Chan (Eds.), *Intelligent Tutoring Systems, 8th International Conference, ITS 2006* (pp. 278-287). Berlin: Springer.

Brooks, C., Winter, C. M., Greer, J., & McCalla, G. (2004). The massive user modelling system (MUMS). In J. C. Lester, R. M. Vicari & F. Paraguaçu (Eds.), *Intelligent Tutoring Systems, 7th International Conference, ITS 2004* (pp. 635-645). Berlin: Springer.

Brusilovsky, P. (2004). *KnowledgeTree: A distributed architecture for adaptive e-learning*. Paper presented at the 13th International World Wide Web Conference, Alternate Track Papers & Posters.

Bull, S., & Kay, J. (2007). Student Models that Invite the Learner In: The SMILI Open Learner Modelling Framework. *International Journal of Artificial Intelligence in Education, 17*(3), 89-120.

Bull, S., Brna, P., & Pain, H. (1995). Extending the Scope of the Student Model. *User Modeling and User-Adapted Interaction, 5*(1), 45-65.

Bull, S., Quigley, S., & Mabbott, A. (2006). Computer-Based Formative Assessment to Promote Reflection and Learner Autonomy. *Engineering Education: Journal of the Higher Education Academy Engineering Subject Centre, 1*(1), 1-18.

Buswell, S., Caprotti, O., Carlisle, D.P., Dewar, M. G., & Kohlhase, M. (2004). *The OpenMath Standard* (Standard): The OpenMath Society.

Carbonell, J. R. (1970). AI in CAI: An artificial intelligence approach to computer assisted instruction. *IEEE Transactions on Man Machine Systems, MMS-11*(4), 190-202.

Cook, R., & Kay, J. (1994). The Justified User Model: A Viewable, explained user model. In *Proceedings of the Fourth International Conference on User Modeling* (pp. 145 - 150). Hyannis MA, The MITRE Corporation.

Chan Núñez, M. E. (2004). *Modelo mediacional para el diseño educativo en línea*. Guadalajara, Jalisco: INNOVA, Universidad de Guadalajara.

Devedzic, V. B. (2003). Key issues in next-generation Web-based education. *IEEE Transactions on Systems, Man, and Cybernetics - Part C: Applications and Reviews, 33*(3), 339-349.

Dichev, C., & Dicheva, D. (2005). Contexts in Educational Topic Maps. In C.K. Looi, G. McCalla, B. Bredeweg & J. Breuker (Eds.), *12th International Conference on Artificial Intelligence in Education* (pp. 789–791). Amsterdam: IOS Press.

Flavell, J. H. (1979). Metacognition and Cognitive Monitoring: A New Area of Cognitive-Development. *American Psychologist, 34*(10), 906-911.

Freire, P. (1999). *Psicología del Oprimido*. México City: Editorial Siglo XXI.

Gibbons, A. S., & Fairweather, P. G. (2000). Computer-based instruction. In S. Tobias & J. D. Fletcher (Eds.), *Training & Retraining: A Handbook for Business, Industry, Government, and the Military*: MacMillan Reference Books.

Gonczi, A., & Athanasou, J. (1996). Instrumentación de la educación basada en competencias. Perspectivas de la teoría y la práctica en Australia. In A. Argüelles (Ed.), *Competencia laboral y educación basada en normas de competencia* (pp. 265-288). México: Limusa y Noriega Editores.

IEEE. (2002). *1484.12.1 Draft Standard for Learning Object Metadata.*

Kay, J., & Lum, A. (2004). Ontologies for scrutable student modelling in adaptive e-learning. In L. Aroyo & D. Dicheva (Eds.), *Proceedings of the AH (Adaptive Hypermedia and Adaptive Web-Based Systems) 2004 Workshop on Applications of Semantic Web Technologies* (pp. 292-301). Department of Mathematics and Computer Science, TU/e Technische Universiteit Eindhoven, 2004.

Kobsa, A., & Pohl, W. (1995). The BGP-MS User Modeling System. *User Modeling and User-Adapted Interaction, 4*(2), 59-106.

Kohlhase, M. (Artist). (2005). *OMDoc: An Open Markup Format for Mathematical Documents*

Kohlhase, M. (2006). *OMDoc—An Open Markup Format for Mathematical Documents (version 1.2)*: Springer Verlag.

LeActiveMath Consortium. (2007). Language-Enhanced, User-Adaptive, Interactive eLearning for Mathematics. Retrieved June 22, 2007, from http://www.leactivemath.org

Melis, E., Andrès, E., Büdenbender, J., Frischauf, A., Gogaudze, G., Libbrecht, P., et al. (2001). ActiveMath: A Generic and Adaptive Web-Based Learning Environment. *International Journal of Artificial Intelligence in Education, 12*, 385-407.

Mitrovic, A., & Martin, B. (2007). Evaluating the Effect of Open Student Models on Self-Assessment. *International Journal of Artificial Intelligence in Education, 17*(3), 121-144.

Morales, R., Van Labeke, N., & Brna, P. (2006). Approximate Modelling of the Multi-dimensional Learner. In M. Ikeda, K. Ashley, & T-W. Chan (Eds.), *Intelligent Tutoring Systems, 8th International Conference, ITS 2006* (pp. 555-564). LNCS 4053. Berlin: Springer-Verlag.

Morales, R., Pain, H., Bull, S., & Kay, J. (1999). Open, interactive, and other overt approaches to learner modelling. *AIED Resources, 10*, 1070-1079.

OECD. (2003). *The PISA 2003 Assessment Framework*: Organisation for Economic Co-Operation and Development. Paris, France: OECD Press.

Paiva, A., & Self, J. A. (1995). TAGUS - A User and Learner Modeling Workbench. *User Modeling and User-Adapted Interaction, 4*(3), 197-226.

Picard, R. W., Kort, B., & Reilly, R. (2007). Exploring the Role of Emotion in Propelling the SMET Learning Process. *NSF Project Summary and Description* Retrieved Nov 23, 2007, from http://affect.media.mit.edu/projectpages/lc/nsf1.html

Polson, M. C., & Richardson, J. J. (Eds.). (1988). *Foundations of Intelligent Tutoring Systems*. New Jersey: Lawrence Erlbaum Associates.

Reigeluth, C. M. (1999). *Instructional-Design Theories and Models: A New Paradigm of Instructional Theory*: Lawrence Erlbaum Associates.

Self, J. (1988). Bypassing the intractable problem of student modelling. In C. Frasson (Ed.), *Proceedings of the 1st International Conference on Intelligent Tutoring Systems ITS'88* (pp. 18-24). Montreal, Canada.

Self, J. (1999). The Defining Characteristics of Intelligent Tutoring Systems Research: ITSs Care, Precisely. *International Journal of Artificial Intelligence in Education, 10,* 350-364.

Shafer, G. (1976). *A Mathematical Theory of Evidence*: Princeton University Press.

Tchetagni, J., Nkambou, R., & Bourdeau, J. (2007). Explicit Reflection in Prolog-Tutor. *International Journal of Artificial Intelligence in Education, 17*(3), 169-215.

TopicMaps.org. (2001). *XML Topic Maps (XTM) 1.0* (Specification): TopicMaps.org.

Toulmin, S. (1959). *The Uses of Arguments*: Cambridge University Press.

UDG Virtual. (2004). *El modelo educativo de UDGVirtual.* Guadalajara, Jalisco: Universidad de Guadalajara.

Van Labeke, N., Brna, P., & Morales, R. (2007). Opening up the Interpretation Process in an Open Learner Model. *International Journal of Artificial Intelligence in Education, 17*(3), 305-338.

Vygotsky, L. (1996). *Thought and Language*: Cambridge, MA: MIT Press.

Wenger, E. (1987). *Artificial intelligence and tutoring systems.* California: Morgan Kaufmann.

Zapata-Rivera, J.-D., & Greer, J. (2004). Inspectable Bayesian Student Modelling Servers in Multi-agent Tutoring Systems. *International Journal of Human-Computer Studies, 61*(535-563).

Zapata-Rivera, D., Hansen, E., Shute, V. J., Underwood, J. S., & Bauer, M. (2007). Evidence-based Approach to Interacting with Open Student Models. *International Journal of Artificial Intelligence in Education, 17*(3), 273-303.

ADDITIONAL READING

Anderson, J. R., Boyle, C. F., Corbett, A. T., & Lewis, M. W. (1990). Cognitive Modeling and Intelligent Tutoring. *Artificial Intelligence, 42,* 7-49.

Atif, Y., Benlamri, R., & Berri, J. (2003). Learning objects based framework for self-adaptive learning. *Educational and Information Technologies 8*(4), 345-368. Kluwer Academic Publishers.

Bateman, S., Brooks, C., & McCalla, G. (2006). Collaborative tagging approaches for ontological metadata in adaptive e-learning systems. In D. Dicheva & L. Aroyo (Eds.), *SW-EL'06: Fourth Workshop on Application of Semantic Web Technologies for Adaptive Educational Hypermedia,* Dublin, Eire, June 2006.

Brooks, C., & McCalla, G. (2006). Towards flexible learning object metadata. *International Journal on Continuous Engineering Education and Lifelong Learning 16*(1/2), 50-63.

Brooks, C., Kettel, L. & Hansen, C. (2005). Building a learning object content management system. In *Proceedings of World Conference on E-Learning in Corporate, Government, Healthcare & Higher Education 2005* (pp. 2836-2843). Charlottesville, VA: Association for the Advancement of Computing in Education.

Brooks, C., McCalla, G., & Winter, M. (2005). Flexible learning object metadata. In L. Aroyo & D. Dicheva (Eds.), *Proceedings of Workshop SW-EL'05: Applications of Semantic Web Technologies for E-Learning* (pp. 1-8). International Conference on Artificial Intelligence in Education 2005, Amsterdam, The Netherlands.

Brusilovsky, P., & Nijhavan, H. (2002). A framework for adaptive e-learning based on distributed re-usable learning activities. *Proceedings of World Conference on E-Learning in Corporate, Government, Healthcare & Higher Education 2002* (pp.

154-161). Charlottesville, VA: Association for the Advancement of Computing in Education.

Conati, C., Gertner, A., & VanLehn, K. (2002). Using Bayesian Networks to Manage Uncertainty in Student Modeling. *User Modeling and User-Adapted Interaction, 12*(4), 371-417.

Conlan, O., Hockemeyer, C., Lefrere, P., Wade, V., & Albert, D. (2001). Extending educational metadata schemas to describe adaptive learning resources. *Proceedings of the Twelfth ACM Conference on Hypertext and Hypermedia,* pp. 161-162. Association for Computing Machinery.

Denaux, R., Dimitrova, V., & Aroyo, L. (2004). Interactive ontology-based user modeling for personalized learning content management. In L. Aroyo & D. Dicheva (Eds.), *Proceedings of the AH (Adaptive Hypermedia and Adaptive Web-Based Systems) 2004 Workshop on Applications of Semantic Web Technologies* (pp. 338-347). Department of Mathematics and Computer Science, TU/e Technische Universiteit Eindhoven, 2004.

Dicheva, D., Sosnovsky, S., Gavrilova, T., & Brusilovsky, P. (2005). Ontological web portal for Educational Ontologies. In L. Aroyo & D. Dicheva (Eds.), *Proceedings of Workshop SW-EL'05: Applications of Semantic Web Technologies for E-Learning* (pp. 19-27). International Conference on Artificial Intelligence in Education 2005, Amsterdam, The Netherlands.

Fernandes, E., Madhour, H., Miniaoui, S., & Forte, M. W. (2005). Phoenix tool: a support to semantic learning model. In L. Aroyo & D. Dicheva (Eds.), *Proceedings of the ICALT (International Conference on Advanced Learning Technologies) 2005 Workshop on Applications of Semantic Web Technologies.* Department of Mathematics and Computer Science, TU/e Technische Universiteit Eindhoven, 2005.

Goldrei, S., Kay, J., & Kummerfeld, B. (2005). Exploiting user models to automate the harvesting of metadata for Learning Objects. In P. Brusilovsky, R. Conejo & E. Millán (Eds.), *Proceedings of Workshop on Adaptive Systems for Web-Based Education: Tools and Reusability* (pp. 19-26). International Conference on Artificial Intelligence in Education 2005, Amsterdam, The Netherlands.

Grandbastien, M., Oubahssi, L., & Claes, G. (2003). A process oriented approach for modelling online learning environments. In R. Calvo & M. Grandbastien (Eds.), *Proceedings of Workshop Towards Intelligent Learning Management Systems* (Supplemental Proceedings Volume 4). International Conference on Artificial Intelligence in Education 2003, Sydney, Australia.

Greer, J., & McCalla, G. (1994). *Student Modelling: The Key to Individualized Knowledge-Based Instruction.* Berlin: Springer-Verlag.

Heift, T., & Schulze, M. (2003). Student modeling and *ab initio* language learning. *System 31* (4), 519–535.

Kasai, T., Yamaguchi, H., Nagano, K., & Mizoguchi, R. (2005). A semantic web system for helping teachers plan lessons using ontology alignment. In L. Aroyo & D. Dicheva (Eds.), *Proceedings of Workshop SW-EL'05: Applications of Semantic Web Technologies for E-Learning* (pp. 9-17). International Conference on Artificial Intelligence in Education 2005, Amsterdam, The Netherlands.

Kumar, A. (2005) Rule-based adaptive problem generation in programming tutors and its evaluation. In P. Brusilovsky, R. Conejo & E. Millán (Eds.), *Proceedings of Workshop on Adaptive Systems for Web-Based Education: Tools and Reusability* (pp. 35-43). International Conference on Artificial Intelligence in Education 2005, Amsterdam, The Netherlands.

Lin, F., Holt, P., Leung, S., Hogeboom, M., & Cao, Y. (2004). A multi-agent and service-oriented architecture for developing integrated and intelligent Web-based education systems. In L. Aroyo & D. Dicheva (Eds.), *Proceedings of the ITS*

2004 Workshop on Applications of Semantic Web Technologies. Department of Mathematics and Computer Science, TU/e Technische Universiteit Eindhoven, 2004.

Liu, J., & Greer, J. (2004). Individualized selection of learning object. In L. Aroyo & D. Dicheva (Eds.), *Proceedings of the ITS 2004 Workshop on Applications of Semantic Web Technologies*. Department of Mathematics and Computer Science, TU/e Technische Universiteit Eindhoven, 2004.

Moodie, P., & Kunz, P. (2003). Recipe for an intelligent learning management system (iLMS). In R. Calvo & M. Grandbastien (Eds.), *Proceedings of Workshop Towards Intelligent Learning Management Systems* (Supplemental Proceedings Volume 4). International Conference on Artificial Intelligence in Education 2003, Sydney, Australia.

Muñoz, L.S., & Moreira de Oliveira, J. P. (2004). Applying Semantic Web technologies to achieve personalization and reuse of content in educational adaptive hypermedia systems. In L. Aroyo & D. Dicheva (Eds.), *Proceedings of the AH (Adaptive Hypermedia and Adaptive Web-Based Systems) 2004 Workshop on Applications of Semantic Web Technologies* (pp. 338-347). Department of Mathematics and Computer Science, TU/e Technische Universiteit Eindhoven, 2004.

Nuzzo-Jones, G., Walonoski, J. A., Heffernan, N.T., & Livak, T. (2005). The eXtensible Tutor architecture: a new foundation for ITS. In P. Brusilovsky, R. Conejo & E. Millán (Eds.), *Proceedings of Workshop on Adaptive Systems for Web-Based Education: Tools and Reusability* (pp. 1-7). International Conference on Artificial Intelligence in Education 2005, Amsterdam, The Netherlands.

Santos, O.C., Rodríguez, A., Guadioso, E., & Boticario, J. (2003). Helping the tutor to manage a collaborative task in a web-based learning environment. In R. Calvo & M. Grandbastien (Eds.), *Proceedings of Workshop Towards Intelligent Learning Management Systems* (Supplemental Proceedings Volume 4). International Conference on Artificial Intelligence in Education 2003, Sydney, Australia.

Schaverien, L. (2003). Re-conceiving "intelligence" in learning management systems: tuning learning to theory. In R. Calvo & M. Grandbastien (Eds.), *Proceedings of Workshop Towards Intelligent Learning Management Systems* (Supplemental Proceedings Volume 4). International Conference on Artificial Intelligence in Education 2003, Sydney, Australia.

Specht, M., Kravcik, M., Klemke, R., Pesin, L., & Huttenhain, R. (2002). Adaptive learning environment for teaching and learning in WINDS. In P. De Bra, P. Bruslovsky & R. Conejo (Eds.), Adaptive Hypermedia and Adaptive Web-Based Systems, Second International Conference, AH 2002 (pp. 572-575). Lecture Notes in Computer Science 2347. Berlin: Springer.

Suraweera, P., Mitrovic, A., & Martin, B. (2004). The use of ontologies in ITS domain knowledge authoring. In L. Aroyo & D. Dicheva (Eds.), *Proceedings of the ITS 2004 Workshop on Applications of Semantic Web Technologies*. Department of Mathematics and Computer Science, TU/e Technische Universiteit Eindhoven, 2004.

Trella, M., Carmona, C., & Conejo, R. (2005). MEDEA: an open service-based learning platform for developing intelligent educational systems for the Web. In P. Brusilovsky, R. Conejo & E. Millán (Eds.), *Proceedings of Workshop on Adaptive Systems for Web-Based Education: Tools and Reusability* (pp. 27-34). International Conference on Artificial Intelligence in Education 2005, Amsterdam, The Netherlands.

Winter, M., Brooks, C., & Greer, J. (2005). Towards best practices for Semantic Web student modelling. In C.K. Looi, G. McCalla, B. Bredeweg & J. Breuker (Eds.), *Artificial Intelligence in Education - Supporting Learning through Intelligent and Socially Informed Technology* (pp. 694-701). Amsterdam: IOS Press.

Yacef, K. (2003). Some thoughts on the synergetic effects of combining ITS and LMS technologies for the service of Education. In R. Calvo & M. Grandbastien (Eds.), *Proceedings of Workshop Towards Intelligent Learning Management Systems* (Supplemental Proceedings Volume 4). International Conference on Artificial Intelligence in Education 2003, Sydney, Australia.

Chapter XV
From E-Learning Tools to Assistants by Learner Modelling and Adaptive Behavior

Klaus Jantke
Research Institute for Information Technologies Leipzig, Germany

Christoph Igel
Universität des Saarlandes, Germany

Roberta Sturm
Universität des Saarlandes, Germany

ABSTRACT

Humans need assistance in learning. This is particularly true when learning is supported by modern information and communication technologies. Most current IT systems appear as more or less complex tools. The more ambitious the problems in the application domain are, the more complex are the tools. This is one of the key obstacles to a wider acceptance of technology enhanced learning approaches (e-learning, for short). In computer science, in general, and in e-learning, in particular, we do need a paradigmatic shift from tools of a growing complexity to intelligent assistants to the human user. Computerized assistants that are able to adapt to their human users' needs and desires need some ability to learn. In e-learning, in particular, they need to learn about the learner and to build an internal model of the learner as a basis of adaptive system behavior. Steps toward assistance in e-learning are systematically illustrated by means of the authors' e-learning projects and systems eBuT and DaMiT. These steps are summarized in some process model proposed to the e-learning community.

TECHNOLOGY ENHANCED LEARNING: PROS AND CONS

Technology has always been changing humans' lives, and the impact of science and technology has frequently been even deeper and longer lasting than expected at the beginning of a change. We are currently experiencing substantial changes driven by information and communication technologies, in general, and by the Internet pervading work places and private homes, in particular.

In the area of education ranging from elementary schools through universities to continuing education and life-long learning, information and communication technologies are paving the road for fundamentally new learning experiences.

The pros of e-learning are discussed in many publications, sometimes even organized toward formation of a strategy as in Igel and Daugs (2002), for example. There are convincing summaries of the benefits of technology enhanced learning for the industries. Tom Kelly, CISCO's vice president of worldwide training, circumscribes it as follows:

E-learning is not the answer to every question, but it needs to be applied as broadly as possible. The classroom simply cannot address business issues. If you have to teach 100 people about one topic, you can train 25 people in a classroom at a time and repeat the course four times. But if you have to train 3,000 people every 60 days on a new product, or on a new technology, or on a new market—there's no way that the classroom can work. There's no way to scale. There's no way to have an impact on the company. It is doomed to fail.

(http://fastcompany.com/magazine/39/quick-study.html)

Motivations to get engaged in e-learning are expectations of added value of new media and added value of information and communication technologies like, for instance, independence of time and place—learning anytime, anywhere (Igel & Daugs, 2002).

From a didactic point of view, there are options for new concepts as situated learning and exploratory learning. Strategic options are ways to address wider audiences, off campus vs. on campus, bridging the gap from the academia to distance education and life long learning and, last but not least, new approaches to controlling in education through the exploitation of learning histories and technology-supported cost analysis.

There is an obvious convergence of technologies and media (computers and computer networks, television, audio communication), promising connections of online and off-line media, and emerging mobility in IT services.

In contrast to the pros, there are plenty of cons as well. Who properly works in the area of e-learning, not only as a "technology provider" (This word sounds like an excuse for scientists and engineers who do not care about how to wield the tools they are producing.), but employing e-learning in regular use, rapidly learns about a variety of difficulties. If you do so, you are also facing learners' frustration for several reasons.

Learners' most frequent complaints refer to missing or inappropriate feedback. Learners feel *misunderstood* by computers. In fact, nowadays all human learners *are misunderstood* by their computers, as computers are far from understanding anything—there is no need for a Chinese Room argument (Searle, 1980) to clarify this.

Here, a brief explanation seems to be necessary, as one of the reviewers of this chapter claimed that "the reference to a Chinese Room Argument is irrelevant, because the chapter deals with what current technology can deliver, while the work of Searle deals with the philosophical limits of computers." What a misunderstanding!

The present chapter does *not* deal with current technology, that is, tools in e-learning, but with steps towards future assistant technologies, thereby touching the rather philosophical question for the computers' potentials or limitations *to understand human learners*.

Human teachers are bringing in a virtually infinite background of implicit knowledge and skills when taking care of their students (Damasio, 1999). The teacher's care is highly appreciated especially in difficult learning situations—when there are too many choices and one is lost in the content, when repeatedly reading, watching or listening does not lead to a satisfying result, when something does not work as expected, when the learner's solution to an exercise is wrong, but the learner does not know why, or when it simply gets boring.

What we do need are e-learning computer systems that react appropriately, that is, adaptively to the learner's general needs, to the learner's current problems and to the specific context.

ADAPTIVITY AND SYSTEM'S ASSISTANCE AT WORK

Adaptivity to the learner's needs and desires is the ultimate aim of the authors' work toward a paradigmatic shift from e-learning tools to e-learning assistants. The authors' work relies on their own experience in designing, implementing and using e-learning systems for higher education. The systems DaMiT (http://damit.dfki.de) and eBuT (http://www.bewegung-und-training.de) are in daily use (see descriptions in Igel & Daugs, 2003a, 2003b; Igel & Sturm, 2003; Jantke, Grieser & Memmel, 2004; Jantke, Lange, Grieser, Grigoriev, Thalheim & Tschiedel, 2004a, 2004b).

DaMiT is a system for the domain of *knowledge discovery and data mining* mostly used for studies in computer science and business administration systems. The domain of eBuT is *human movement and training sciences* used in studies of sports science, kinesiology, or medicine. Both systems have been developed independently. They enjoy mutually different strengths and have both their individual peculiarities. The authors' common interest is in their systems' adaptivity as laid out in Jantke (2005), for example. The systems' adaptivity currently available is setting the stage for a transformation from e-learning tools into intelligent learning assistants.

The backbone of any system's adaptivity is its knowledge about the user, that is, the learner. The learner model of eBuT (see Figure 1) has been designed as a multilevel overlay model following Weber (2005). In contrast, the DaMiT learner model is flat in structure, but enjoys a particular feature: expressive learning goals. These fundamentals are not discussed in detail.

Instead, we are going to illustrate the systems' adaptivity at work. Concerning adaptivity, the authors rely on systematic approaches as developed in Specht (1998) and Weber, Kuhl, and Weibelzahl (2001), among others.

A first appearance of an e-learning system's adaptivity is guiding the learner's navigation through the system's content. In eBuT, this is based upon the top level information of the multilevel overlay model.

The navigation overview on the left hand side informs the learner about pages already visited (bracket on the left side as in "[+", e.g.) and those not yet seen (annotated like "+]"). The arrow is pointing to the present page "Stretch reflex." Derived from the learner model, there does appear some link To the Exercises on top of the page understood as a suggestion to the learner.

The DaMiT system is offering a different version of assistance on the level of navigation. Learners may have preferences of more or less succinct presentations. Those who prefer more examples and illustrations and are willing to spend more time with their studies get extra pages offered. There are additional case studies as well as animated illustrations, for example. To say it in terms of the book metaphor, the content offered to learners who prefer a more succinct presentation contains less pages. However, the learner has always the freedom to chance the presentation style from what is called *example-oriented* to *theory-oriented* and vice versa.

Figure 1. Inspection of a learner model in eBuT containing bookkeeping and recommendations

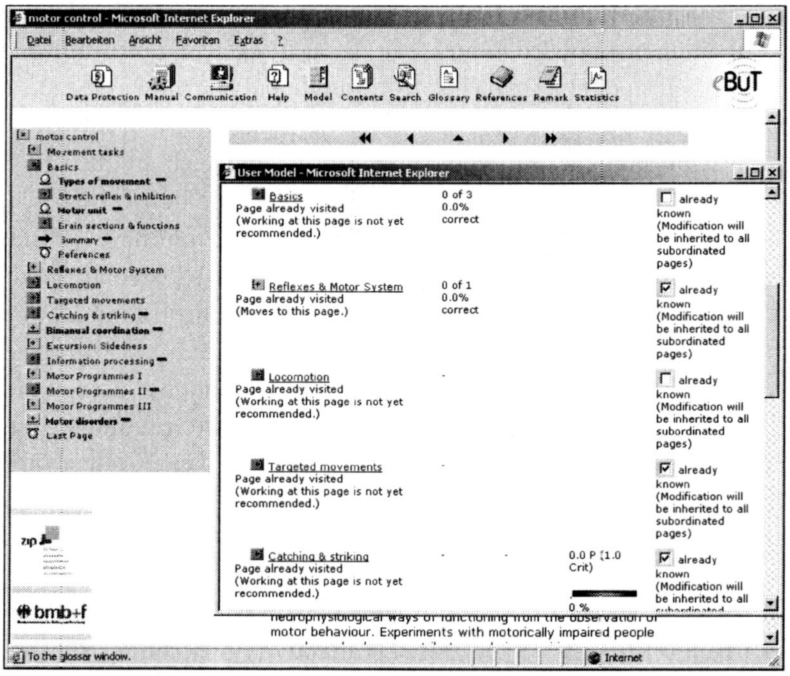

Figure 2. Navigation advice in eBuT adapted to the state of the learner model

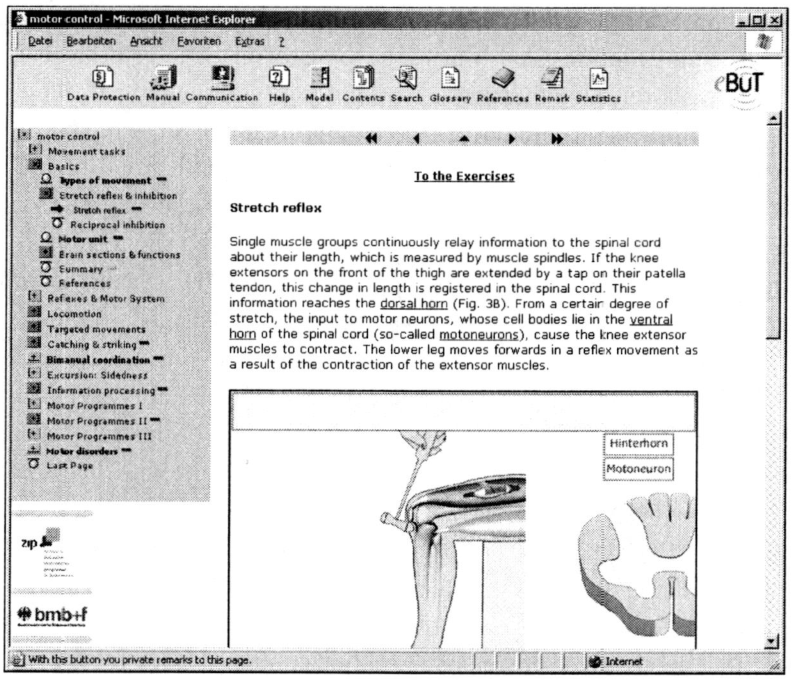

Figure 3. Navigation advice in eBuT adapted to the state of the learner model

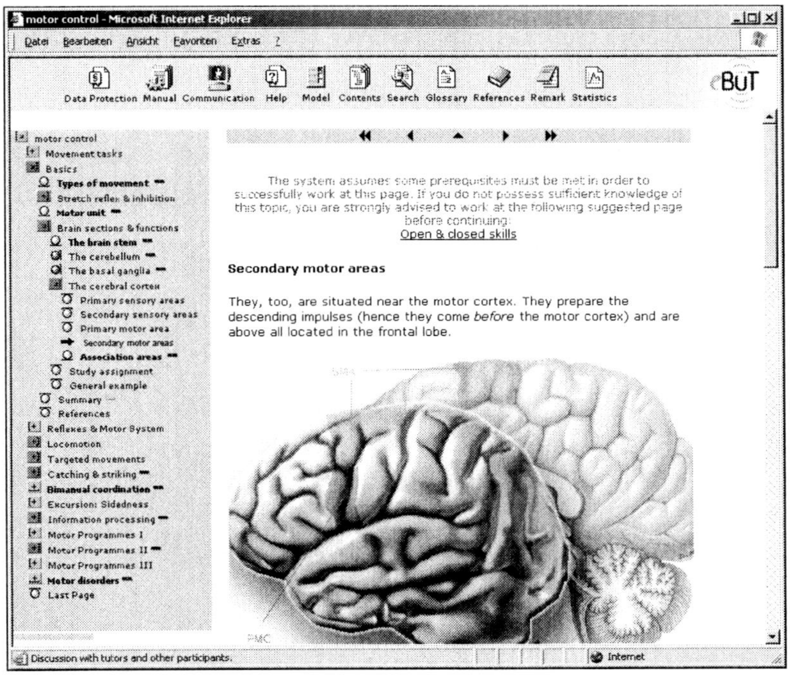

Figure 3, displaying another screenshot from the eBuT system, there appears a warning (in red). From the system's analysis of the learner model's top level entries, it derives the "belief" that the learner might have a lack of prerequisites. The system's assistance consists in directing the learner straight to suitable background material. A closer inspection of Figure 3 exhibits that the learner has left out several topics preceding the one currently visited. Those are shown as red icons (in black and white print identifiable by the bracket on the right as in "+]") above the arrow pointing to the page displayed. This system reacts accordingly.

The reader may easily recognize that the assistant system has to rely on hypothetical knowledge about its human user. Leaving out some learning material does not necessarily mean that one is not sufficiently familiar with the content. However, the system has to make its guesses that may be revised later, if necessary.

So far, the system's adaptivity consists in guiding the learner's navigation according to the system's knowledge about the learner and, derived from this knowledge, the system's belief about the learner's needs and desires. Taking into account that the system may be mistaken, the final decision about the navigation is left to the human user.

Another functionality of an e-learning system's assistance may be to offer one and the same content in different forms according to the learner's preference or even to the learner's mood.

The authors' experience has shown that a larger number of learners enjoy changing the views at learning content. Reading some definition in a strictly mathematical form and in another more explanatory formulation, for instance, frequently leads to a deeper understanding.

In the DaMiT system, a large amount of material is available in different variants enabling the learner to view it from different perspectives.

Figure 4. A definition within the DaMiT system in formal and informal presentation

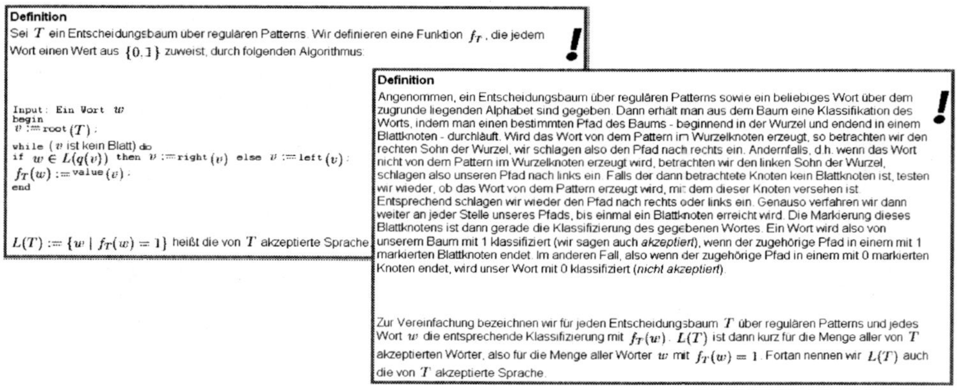

Figure 4 is displaying two cutouts from two dual presentation pages showing a certain definition in its formal variant (left cutout) and in its informal variant (right cutout). It is worth to be mentioned that the cutouts shown are not complete pages of the DaMiT presentation. In DaMiT, a page that appears on the learner's screen usually consists of several smaller units. Modularity is crucial to the systems ability to assemble slightly varying presentations dynamically.

It is already known for decades (Hull, 1943; Thorndike, 1913) that the effect of exercising depends substantially on the feedback provided to the learner. Responding to a learner's efforts in solving an exercise is a key assistance functionality.

The eBuT system is offering a variety of feedback forms. The screenshot on the left displays the systems explanation why the learner's answers are incorrect. The screenshot on the right shows an even more elaborate attempt of the eBuT system to assist the human learner. Background information is offered.

There is an obvious problem with offering variants of system's response to the learners' input in dependence on internally stored knowledge. The varying learning paths have to be anticipated at system design and content development time. The authors favor didactic design through storyboarding as outlined in Jantke and Knauf (2005).

The examples drawn from DaMiT and eBuT sketched in the present chapter may be seen as first steps toward intelligent systems' assistance. In fact, they are only representing features of adaptive tools. The stage is set for more system intelligence. It is an exciting task to transform the current state of the art into the next generation of e-learning systems—*intelligent assistants.*

TECHNOLOGIES FOR SYSTEMS' ADAPTIVITY AND ASSISTANCE

After we have seen adaptivity in e-learning at work, it is worth to ask for the technologies behind this systems' behavior. The problem to be investigated later on is how to use and to extend these technologies for the transformation to systems' assistance. Another problem is whether one may need new technologies.

It is obviously fundamental to equip an e-learning system with knowledge about the learner. Database and user modeling technologies are invoked. A crucial conceptual question is what to model about a human learner, which properties to ascribe to a learner and how to acquire the necessary information during the learner's interaction with the computer system. There are some novelties. In certain domains, one may exploit additional knowledge as demonstrated in

Figure 5. Variants of system's response to forced-choice questions in eBuT

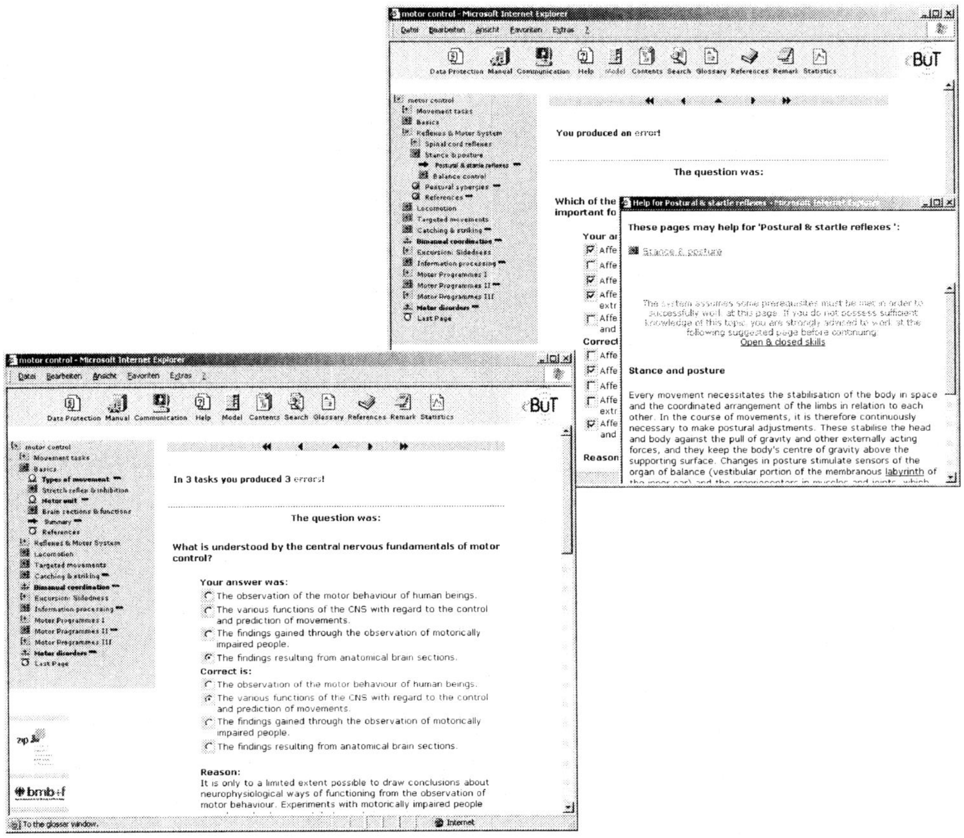

Nébel (2005), where the author exploits the fact that the learners he is addressing are also patients within a particular medical treatment. In Jantke, Grieser, and Lange (2004), the authors develop query scenarios for learner modeling without the learner's awareness of being modeled.

If expressive learner models are available and the learner's current situation is reasonably reflected by the e-learning system, one may ask how to assist the learner. The problem area begins with didactic issues beyond technologies. But didactics and technologies cannot be completely separated. The eBuT system demonstrates how concepts from media didactics Weber (2005) are related to and implemented by representational decisions (Igel & Daugs, 2003b).

Adaptivity means—as illustrated in some detail previously—to present the system's content in varying order and form and to approach the learner with different opportunities to act. For doing so, the right digitalized material must be found in the right moment to be presented in the right way.

Whatever "learning objects" are (there does not exist any consensus in the community), they have to be annotated suitably. Annotations require decisions about metadata concepts. Which metadata are required depends very much on the intended functionality. XML provides the technology of choice. After the conceptual decisions about (hierarchies of) learning objects and metadata, one may represent the learning content. (Discussion about authorship, digital rights, getting students involved, integrating research and e-learning content and the like are suppressed here.) accordingly and store it in some relational data base, for example. The decision about the underlying data base schema is another issue.

The crux beyond all the technicalities discussed so far is that variants of presentation require available variants of material. When a human teacher—on the fly—in response to the students' needs (perhaps, recognizing that they are getting tired or bored) effortlessly decides to change some presentation, for instance, by repeating a certain explanation in other words, this relies on competencies and so-called soft skills acquired and trained over years.

For a computerized assistant, this requires (1) to have the different material available (two or more variants must be prepared) and (2) to have some control implemented to change the presentation dynamically. The crux is to develop those variants with a certain vision of their use under some particular didactics in mind.

SYSTEMS' INTELLIGENCE IN E-LEARNING: PROS AND CONS

It is the authors' strong belief that so-called *systems' intelligence* is, to some extent, an ultimate criterion of success for technology enhanced learning. Learners do need care and are usually frustrated when being treated inappropriately. The learners' mood is a substantial factor of the learning success (Bransford, Brown, & Cocking, 2003; Davis, Sumara, & Luce-Kapler, 2000). There is no more need to argue in favor of intelligent assistance to human learners.

The crux is that machine intelligence is expensive (Jantke, 2004b). Both the DaMiT project and the eBuT project, though not yet resulting in intelligent computerized assistants, let the developers to the limits. For illustration, consider variants of content as shown in Figure 4. To offer those alternatives requires to design, produce, and integrate multiple variants of learning objects. The DaMiT system does contain hundreds of units in multiple forms.

The next inevitable step is to develop strategies for the system's adaptive behavior and to implement them. Evaluation is another inevitable issue not discussed here in more detail. To stick to the issue of designing the systems behavior, one has to take into account that an intelligent assistant for e-learning is more than just an IT system. The high level design of such a system requires to anticipate the intended human-machine interactions. The first author's recent approaches to attack the high level design problem in e-learning lead to some storyboard concept (Jantke & Knauf, 2005). Storyboards are understood as representations of a community of learners' potential learning experiences. As such, they go beyond the limits of conventional software engineering.

Needless to mention that not only multiple content production is expensive, storyboarding is an ambitious and time-consuming process as well.

The cons briefly mentioned above are possibly not that much surprising. As a consequence of the present chapter's discussion, the authors suggest to develop a program for gradually introducing intelligent systems' assistance into e-learning. Such a program has to cover a large variety of issues, needs competencies from different disciplines, and should be attacked within a concerted endeavor of a sufficiently strong community.

TRANSFORMATION STEPS FROM LEARNING TOOLS TO ASSISTANTS

The area of e-learning is still having its teething troubles. Notions and notations are under development. There is not much agreement about what should be accepted as an e-learning system and what should not. A large number of developers decided to begin with simple approaches and to offer elementary services with the intention to go first steps, at least. The reluctance to employment of top level technologies has many good reasons. Among them, the missing standards and the insufficient support by development tools are two prominent arguments.

When discussing the paradigmatic shift from e-learning tools to e-learning assistants, one has to take into account the remarkable number of simpler systems that have just been invented. Besides introducing innovative assistants, we have to think about transformation strategies leading from tools to assistants.

Transformation processes like the one under consideration may be, at least, seen from two different perspectives: top-down and bottom-up. It is not easy to say which way is more promising. Stanislaw Lem when pondering about the development of Artificial Intelligence in his book *Die Technologiefalle* circumscribed the problem with the following words: "Die Möglichkeiten sind so weit wie der Ozean, und wir haben weder einen ordentlichen Kompaß noch eine Karte" (p. 261), roughly saying, *the space of possibilities is as wide as the ocean, but we neither have a compass nor a map.*

Especially when going to develop a new e-learning solution from scratch, a top-down approach that starts with some carefully developed storyboard seems highly desirable. But this shall not be the focus of the present chapter. An in-depth discussion of the authors' perspectives at (or dreams of) a new development from scratch had to begin with intensive investigations of storyboard concepts and technologies (Jantke & Knauf, 2005). This is left to another publication.

The present chapter, instead, is intended to lay out some process model toward a bottom-up introduction of intelligent systems' assistance into e-learning (see Figure 6). The paradigmatic shift announced will take place, but slowly step by step.

This is a rough process model which may be completed, refined and extended. A future version might fill pages and may be accompanied by its manual. Several aspects are obviously left out. For instance, there is no reasoning about available resources and the related resource allocation is suppressed. Curricular aspects are completely missing in this first approach.

Figure 6. Top level of the transformation process model

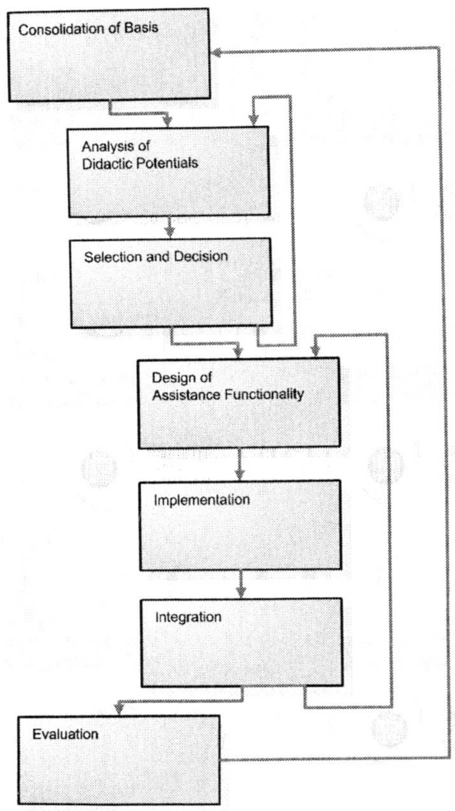

The authors confine themselves to a brief discussion of the core steps. As said earlier, both systems eBuT and DaMiT are not yet assistant systems. They are both quite successfully used in technology enhanced learning and enjoy didactically driven learner adaptivity, to some extent. But they still need to be transformed from tools into assistants.

- **Consolidation of basis** means to summarize what you have available for advancing your system and service. This is a point badly underestimated in the academia. Universiti[es] suffer from a continuous loss of competen[ce] when students are finishing their stud[ies] and leaving the institute. It might be [that] you have great applets, but the source[s are] gone, for example.

- **Analysis of didactic potentials** addresses the question where to begin. Which are the points that promise most valuable improvements? In DaMiT, for instance, one of these points is surely using the expressive learning goals to better serve learners with different intentions adaptively.
- **Selection and decision** is an inevitable administrative step because the transformation of tools into programs may be performed in literally innumerably many ways.
- **Design of assistance functionality** is the crucial creative step from tool functionality to system assistance. In DaMiT, for instance, we have very expressive interactive applets for exploratory learning. One of the applets allows the learner to pose data mining problems to the computer system which in turn tries to solve the learning task. The goal is to enable learners to develop a feeling for the complexity of learning tasks. Currently, this applet does not adapt to the human's learning goal. Some learner not interest in in-depth studies, but in getting an overview, might better be served by an illustrative case study than by her/his own time-consuming exploration.
- **Implementation** is an obviously essential nd complex task in performing the trans- rmation.
- **egration** means to relate the novel tionality to the learning environment. ans much more than just plugging in mplementation. Among other aspects, ossibilities of user interaction may new potentials of learner modeling s, lead to some additional procedures ng the learner model.
- **ion** is widely accepted to be inevi- wever, there are several problems valuation of e-learning systems. lar, when taking an incremental s sketched by the present process nains unclear to which granularity of system and service changes evaluation activities should be applied.

To sum up, the present process model comprises the authors' approach to make eBuT and DaMiT true assistant systems. This will be a laborious process, but it will lead us to the next generation of e-learning systems.

SUMMARY AND CONCLUSION

The authors admit that several aspects of the problem under consideration have been simply left out. The field ranges from role concepts, role adaptivity, and rights management through presentation generation technologies like the stored procedures of the DaMiT system to concerns on privacy issues and data security.

Other issues like storyboarding and metadata, which are deemed to be of a particular importance, are discussed in some detail, but not truly worked out.

Storyboarding—at least in its ambitious form favoured by the authors—is not yet mature enough. When submitting this chapter, the source, Jantke and Knauf (2005), has been just about one month old.

An area of research and development in its own right is established by the vision of assistant systems that are able to practice didactics for the benefit of human learners. A deeper discussion is beyond the limits of the present chapter.

As said above, among the many prerequisites of intelligent systems' assistance in e-learning, there are metadata concepts to annotate learning objects. A basic problem is that the community's agreement about metadata and the development of standards is far behind the needs. The authors experienced the necessity to extend available standards for required applications in DaMiT and eBuT. For illustration, the DaMiT system has an integrated e-payment, but none of the existing metadata standards for e-learning has concepts

When discussing the paradigmatic shift from e-learning tools to e-learning assistants, one has to take into account the remarkable number of simpler systems that have just been invented. Besides introducing innovative assistants, we have to think about transformation strategies leading from tools to assistants.

Transformation processes like the one under consideration may be, at least, seen from two different perspectives: top-down and bottom-up. It is not easy to say which way is more promising. Stanislaw Lem when pondering about the development of Artificial Intelligence in his book *Die Technologiefalle* circumscribed the problem with the following words: "Die Möglichkeiten sind so weit wie der Ozean, und wir haben weder einen ordentlichen Kompaß noch eine Karte" (p. 261), roughly saying, *the space of possibilities is as wide as the ocean, but we neither have a compass nor a map.*

Especially when going to develop a new e-learning solution from scratch, a top-down approach that starts with some carefully developed storyboard seems highly desirable. But this shall not be the focus of the present chapter. An in-depth discussion of the authors' perspectives at (or dreams of) a new development from scratch had to begin with intensive investigations of storyboard concepts and technologies (Jantke & Knauf, 2005). This is left to another publication.

The present chapter, instead, is intended to lay out some process model toward a bottom-up introduction of intelligent systems' assistance into e-learning (see Figure 6). The paradigmatic shift announced will take place, but slowly step by step.

This is a rough process model which may be completed, refined and extended. A future version might fill pages and may be accompanied by its manual. Several aspects are obviously left out. For instance, there is no reasoning about available resources and the related resource allocation is suppressed. Curricular aspects are completely missing in this first approach.

Figure 6. Top level of the transformation process model

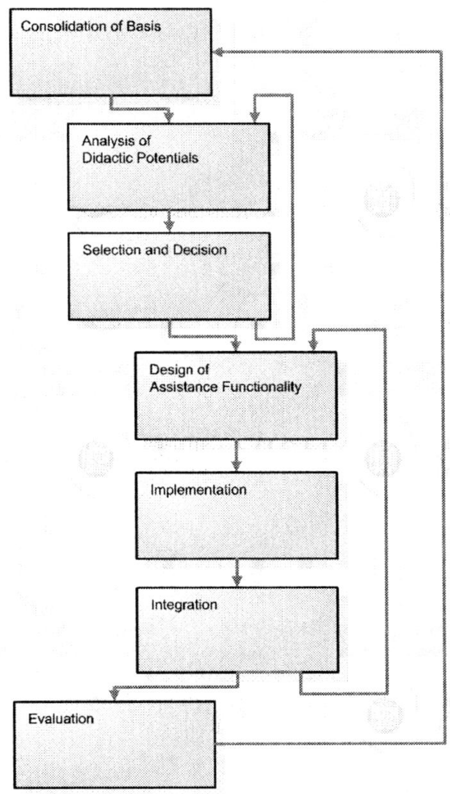

The authors confine themselves to a brief discussion of the core steps. As said earlier, both systems eBuT and DaMiT are not yet assistant systems. They are both quite successfully used in technology enhanced learning and enjoy didactically driven learner adaptivity, to some extent. But they still need to be transformed from tools into assistants.

- **Consolidation of basis** means to summarize what you have available for advancing your system and service. This is a point badly underestimated in the academia. Universities suffer from a continuous loss of competency when students are finishing their studies and leaving the institute. It might be that you have great applets, but the sources are gone, for example.

- **Analysis of didactic potentials** addresses the question where to begin. Which are the points that promise most valuable improvements? In DaMiT, for instance, one of these points is surely using the expressive learning goals to better serve learners with different intentions adaptively.
- **Selection and decision** is an inevitable administrative step because the transformation of tools into programs may be performed in literally innumerably many ways.
- **Design of assistance functionality** is the crucial creative step from tool functionality to system assistance. In DaMiT, for instance, we have very expressive interactive applets for exploratory learning. One of the applets allows the learner to pose data mining problems to the computer system which in turn tries to solve the learning task. The goal is to enable learners to develop a feeling for the complexity of learning tasks. Currently, this applet does not adapt to the human's learning goal. Some learner not interest in in-depth studies, but in getting an overview, might better be served by an illustrative case study than by her/his own time-consuming exploration.
- **Implementation** is an obviously essential and complex task in performing the transformation.
- **Integration** means to relate the novel functionality to the learning environment. It means much more than just plugging in some implementation. Among other aspects, new possibilities of user interaction may provide new potentials of learner modeling and, thus, lead to some additional procedures of feeding the learner model.
- **Evaluation** is widely accepted to be inevitable. However, there are several problems with the evaluation of e-learning systems. In particular, when taking an incremental approach as sketched by the present process model, it remains unclear to which granularity of system and service changes evaluation activities should be applied.

To sum up, the present process model comprises the authors' approach to make eBuT and DaMiT true assistant systems. This will be a laborious process, but it will lead us to the next generation of e-learning systems.

SUMMARY AND CONCLUSION

The authors admit that several aspects of the problem under consideration have been simply left out. The field ranges from role concepts, role adaptivity, and rights management through presentation generation technologies like the stored procedures of the DaMiT system to concerns on privacy issues and data security.

Other issues like storyboarding and metadata, which are deemed to be of a particular importance, are discussed in some detail, but not truly worked out.

Storyboarding—at least in its ambitious form favoured by the authors—is not yet mature enough. When submitting this chapter, the source, Jantke and Knauf (2005), has been just about one month old.

An area of research and development in its own right is established by the vision of assistant systems that are able to practice didactics for the benefit of human learners. A deeper discussion is beyond the limits of the present chapter.

As said above, among the many prerequisites of intelligent systems' assistance in e-learning, there are metadata concepts to annotate learning objects. A basic problem is that the community's agreement about metadata and the development of standards is far behind the needs. The authors experienced the necessity to extend available standards for required applications in DaMiT and eBuT. For illustration, the DaMiT system has an integrated e-payment, but none of the existing metadata standards for e-learning has concepts for the representation of payment information. One can take it for granted that the transformation from e-learning tools to e-learning assistants will bring with it further needs to extend current metadata standards.

Beyond all those topics in technology enhanced learning left out or discussed only in a brief, the authors have put most emphasis on some process model for introducing intelligent systems' assistance into e-learning. Well-prepared by means of the state of the art report, the reader—hopefully—should have got an impression of how to apply this process model to the authors' systems and services DaMiT and eBuT. In some sense, the authors advocate an evolutionary process towards more system assistance in technology enhanced learning.

Next steps of research and development will be (1) a completion and more explicit representation of the process model and (2) an application of the process model to DaMiT and eBuT.

In such a way, the transformation from e-learning tools to intelligent systems' assistants will be exemplified. Both steps shall be deeply dovetailed. The authors' application efforts will help to evaluate and revise the process model. In turn, the applications may benefit again.

ACKNOWLEDGMENT

The authors gracefully acknowledge several years of an enjoyable and fruitful cooperation with many colleagues and friends within the joint e-learning projects (1) DaMiT: http://damit.dfki.de, and (2) eBuT: http://www.bewegung-und-training.de. Readers are invited to pay a visit to these service pages in the Internet.

REFERENCES

Bransford, J. D., Brown, A. L., & Cocking, R. R. (Eds.). (2003). *How people learn: Brain, mind, experience, and school.* National Academy Press.

Damasio, A. (1999). *The feeling of what happens: Body and emotion in the making of consciousness.* Hartcourt.

Davis, B., Sumara, D., & Luce-Kapler, R. (2000). *Engaging minds: Learning and teaching in a complex world.* Lawrence Erlbaum Associates.

Flechsig, K.-H. (1996). *Kleines Handbuch didaktischer Modelle (Small manual of didactical models).* Eichenzell: Neuland.

Hull, C. L. (1943). *Principles of behavior.* New York: Appleton-Century-Crofts.

Igel, C., & Daugs, R. (2002). Mehrwertpotenziale Internetbasierter Lehre (Added value capabilities of Internet-based teaching). In K. P. Jantke, W. S. Wittig, & J. Herrmann (Eds.), *Vom e-Learning bis e-Payment: Das Internet als sicherer Marktplatz (From e-learning to e-payment: The Internet as a safe marketplace)* (pp. 8–19). Berlin: infix.

Igel, C., & Daugs, R. (2003a). eLearning in der Bewegungs- und Trainingswissenschaft: Das Engineering des BMBF-Projektes "eBuT" (eLearning in movement and training science: The engineering of the project eBut backed by the Federal Ministry of Education and Resarch). *dvs Informationen, 18*(3), 5–8.

Igel, C., & Daugs, R. (2003b). Zur Individualisierung Internetbasierter Lehr-Lern-Prozesse: Didaktische Überlegungen und technologische Entwicklungen im BMBF-Projekt "eBuT" (Individualization of Internet-based teaching-learning processes: Didactical considerations and technological developments in the eBUT). In U. Beck & V. Sommer (Eds.), *Learntec 2003: 11. Europäischer Kongress und Fachmesse für Bildungs- und Informationstechnologie* (pp. 253–258). Karlsruhe: Holler Verlag.

Igel, C., & Daugs, R. (Eds.). (2005). *eLearning in der Sportwissenschaft: Strategien, Konzeptionen, Perspektiven (eLearning in sports science: Strategies, conceptual design, prospects).* Schorndorf: Hofmann.

Igel, C., & Sturm, R. (2003). Server-Architektur, Autorensystem, Datenbanken, Assets: Die Informationsinfrastruktur des Projektes "eBuT" (Server architecture, authoring tool, databases, assets: The information infrastructure of the eBut). *dvs Informationen, 18*(3), 9–13.

Jank, W., & Meyer, H. (2002). *Didaktische Modelle (Didactical models).* Frankfurt a.M.: Cornelsen.

Jantke, K. P. (2003, June 13). Knowledge discovery & data mining: Lehren und Lernen im Internet (Knowledge discovery & dat mining: Teaching and learning in the Internet). In *Köthener Informatik-Tag.* Köthen: FH Anhalt.

Jantke, K. P. (2004a, June 3-4). Neue Technologien: Potentiale und Probleme illustriert an Anwendungen des e-Learning (eingeladener Hauptvortrag) (New technologies: Potentials and problems illustrated on eLearning applications – invited speech). In *Wismarer Wirtschaftsinformatik-Tage, WIWITA 2004.*

Jantke, K. P. (2004b, June 3-4). ROI: Das unlösbare Problem des e-Learning (ROI: The unsolvable problem of eLearning). In *Wismarer Wirtschaftsinformatik-Tage, WIWITA 2004.*

Jantke, K. P. (2005). Informatik und Künstliche Intelligenz: Beiträge zur Adaptivität einer kommenden Generation intelligenter eLearning-Systeme (Information technology and artificial intelligence: Contributions on adptivity of a coming generation of intelligent eLearning systems). In C. Igel & R. Daugs (Eds.), *eLearning in der Sportwissenschaft: Strategien, Konzeptionen, Perspektiven (eLearning in sports science: Strategies, conceptual design, prospects)* (pp. 49–70). Schorndorf: Hofmann.

Jantke, K. P., Degel, G., Grieser, G., Memmel, M., Rostanin, O., & Tschiedel, B. (2004, September 29 - October 1). Technology enhanced dimensions in e-learning. In M.E. Auer & U. Auer (Eds.), *International Conference on Interactive Computer Aided Learning, ICL 2004* (CD). Villach, Austria.

Jantke, K. P., Grieser, G., & Lange, S. (2004, September 29 - October 1). Adaptation to the learners' needs and desires by induction and negotiation of hypotheses. In M.E. Auer & U. Auer (Eds.), *International Conference on Interactive Computer Aided Learning, ICL 2004* (CD), Villach, Austria.

Jantke, K. P., Grieser, G., & Memmel, M. (2004, October 4-6). DaMiT: Data Mining lernen und lehren (Learning and teaching data mining). In *Lernen, Wissensentdeckung und Adaptivität (Learning, Knowledge detection and adaptivity)* (LWA-2004), Fachgruppentreffen Maschinelles Lernen (FGML). Berlin.

Jantke, K. P., & Knauf, R. (2005, January 3-6). Didactic design through storyboarding: Standard concepts for standard tools. In *Proceedings of the First International Workshop on Dissemination of E-Learning Technologies and Applications,* Cape Town, South Africa.

Jantke, K. P., Lange, S., Grieser, G., Grigoriev, P., Thalheim, B., & Tschiedel, B. (2004a, April 14-17). Learning by doing and learning when doing. In I. Seruca, J. Filipe, S. Hammoudi, & J. Cordeiro (Eds.), *Proceedings of the International Conference on Enterprise Information Systems* (Vol. 5, pp. 238–241), Porto, Portugal. INSTICC.

Jantke, K. P., Lange, S., Grieser, G., Grigoriev, P., Thalheim, B., & Tschiedel, B. (2004b, September 27-30). Work-integrated e-learning: The DaMiT approach. In O. Sawodny & P. Scharff (Eds.), *Proceedings of the 49 Internationales Wissenschaftliches Kolloquium, TU* (Vol. 2, pp. 333–339). Shaker Verlag.

Jantke, K. P., & Lunzer, A. (2005). Search, comparison and evaluation in exploratory e-learning with subjunctive interfaces. In *Proceedings of the 3rd Conference on Professional Knowledge Management, 1st Workshop on Learner-Oriented*

Knowledge Management and KM-Oriented E-Learning, Kaiserslautern, Germany.

Jantke, K. P., Memmel, M., Rostanin, O., & Rudolf, B. (2004, November 1-5). Media and service integration for professional e-learning. In *Proceedings of the E-Learn 2004, World Conference on E-Learning in Corporate, Government, Healthcare & Higher Education,* Washington, DC.

Jantke, K. P., Memmel, M., Rostanin, O., Thalheim, B., & Tschiedel, B. (2003). Decision support by learning-on-demand. In *CAiSE Workshop 2003,* Klagenfurt, Österreich.

Klein, B., & Weber, G. (2002, March 3-5). Die Realisierung von Adaptivität mit dem Internet-Autorensystem NetCoach (The realization of adaptivity with the Internet authoring tool NetCoach). In U. Rinn & J. Wedekind (Eds.), *Referenzmodelle netzbasierten Lehrens und Lernens (Models of reference on net-based teaching and learning)* (pp. 101–118). Münster: Waxmann.

Nébel, I.-T. (2005). Patient and learner adaptation in e-learning by induction based on medical context. In R. Kaschek (Ed.), *Perspectives of Intelligent Systems' Assistance, International Workshop,* Palmerston North, New Zealand.

Rothwell, W. J., & Kazanas, H. C. (2004). *Mastering the instructional design process: A systematic approach* (3rd ed.). Pfeiffer.

Searle, J. R. (1980). *Mind, brains, and programs: Vol. 3 of The Behavioral and Brain Sciences.* Cambridge University Press.

Specht, M. (1998). *Adaptive Methoden in computerbasierten Lehr/Lernsystemen (Adaptive methods in computer-based teaching-learning systems).* Doctoral thesis, Universität Trier, FB Psychologie.

Tergan, S.-O., & Schenkel, P. (Eds.). (2004). *Was macht E-Learning erfolgreich? Grundlagen und Instrumente der Qualitätsbeurteilung (How does eLearning become successful? Basics and tools of quality-assessment).* Springer.

Thorndike, E. L. (1913). *Educational psychology* (Vol. 1 & 2). New York: Columbia University Press.

Weber, G. (1996). Episodic learner modelling. *Cognitive Science, 20,* 195–236.

Weber, G. (1999). Adaptive learning systems in the World Wide Web. In *User Modeling; Proceedings of the Seventh International Conference UM'99* (pp. 371–378). Springer.

Weber, G. (2005). Mediendidaktik: Varianten virtueller Lehr-/Lernformen (Versions of virtual teaching-learning forms). In C. Igel & R. Daugs (Eds.), *eLearning in der Sportwissenschaft: Strategien, Konzeptionen, Perspektiven (eLearning in sports science: Strategies, conceptual design, prospects)* (pp. 71-98). Schorndorf: Hofmann.

Weber, G., Kuhl, H.-C., & Weibelzahl, S. (2001). Developing adaptive Internet based courses with the authoring system NetCoach. In S. Reich, M.M. Tzagarakis, & P.M.E. De Bra (Eds.), *Hypermedia: Openness, structural awareness and adaptivity* (pp. 226–238). Springer.

This work was previously published in Intelligent Assistant Systems: Concepts, Techniques and Technologies, edited by R. Kaschek, pp. 212-231, copyright 2007 by IGI Publishing, formerly known as Idea Group Publishing (an imprint of IGI Global).

Chapter XVI
Using Emotional Intelligence in Personalized Adaptation

Violeta Damjanovic
Salzburg Research, Austria

Milos Kravcik
Open University Nederland, The Netherlands

ABSTRACT

The process of training and learning in Web-based and ubiquitous environments brings a new sense of adaptation. With the development of more sophisticated environments, the need for them to take into account the user's traits, as well as the user's devices on which the training is executed, has become an important issue in the domain of building novel training and learning environments. This chapter introduces an approach to the realization of personalized adaptation. According to the fact that we are dealing with the stereotypes of e-learners, having in mind emotional intelligence concepts to help in adaptation to the e-learners real needs and known preferences, we have called this system eQ. It stands for the using of the emotional intelligence concepts on the Web.

INSIDE CHAPTER

The process of training and learning in Web-based and ubiquitous environments brings a new sense of adaptation. With the development of more sophisticated environments, the need for them to take into account the user's traits, as well as a user's devices on which the training is executed, and to place them within the context of the training activities, has become an important issue in the domain of building novel training and learning environments. Personalized adaptation represents a key aspect in technology enhanced learning and training communities. Different users could have different learning needs and preferences, and they could have different knowledge levels, as well as different opportunities to use certain training methods related to the fact that both users and theirs labs are placed in physical world. The chapter presents an approach to the realization of personalized adaptation according to the individual user's traits, such as: personality factors, cognitive factors, learning styles, and personality types (stereotypes) on one side, and user's devices on which the training is executed on the other side. At the same time, we are interested in how to manage teaching resources when the e-learners have different emotions, perceptions, and reactions. Because that we are dealing with the stereotypes of e-learners, having in mind emotional intelligence concepts to help in adaptation to the e-learners real needs and known preferences, we have named this system eQ, which stands for the using of emotional intelligence on the Web (electronic emotional intelligence). There are several key paradigms being used in the conceptual design of the eQ system: (1) this approach is based on using a multiagent system with the belief-design-intention agent rational model, (2) the eQ system is initially defined by considering component-based definition of the adaptive educational hypermedia system, (3) the eQ system uses the FOSP adaptive learning strategy, and (4) the main aim of the eQ system is to improve the adaptation processes in the Semantic Web and Grid environment.

INTRODUCTION

The history of learning can be followed back to ancient Greece, where Socrates used tutorial learning. Plato established one of the earliest known organized schools in Western civilization, the Academy in Athens, and further developed the form of live dialogue. Aristotle considered learning by doing as an efficient way of education. Already, in the 17th century Comenius wrote that learning has to be adjusted to the learner's abilities. Each person learns differently and needs to develop their own learning skills in their own way. Looking into the past we can see that ideas about how to learn are not new. However, what is new are the circumstances and opportunities. The existing school system is suitable for the industrial age, when manufacturing processes were performed in a routine way. The knowledge age demands higher skilled jobs based on critical thinking, creativity, collaboration, and interpretation abilities. Additionally, the percentage of "knowledge workers" is rapidly increasing and 50% of all employee skills become outdated in three to five years (Moe & Blodgett, 2000). Therefore, using only traditional methods cannot cover today's educational needs. Many relevant authorities have recognized the new demands on one hand and new potential on the other. In the following we mention some of them.

Peter Drucker sees new horizons. *"For the first time substantial and rapidly growing number of people have choices. For the first time, they will have to manage themselves. And society is totally unprepared for it."* He cites Plutarch in Drucker (1989), saying that education requires a focus on the strengths and talents of learners:

Any teacher of young artist—musicians, actors, painters—knows this. So does any teacher of young athletes. But schools do not do it. They focus instead on a learner's weaknesses. One cannot build performance on weaknesses, even corrected ones; one can build performance only on strengths. And these the schools traditionally ignore, in fact, consider more or less irrelevant. Strengths do not create problems—and schools are problem-focused.

Alfred Bork (2001) considers current and new paradigms concerning technology and learning. The current main learning paradigm, called *information transfer* or *classroom-teacher paradigm*, envisions the primary aim of learning as the acquisition of information. Its major auxiliary learning technology is the textbook. The author argues that we need much better learning for all and this learning has to be affordable for the individual and the world. Therefore, he predicts a future paradigm—*tutorial learning.* It sees learning as fully active, focusing on the student as learner rather than on authority figures giving information. *Tutorial learning* refers to the type of learning that takes place between a highly skilled tutor and the student, or a small group of students. The main problem related to this form of learning was that there were few good tutors, and it is a very expensive way of learning. But what makes the difference now is the available technology to rebuild learning and make it more interactive, individualized, and adaptive. *"For the first time we have the possibility of educating everyone on earth to each person's full potential."*

Wayne Hodgins (2005) presents the grand vision of *meLearning* that will provide personalized learning experiences to every person on the planet every day. When the learner is ready, the "teacher" will appear.

Roger C. Schank (2002) revises the concept *intelligence*. In the past, education and intelligence was built on accumulation of facts and ability to cite opinions of others. Today in school, pupils learn how to answer instead of how to query. The easier it is to get information, the lower its value. But the value of good questions increases. In a scenario from the future, when an issue arises, one can easily get related opinions of relevant authorities in a preferred form. If it is not enough, one can discuss the problem with other (suitable) people (all over the world) who are just dealing with a similar issue or with currently available instructors. In the future, intelligence will mean ability to reach the boundaries of the knowledge base.

Each person learns differently and needs to develop own learning skills in his or her own way. This is a reason why we explore using *emotional intelligence* (eQ) in learning on the Web (Web-based learning).

The main technological challenges and requirements for the next generation Web and Grid systems can be fulfilled by using emerging technologies, such as:

- **The Semantic Web:** This represents the idea of having data on the Web defined and linked in a way that can be used for more effective discovery, automation, semantic integration, metadata annotation, and reuse across various applications (W3C, 2001).
- **The Semantic Grid:** This attempts to extend the Semantic Web approaches and solutions to take into account Grid characteristics.
- **Knowledge Grid:** This offers high-level tools and techniques for distributed knowledge extraction from data repositories on the Grid.
- **Adaptive Web systems:** These are able to adjust to different user requirements and to manage sources of heterogeneity.
- **Peer-to-peer (P2P) architecture:** This considers a set of protocols, a computing model, and a design philosophy for distributed, decentralized, and self-organizing systems.
- **Ubiquitous computing (pervasive computing):** This describes distributed computing devices, such as personal devices, wearable computers, and sensors in the environment, as well as the software and hardware infrastructures needed to support applications on these computing devices.

Adaptation represents an important factor in building intelligent educational systems, with the aim to facilitate learning processes and to improve the learning efficiency through adjustment to real user needs. On one side, there are methods and techniques of adaptive hypermedia (AH) systems, as well as user modelling and personalization/adaptation methods, such as Brusilovsky (2001, 2003):

- **"pre-Web" generation of AH systems:** They explore adaptive presentation and adaptive navigation support and are concentrate on modelling user knowledge and goals.

- **"Web" generation of AH systems:** They explore adaptive content selection and adaptive recommendation based on modelling user interests.
- **"Mobile" generation of AH systems:** They explore using of known adaptation technologies with the aim to adapt to both an individual user and a context of his/her work.

On the other side, there is an opportunity for using new technologies and standards, such as metadata, Semantic Web, Web services, Semantic Web services, as well as the Semantic Grid. Development of the Semantic Grid has led to new achievements, such as OWL (Web Ontology Language) for expressing ontologies in a way that supports interoperability between systems. A key motivation for the semantic interoperability is the need to assemble new applications, as well as new tools and equipment for cooperation in order to provide the requisite global behaviour, without manual intervention (De Roure & Hendler, 2004).

In this chapter, we explore the impact of using AH systems in the Semantic Grid environment with the aim to point out certain potentials in further learning on the Web, as well as to show the way to increase learning efficiency. The Semantic Grid must be able to interoperate with a large-scale spectrum of current and emerging hardware and software technologies, on one side, and with a different user's profiles on the other side. Different users prefer different presentation forms: some prefer multimedia contents (graphical material and hypertext documents, simulations, presentations); others use traditional web pages (questionnaires, exercises, research study).

This chapter presents an approach to the realization of personalized adaptation according to the individual user's traits, such as: (1) personality factors, (2) cognitive factors, (3) learning style, and (4) personality types (stereotypes). Different users could have different learning needs and preferences, different knowledge levels, and different opportunities to use certain training methods and equipment.

The chapter first provides an overview of personalized adaptation and the adaptive educational hypermedia systems. In addition, this chapter explains the role of context, content, and adaptation management parts in building multiagent systems for personalized adaptation. Then, the key paradigms of the eQ agent system are discussed in detail. In the following section, implementation of our eQ agent system is presented. Chapter five explains fine art professional training, ACCADEMI@VINCIANA, and two examples of using eQ agent system in improving the adaptation process in the Semantic Web and Grid environment: (1) e-learner is a preschool child, and (2) e-learner is an expert in the domain of painting technologies. The last section contains some conclusion remarks.

USING PERSONALIZED ADAPTATION IN LEARNING

We can see certain similarities and parallels between the delivery processes in art and education, especially in their two forms, artefact and experience. This can illustrate the difference between learning objects and learning design, as well as the various degree of adaptation provided by different media.

In both areas artefacts are produced by authors—writers produce books, painters produce paintings, and composers produce compositions. On the other side, domain experts with pedagogical background write textbooks. These artefacts typically require active processing from their users, interpretation, and usually a require a higher degree of imaginative involvement to integrate the message into their minds.

Another form of delivery is experience—books and scenarios are interpreted by actors in plays and movies, and musicians interpret compositions in concerts. Also, traditional (*objectivist*) teaching is based mostly on the interpretation of textbooks by teachers and trainers. In these cases, the audience's mental processing is usually more passive as some abstract dimensions of the original artefact become concrete and therefore do not need so much imagination to be activated; typically the interpretation is more unambiguous.

In both art and education there is a transformation process between the artefact and experience. In art it is controlled by directors or conductors during rehearsals. Teachers are educated how to interpret textbooks during their pedagogical study. In modern (*constructivist*) forms of teaching they overtake the mediator or guide role and the performers are learners themselves instead of teachers, resulting in a very active participation, possibly fully embedded in the learning experience (e.g., field trips).

Personalized adaptation represents a key aspect in technology enhanced learning and training communities. This implies the requirement of a reactive and decentralized platform that can make informed decisions about how to respond to changes of the user's preferences, device capability, enterprise policy, and many other environmental factors. Roughly speaking, the main aim of personalized adaptation is to support ubiquitous, decentralized, agent-based systems and devices for learning, training, and doing well in different environments.

Development of a sharable digital library of learning and training resources can be useful in various systems, such as computer-based training systems, interactive learning environments, intelligent computer-aided instruction systems, distance learning systems, and collaborative learning environments. At the same time, there are different resources types, such as graphical material and hypertext documents, simulations, questionnaires, exercises, presentations, research study, experiments, and much more.

In this chapter, we propose using concepts of emotional intelligence (eQ) with the aim to achieve adaptivity in the domain that can be collectively referred to as a "context" in professional learning and training environments. More recently, the notion of eQ has attracted increased attention as one of the prerequisites for improving student's learning. Starting from the preliminary definition of eQ, originally proposed in Salovey and Mayer (2000), we describe eQ as *"a person's ability to understand learning emotions and to act appropriately based on this understanding."*

eQ represents an essential part of effective communication and adaptability, especially in the field of education, to support the user being more emotionally and socially intelligent, and to reduce negative behaviours. Web environment represents the perfect place to measure eQ skills and offer new suggestions for practicing these skills. The process for developing eQ online (Bradberry & Greaves, 2003) is shown in Figure 1, as well as in context management part of Figure 5.

The Role of Context, Content, and Adaptation Management

Based on experience from the development of adaptive educational hypermedia authoring tools

Figure 1. The process for developing eQ online

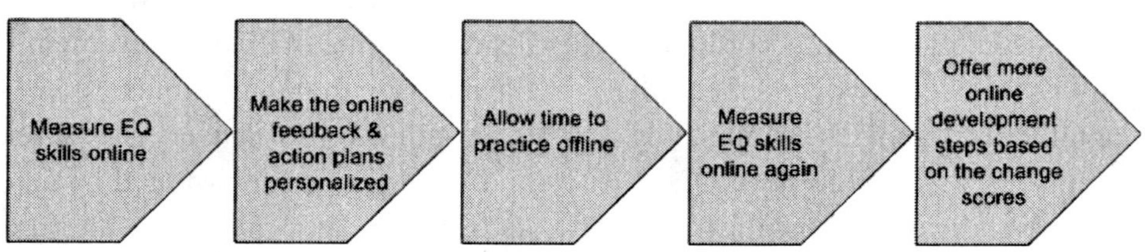

(Kravcik, Specht, & Oppermann, 2004), the authors suggest that an efficient AH system should contains the following three parts:

- Context management
- Content management
- Adaptation management

Some of the more significant roles of each of these parts are discussed.

Context Management

Context management includes user modelling, enabling reusability, and sharing of the user model by various adaptive applications and user devices. In other words, context managers can be used to collect, collate, and process context information about users. The goal of this part is to design and implement a mechanism by which context information can be updated and distributed. Context management must be able to detect modification and addition of user's characteristics, and it must have location awareness module, as well as a component that provides data about enterprise policy (Robinson, 2000).

The approach represented here is based on modelling stereotypical models of user individual traits for adaptation. These individual traits include the following:

- Personality factors (extrovert, introvert)
- Cognitive factors (perceptual processing, phonological awareness, ability to maintain attentional focus)
- Learning styles (moving, touching, doing, auditory, visual)
- Personality types (conventional, social, investigative, artistic, realistic, and enterprising personality)
- Information about user's devices

All of these individual traits could be extracted by using specially designed psychological tests that perform multiagent systems represented as a distributed test-sensor system. The ontology for adaptation is made from context information about users, as well as about user's devices. This ontology is based on using the IEEE PAPI (Public and Private Information) Standard, which represents (IEEE PAPI, 2001):

A data interchange specification that describes learner information for communication among cooperating systems.

Figure 2. An extension of the IEEE PAPI learner preference information (IEEE 1484.2.24)

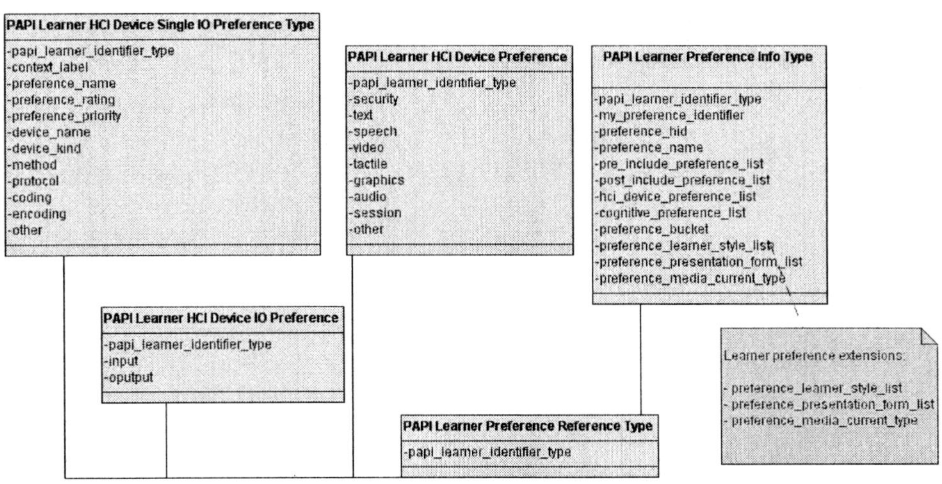

Figure 3. An extension of the IEEE PAPI learner portfolio information (IEEE 1484.2.26)

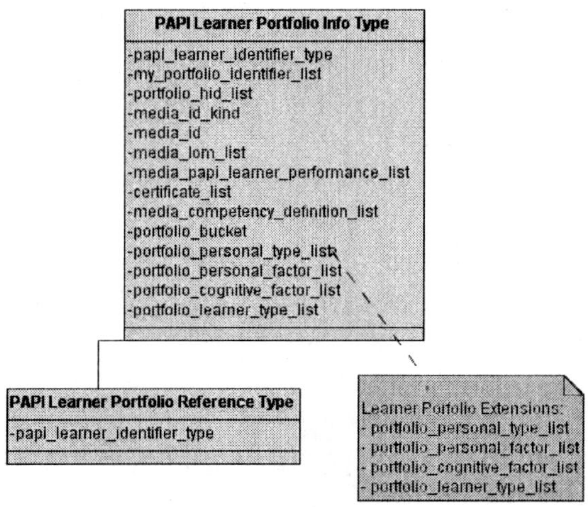

The IEEE PAPI Standard is extended to the parts that are related to the learner *preference information* (IEEE 1484.2.24), as well as the learner *portfolio information* (IEEE 1484.2.26) (shown in Figure 2, as well as Figure 3). These extensions are made with the aim of enabling using eQ concepts during the learning processes on the Web.

Content Management

The content management part maintains the domain model (learning objects with metadata, semantic concept networks/ontologies) and supports the authoring process (separation of content and layout, their reusability, semi-automatic annotation) (Kravcik, 2004). As an example of professional training domain, we have represented the ontology ACCADEMI@VINCIANA. This ontology involves solid team of experts from the area of fine art conservation and restoration, as well as physics and chemistry. It has three main parts, with the knowledge supporting the following (Damjanovic, Kravcik, & Devedzic, 2005):

- Learning about fine art painting methods and materials (education: painting methods and materials, conservation treatments, preventive conservation strategies, restoration, reproduction)
- Training on fine art painting methods and materials (education, classical painting technology analysis, painting damage diagnosis)
- Art Fraud E-detection (author identification, original expertise, fraud detection)

The ontology ACCADEMI@VINCIANA has several dimensions concerning professional training's intentions. First, this ontology describes three fundamental painting components, as well as their role in the construction of painting. These components could be explained as follows: colours (represent main artistic instrumentation), ground (represents the base, the underlay of painting), and binder (represents an important factor to firm adherence of colours to the ground). Second, this ontology observes fundamental aspects for analyzing painting methods and techniques. These aspects can be considered as follows (Kraigher-Hozo, 1991):

- **Purpose and usage:** icon, miniature, illumination, altar painting,
- **Ground material:** stone, tree, glass, ivory, parchment, canvas, paper, cardboard,
- **Binder and colours:** chalk, carbon, aquarelle, pastel, tempera, oil, encaustic,
- **Painting tools:** quill, cane, brush, air brush, artistic knife, aerograph,
- **Painting methods and techniques:** proplasmos, glykasmos, verdaccio, puntegiaro, trattegiaro, fa presto, impasto, alla prima, collage, frottage.

Third, ACCADEMI@VINCIANA ontology can be divided into the following two categories of trainings (Kraigher-Hozo, 1991) (shown in Figure 4):

- Trainings made by using physical methods

Figure 4. One part of the domain ontology - ACCADEMI@VINCIANA

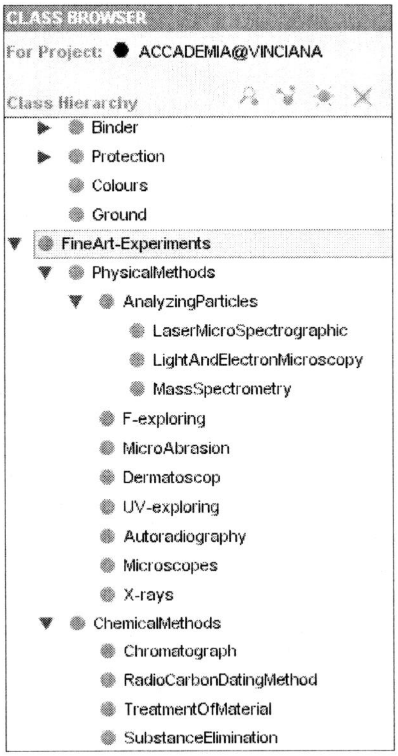

- Trainings made by using chemical methods

Trainings made by using Physical Methods

This includes trainings that could be performed by using (Kraigher-Hozo, 1991):

- **Dermatoscope:** For non-invasive diagnosis
- **Micro abrasion equipments:** For drilling micron level holes, and cutting or marking fragile or otherwise difficult materials
- **Microscopes:** For histological analyzing of paintings
- **Exploring the nanostructures of painting materials with X-rays:** This method show solid results in uncovering fraud, as well as in exploring the way of building paintings
- **UV exploring:** It can be used to learn the process of building paintings up to the identification of original
- **Fluorescent microscope (F-exploring):** It can be used to explore homogeneity of varnish and other transparent layers
- **Analyzing particles (protons, neurons):** ESA (Emission Spectral Analyze) (laser), Laser micro spectrographic analysis, Light and electron microscopy (scanning), Mass spectrometry, DBA (*Debye-Scherrer* Analyze) (analyzing small particles);
- **Autoradiography:** It can be useful for microscopic fluorescent measurements.

Trainings made by using Chemical Methods

This includes trainings that could be performed by using (Kraigher-Hozo, 1991):

- Microchemistry approach with pigments identification, emission spectral analysis, the iodine probe, DBA …
- **Chromatograph:** Substance that reacts on certain components (for example, if the reagent is protein, substance will be coloured red).
- **Exploring substance elimination:** Binders have different behaviours when they are heated in water (wax is smelted at 60°C, oil at 160°C).
- **Different treatments of certain material:** Burning samples, exposing samples to the rays of the sun or to the X-rays, high temperature, …
- **Radio carbon dating method:** One of the most widely used and best known absolute dating methods, based on the decay rate and half-time of C-14 (an unstable isotope of carbon).

All of these physical and chemical methods and devices could be used to explore and make artistic trainings with the aim to learn about painting methods and materials, as well as to explore and diagnose conservation strategies, originality, author identification, forgery, and much more (Damjanovic, Kravcik, & Devedzic, 2005).

Adaptation Management

Adaptation can be thought of as the behaviour of an entity in response to both changes in context management and needs in content management part. The adaptation manager could be used directly by an application that pushes relevant information to a user based on the user's stereotype and the user's learning and training needs. In this chapter, the adaptation manager decides to modify presentation content by using the FOSP (filter-order-select-present) adaptive learning strategy (Kravcik, 2004) that will be discussed in detail.

Figure 5 shows the conceptual design of the eQ agent system (Damjanovic, Kravcik, & Devedzic, 2005). *Context management part* is related to the first level of personalized adaptation in which using eQ concepts are made. The process for developing eQ online includes the following:

1. Measure eQ skills online
2. Make the online feedback and action plans personalized
3. Allow time to practice offline
4. Measure eQ skills online again
5. Offer more online development steps based on the change scores

Content management part includes learning objects (LOs), semantic metadata about learning materials, and training devices. *Adaptation management part* consists of the eQ agent system, which performs the proposed FOSP adaptive strategy.

Figure 5. Conceptual design of the eQ agent system

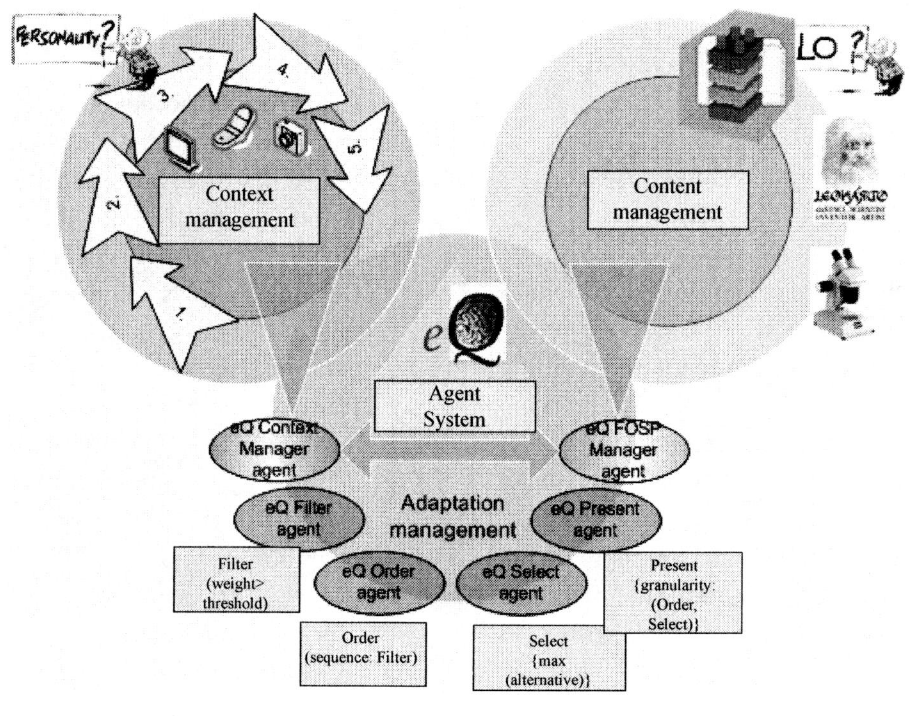

Adaptive Educational Hypermedia Systems

Development of the AH systems can be roughly divided into three generations of research (Brusilovsky, 2004):

- The first generation describes pre-Web hypertext and hypermedia (before 1996).
- The second generation is devoted to the Web-based AH systems (between 1996 and 2002).
- The third generation explores advanced developing technologies for "open corpus AH" and developing a component-based architecture for assembling adaptive Web-based educational systems (since 2002).

Recently, the impacts of many technology trends in further development of the AH systems can be noticed. These impacts can be considered as developing comprehensive frameworks for adaptive Web-based education, developing more intelligent educational material by using learning object metadata (LOM), and exploring the ideas of the Semantic Web for content representation and resource discovery.

The main characteristics of the AH system is their ability of adaptation to the following (Brusilovsky, 2001):

- **User characteristics:** User goals/tasks, knowledge, background, hyperspace experiences, preferences, interests, and individual traits. When we consider learning processes, we should observe some pedagogical attributes of learners, such as: teaching style, interaction style, grade level, and mastery level.
- **User environment:** Encompasses all aspects of the user environment that are not related to the users themselves, such as location, computing platform, bandwidth, and so on. Environment variables specify search paths for files, directories for temporary files, application-specific options, and other similar information.

The user characteristics might be determined by modelling users or by modelling groups of users with similar requirements (stereotypes). So, user models may be individual or stereotypical (Henze & Nejdl, 2003). In this chapter, we explore adaptation to the user's individual traits (personality factors, cognitive factors, learning styles, personality types). As it has been mentioned in Brusilovsky (2001), many researchers agree on the importance of modelling and using individual traits for adaptation, but there is little agreement on which features can and should be used, or how to use them.

One of the most popular kind of AH system is that one dedicated to the learning on the Web, known as the Adaptive Educational Hypermedia (AEH) system. Notable definitions of the AH, as well as AEH systems, could be mentioned:

AH system (Brusilovsky, 1996): *"By adaptive hypermedia systems we mean all hypertext and hypermedia systems which reflect some features of the user in the user model and apply this model to adapt various visible aspects of the system to the user."*

AEH system (Henze & Nejdl, 2003): *"An adaptive education hypermedia system is a quadruple."*

$$(DOCS, UM, OBS, AC) \qquad (1)$$

Each component represented in (1) can be briefly described as follows (Henze & Nejdl, 2003):

- **DOCS** (**DOC**ument **S**pace): A finite set of first-order logic (FOL) sentences with constant symbols for describing documents (and knowledge concepts), and predicates for defining relations between these (and other) constant symbols.

- **UM** (**U**ser **M**odel): A finite set of FOL sentences with constant symbols for describing individual users (user groups), and user characteristics, as well as predicates and formulas for expressing whether a characteristic applies to the user.
- **OBS** (**OBS**ervation): A finite set of FOL sentences with constant symbols for describing observation, and predicates for relating users, documents/concepts, and observations.
- **AC** (**A**daptation **C**omponent): A finite set of FOL sentences with formulas for describing adaptive functionality (rules for adaptive functionality, rules for adaptive treatment)."

Our approach is based on modelling stereotypical models of user's individual traits for adaptation. We have used the *Jung/Briggs-Myers* typology of personality (Berens, 2002) in modelling the following basic personality types (stereotypes) (shown in Figure 6): (1) conventional personality, (2) social personality, (3) investigative personality, (4) artistic personality, (5) realistic personality, and (6) enterprising personality.

Individual traits can be extracted by using specially designed psychological tests. Moreover, several studies that have explored the use

Figure 6. Personality types (stereotypes)

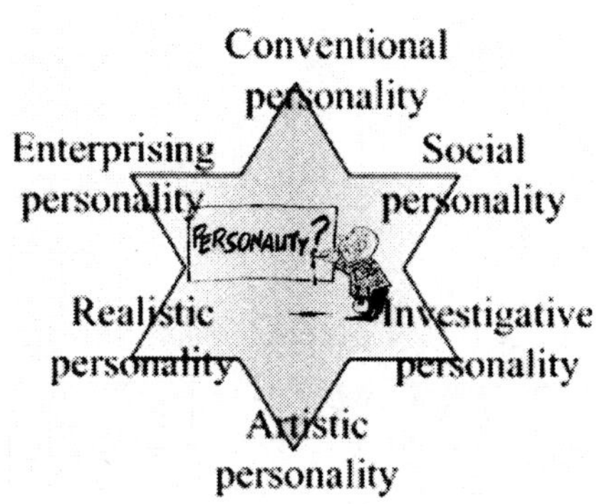

of individual traits in adaptation to the different user profiles (stereotypes) have concluded without finding any significant differences (Brusilovsky, 2001). As a possible solution, there is a need to have a certain relation between user traits on one side, and possible interface settings on the other side. It can be realized through building a repository of different metadata for adaptation that can be used, together with different catalogues of metadata, for education.

Current researches about the use of educational metadata are concentrated on applications of LOM standards (e.g., IEEE LOM). The main purpose of these standards is to improve reusability of LOs. LOM standards are supported by many LOs repositories (e.g., ARIADNE). LOs repositories represent an important research topic, which is connected through peer-to-peer (P2P) networks (e.g., Edutella). ELENA project is a closely related system that tries to employ ontology-based reasoning in adaptive Web-based systems (Dolog, Henze, Nejdl, & Sintek, 2003). This system uses user model ontology, and its purpose is to improve the level of personalization when a user searches for LO in open hypermedia space. However, none of those systems have explored the potentials of emotional intelligence in the Semantic Web environment.

We can start from the above explained definition of AEH system (definition 1). We will consider an artistic personality type with an introverted perception, with the aim to suggest users (learners) in which online experiments they could participate. The adaptive dimension of the eQ agent system will be discussed in the upcoming subsections (Damjanovic, Kravcik, & Gasevic, 2005).

eQ System: Document Space (DOCS)

The document space consists of:

- A set of n atoms (n corresponds to the number of online experiments)

- A set of m atoms (m corresponds to the equipment needed to execute an online experiment)

$$OE_1, OE_2, .., OE_n, EQP_1, EQP_2, .., EQP_m \quad (2)$$

In addition, the document space includes a set of predicates about specific equipment requirements for doing an online experiment:

$$e\_request1(EQPi, EQPj) \text{ for certain } EQPi \neq EQPj \quad (3)$$

Sometimes, the online experiments can be finished in different ways and by using different equipment. This kind of dependence between online experiments and equipment needed can be expressed by the needEquipment predicate:

$$\forall OE\ \exists EQP\ needEquipment(OE, EQP) \quad (4)$$

The above constraint (definition 4) is useful in the Semantic Grid environment for resource sharing among dynamic collections of individuals, institutions, and Web resources.

eQ System: Observation (OBS)

eQ has one atom for the observation of the participation of users in certain online experiments. It is based on using the user psychological facts, called facts. In addition, eQ has a predicate observe:

$$observe(OE, P, facts) \text{ for certain } OE, P \quad (5)$$

P represents user (learner) personality type.

eQ System: User Model (UM)

User model represents an important part of any AEH system. User model models user features and user preferences, which can be described as follows (Henze & Nejdl, 2003):

- User features describe the ability of user to exploit some of the effects. For example, it is a user's knowledge and experience about the effects they consider.
- User preferences describe to what extent the user is eager to make use of some effects. For example, it is a user's subjective mark of the effects they prefer or dislike.

User model characterizes a learner and learner's knowledge/abilities, so the other systems can access and update this information in a standard way. Participation of users (learners) in some online experiment can be convenient to the user when user personality type satisfies a set of psychological requests, such as: introverted, extroverted, and so on. For example, if we have an artistic personality with introverted perception, implying the usage of the keywords inner_world, ideas, images, memories, reflection, depth, then the rule for processing the above observation (definition 5) can be expressed in the following way:

$$\begin{aligned}&\forall OEi\ \forall Pj\\ &observe(OEi, Pj, inner\_world) \vee\\ &observe(OEi, Pj, ideas) \vee\\ &observe(OEi, Pj, images) \vee\\ &observe(OEi, Pj, memories) \vee\\ &observe(OEi, Pj, reflection) \vee\\ &observe(OEi, Pj, depth)\\ &\Rightarrow type(OEi, Pj, artistic\_personality) \quad (6)\end{aligned}$$

eQ System: Adaptation Component (AC)

People with artistic personality and introverted perception are energized when they are involved with the ideas, images, memories, and reactions that are a part of their inner world. Introverts often prefer solitary activities and feel comfortable being alone, or spending time with one or two others with whom they feel an affinity. Based on these facts, the eQ adaptation component uses certain defined symbols to represent a suggestion to the user in order for their participations in certain online experiments. In addition, eQ adaptation component uses some keywords for representing a proposal about instruments needed in doing the experiment.

Now, we can explain the use of the following predicates of the eQ adaptation component: use_instrument and suggest_participant.

∀OEi ∀Pj
∀EQPk (observe(OEi, Pj, ideas)
⇒ type(OEi, Pj, artistic_personality)
⇒ EQPj e_request(EQPi, EQPj))
∧ ¬suggest_participant(Pj, OEi, big_experiment)
⇒ suggest_participant(Pj, OEi, small_experiment)
(7)

According to the fact about resource sharing on the Semantic Grid, we define a predicate called use_instrument:

∀OEi ∃EQPk
∀Pj (observe(OEi, Pj, ideas)
⇒ type(OEi, Pj, artistic_personality)
⇒ EQPj e_request(EQPi, EQPj))
∧ ¬use_ instrument (Pj, OEi, manual)
⇒ use_ instrument (Pj, OEi, digital) (8)

Summary and Implications

One of the key challenges in today's Web environment is the need to deal with data and knowledge resources that are distributed, heterogeneous, and dynamic, based on using effective open, distributed, and knowledge-based solutions. This knowledge-oriented and semantics-based approach to the Web brings new paradigms to exploit techniques and methodologies from intelligent software agents and Web services representing components of the social networking and interacting in a ubiquitous and pervasive manner. These challenges are addressed in the eQ agent system we have proposed for dealing with personalized adaptation in the Semantic Web and Grid learning and training environment, which will be presented in the next section.

THE KEY PARADIGMS OF THE EQ AGENT SYSTEM

E-learning and training should provide advanced knowledge sharing and collaboration between both user profiles and user needs. This means that e-learning courses and trainings can be assembled dynamically from different repositories of LOs and tailored according to the user profiles and their learning needs.

In this chapter, we explore several key paradigms being used in conceptual design of proposed eQ agent system for personalized adaptation.

- First, this approach is based on using a multiagent system with the Belief-Desire-Intention (BDI) agent rational model.
- Second, this system is initially defined by considering the component-based definition of the AEH systems represented in Henze & Nejdl (2003).
- Third, this system uses the FOSP adaptive strategy proposed in Kravcik (2004).
- Finally, because we are dealing with the stereotypes of users, having in mind eQ concepts to help in adaptation to the user's real needs and known preferences, we have named this system eQ.

eQ stands for using eQ concepts on the Web, or using electronic eQ (Damjanovic, Kravcik, & Gasevic, 2005). In that way, we could determine the eQ agent system as a distributed test-sensor system, with the main aim to infer about user stereotypes, to recognize them, and to offer the personalized information and content wherever it happens, in online, offline, or virtual training labs.

eQ System: Multiagent System with the BDI Rational Model

Multiagent systems (MAS) are widely seen as the most promising technology for developing complex distributed software systems in the years to come. The most important reasons for using MAS when designing a system can be described as follows (Stone, 1997):

- Domains with different (possibly conflicting) goals and information, where MAS is needed to handle their interactions
- Having MAS could provide a method for parallel computation by assigning different tasks or abilities to different agents
- Full robustness of system and applications
- An easy way to add new agents (scalability)
- The modularity of MAS and simpler programming
- Exploring intelligence according to the need to deal with social interactions

eQ system represents MAS being developed to support a decentralized approach in both Web-oriented and ubiquitous environments. eQ uses embedded BDI rational model, in which the proposed FOSP adaptive learning strategy can be implemented. The BDI paradigm is based on the early philosophical work of Bratman regarding rational action theory (Bratman, 1987). Their primary contribution is the integration of the various aspects of BDI agent research, such as theoretical foundation from both a quantitative decision-theoretic perspective and a symbolic rational agency perspective, to the system implementation and building applications that are used as a practical BDI architecture.

eQ agents considers information about the user (user group), represented as instances from the ontology for adaptation, and according to the user stereotypes, user types (schoolchildren or experts), personality factors, cognitive factors, and learning styles, they find appropriate educational resources. Using the eQ agent system, personalized adaptation mechanisms pass by two phases: (1) personalized adaptation based on using contextual management, and (2) additional personalized adaptation based on using the proposed FOSP adaptive strategy.

eQ System: System Defined as an AEH System

A decentralized user model (UM) could be formed in continual following of the user's physical movements, as well as the user's history of preferences from the ontology for adaptation. For example, participation of user Pj in certain online training OEi could be done when the user's personality type satisfies a set of psychological requests, such as introverted, extroverted, and so forth An example is described in subsection 2.2.

eQ System: Using the FOSP Adaptive Strategy

Learning strategies represent techniques and methods that include techniques for accelerated learning, using certain environments for learning, graphic tools, emotional intelligence, and the other most widely implemented methods of helping learners to learn more successfully. These strategies are most successful when they are implemented and used in the collaborative learning environments in which each pair of learner/teacher is a part of a well-planned learning system. There must also be efficient methods of feeding that information back into the system so that there will be continued progress in teaching and learning. Nowadays, this process is well known as reusability of teaching resources that can be achieved at various levels. In addition, these strategies are most effective when they are applied in positive, supportive environments where there is recognition of the emotional, social, and physical needs of learners and where individual strengths are recognized, nurtured, and developed. This is one reason we explore use of eQ concepts in this chapter.

A novel method for specification of adaptation strategies in AH systems, which should support efficient collaborative authoring, is known as the FOSP method. The FOSP method is based on using a pattern identified in the adaptation process that consists of four operations (Kravcik, 2004):

1. Filter
2. Order
3. Select
4. Present

The main idea is to separate the partial results produced by different authors in such a way that they can be reused. FOSP method consists of the following three levels shown, in Figure 7:

Level 1: Operations:

- Filter (selects just those components that have their weight greater than threshold)
- Order (sorts the selected components according to the sequence value)
- Select (chooses that one component with the highest alternative value)
- Present (displays the components, taking into account the granularity value)

Level 2: Functions:

- Weight (the relevancy of the pedagogical role for the learning style)
- Sequence (the presentation order of the role for the learning style)
- Alternative (the relevancy of the media type for the learning style)
- Threshold (the threshold for the object display based on the learning style)
- Granularity (the max number of objects presented for the context)

Level 3: Sets:

- role, style, media, and context

This can be explained in the following way (Kravcik, 2004):

When a teacher wants to teach a learner certain new knowledge or skill, he usually first decides what types of learning resources are suitable for the particular user, for example for one learner it can be a definition and an example, for another a demonstration and an exercise. Then he should order the resources, that is decide whether to start with the definition or the example. Each learning resource can have alternative representations, so the teacher has to select the most suitable one—narrative explanation, image, animation, video, and so forth.

But, how to manage teaching resources when the learners have different emotions, perceptions, and reactions? In this chapter, we propose using the eQ agent system with the FOSP adaptation strategy, shown in Figure 7.

The aim of each of the above-mentioned levels in creating a flexible and ontology-powered agent system to support better adaptation and e-learning mechanisms will be discussed in detail. In order to explain the FOSP method, we define new document space that includes the sets of the following atoms (Damjanovic, Kravcik, & Gasevic, 2005):

- A set of r atoms (the pedagogical role of the object [e.g., definition, example, demonstration]),

Figure 7. Introduction of the eQ agent system into the FOSP method

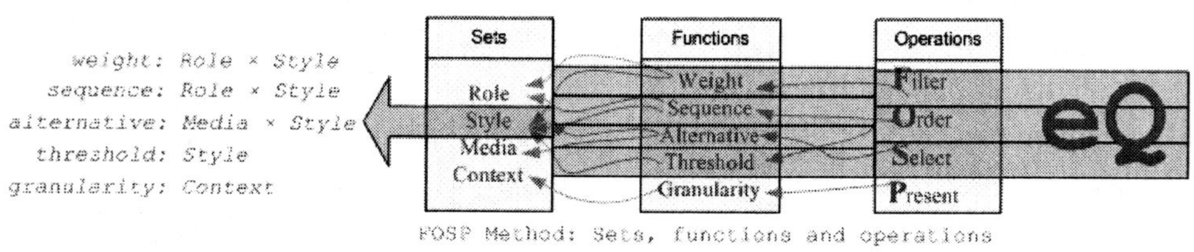

- A set of t atoms (the media type [e.g., text, image, audio, video, animation]),
- A set of c atoms (the usage context [e.g., multimedia desktop, mobile device]):

$R_1, R_2, .., R_r, MT_1, MT_2, .., MT_t, UC_1, UC_2, .., UC_c$ (2')

All of these atoms explained in (2') can be associated with those ones that are explained in (2). Further, the document space includes a set of predicates about media type and usage context need in e-learning (definitions 3' and 3'' can be also associated with predicate e_request1 explained in definition 3):

e_request2(MT_k, MT_l) for certain $MT_k \neq MT_l$ (3')

e_request3(UC_e, UC_f) for certain $UC_e \neq UC_f$ (3'')

Apart from the above explained pedagogical role, media type, and usage context, FOSP method considers one more type—the learner learning style (e.g., intuitive, sensitive, active, reflective). It can be represented as a set of l atoms (l corresponds to the learning style) (shown in 2''):

$L_1, L_2, .., L_l$ (2'')

Learning style can be: (1) haptic (moving, touching, and doing), (2) auditory (sound, music), and (3) visual (learning from pictures). Learning style is a subset of the learner personality type. At the same time, one personality type can use more learning styles. For example, if we have an artistic personality with introverted perception, the main motivation factor of this personality is in relation to her/his creativity. So, an artistic personality can use auditory or visual learning style. Now, the definition 6 can be extended in the following way:

$\forall$Pj $\exists$Ll
observe_deep(observe, Ll, sound) $\vee$
observe_deep(observe, Ll, music)
$\Rightarrow$ person(observe, Li, auditory) (6')

The definition 5 can be expressed in the following way:

observe_deep(OE, P, L, facts_style)
for certain OE, P, L (5')

This definition can be substituted with the following:

observe_deep(observe, L, facts_style)
for certain OE, P, L (5'')

Based on the adaptive strategy proposed in Kravcik (2004) we explain the FOSP functions (Damjanovic, Kravcik, & Gasevic, 2005):

- The weight function—it represents the relevancy of the pedagogical role for the learning style:

weight: Role × Style → Integer (9)

$\forall$R $\forall$L
observe_deep(R, observe, L, facts_style)
$\Rightarrow$ weight(R, L, Relevancy) (10)

- The sequence function—it defines the presentation order of the role for the learning style:

sequence: Role × Style → Integer (11)

$\forall$R $\forall$L
observe_deep(R, observe, L, facts_style)
$\Rightarrow$ sequence(R, L, Order) (12)

- The alternative function—it expresses the relevancy of the media type for the learning style:

alternative: Media × Style → Integer (13)

$\forall$MT $\forall$L
observe_deep(MT, observe, L, facts_style)
$\Rightarrow$ alternative(MT, L, MT_Relevancy) (14)

- The threshold function—it sets the threshold for the object display based on the learning style:

threshold: Style → Integer (15)

∀UC ∀L
observe_deep(UC, observe, L, facts_style)
⇒ threshold(UC, L, threshold_set) (16)

- The granularity function—it specifies the max number of objects presented for the context:

granularity: Context → Integer (17)

∀UC ∀L
observe_deep(UC, observe, L, facts_style)
⇒ granularity(R, L, max_number) (18)

eQ System: New Adaptation Component

Specification of adaptation strategy by using the FOSP method consists of the following operations (Damjanovic, Kravcik, & Gasevic, 2005):

- Filter—for the current object it selects just those components that have their weight greater than threshold:

∀R ∀L observe_deep(R, observe, L, facts_style)
⇒ weight(R, L, Relevancy)
> (∀UC ∀L observe_deep(UC, observe, L, facts_style)
⇒ threshold(UC, L, threshold_set))
⇒Filter(component) (19)

- Order—this sorts the selected components according to the sequence value:

∀R ∀L observe_deep(R, observe, L, facts_style)
⇒ sequence(R, L, Order)
⇒Order(component) (20)

- Select—from the alternative components it chooses the one with the highest alternative value:

∀MT ∀L observe_deep(MT, observe, L, facts_style)
⇒ alternative(MT, L, MT_Relevancy)
∧ max(alternative)
⇒Select(component) (21)

- Present—it displays the components, taking into account the granularity value:

∀UC ∀L
observe_deep(UC, observe, L, facts_style)
⇒ granularity(R, L, max_number)
⇒Present(component) (22)

Summary

In practice, defining a pedagogic strategy for learners with a certain learning style means the instruction designer needs to specify the functional values of weight, sequence, alternative, threshold, and granularity for different types of LOs (i.e., content objects) (Kravcik, 2004). But it is not necessary to define all values. If no value is specified, a default one will be applied: 0 for weight, the minimum value for threshold and the maximum one for granularity. This approach is compliant with the established standards and recommendations, including the adaptive hypermedia application model (AHAM) reference model for adaptive hypermedia. Specification of adaptation strategies separating the content, declarative, and procedural knowledge in adaptive courses is quite natural, and similar approaches have been successfully applied in related areas, for instance in electronic documents generally.

IMPLEMENTATION OF THE EQ AGENT SYSTEM

Nowadays, there are different agent's methodologies and frameworks based on using the BDI rational model, such as JACK, Jason, Nuin, Jam, 3APL, SPARK, Gaia, and Jadex. Each of these methodologies/frameworks considers different types of goals: *query, perform, achieve, maintain, cease, avoid, optimize, test, preserve*. We have chosen to use the Jadex platform, which supports reasoning by exploiting the BDI model, and is realized as an extension to the widely used JADE middleware platform (Braubach, Pokahr, & Lamersdorf, 2004). Jadex supports the development of rational agents on top of the FIPA-compliant JADE platform, and supports *achieve*, *maintain*, *query*, and *perform* goal types (Braubach, Pokahr, Moldt, & Lamersdorf, 2004).

The Jadex BDI model considers three types of attitudes of agent rational behaviours: (1) belief (goals), (2) desire, and (3) intention. Beliefs represent the information about agent's internal, as well as external states, and provide domain-dependent abstraction of entities. The motivational attitudes of agents are captured by goals, which represent a central concept of the Jadex BDI architecture. And, last but not least, plans are the means by which agents achieve their goals.

All triggering events and beliefs must be specified in the agent definition file (ADF), whose role is to let the agents know what kind of event they must handle. Figure 8 shows one part of the eQ agent system's belief base defined in the ADF.

Figure 8. ADF belief-base

```
<beliefs>
<!-- FILTER agent -->
<beliefref name="eQFAgent" class="String"
    exported="true"><abstract/>
</beliefref>    <!-- ... -->  </beliefs>
<goals>
<!-- Perform filter operations -->
<performgoal name="filter_op" exported="true">
<dropcondition>  $beliefbase.mission  </
dropcondition>
</performgoal> <!-- ... -->  </goals>
<plans>
<!-- Filter operation -->
<plan name="weight"> <body>new FilterPlan()</
body>
<trigger> <goal ref="filter_op"/> </trigger>
</plan> <!-- ... -->  </plans>
```

All important agent startup properties, such as an agent name, agent implementation class, packages, and others, are possible to define in the ADF.

FINE ART PROFESSIONAL TRAINING: ACCADEMI@VINCIANA

The main idea presented here is to implement a novel art academy based on using the Semantic Web and Grid possibilities, on one side, and better personalized adaptation methods based on using eQ concepts with the proposed adaptation strategy, on the other side.

Personalized Adaptation in Fine Art Professional Training

When the user starts application for fine art professional training and learning, this application automatically recognizes both user's individual traits and user's devices on which this application is executed (Damjanovic, Kravcik, & Devedzic, 2005). All information about the user's characteristics is contained within the ontology for adaptation (context information), extracted by distributed personality test-sensors. An eQ Context Manager Agent finds all context facts about observed user and sends these results to the eQ FOSP Manager Agent, with the aim to perform personalized adaptation and to present adapted content information to the user. eQ Context Manager Agent has a location awareness module whose role is to support changes in the user's device attribute values. For example, the user starts using training application on the laptop, and then migrates to a PDA. This means that the content information has to be additionally adapted, and the eQ FOSP Manager Agent has to perform some kind of filtering which shrinks the images to a size that fits nicely on the screen of the PDA.

All points of the considered eQ agent system, which uses the FOSP method for personalized

Figure 9. eQ Agent System uses three levels of the FOSP method: Operations, functions, and sets

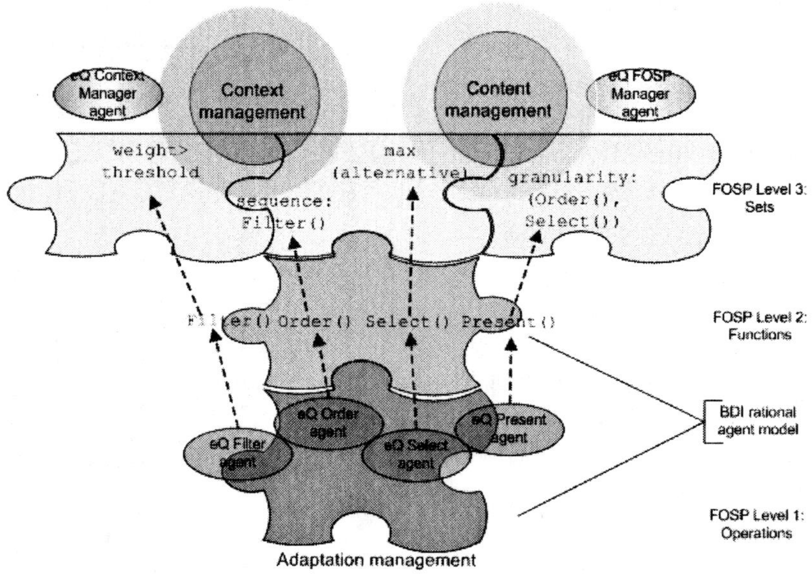

adaptation, are shown in Figure 9. Levels one and two can be directly implemented through the eQ BDI reasoning engine, as shown in Figure 9. This means all triggering events and beliefs must be specified in the Agent Definition File (ADF), whose role is to let the agents know what kinds of events they must handle.

Practical Results

We represent two examples of using the eQ agent system for improving the adaptation processes in the Semantic Web and Grid environment: (1) e-learner is a preschool child, and (2) e-learner is an expert in the domain of painting technologies. The main difference between both of these learner's profiles represents their ability to organize and use knowledge. Experts have a notable level of experience and knowledge, different from beginners (preschool child). Knowledge and experience of experts can be distinguished in the way they have organized knowledge, as well as the way they represent and interpret information about their environment. According to the way in which the knowledge is organized, experts remember information, infer about certain facts and categories from the organized knowledge, and solve different problems by using existing knowledge.

User identification means considering a huge number of criteria and characteristics from the ontology for personalized adaptation. In order to explain as simply as possible the role of the eQ agent system in achieving better personalized adaptation, we consider minimum criteria required from the FOSP adaptation method. That means joining both the ontology for personalized adaptation and the domain ontology - ACCADEMI@VINCIANA, based on finding the pair of values, such as: (1) learning style – style, (2) learner type – role, (3) media type – media, (4) presentation form – form. The eQ BDI agent rational mechanism executes the FOSP adaptation method based on using all of these pairs of values from ontologies. As a result, different e-learners get adapted and personalized educational contents.

Firstly, we can define the FOSP Level 3 (Sets) for both examples (shown in Table 1).

The FOSP adaptive strategy is executed based on using the definitions (9-22). If we suppose that there are the following educational resources from the domain ontology ACCADEMI@VIN-

Table 1. Learner's characteristics at the FOSP Level 3 – Sets

	A) e-learner is a preschool child		B) e-learner is an expert	
Attribute name	**Instance value - Ontology for adaptation**	**Instance value - Domain ontology**	**Instance value - Ontology for adaptation**	**Instance value - Domain ontology**
Learner type (LT)	Beginner	Preschool child	Expert	Expert
Learning style (LS)	Visual	Visual	Visual	Video; Audio; Speech; Text
Media type (MT)	Computer	Computer	Computer; PDA; online experiments	Computer; PDA; online experiments
Presentation form (PF)	Video	Video	Video	Video; online experiments; docs + pictures

Table 2. Characteristics of the educational resources

	A) e-Learner is a preschool child			B) e-Learner is an expert		
Instance name	**Learner type (Role)**	**Learning style**	**Media type**	**Learner type (Role)**	**Learning style**	**Media type**
Techniques	Beginner (5); Expert (5)	Video (5); Audio (5); Text (1)	Computer (5); Mobile (2)	Beginner (5); Expert (5)	Video (4); Audio (5); Text (5)	Computer (5); Mobile (2)
Materials	Beginner (3); Expert (5)	Video (3); Audio (2); Speech (1); Text (1)	Computer (5); Mobile (2)	Beginner (3); Expert (5)	Video (4); Audio (5); Speech (3); Text (5)	Computer (5); Mobile (3)
Fundamentals	Beginner (2); Expert (5)	Video (3); Audio (2); Speech (1); Text (1)	Computer (5)	Beginner (2); Expert (5)	Video (4); Audio (5); Speech (3); Text (5)	Computer (5)
Experiments	Beginner (1); Expert (5)	Video (3); Audio (2); Speech (1); Text (1)	Computer (5); PDA (3); Mobile (1)	Beginner (1); Expert (5)	Video (5); Audio (5); Speech (4); Text (4)	Computer (5); PDA (3); Mobile (2)

CIANA, such as (1) *techniques*, (2) *materials*, (3) *fundamentals*, and (4) *experiments*, then the characteristics of the ontology resources could be represented. Therefore, we define the importance indexes of educative resources for both examples of e-learners (shown in Table 2).

Now, we execute the FOSP functions: weight, sequence, alternative, threshold, and granularity. This execution is based on using the component-based definition of the AEH system by using the values that came from both Table 1 and Table 2.

- **The FOSP weight function:** We can suppose that the user is a **beginner** with the **visual learning style**, which uses a **computer** to access the educational resources. The FOSP adaptive strategy executes weight function for different values of resources. For example, in the case that the educational resource is *techniques*, the value of weight function is:

weight: Role × Style → Integer, or

weight: (5 × 5 → 25)

In the case that the educational resource is *experiments*, the value of weight function is:

weight: (1 × 3 → 3)

If the educational resource is *materials*, the value of weight function is:

weight: (3 × 3 → 9)

And, if the educational resource is *fundamentals*, the value of weight function is:

weight: (2 × 3 → 6)

Based on these results, we conclude that the course about painting techniques that represent the best educational material fits in with the learner who is a beginner who uses a visual learning style and the computer as a device to access the educational materials. The next courses could be the following: the course about painting materials,or the course about fundamental elements of painting technology, while the course about painting experiments would not fit in with the beginner's profile.

- **The FOSP sequence function:** Using the definition (11) with the different values of the educational resources, the FOSP sequence function calculates the next order of these resources: (1) *techniques*, (2) *materials*. Now, the FOSP alternative function is executed.
- **The FOSP alternative function:** For example, in the case that the educational resource is *techniques*, the value of alternative function is:

alternative: Media × Style → Integer, or
alternative: (5 × 5 → 25)

In the case that the educational resource is *materials*, the value of alternative function is:

alternative: (5 × 3 → 15)

We conclude that the course about painting techniques represents the better solution for the beginning learner. At the same time, the course about painting materials represents an alternative solution for the beginner.

- **The FOSP threshold function:** Using the definition (15) with the different values of the educational resources, the FOSP threshold function calculates the next order of these resources: (1) *techniques*, (2) *materials*.
- **The FOSP granularity function:** The FOSP granularity function specifies the max number of objects presented for the context. For example, the course about painting

Table 3. The results of the FOSP functions

	A) e-learner is a preschool child					B) e-learner is an expert				
Instance name	weight	sequence	alternative	threshold	granularity	weight	sequence	alternative	threshold	granularity
Techniques	25	1	25	5	8	20 / 25	2	20 / 25	4 / 5	8
Materials	9	2	15	3	2	20 / 25	3	20 / 25	4 / 5	2
Fundamentals	6	-	-	-	4	20 / 25	4	20 / 25	4 / 5	4
Experiments	3	-		-	2	25 / 25	1	25 / 25	5 / 5	2

techniques includes 8 sub courses, while the course about painting materials includes just 2 smaller sub courses.

All results of the FOSP functions are shown in Table 3.

Now, we execute the FOSP operations: Filter, Order, Select, and Present, based on the results of the FOSP functions shown in Table 3. The results of the FOSP operations are adapted to the specific user's profiles.

In a case when the e-learner is a preschool child, result of Present operation includes components of the educative resource – *techniques*: (1) Tempera, (2) Wash Painting, (3) Aquarelle, (4) Oil Painting, (5) Varnish Painting, (6) Encaustic, (7) Gilding, and (8) Drawing.

When the e-learner is an expert in the domain of painting technologies, the eQ agent system offers components of the educative resource—*experiments* that include the following components: (1) physical methods and (2) chemical methods.

Summary

The important characteristics for considering user stereotypes could be extended with the aim to give more precise and adapted results of the educational processes. It means that new instances from the ontology for personalized adaptation should be considered, including those instances made as a result of the IEEE PAPI Standard extension. Moreover, we could achieve usage of the eQ agent system in the Semantic Grid environment by introducing instances that represent instruments needed for doing online experiments. This kind of environment could be used to execute specialized experiments about painting technologies and materials. Then, the experts can use expensive, but distributed scientific devices, in an ubiquitous and pervasive manner. They can share the results with other practical scientists, remote colleagues, and students, as well as members of various online societies (physics, chemistry, government, police…).

CONCLUSION

The process of training and learning in Web-based and ubiquitous environments brings a new sense of adaptation. E-learning needs to use new technologies in order to provide advanced knowledge sharing and collaboration between different user's profiles and different user's needs. Thus, the Semantic Grid can be used for the creation of new scientific results, new business, and even new research disciplines.

With the development of more sophisticated environments, the need for them to take into account the user's traits and user's devices on which the training is executed, and to place them within the context of the training activities, has become an important issue in the domain of building novel training and learning environments. Hence, our approach for achieving adaptivity is based on using the eQ concepts, MAS, AEH systems, and the BDI rational agent's paradigm in the Semantic Web and Grid environment. The benefits of taking the proposed approach are numerous, and can be characterized as follows:

- **Collaboration** with other students, teachers, tutors, experts
- **Knowledge-based:** It includes domain knowledge representation in the form of ontologies, as well as knowledge about the learner and his/her social and emotional context.
- **Ubiquitous:** The capability to support multiple pedagogical models and to automatically adopt them.

In this chapter, an example of fine art professional training illustrates the potential benefits of using personalized adaptation in professional training environments. As the potential benefits, we can mention the following:

- Adaptation by focusing on the main subjects from the domain of artistic training (paint-

ers, conservators, restorers, technologists, fraud investigators)
- Using all available resources (learning materials, training devices) wherever the user is physically located
- Exploring ancient and current technologies with the aim of finding better solutions
- Analyzing generated results and deciding about using preventive painting strategies
- Collaboration with the aim of achieving the original expertise and art fraud investigation

In addition, we can stress the possibility to envisage Semantic Grid, which behaves like a constantly evolving organism, with ongoing, autonomous processing rather than on-demand processing (De Roure, Jennings, & Shadbolt, 2005). Thus, the Semantic Grid becomes an *organic Grid* which itself can generate new processes and new knowledge, manifest in the physical world through ambient intelligence vision.

ACKNOWLEDGMENT

This research is linked to the Network of Excellence (NoE) in Professional Learning – ProLearn, Work package WP1: Adaptive Personalized Learning.

REFERENCES

Berens, L.V. (2002). Multiple models of personality types. *Australian Psychological Type Review, 4*(1-2), 9-14.

Bork, A. (2001). Tutorial learning for the new century. *Journal of Science Education and Technology, 10*(1), 57-71.

Bradberry, T., & Greaves, J. (2003). *Can you develop emotional intelligence online?* TalentSmart Inc. Retrieved October 15, 2006, from http://www.talentsmart.com/media/uploads/pdfs/Can%20You%20Develop%20Emotional%20Intelligence%20Online.pdf

Bratman, M.E. (1987). *Intentions, plans, and practical reason.* Cambridge, MA: Harvard University Press.

Braubach, L., Pokahr, A., & Lamersdorf, W. (2004). Jadex: A short overview. In *Proceedings of the Net.ObjectDays 2004 Conference, Agent-Expo* (pp. 195-207).

Braubach, L., Pokahr, A., Moldt, D., & Lamersdorf, W. (2004). Goal representation for BDI agent systems. In *Proceeding of the Second International Workshop on Programming Multiagent Systems (PROMAS-2004)* (pp. 9-20).

Brusilovsky, P. (1996). Methods and techniques of adaptive hypermedia. *User Modelling and User-Adapted Interaction, 6*(2-3), 87-129.

Brusilovsky, P. (2001). Adaptive hypermedia. *User Modelling and User-Adapted Interaction, 11*(1-2), 87-110.

Brusilovsky, P. (2003). From adaptive hypermedia to the adaptive Web. In J. Ziegler & G. Szwillus (Eds.), *Proceedings of Mensch & Computer 2003: Interaktion in Bewegung* (pp. 30-33). Stuttgart, Germany.

Brusilovsky, P. (2004). Adaptive educational hypermedia: From generation to generation. In M. Grigoriadou et al. (Eds.), *Proceedings of the 4th Hellenic Conference with International Participation in Information and Communication Technologies in Education* (pp. 19-33). New Technologies Publications.

Damjanovic, V., Kravcik, M., & Devedzic, V. (2005). An approach to the realization of personalized adaptation by using eQ agent system. In *Proceedings of UM'2005 Workshop on Personalized Adaptation on the Semantic Web (PerSWeb'05)* (pp. 116-125).

Damjanovic, V., Kravcik, M., & Gasevic, D. (2005). eQ through the FOSP method. In *Proceedings of the ED-MEDIA 2005 World Conference on Educational Multimedia, Hypermedia and Telecommunications* (pp. 3080-3088). Montreal, Canada.

De Roure, D., & Hendler, J.A. (2004). E-science: The grid and the Semantic Web. *IEEE Intelligent Systems, 19*(1), 65-71.

De Roure, D., Jennings, N.R., & Shadbolt, N.R. (2005). The semantic grid: Past, present and future. *Proceedings of the IEEE, 93*(3), 669-681.

Dolog, P., Henze, N., Nejdl, W., & Sintek, M. (2003). Towards the adaptive semantic Web. In *Proceedings of Principles and Practice of Semantic Web Reasoning, International Workshop, PPSWR 2003,* Mumbai, India.

Drucker, P. (1989). *New realities.* New York: Harper & Row.

Henze, N., & Nejdl, W. (2003). *Logically characterizing adaptive educational hypermedia systems.* In *Proceeding of the International Workshop of Adaptive Hypermedia and Adaptive Web-based Systems (AH 2003),* Budapest, Hungary.

Hodgins, W. (2005). *Grand challenges for learning objects.* Presentation at Learntec, Karlsruhe, Germany.

IEEE PAPI. (2001). IEEE 1484.2.1, Standard for Learning Technology - Public and Private Information (PAPI) for Learners (PAPI Learner) - Core Features.

Kraigher-Hozo, M. (1991). *Painting / Painting methods / Materials.* Sarajevo: Svjetlost Publications.

Kravcik, M. (2004). The specification of adaptation strategy by FOSP method. In *Proceedings of AH2004 Conference,* Eidhoven, The Netherlands.

Kravcik, M., Specht, M., & Oppermann, R. (2004). Evaluation of WINDS authoring environment. In *Proceedings of the Adaptive Hypermedia 2004 Conference* (pp. 166-175). Eidhoven, The Netherlands.

Moe, M., & Blodgett, H. (2000). *The knowledge Web.* Merrill Lynch.

Robinson, R. (2000). *Context management in mobile environments.* PhD thesis, University of Queensland, Australia.

Salovey, P., & Mayer, J.D. (2000). Emotional intelligence. *Imagination, Cognition and Personality, 9*(3), 185-911.

Schank, R.C. (2002). Are we going to get smarter? In J. Brockman (Ed.), *The next fifty years: Science in the first half of the twenty-first century* (pp. 206-215). New York: Vintage.

Stone, P. (1997). *Multiagent systems.* Retrieved October 15, 2006, from http://www-2.cs.cmu.edu/afs/cs/usr/pstone/public/papers/97MAS-survey/node2.html

W3C. (2001). *Semantic Web.* Retrieved October 15, 2006, from http://www.w3.org/2001/sw/

APPENDIX I: CASE STUDY

Fine Art Professional Training

The application for fine art professional training recognizes the user with the "artistic personality" (personality type), "introverted perception" (personality factor), "visual" learning style, in which the user type is an "expert" that explores "art fraud" and uses a "PDA" (user device). Thus, the first level of *contextual* personalized adaptation is finished. Now, the content is adapted for that user, which is the task of the eQ FOSP Manager Agent. This agent supervises four other eQ agents, who, one after the other, performs the main operations of the FOSP adaptive strategy (Filter, Order, Select, and Present). The eQ Filter Agent starts to perform Filter operation by selecting just those components that have their weight function greater than threshold function. Both of these functions are related to the semantically annotated FOSP sets that represent content from both the ontology for personalized adaptation and the domain ontology. The eQ Filter Agent sends the filtered components as results to the next agent—eQ Order Agent, which performs Order operation by sorting the selected (filtered) components according to the sequence value. It sends a sequence of the selected components to both the eQ Select Agent and the eQ FOSP Manager Agent. The eQ Select Agent performs Select operation by selecting the component with the highest alternative value, and finally, the eQ Present Agent performs Present operation according to having the granularity value from the sets of the selected or the alternative components. All values of considered FOSP functions, such as threshold, weight, alternative, sequence, and granularity, are related to the ontology concepts, such as Role, Style, Media, and Context (FOSP sets).

Fine art professional trainings based on the use of physical methods could be realized with different optical tools (microscopes, dermatoscopes, micro-abrasion equipment, equipment for UV and F exploring, cameras). In the case of the above explained user, the eQ Present Agent brings some physical methods as a result. Actually, it means that the eQ Present Agent offers trainings by using X-ray, UV exploring, and F-exploring as training methods that could be used to achieve art fraud investigation.

Questions

1. How can the results of the eQ agent system be executed in the case of using different typology of personality in modelling user stereotypes than *Jung/Briggs-Myers* typology?
2. What kind of typology of personality would you use in modelling user stereotypes?

APPENDIX II: USEFUL URLS

Pervasive Computing Reading Group – Papers, Related Conferences, & Journals
http://www.cs.utah.edu/~sgoyal/pervasive/

IEEE Pervasive Computing - A catalyst for advancing research and practice in ubiquitous computing
http://www.computer.org/portal/site/pervasive//

Emotional Intelligence – White Papers, Case Studies
http://jobfunctions.bnet.com/search.aspx?scname=Emotional+Intelligence&dtid=1

Web site on Emotions, Emotional Intelligence, Learning & more
http://eqi.org/toc2.htm

IEEE PAPI Standards – PAPI Learner, Drafts, and Specifications
http://edutool.com/papi/

Jadex – BDI Agent System
http://vsis-www.informatik.uni-hamburg.de/projects/jadex/

W3C Workshop on Metadata for Content Adaptation
http://www.w3.org/2004/06/DI-MCA-WS/

ProLearn Project (Professional Learning) Research Activities
http://www.prolearn-project.org/index.html

APPENDIX III: FURTHER READING

De Roure, D., & Hendler, J.A. (2004). E-science: The grid and the Semantic Web. *IEEE Intelligent Systems, 19*(1), 65-71.

De Roure, D., Jennings, N.R., & Shadbolt, N.R. (2005). The semantic Grid: Past, present and future. *Proceedings of the IEEE, 93*(3), 669-681.

Dolog, P., Henze, N., Nejdl, W., & Sintek, M. (2003). *Towards the adaptive semantic Web.* Proceedings of the PPSWR 2003 Workshop, Mumbai, India.

Henze, N., & Nejdl, W. (2003). Logically characterizing adaptive educational hypermedia systems. In *Proceedings of the International AH 2003Workshop,* (pp. 15-28). Budapest, Hungary.

Salovey, P., & Mayer, J.D. (2000). Emotional intelligence. *Imagination, Cognition and Personality, 9*(3), 185-911.

This work was previously published in Ubiquitous and Pervasive Knowledge and Learning Management: Semantics, Social Networking and New Media to Their Full Potential, edited by M. Lytras & A. Naeve, pp. 158-198, copyright 2007 by IGI Publishing, formerly known as Idea Group Publishing (an imprint of IGI Global).

Section V
Security, Privacy, and Personalization

Chapter XVII
Technical Solutions for Privacy-Enhanced Personalization

Yang Wang
University of California, Irvine, USA

Alfred Kobsa
University of California, Irvine, USA

ABSTRACT

This chapter presents a first-of-its-kind survey that systematically analyzes existing privacy-enhanced personalization (PEP) solutions and their underlying privacy protection techniques. The evaluation is based on an analytical framework of privacy-enhancing technologies, an earlier work of the authors. More specifically, we critically examine whether each PEP solution satisfies the privacy principles and addresses the privacy concerns that have been uncovered in the context of personalization. The chapter aims at helping researchers better understand the technical underpinnings, practical efficacies and limitations of existing PEP solutions, and at inspiring and developing future PEP solutions by outlining several promising research directions based on our findings.

INTRODUCTION

Privacy and personalization are currently at odds (Kobsa, 2002, 2007a, 2007b; Teltzrow & Kobsa, 2004; Wang & Kobsa, 2006). For instance, online shoppers who value that an online bookstore can give them personalized recommendations based on what books they bought in the past may wonder whether their purchase records will be kept truly confidential in all future. Online searchers who are pleased that a search engine disambiguates their queries and delivers search results geared towards their genuine interests may feel uneasy that this entails recording all their past search terms. Students who appreciate that a personalized tutoring system can provide individualized instruction based on a detailed model of each student's understanding of the different learning concepts may wonder whether anyone else besides the system will have access to these models of what they know and don't know.

Various technical solutions have been proposed to safeguard users' privacy while still providing satisfactory personalization, e.g., on web retail or product recommendation sites. Technical solutions for privacy protection represent a special kind of so-called Privacy-Enhancing Technologies (PETs). In (Wang & Kobsa, forthcoming), we propose an evaluation framework for PETs that considers the following dimensions:

1. **What high-level principles the solution follows:** We identify a set of fundamental privacy principles that underlie various privacy laws and regulations and treat them as high-level guidelines for enhancing privacy.
2. **What privacy concerns the solution addresses:** We analyze privacy solutions along major privacy concerns that were identified in the literature.
3. **What basic privacy-enhancing techniques the solution employs:** We look at the technical characteristics of privacy solutions, to critically analyze their effectiveness in safeguarding privacy and supporting personalization.

The rest of this chapter is organized as follows. Firstly, we describe and categorize major privacy principles from privacy laws as well as other desirable principles in the context of privacy protection (we thereby largely follow (Wang & Kobsa, forthcoming)). Secondly, we discuss privacy concerns and how different privacy principles address them. Thirdly, as the central contribution of this chapter, we describe the techniques that have been used in the main types of privacy-enhanced personalization solutions, and how they relate to the major privacy concerns and privacy principles. Fourthly, we discuss findings from this analysis. Finally, we conclude with future research directions.

PRIVACY PRINCIPLES

Privacy legislation and regulation is usually based on more fundamental privacy principles. In our framework, we select a comprehensive set of major principles from our survey of over 40 international privacy laws and regulations (Kobsa, 2007b; Wang, Zhaoqi, & Kobsa, 2006). Any principle manifested in these privacy laws and regulations was included in our framework if it has impacts on how web-based personalized systems operate. Besides, we also define or identify other principles/properties that are desirable for privacy enhancement and personalization. Additional principles may possibly need to be added in the future, as new personalization technologies with new privacy threats emerge or the concept of privacy evolves. Below we list our principles, grouped by their provenance.

Privacy Principles from Privacy Laws, Regulations and Recommendations

1. **Notice/Awareness:**
    - **Clarity:** *Make these privacy policy statements clear, concise, and conspicuous to those responsible for deciding whether and how to provide the data* (Kobsa, 2007b; USACM, 2006);
    - **Notice upon collection:** *Whenever any personal information is collected, explicitly state:*
        - *the precise purpose of the collection,*
        - *all the ways in which the information might be used,*
        - *all the potential recipients of the personal data,*
        - *how long the data will be stored and used;* (USACM, 2006)
2. **Minimization:** *Before deployment of new activities and technologies that might impact personal privacy, carefully evaluate them for their necessity, effectiveness, and*

proportionality: the least privacy-invasive alternatives should always be sought (USACM, 2006).

3. **Purpose specification:** *The purposes for which personal data are collected should be specified not later than at the time of data collection and the subsequent use limited to the fulfillment of those purposes or such others as are not incompatible with those purposes and as are specified on each occasion of change of purpose* (OECD, 1980).
4. **Collection limitation:** *There should be limits to the collection of personal data and any such data should be obtained by lawful and fair means [...]* (OECD, 1980).
5. **Use limitation:** *Personal data should not be disclosed, made available or otherwise used for purposes other than those specified* (OECD, 1980).
6. **Onward transfer:** Personal data should not be transferred to a third country/party if it does not ensure an adequate level of protection (EU, 1995; FTC, 2000c)
7. **Choice/Consent:** *Where appropriate, individuals should be provided with clear, prominent, easily understandable, accessible and affordable mechanisms to exercise choice in relation to the collection, use and disclosure of their personal information* (APEC-FIP, 2004). The two widely adopted mechanisms are:
    - **Opt-in:** *requires affirmative steps by the consumer to allow the collection and/or use of information* (FTC, 2000a);
    - **Opt-out:** *requires affirmative steps to prevent the collection and/or use of such information* (FTC, 2000a).
8. **Access/Participation:** An individual should have right to:
    - *know whether a data controller has data relating to her* (OECD, 1980),
    - *inspect and make corrections to her stored data* (USACM, 2006)
9. **Integrity/accuracy:** *A data controller should ensure the collected personal data is sufficiently accurate and up-to-date for the intended purposes and all corrections are propagated in a timely manner to all parties that have received or supplied the inaccurate data* (USACM, 2006).
10. **Security:** *Personal data should be protected by reasonable security safeguards against such risks as loss or unauthorized access, destruction, use, modification or disclosure of data* (OECD, 1980).
11. **Enforcement/Redress:** Effective privacy protection must include mechanisms for enforcing the core privacy principles. At a minimum, the mechanisms must include (FTC, 2000b):
    - **Recourse mechanisms for customers:** *readily available and affordable independent recourse mechanisms by which an individual's complaints and disputes can be investigated and resolved and damages awarded where the applicable law or private sector initiatives so provide;*
    - **Verification mechanisms for data controllers:** follow-up procedures for verifying that the attestations and assertions businesses make about their privacy practices are true and that privacy practices have been implemented as presented;
    - **Remedy mechanisms:** obligations arising out of failure to comply with these principles by organizations announcing their adherence to them, and consequences for such organizations.

Anonymity-Related Principles from the Security Literature

12. **Anonymity:** Anonymity means that users cannot be identified nor be tracked online.
13. **Pseudonymity:** Pseudonymous users also

cannot be identified, but can be tracked by their unique "aliases" or "personae".

14. **Unobservability:** A data controller cannot recognize that a system/website is being used/visited by a given user.
15. **Unlinkability:** A data controller cannot link two interaction steps of the same user.
16. **Deniability:** Deniability means that users are able to deny some of their characteristics or actions (e.g., a visit to a particular website), and others cannot validate the veracity of this denial.

Other Desirable Principles for Privacy Enhancement, Mostly from Human-Computer Interaction Research

17. **User preference:** Different users can have different privacy preferences. A data controller should tailor its privacy practices to each individual user's preferences.
18. **Negotiation:** This principle calls for the support of negotiation between users and websites so that they can agree on the privacy practices that the website can follow.
19. **Non-intrusiveness:** Non-intrusiveness means that users have control over incoming information. Popup ads and junk e-mails are typical example for intrusiveness.
20. **Ease of adoption:** This principle considers how easy it is for organizations to implement a given privacy protection solution, for instance, whether the solution relies on special or unusual protocols or proprietary technologies, or on technologies that are not readily available.
21. **Ease of compliance:** An increasing number of legal privacy duties have been imposed on data controllers, such as to monitor and provide audit trails of their factual privacy practices. This principle is concerned with the ease of meeting such legal requirements by adopting a specific privacy protection solution.
22. **Usability:** A privacy protection solution should be easy on users, e.g., user involvement should be reasonable.
23. **Responsiveness:** The privacy protection solution should respond promptly to changes of a user's privacy decisions.

Desirable Principle for Personalization

24. **Personalization quality:** This principle is concerned with maximizing the personalization quality and associated benefits.

PRIVACY CONCERNS

There exist various approaches to categorize privacy (Camp & Osorio, 2003; Solove, 2006; Wang, Lee, & Wang, 1998), and they seem to have three main themes in common: the protection of people's identities, people's right to seclusion, and their right to control their data (such as to decide what data can be collected or disclosed for what purpose, how their data will be used, with whom the data may be shared, etc.). In Table 1, we categorize the 24 identified principles by the type of privacy protection that they afford. Notice that the general category contains principles that afford all three types of privacy protection.

A web personalization process is typically comprised of three tasks (Kobsa, Koenemann and Pohl, 2001):

1. **Acquisition:** This task involves: (1) gathering information about users' characteristics, computer usage behavior and the usage environment, and (2) building a user model, a usage model and an environment model.
2. **Representation and secondary inference:** This task consists in expressing the content of the user model and usage model in a formal system, allowing further access and processing.

Table 1. Categorization of principles based on the type of privacy protection

Principle \ Privacy	General	Protection of Identity	Seclusion	Control over data
Notice/Awareness	X			
Minimization				X
Purpose specification				X
Collection limitation				X
Use limitation				X
Onward transfer				X
Choice/Consent	X			
Access/Participation				X
Integrity/accuracy				X
Security				X
Anonymity		X		
Pseudonymity		X		
Unobservability		X		
Unlinkability		X		
Deniability		X		
Enforcement/Redress	X			
User preference	X			
Negotiation	X			
Seclusion			X	
Ease of adoption	X			
Ease of compliance	X			
Usability	X			
Responsiveness	X			
Personalization quality	X			

3 **Production:** This task is concerned with the adaptation of content, presentation, modality and structure of information conveyed to the user, based on the user, usage and environment models.

Another way of understanding web personalization is to dissect it in terms of higher-level system activities that it may entail, such as tracking user interactions with websites, creating user profiles based on the interaction logs, generating personalized recommendations to users based on their logs and profiles, and contacting users with personalized recommendations for potential purchases. These activities may cause different privacy concerns at varying degrees of likelihood. For instance, sharing users' personal data with third parties will be *very likely* to cause concerns over improper transfer of personal data, while it will be *likely* to engender concerns over unwanted solicitation (e.g., that third parties use the shared personal information to advertise their products to them).

Wang et al. (H. Wang, Lee, & Wang, 1998) present a taxonomy of privacy concerns in Internet marketing including improper access, improper collection, improper monitoring, improper analysis, improper transfer, unwanted solicitation and improper storage. These concerns as well as improper merge (of data) also seem to apply to web personalization. Table 2 that is based on (Teltzrow & Kobsa, 2004; Wang, Lee, & Wang, 1998) shows what privacy concerns (columns) are *very likely* or *likely* to arise from web personalization activities (rows). Table 3 depicts what privacy concerns (columns) might be involved in the tasks of a web personalization process (rows).

TECHNICAL SOLUTIONS FOR PRIVACY-ENHANCED PERSONALIZATION

Our framework for evaluating the effectiveness of technical solutions for safeguarding privacy whilst supporting meaningful personalization assesses privacy solutions along three different dimensions: (1) what high-level privacy principles the solution follows, (2) what privacy concerns it addresses, and (3) what basic privacy-enhancing

Table 2. Potential privacy concerns in potential web personalization activities

	Control over data							Seclusion	Protection of identity
	Improper acquisition			Improper use			Improper storage	Unwanted solicitation	Identity fraud/theft
	Improper access	Improper collection	Improper monitoring	Improper analysis	Improper merge	Improper transfer			
Tracking		XX	XX						
Profiling		X	X	X	X	X			X
Cross-website recommendation		X	X	X	XX	XX	X	X	
Single-website recommendation		X	X	X	X	X	X	X	
Third-party data sharing				XX	X	XX	X	X	X
Direct mailing				X				XX	

XX: *Very likely* X: *Likely*

Table 3. Potential privacy concerns in web personalization proces

	Control over data							Seclusion	Protection of identity
	Improper acquisition			Improper use			Improper storage	Unwanted solicitation	Identity fraud/theft
	Improper access	Improper collection	Improper monitoring	Improper analysis	Improper merge	Improper transfer			
Acquisition	X	X	X			X	X		X
Representation & secondary inference				X	X		X		X
Production				X	X	X		X	

techniques it employs. In the preceding sections, we identified 24 major principles and 3 major privacy concerns and presented their relationship to each other. In this section we discuss the major privacy-enhancing personalization solutions that have been proposed today, what basic privacy-enhancing techniques they employ, and how these solutions relate to the described principles and privacy concerns.

Pseudonymous Personalization

Pseudonymous personalization allows users to remain anonymous with regard to the personalized system and the whole network infrastructure, whilst enabling the system to still recognize the same user in different sessions so that it can cater to her individually. Most of these techniques allow a user to have more than one pseudonym/account/role/persona, so that the user can keep apart different aspects of their online activities (e.g., work versus entertainment).

The Janus Personalized Web Anonymizer (Gabber, Gibbons, Matias, & Mayer, 1997) serves as a proxy between a user and a web site. For each distinct user-website pair, it utilizes a cryptographic function to automatically generate a different alias (typically a user name, a password and an e-mail address) for establishing an anonymous account at the website. Janus also supports anonymous e-mail exchanges from a website to a user, and filters the potentially identifying information of the HTTP protocol to preserve user privacy.

Arlein et al. (Arlein, Jai, Jakobsson, Monrose, & Reiter, 2000) suggest an infrastructure that enables global user profiles to be maintained and accessed by different merchants. Users can control their data disclosure by grouping their information into profiles pertaining to different personae and can selectively authorize merchants to access these profiles. The infrastructure includes a persona server to assist users manage their personae. The persona server is separate from the profile database, so as to prevent linking different profiles of the same user. Besides, the infrastructure also has a tainting-based access control mechanism that allows merchants to designate which data about user interaction at their sites can be accessed by other merchants.

Ishitani et al. (Ishitani, Almeida, & Wagner, 2003) implemented a system called Masks (Managing Anonymity while Sharing Knowledge to Servers). The system consists of both server-side and client-side components, namely the Masks server and the privacy and security agents (PSAs). The Masks server, acting as a proxy between users and websites, manages masks (temporary group identifications that are associated with specific topics of interest) and assigns them to users. This enables user information to be collected under those masks and enables the users to receive group-based personalization. The PSAs runs with users' web browsers and allows users to configure the masks as well as other functionalities such as blocking and filtering cookies and web bugs.

Kobsa and Schreck (Kobsa & Schreck, 2003) propose a reference architecture for pseudonymous yet fully personalized interaction. The architecture includes a MIX network between applications and user modeling servers, supports standard anonymization techniques between clients and applications, offers a choice of encryption at the application and the transport layers, and a hierarchical role-based access control model. One privacy enhancement of this architecture over other anonymization or pseudonymization techniques is that it hides both the identities of the users and the location of the user modeling servers in the network.

Hitchens et al. (Hitchens, Kay, Kummerfeld, & Brar, 2005) present an architecture that allows users to easily create their personas (a subset of a user model), and to selectively share these authenticated pseudonymous personas with certain service providers (via user defined preferences). Service providers can use the information contained in the personas to tailor their services to users.

Table 4. Pseudonymous personalization systems and their characteristics

System / Characteristics	*Janus*	*Global user profile infrastructure*[1]	*Masks*	*Pseudonymous personalization reference architecture*[2]	*Personas architecture*[3]
GENERAL					
Alias-to-website cardinality	1:1	m:n	m:n	m:n	m:n
User control		+	+	+	+
Personalization	*Single site single user*	*From single site single user to cross-site single user*	*Group based*	*Cross-site single user*	*From single site single user to cross-site single user*
PROCEDURAL ANONYMITY					
Sender/user anonymity	+	+	+	+	+
Receiver/website anonymity		+			
UMS anonymity				+	
CONTENT-BASED ANONYMITY					
Content-based anonymity				+	
LINKABILITY					
Linkability for a single pseudonym	+	+	+	+	+
Unlinkablity of pseudonyms for a user	+	+	+		+

+: Support

[1] *(Arlein, Jai, Jakobsson, Monrose, & Reiter, 2000; Kobsa, 2002, 2007b; Teltzrow & Kobsa, 2004)*
[2] *(Kobsa, 2007b; Kobsa & Schreck, 2003)*
[3] *(Hitchens, Kay, Kummerfeld, & Brar, 2005; Kobsa, 2007b)*

Table 4 presents an analysis of the aforementioned pseudonymous personalization systems along the following characteristics:

1. **Alias-to-website cardinality:** The alias-to-website cardinality describes the relationship between the number of aliases pertaining to a user and the number of websites at which the alias(es) may be used. For example, a cardinality of 1:1 means that each user will have exactly one alias for every website, while 1:n means that a user has one global alias/profile for all websites, and m:n means that a user can have an arbitrary number of aliases for any number of websites.
2. **User control:** User control denotes whether the system allows users to control the usage of their alias/profile at different websites.
3. **Personalization:** This factor evaluates to what extent the websites can provide personalized services to users. For example, a site can provide personalized services using the user's interaction logs with this site, or it could use the logs from multiple sites.
4. **Sender anonymity:** Sender anonymity indicates whether or not users are identified in the interactions.
5. **Receiver anonymity:** Receiver anonymity indicates whether websites are identified in the interactions.
6. **User Modeling Server (UMS) anonymity:** UMS anonymity indicates whether or not user modeling servers (or more general, the repositories that store the user models/profiles) are kept anonymous.

7. **Content-based anonymity:** Content-based anonymity prevails when no identification by means of the exchanged data is possible.
8. **Linkability for a single pseudonym:** This characteristic indicates whether or not a user's interaction steps or sessions with one or multiple websites can be linked using one pseudonym of hers
9. **Unlinkability of pseudonyms for a user:** This characteristic indicates whether or not multiple pseudonyms pertaining to the same user can be linked.

At first sight, pseudonymous personalization seems to be a panacea for all privacy problems because it seems to protect identity and, in most cases, privacy laws do not apply any more when the interaction is anonymous. However, anonymity is currently difficult and/or tedious to preserve when payments, physical goods and non-electronic services are being exchanged. It harbors the risk of misuse, and it hinders vendors from cross-channel marketing (e.g. sending a product catalog to a web customer by mail). Besides, users may still have additional privacy preferences such as not wanting to be profiled even when done pseudonymously only, to which personalized systems need to adjust. Moreover, Rao et al. (Rao & Rohatgi, 2000) point out that pseudonymity, or more broadly, hiding explicit identity information (e.g., name, e-mail address) is not sufficient to guarantee privacy. They demonstrate using a technique from stylometry (a field of linguistics that uses syntactic and semantic information to ascribe identity or authorship to literary works), and principal component analysis of function words, to attack pseudonymity. Similar findings were made for of database entries (Sweeney, 2002), web trails (Malin, Sweeney, & Newton, 2003), query terms (Nakashima, 2006), and ratings.

Distributed Personalization

Distributed personalization for safeguarding users' privacy has so far primarily been investigated in the domain of collaborative filtering (CF). Collaborative filtering is a popular technique for generating personalized recommendations using other users' preferences. The underlying assumption is that a user will prefer things that similar users like. In general, CF techniques use weighted combinations of nearest neighbor ratings to make predictions based on a user's preferences. A number of algorithms exist to determine proximity, including correlation between users, vector similarity methods, Bayesian clustering and Bayesian networks.

In recommender systems based on CF techniques, distribution may affect two aspects: the storage of personal profiles, and computation aspects (such as neighborhood formation and prediction generation). One argument why distribution leads to better privacy protection is that users may have better control over their own data if they are stored at the client side as compared to a central (user modeling) server. What is more important though is that CF computation is performed in a distributed and cooperative fashion rather than centrally. Personalization either takes places at the client side using merely the user's data, or is realized by specific privacy-preserving collaborative filtering schemes such as the ones described below.

Yenta (Foner, 1997) is a multi-agent distributed matchmaking system that learns about users by finding sets of keywords that characterize a user's interests. It matches users with similar interests by comparing their keywords without disclosing their identities. If a match is found, the Yenta clients can discretely negotiate to decide whether the matched users would like to reveal their identities to each other. Yenta utilizes anonymity/pseudonymity and encryption in protecting users' privacy.

Olsson (Olsson, 1998) describes a decentralized social filtering model that is built on interactions between collaborative software agents performing content-based filtering. This system is similar to Yenta but differs in its way of measuring similarity between different users via trust rather than interests as in Yenta.

Canny (Canny, 2002a, 2002b) outlined a peer-to-peer collaborative filtering model in which users' profiles are all stored at the client side so that users can fully control their data. The underlying multi-party computation scheme allows a community of users to compute an aggregate of their data (i.e., a singular value decomposition (SVD) model of the user-item matrix) based solely on vector addition so that individual data will not be disclosed. This non-disclosure property is achieved by using techniques including ElGamal encryption, homomorphic encryption and Zero Knowledge Proofs.

Miller et al. (Miller, Konstan, & Riedl, 2004) propose a peer-to-peer CF algorithm called PocketLens. For each individual user, PocketLens first searches for neighbors in the P2P network, then incrementally updates the user's individual item-item similarity model by incorporating one neighbor's ratings at a time (the neighbor's ratings will be discarded after updating the model), and finally generates recommendations based on the model. The paper also compares and discusses five implementation frameworks:

- a central server architecture where the key data is stored on a central server while the computations are performed at each individual node;
- a random discovery architecture that allows users to remain anonymous and uses Gnutella's ping/pong mechanism for finding neighbors;
- a transitive traversal architecture that allows clients to share their neighborhood lists by query flooding and thus enables neighborhood formation via a form of transitivity;
- a content-addressable architecture that adopts P2P file sharing networks, e.g., Chord, which places a deterministic overlay routing system over the network and provides a scalable and distributed lookup function (the II-Chord implementation described in the paper uses the network basically as a distributed storage mechanism to collaboratively build and maintain the item-item matrix); and
- a secure blackboard architecture that leverages the secure operations used in a secure online voting protocol and in Canny's work (Canny, 2002a, 2002b), whereby each client writes encrypted partial results to a Write Once Read Many (WORM) blackboard and the final model is generated by incorporating those partial profiles.

Gilburd et al. (Gilburd, Schuster, & Wolff, 2004) introduce a k-TTP (trusted third party) model which suggests that privacy is preserved as long as no participant of a distributed (joint) computation learns statistics of a group with less than k members. This is less restrictive than an ordinary TTP model in the sense that it does not protect unauthorized access to statistics of individual users if less than k members participate in a joint computation, and is thus more flexible. The authors demonstrate that k-TTP enables more scalable distributed computation schemes. While the paper illustrates the idea of k-TTP by an association-rule mining algorithm, the same idea could be applied to personalization techniques such as collaborative filtering. Berkovsky et al.'s idea of super-peers echoes the same aggregation spirit (Berkovsky, Eytani, Kuflik, & Ricci, 2006).

Privacy-Preserving Collaborative Filtering

The aim of work in this area is to apply and extend privacy-preserving data mining techniques in the area of collaborative filtering. The common approach for achieving privacy preservation in data mining tasks is to replace each message exchange in an ordinary distributed data mining algorithm with a cryptographic primitive that provides the same information without disclosing the data of the individual participants. The research challenge here is to enable users to contribute their information for CF purposes without compromising their privacy (e.g., through exposure of their personal data). Here, privacy-preserving CF is treated as a secure multiparty computation problem where users and different websites jointly conduct CF computations based on their private data. These parties could be mutually untrusted, or even competitors. Typical ways of privacy preservation include decentralization, encryption, aggregation, perturbation and obfuscation.

Encryption

In this type of work, CF computation is based on encrypted user data. An example is the abovementioned work of (Canny, 2002a), which describes a secure multi-party computation scheme that allows a community of users to compute an aggregate of their data without disclosing individual data by using homomorphic encryption and ElGamal encryption. More specifically, a combination of ElGamal encryption and homomorphic encryption allows vectors to be added by multiplying the encrypted addends, and the final result to be decrypted. Individual addends can be verified as valid data using zero knowledge proofs. The resultant aggregate SVD model can then be used to generate personalization.

Randomized Perturbation

*Pol*at and Du (Polat & Du, 2003, 2005a, 2005b) demonstrate the usage of randomized perturbation techniques (adding random numbers from a given range to the original data) in disguising the original user ratings before feeding them into CF algorithms based on correlation and singular value decomposition. The CF system thereby does not know the exact values of the original ratings, yet is still able to compute reasonably accurate recommendations. The underlying reason is that the CF algorithms often use aggregations like scalar products and sums, and that the perturbations tend to cancel themselves out.

Aggregation

In this privacy-protecting approach (e.g., (Canny, 2002a)), users' personal data are aggregated in such a way that an individual's data cannot be identified.

Community Model

In this approach, CF computation (e.g., model generation) is carried out collaboratively by a community of clients. The difference to aggregation techniques is that a community model may not generate an aggregate model and may still reveal individual user's data, e.g., in the II-Chord implementation of PocketLens (Miller, Konstan, & Riedl, 2004). Both aggregate and community model can also be considered as examples of distributed personalization, since they either store personal profiles or perform CF computation in a distributed manner.

Obfuscation

Another way of disguising users' personal data is via obfuscation. Berkovsky et al. (Berkovsky, Eytani, Kuflik, & Ricci, 2005) describe a decentralized CF model in which user profiles are stored at the client side. In this approach, some of the personal data is replaced by some other data (which is either constant or drawn from some distribution). The authors demonstrate that relatively large parts of the user profile can be obfuscated while CF can still generate reasonably accurate recommendations. In their follow-up work (Berkovsky, Eytani, Kuflik, & Ricci, 2006), they propose a decentralized recommendation generation scheme that is based on a hierarchical neighborhood topology. More specifically, users (peers) are organized into groups managed by super-peers. To enhance privacy, the super-peers choose only a random subset of their peers to form the neighborhood of similar users. To protect individual peers' privacy within a peer-group, the obfuscation techniques can be used and also only a subset of peers can be queried.

Scrutable Personalization

Kay et al. (Kay, 2006; Kay, Kummerfeld, & Lauder, 2003) suggest putting scrutability into user modeling and personalized systems. By scrutability the authors mean that users can understand and control what goes into their user model, what information from their model is available to different services, and how the model is managed and maintained. Their user modeling system Personis applies three privacy-enhancing mechanisms to control the protection of each unit of personal information ("evidence") in the user model (Kay, Kummerfeld, & Lauder, 2003):

- expiration dates and purging of older evidence,
- compaction, for replacing a set of evidence from a single source with an aggregate, and
- morphing, which replaces an arbitrary collection of evidence.

For controlling the usage of evidences from the user model, Personis allows users to restrict the evidences that are available to applications, and the methods that may generate a user model and operate on it. Despite the desirability of scrutability from a privacy point of view, its implementation and control is currently very challenging, due to users' lack of understanding of these notions and of effective and efficient user interfaces to support them. Moreover, scrutability may reveal the personalization methods that a website uses, which may pose a problem in application areas in which those are considered to be competitive advantages and therefore confidential (e.g., in online retail websites).

Task-Based Personalization

Herlocker and Konstan (Herlocker & Konstan, 2001) propose a content-independent task-focused recommendation scheme. The scheme assumes that a traditional recommender system may already possess historical ratings data, and that recommendation is possible with data that pertain to the current session or specific task only (e.g., buying a martial arts DVD) rather than collecting a comprehensive profile of the user across multiple sessions. The system builds an item-item association model based on the legacy ratings, and uses the model to generate recommendations. The privacy improvement is that users do not need to disclose their historical ratings while still being able to receive task-focused recommendations. Cranor (Cranor, 2003) also supports task or session based personalization as a way to reduce privacy risks and make privacy compliance easier. However, the price is that the recommendations are not truly personalized, i.e., all users may receive the same recommendations for the same task.

Tailoring Personalization to Users' Privacy Constraints

Wang et al. (Wang, Kobsa, van der Hoek, & White, 2006) propose a user modeling server architecture that encapsulates different user modeling components (UMCs) and, at any point during runtime, ascertains that only those components can be operational that are in compliance with the currently prevailing privacy constraints (including privacy legislation, regulations and users' personal privacy preferences). Moreover, the architecture can also dynamically select the component with the optimal anticipated personalization effects among those that are currently permissible (Kobsa, 2003). Each user has their own tailored instance of the UMC pool, containing only those UMCs that meet the privacy requirements for the respective user (users with identical UMC pool instances share the same instance). An advantage of this approach is its capability to reconfigure the architecture immediately to cater to users' changes of privacy preferences at any time (we denote this capability as dynamism support). This approach directly addresses the principles of enforcement, ease of compliance and responsiveness.

Analysis of Technical Solutions for Privacy-Enhanced Personalization

We have seen that different privacy enhancing solutions for personalized systems often implement several basic techniques. Table 5 gives a summary of the techniques used in the discussed systems. Table 6 shows how well a set of representative privacy protection solutions from the ones discussed above meet the privacy principles described earlier. Table 7 presents how these solutions address the privacy concerns in web personalization described earlier. The following observations can be made:

First, several solutions aim for a balance between privacy and personalization. Examples include pseudonymous personalization, scrutable personalization and dynamic personalization. They all address a handful of privacy concerns and achieve at least reasonably good personalization.

Table 5. Basic privacy protection techniques used in privacy-enhanced personalization solutions

System \ Technique	A/P	En	SD	CD	Ag	CM	Pe	Ob	ScS	TP	DS
Yenta	X	X	X	X							
Trust-based Social Filtering (Olsson 1998)			X	X							
PocketLens Central Server				X							
PocketLens Random Discovery	X		X	X							
PocketLens Transitive Traversal	X		X	X							
PocketLens II-Chord			X	X		X					
PocketLens Secure Blackboard		X	X	X	X	X					
k-TTP		X	X	X	X	X					
Privacy Preserving CF (Canny 2002a)		X	X	X	X	X					
Factor Analysis-CF (FA-CF) (Canny 2002b)		X	X	X	X	X					
Random Perturbation-CF							X				
Privacy Enhancing CF (Berkovsky et al. 2005)			X	X				X			
Hierarchical Neighborhood Topology-CF (HNT-CF) (Berkovsky et al. 2006)			X	X	X			X			
Personis			X	X	X		X		X		
Task-based Personalization										X	
Privacy-Tailored Personalization											X

A/P: Anonymity/pseudonymity   En: Encryption   SD: Storage distribution
CD: Computation distribution   Ag: Aggregation   CM: Community model
Pe: Perturbation   Ob: Obfuscation   ScS: Scrutability support
TP: Task-based personalization   DS: Dynamism support

Table 6. An analysis of privacy protection solutions in Web personalization

Principle \ Solution	Pseudonymous UMS	Yenta	PocketLens—II-Chord	Canny's FA-CF	HNT-CF	Task-based CF	Personis	Privacy-tailored personaliztion
GENERAL								
Notice/Awareness							++	
Choice/Consent		+	+	+	+		+	+
Enforcement/Redress	+	+		+			+	++
User preference							+	++
Negotiation		+						
Ease of adoption	–			–				+
Ease of compliance								++
Usability							–	
Responsiveness								++
Personalization quality	++	+	++	+	++	+	+	++
IDENTITY								
Anonymity	++		+					
Pseudonymity	++	+		++	+		+	
Unobservability	++		+	+	+			
Unlinkability			+	++				
Deniability					+			
SECLUSION								
Seclusion								
DATA								
Minimization				+	+	++		++
Purpose specification							+	+
Collection limitation							+	
Use limitation	+						+	++
Onward transfer								
Access/Participation							++	
Integrity/accuracy							+	
Security	+	+		+	+			

++*: Strong support*
+*: Support*
–*: Negative impact*

Table 7. How existing solutions address privacy concerns in web personalization

	Control over data							Seclusion	Protection of identity
	Improper acquisition			Improper use			Improper storage	Unwanted solicitation	Identity fraud/theft
	Improper access	Improper collection	Improper monitoring	Improper analysis	Improper merge	Improper transfer			
Pseudonymous UMS		++	++					+	++
Yenta	+	++	+	+	+	+	+		++
PocketLens + H-Chord	+	++	+	+	+	+	+		
Canny's FA-CF	+	+	+	+	+	+	+		++
HNT-CF	+	+	+	+	+	+	+		++
Task-based personalization		+	+	+	+	+			+
Personis	++	++	++	++	++	++	++	+	+
Privacy-tailored personalization				++	++		++		+

++: *Effective*
+: *Partially effective*

Second, none of the solutions in Table 5 uses all available privacy-enhancing techniques. We believe more comprehensive future solutions will need to incorporate a variety of basic privacy enhancing techniques.

Third, none of the solutions in Table 7 addresses all privacy concerns, except Personis which relies on a "user empowerment" strategy. However, Personis does not address all the concerns effectively. For example, it does not provide comprehensible and effective user interfaces even though most users do not possess mental models of the operation of user modeling systems.

Finally, we find that principles such as onward transfer, enforcement, user preference, negotiation, ease of compliance and responsiveness are currently insufficiently observed. Taking "onward transfer" as an example, no current privacy-enhancing solution in web personalization allows "sticky" privacy policies that travel with data so that, e.g., user data cannot be copied and transferred by an entity that is only allowed to read the data. Techniques used in Digital Rights Management (DRM) (Rosenblatt, Trippe, & Mooney, 2001) may be adapted for this purpose.

DISCUSSION

We discuss the major findings of our survey from two points of views, namely the one of users and of websites.

Users

User would like to enjoy personalized services of websites while at the same time have their individual privacy needs respected (Kobsa, 2007a). The traditional strategy for addressing users' privacy needs is through expression and enforcement – users specify their privacy needs which are then translated into formal expressions and finally enforced in technical solutions.

There are several problems with this strategy. First, privacy decisions (e.g., whether to disclose one's telephone number in a particular situation) are inherently contingent and situated. As Dourish and colleagues (DiGioia & Dourish, 2005; Dourish & Anderson, 2006) point out, the artificial separation of configuration and action may be overly rigid or ineffective. Second, it is a known fact that users' actual behaviors may diverge from their stated privacy attitudes or preferences (Spiekermann, Grossklags, & Berendt, 2001). Third, we observe that currently available technical privacy languages fall short of expressing users' highly flexible and nuanced privacy needs. This may well be an inevitable "social-technical gap" (Ackerman, 2000) between human activities/decisions and what we can support technically. Forth, even if users' privacy decisions could be accurately translated into enforceable specifications, we notice that the majority of existing solutions lack enforcement mechanisms that respond to users' unpredictable changes of privacy decisions in an effective manner.

We see three emerging ways of alleviating or solving these problems:

1. by empowering users to make informed decisions (e.g., by giving them insights into the consequences of their actions through visualizations of system states and events, by enabling them to carry out their privacy decisions rather than merely expressing them through integration of configuration and action (de Paula et al., 2005), or by providing scrutability support in user models (Kay, 2006));
2. by supporting the negotiation between users and websites to reach a consensus on the privacy practices of websites (e.g., (Buffett, Jia, Liu, Spencer, & Wang, 2004; Preibusch, 2006)); and
3. by enabling run-time system variability (Wang, Kobsa, van der Hoek, & White, 2006) as a way to address the responsiveness principle that directly relates to the enforcement problem.

Websites

One of the pressing challenges that websites face today is the need to provide competitive value-added personalized services to its users while complying with a growing number of regulatory privacy requirements. From our survey, we recognize deficiencies in the area of compliance (see Table 7). More specifically, we witness that compliance-related principles such as enforcement and ease of compliance are mostly not addressed, with the exception of a few solutions based on the abovementioned "expression and enforcement" strategy such as in the IBM Tivoli privacy manager (IBM, 2003). From the previous section we can infer though that this approach may run into problems when users become involved.

In the light of this, we coarsely categorize regulatory privacy requirements into two types. The first type consists of requirements that can be met without user involvement (we call them "website-exclusive" requirements). An instance of this type is "*usage data must be erased immediately after each session*" (except for very limited purposes) (DE-TML, 2007). The second type consists of requirements that may include privacy decisions of the user (we call them "user-involving" requirements). Examples are "*users must be able to withdraw their consent to the processing of traffic and location data at any time* (EU, 2002)", and "*value-added (e.g. personalized) services based on traffic or location data require the anonymization of such data or the user's consent* (EU, 2002)".

Since "user-involving" requirements can be fulfilled by users' involvement (giving their consent), we believe that this type of privacy requirements might also be well addressed by using some of the alternatives to the expression and enforcement approach that were discussed in the previous section. We expect new solutions to emerge in the future that follow these alternate directions.

In contrast, the traditional strategy of expression and enforcement is by and large appropriate and effective for fulfilling the website-exclusive obligations. First, because of its website-exclusiveness, the user empowerment alternative is obviously irrelevant. Second, the separation of expression and enforcement is no longer a problem here, for three reasons: (1) website-exclusive requirements are usually unambiguous and rigid, and thus amenable to accurate formal expressions; (2) there are tools available that can automatically translate textual requirements into specifications in formal languages like P3P (e.g., IBM's Sparcle (Karat, Karat, Brodie, & Feng, 2005)); and (3) once put into effect, privacy laws and regulations are fairly stable, and changes are normally known a few months before they become effective.

While expression can become much easier with support through tools like Sparcle, enforcement is still quite challenging, for the following reasons.

- An effective enforcement mechanism needs to cover the whole lifecycle of user data from collection to usage to transfer, etc.
- In centralized user modeling systems (which collect and supply user information from and to different websites for usually different purposes), the complexities of defining different permissible purposes for collecting and using personal data must be addressed. What is more, since privacy laws can also affect the permissibility of personalization methods used to process user data, the enforcement may involve substituting methods in the user modeling systems at runtime (Wang, Kobsa, van der Hoek, & White, 2006).
- For legacy systems it is likely that privacy had been disregarded during their design and implementation. As with usability, research has revealed though that privacy and security cannot be an afterthought in system design (de Paula et al., 2005; Dourish & Anderson, 2006; Dourish, Grinter, Dalal, Flor, & Joseph, 2004). The support of the enforcement of privacy in legacy systems is therefore likely to be very hard.

SUMMARY AND FUTURE RESEARCH DIRECTIONS

Privacy and web personalization are in tension with each other. The more user data websites collect and utilize, the better are generally the personalized services they provide but the more potential privacy concerns may arise. With the enactment of privacy legislation and regulations worldwide, the conflict is even more acute because personalized websites are obliged to comply with their provisions, which often have remarkable impacts on how personalization may be performed.

In analyzing technical solutions for privacy-enhancing personalization, we propose and apply a multi-faceted approach, consisting of privacy guidelines, privacy concerns, and privacy-enhancing characteristics of these solutions. We relate these facets to each other and reveal trends and identify deficiencies.

Based on our study of existing privacy-enhancing personalization solutions, we suggest the following directions for future research:

- We advocate more recognition of the importance of privacy in web personalization research and practice, and argue that privacy needs be treated as first-class design requirements since (1) regulatory privacy requirements and users' privacy concerns have significant impacts on personalization and its possible benefits, and (2) privacy, like security and usability, is extremely difficult if not impossible to achieve after a system has already been built. Therefore, privacy should be taken into serious consideration from the early onsets of the development process.

- Further research is needed to improve the expression and enforcement approach. With regard to the expression of privacy constraints, two things are desirable. First, a formal language is needed that can sufficiently express potential privacy constraints. As discussed in (Wang & Kobsa, forthcoming), XACML (OASIS, 2005) seems to come close to this vision. However, further studies need to confirm this or/and uncover deficiencies. Secondly, potential privacy constraints should be captured and expressed as they arise, preferably in real time. Users' privacy concerns usually emerge as they interact with a web-based personalized system. Designers of privacy enhanced web personalization should not assume that users can and would express their privacy concern in a formal privacy language. A hybrid approach of "user empowerment" and "expression and enforcement" might be promising in which users become empowered to act on their contingent privacy needs and possibly also express them in a user-friendly fashion (e.g., in natural language). Thereafter, the system would compile this information into formal expressions that can be executed and enforced. Systematic enforcement is also largely neglected in privacy enhancement in web personalization. Solutions like the IBM Tivoli Privacy Manager need to be adopted.
- While compliance has long been technically framed and treated as a server-side problem, solutions that follow the user empowerment strategy (such as Personis) bear great potential. How to appropriately empower users in the context of web personalization is still an open question, e.g. in light of the fact the users may not be technically savvy. Techniques such as visualization may be useful in this regard.
- Users' privacy needs have been studied predominately in the domain of E-commerce. However, web personalization can also take place in, e.g., E-learning or Ubiquitous Computing, and research is needed to uncover users' privacy needs in these domains as well. Besides, since users' privacy needs and preferences are inherently dynamic and contingent, users' *individual* privacy needs must be taken into account. Solutions that allow for tailored privacy in personalization at runtime seem promising in this regard (Wang & Kobsa, 2007).
- Another promising future direction is usable personal privacy management tools that can help users manage and keep track of the disclosure and usage of their personal information (e.g., by indicating which organization knows what about the user and employs this information for what purposes).

REFERENCES

Ackerman, M. S. (2000). The Intellectual Challenge of CSCW: The Gap between Social Requirements and Technical Feasibility. Human-Computer Interaction, 15 (2), 179-203.

APEC-FIP. (2004). APEC Privacy Framework (No. 2004/AMM/014rev1): Asia-Pacific Economic Cooperation. from http://www.apecsec.org.sg/.

Arlein, R. M., Jai, B., Jakobsson, M., Monrose, F., & Reiter, M. K. (2000). Privacy-Preserving Global Customization. In proceedings of the 2nd ACM Conference on Electronic Commerce (pp. 176-184). Minneapolis, MN.

Berkovsky, S., Eytani, Y., Kuflik, T., & Ricci, F. (2005). Privacy-Enhanced Collaborative Filtering. In proceedings of the PEP05, UM05 Workshop on Privacy-Enhanced Personalization (pp. 75-84). Edinburgh, UK.

Berkovsky, S., Eytani, Y., Kuflik, T., & Ricci, F. (2006). Hierarchical Neighborhood Topology for Privacy-Enhanced Collaborative Filtering In proceedings of the PEP06, CHI06 Workshop on Privacy-Enhanced Personalization (pp. 6-13). Montreal, Canada.

Buffett, S., Jia, K., Liu, S., Spencer, B., & Wang, F. (2004). Negotiating Exchanges of P3P-Labeled Information for Compensation. Computational Intelligence, 20 (4), 663-677.

Camp, J., & Osorio, C. (2003). Privacy-Enhancing Technologies for Internet Commerce. In O. Petrovic, M. Ksela, M. Fallenböck & C. Kittl (Eds.), Trust in the Network Economy (pp. 317-331). Wien: Springer.

Canny, J. (2002a). Collaborative Filtering with Privacy. In proceedings of the IEEE Conference on Security and Privacy (pp. 45- 57). Oakland, CA.

Canny, J. (2002b). Collaborative Filtering with Privacy via Factor Analysis. In proceedings of the 25th Annual International ACM SIGIR Conference on Research and Development in Information Retrieval (SIGIR 2002) (pp. 238 - 245). Tampere, Finland.

Cranor, L. F. (2003). 'I Didn't Buy it for Myself': Privacy and Ecommerce Personalization. In proceedings of the 2003 ACM Workshop on Privacy in the Electronic Society. Washington, DC.

de Paula, R. r., Ding, X., Dourish, P., Nies, K., Pillet, B., Redmiles, D. F., et al. (2005). In the Eye of the Beholder: A Visualization-based Approach to Information System Security. International Journal of Human-Computer Studies, 63 (1-2), 5-24.

DE-TML. (2007). German Telemedia Law. from http://www.gesetze-im-internet.de/tmg/.

DiGioia, P., & Dourish, P. (2005). Social Navigation as a Model for Usable Security. In proceedings of the Symposium on Usable Privacy and Security SOUPS 2005 (pp. 101-108). Pittsburgh, PA.

Dourish, P., & Anderson, K. (2006). Collective Information Practice: Exploring Privacy and Security as Social and Cultural Phenomena. Human-Computer Interaction, 21 (3), 319-342.

Dourish, P., Grinter, R. E., Dalal, B., Flor, J. D. d. l., & Joseph, M. (2004). Security Day-to-Day: User Strategies for Managing Security as an Everyday, Practical Problem. Personal Ubiquitous Computing, 8 (6), 391-401.

EU. (1995). Directive 95/46/EC of the European Parliament and of the Council of 24 October 1995 on the Protection of Individuals with Regard to the Processing of Personal Data and on the Free Movement of such Data. Official Journal of the European Communities (23 November 1995 No L. 281), 31ff. from http://158.169.50.95:10080/legal/en/dataprot/directiv/directiv.html.

EU. (2002). Directive 2002/58/EC of the European Parliament and of the Council Concerning the Processing of Personal Data and the Protection of Privacy in the Electronic Communications Sector. from http://register.consilium.eu.int/pdf/en/02/st03/03636en2.pdf.

Foner, L. N. (1997). Yenta: A Multi-Agent Referral-Based Matchmaking System. In proceedings of the International Conference on Autonomous Agents (pp. 301-307). Marina del Rey, CA.

Frankowski, D., Cosley, D., Sen, S., Terveen, L., & Riedl, J. (2006). You Are What You Say: Privacy Risks of Public Mentions. In proceedings of the 29th Annual International ACM SIGIR Conference on Research and Development in Information Retrieval (pp. 565-572). Seattle, WA.

FTC. (2000a). Online Profiling: A Report to Congress. from http://www.ftc.gov/os/2000/07/onlineprofiling.pdf.

FTC. (2000b, May 2000). Privacy Online: Fair Information Practices in the Electronic Marketplace. A Report to Congress. from http://www.ftc.gov/reports/privacy2000/privacy2000.pdf.

FTC. (2000c). The Seven Safe Harbor Principles. from http://europa.eu.int/comm/internal_market/en/media/dataprot/news/shprinciples.pdf.

Gabber, E., Gibbons, P. B., Matias, Y., & Mayer, A. (1997). How to Make Personalized Web Browsing Simple, Secure, and Anonymous. In Financial Cryptography'97 (Vol. 1318). Berlin - Heidelberg - New York: Springer Verlag.

Gilburd, B., Schuster, A., & Wolff, R. (2004). k-TPP: A New Privacy Model for Large-Scale Distributed Environments. In proceedings of the 10th ACM SIGKDD International Conference on Knowledge Discovery and Date Mining (KDD'04) (pp. 563-568). Seattle, WA.

Herlocker, J., & Konstan, J. (2001). Content-Independent Task-Focused Recommendation. IEEE Internet Computing, 5 (6), 40 - 47.

Hitchens, M., Kay, J., Kummerfeld, B., & Brar, A. (2005). Secure Identity Management for Pseudo-Anonymous Service Access. In proceedings of the Security in Pervasive Computing: Second International Conference (pp. 48-55). Boppard, Germany.

IBM. (2003). IBM Tivoli Privacy Manager for E-Business. from http://www-306.ibm.com/software/ tivoli/products/privacy-mgr-e-bus/.

Ishitani, L., Almeida, V., & Wagner, M., Jr. (2003). Masks: Bringing Anonymity and Personalization Together. IEEE Security & Privacy Magazine, 1 (3), 18-23. from DOI 10.1109/MSECP.2003.1203218.

Karat, J., Karat, C.-M., Brodie, C., & Feng, J. (2005). Privacy in Information Technology: Designing to Enable Privacy Policy Management in Organizations. International journal of Human-Computer Studies, 63, 153-174. from DOI 10.1016/j.ijhcs.2005.04.011.

Kay, J. (2006). Scrutable Adaptation: Because We Can and Must. In Adaptive Hypermedia and Adaptive Web-Based Systems (pp. 11-19): Springer Berlin / Heidelberg.

Kay, J., Kummerfeld, B., & Lauder, P. (2003). Managing private user models and shared personas. In proceedings of the Workshop on User Modelling for Ubiquitous Computing, 9th International Conference on User Modeling (pp. 1-11).

Kobsa, A. (2002). Personalization and International Privacy. Communications of the ACM, 45 (5), 64-67. from DOI 10.1145/767193.767196.

Kobsa, A. (2003). A Component Architecture for Dynamically Managing Privacy in Personalized Web-based Systems. In proceedings of the Privacy Enhancing Technologies: Third International Workshop (Vol. LNCS 2760, pp. 177-188). Dresden, Germany. from DOI: 10.1007/b94512.

Kobsa, A. (2007a). Privacy-Enhanced Personalization (cover article). Communications of the ACM, 50 (8), 24-33. from DOI 10.1145/1278201.1278202.

Kobsa, A. (2007b). Privacy-Enhanced Web Personalization. In P. Brusilovsky, A. Kobsa & W. Nejdl (Eds.), The Adaptive Web: Methods and Strategies of Web Personalization (pp. 628-670): Springer-Verlag. from DOI 10.1007/978-3-540-72079-9_21.

Kobsa, A., J. Koenemann and W. Pohl. (2001). Personalized Hypermedia Presentation Techniques for Improving Online Customer Relationships. The Knowledge Engineering Review, 16 (2), 111-155. from DOI 10.1017/S0269888901000108.

Kobsa, A., & Schreck, J. (2003). Privacy through Pseudonymity in User-Adaptive Systems. ACM Transactions on Internet Technology, 3 (2), 149-183. from DOI 10.1145/767193.767196.

Malin, B., Sweeney, L., & Newton, E. (2003). Trail Re-Identification: Learning Who You Are From Where You Have Been (Technical Report No. LIDAP-WP12). Pittsburgh, PA: Carnegie Mellon University, Laboratory for International Data Privacy. from http://privacy.cs.cmu.edu/people/sweeney/trails1.pdf.

Miller, B., Konstan, J., & Riedl, J. (2004). PockLens: Toward a Personal Recommender System. ACM Transactions on Information Systems, 22 (3), 437-476.

Nakashima, E. (2006). AOL Search Queries Open Window Onto Users' Worlds. from http://www.washingtonpost.com/wp-dyn/content/article/2006/08/16/AR2006081601751_pf.html.

OASIS. (2005). eXtensible Access Control Markup Language (XACML), Version 2.0; OASIS Standard, February 1, 2005. .

OECD. (1980). Recommendation of the Council Concerning Guidelines Governing the Protection of Privacy and Transborder Flows of Personal Data. from http://www.oecd.org/dsti/sti/it/secur/prod/PRIV-EN.HTM.

Olsson, T. (1998). Decentralised Social Filtering based on Trust. In proceedings of the The AAAI-98 Recommender Systems Workshop (Working Notes) (pp. 84-88). Madison, Wisconsin.

Polat, H., & Du, W. (2003). Privacy-Preserving Collaborative Filtering Using Randomized Perturbation Techniques. In proceedings of the Third IEEE International Conference on Data Mining (ICDM'03) (pp. 625-628). Melbourne, FL.

Polat, H., & Du, W. (2005a). Privacy-Preserving Collaborative Filtering. The International Journal of Electronic Commerce (IJEC), 9 (4), 9-35.

Polat, H., & Du, W. (2005b). SVD-based Collaborative Filtering with Privacy. In proceedings of the 20th ACM Symposium on Applied Computing (pp. 791-795). Santa Fe, NM.

Preibusch, S. (2006). Personalized Services with Negotiable Privacy Policies. In proceedings of the PEP06, CHI 2006 Workshop on Privacy-Enhanced Personalization (pp. 29-38). Montreal, Canada.

Rao, J. R., & Rohatgi, P. (2000). Can Pseudonymity Really Guarantee Privacy? In proceedings of the 9th USENIX Security Symposium (pp. 85–96).

Rosenblatt, W., Trippe, W., & Mooney, S. (2001). Digital Rights Management: Business and Technology. Indianapolis, IN: Hungry Minds, Inc.

Solove, D. (2006). A Taxonomy of Privacy. University of Pennsylvania Law Review, 154 (3), 477-564.

Spiekermann, S., Grossklags, J., & Berendt, B. (2001). Stated Privacy Preferences versus Actual Behaviour in EC Environments: a Reality Check. In proceedings of the WI-IF 2001: the 5th International Conference Wirtschaftsinformatik - 3rd Conference Information Systems in Finance (pp. 129-148). Augsburg, Germany.

Sweeney, L. (2002). k-Anonymity: A Model for Protecting Privacy. International Journal on Uncertainty, Fuzziness, and Knowledge-based Systems, 10 (5), 557-570. from DOI 10.1142/S0218488502001648.

Teltzrow, M., & Kobsa, A. (2004). Impacts of User Privacy Preferences on Personalized Systems: a Comparative Study. In C.-M. Karat, J. Blom & J. Karat (Eds.), Designing Personalized User Experiences for eCommerce (pp. 315-332). Dordrecht, Netherlands: Kluwer Academic Publishers. from DOI 10.1007/1-4020-2148-8_17.

USACM. (2006). USACM Policy Recommendations on Privacy. New York, NY: U.S. Public Policy Committee of the Association for Computing Machinery. from http://www.acm.org/usacm/Issues/Privacy.htm.

Wang, H., Lee, M. K. O., & Wang, C. (1998). Consumer Privacy Concerns about Internet Marketing. Communications of the ACM, 41 (3), 63-70.

Wang, Y., & Kobsa, A. (2006). Impacts of Privacy Laws and Regulations on Personalized Systems. In proceedings of the PEP06, CHI06 Workshop on Privacy-Enhanced Personalization (pp. 44-46). Montréal, Canada. http://www.ics.uci.edu/~kobsa/papers/2006-PEP-wang-kobsa.pdf

Wang, Y., & Kobsa, A. (2007). Respecting Users' Individual Privacy Constraints in Web Personalization In proceedings of the UM07, 11th International Conference on User Modeling (pp. 157–166). Corfu, Greece. from DOI 10.1007/978-3-540-73078-1.

Wang, Y., & Kobsa, A. (forthcoming). Privacy-Enhancing Technologies. In M. Gupta & R. Sharman (Eds.), Social and Organizational Liabilities in Information Security: IGI Global.

Wang, Y., Kobsa, A., van der Hoek, A., & White, J. (2006). PLA-based Runtime Dynamism in Support of Privacy-Enhanced Web Personalization. In proceedings of the 10th International Software Product Line Conference (pp. 151-162). Baltimore, MD. from DOI 0.1109/ SPLINE.2006.1691587.

Wang, Y., Zhaoqi, C., & Kobsa, A. (2006). A Collection and Systematization of International Privacy Laws, with Special Consideration of Internationally Operating Personalized Websites. from http://www.ics.uci.edu/~kobsa/privacy/intl-privlawsurvey.html.

ADDITIONAL READING

Agrawal, D., & Aggarwal, C. C. (2001). *On the Design and Quantification of Privacy Preserving Data Mining Algorithms.* In proceedings of the 20th ACM SIGACT-SIGMOD-SIGART Symposium on Principles of Database System (pp. 247–255). Santa Barbara, CA.

Agrawal, R., & Srikant, R. (2000). *Privacy-Preserving Data Mining.* In proceedings of the ACM-SIGMOD 2000 Conference on Management of Data (pp. 439-450). Dallas, TX.

Ashrafi, N., & Kuilboer, J.-P. (2005). Privacy Protection via Technology: Platform for Privacy Preferences (P3P). *International Journal of E-Business Research, 1*(2), 56-69. from http://www.igi-online.com/details.asp?ID=7675.

Blarkom, G. W. v., Borking, J. J., & Verhaar, P. (2003). PET. In G. W. v. Blarkom, J. J. Borking & J. G. E. Olk (Eds.), *Handbook of Privacy and Privacy-Enhancing Technologies: The Case of Intelligent Software Agents* (pp. 33-53): College bescherming persoonsgegevens.

Borking, J., & Raab, C. (2001). Laws, PETs and Other Technologies for Privacy Protection. *Journal of Information, Law and Technology*(1). from http://www2.warwick.ac.uk/fac/soc/law/elj/jilt/2001_1/borking/.

Boyens, C., & Günther, O. (2002). *Trust Is not Enough: Privacy and Security in ASP and Web Service Environments.* In proceedings of the Advances in Databases and Information Systems, 6th East European Conference (Vol. 2435). Bratislava, Slovakia.

Burkert, H. (1997). Privacy-Enhancing Technologies: Typology, Critique, Vision. In P. E. Agre & M. Rotenberg (Eds.), *Technology and Privacy: The New Landscape* (pp. 126-143). Boston, MA: MIT Press.

Cassel, L. N., & Wolz, U. (2001). *Client Side Personalization.* In proceedings of the DELOS Workshop: Personalisation and Recommender Systems in Digital Libraries.

Ceri, S., Dolog, P., Matera, M., & Nejdl, W. (2004). Model-Driven Design of Web Applications with Client-Side Adaptation. In N. Koch, P. Fraternali & MartinWirsing (Eds.), *Web Engineering: 4th International Conference, ICWE 2004* (pp. 201-214). Berlin–Heidelberg: Springer Verlag.

Chellappa, R. K., & Sin, R. (2005). Personalization versus Privacy: An Empirical Examination of the Online Consumer's Dilemma. *Information Technology and Management, 6*(2-3), 181-202. from DOI 10.1007/s10799-005-5879-y.

Coroama, V., & Langheinrich, M. (2006). *Personalized Vehicle Insurance Rates: A Case for Client-Side Personalization in Ubiquitous Com-*

puting. In proceedings of the PEP06, CHI 2006 Workshop on Privacy-Enhanced Personalization (pp. 56-59). Montreal, Canada.

Cranor, L. F., & Reidenberg, J. R. (2002). *Can User Agents Accurately Represent Privacy Notices?* In proceedings of the 30th Research Conference on Communication, Information and Internet Policy. Alexandria, VA.

Dornbach, P., & Németh, Z. (2003). Privacy Enhancing Profile Disclosure. In R. Dingledine & P. Syverson (Eds.), *PET 2002* (Vol. LNCS 2482, pp. 85–98). Heidelberg, Germany: Springer-Verlag.

Foner, L. N. (1999). *Political Artifacts and Personal Privacy: The Yenta Multiagent Distributed Matchmaking System.* Massachusetts Institute of Technology.

Gandon, F. L., & Sadeh, N. M. (2004). Semantic Web Technologies to Reconcile Privacy and Context Awareness. *Web Semantics: Science, Services and Agents on the World Wide Web, 1,* 241–260. from http://dx.doi.org/10.1016/j.websem.2003.07.008.

Garfinkel, S. L., Juels, A., & Pappu, R. (2005). RFID Privacy: an Overview of Problems and Proposed Solutions. *IEEE Security & Privacy Magazine, 3*(3), 34-43. from DOI 10.1109/MSP.2005.78.

Goldberg, I., Wagner, D., & Brewer, E. (1997). *Privacy-Enhancing Technologies for the Internet.* In proceedings of the 42nd IEEE Spring COMPCON. San Jose, CA.

Goldberg, I. A. (2003). Privacy-Enhancing Technologies for the Internet, II: Five Years Later. In R. Dingledine & P. Syverson (Eds.), *Privacy Enhancing Technologies – Second International Workshop, PET 2002* (pp. 1-12). Berlin - Heidelberg: Springer Verlag.

ICPP-SNG. (2003). *Identity Management Systems (IMS): Identification and Comparison Study* (Report 2003-09-07): Independent Centre for Privacy Protection (ICPP) Schleswig-Holstein and Studio Notarile Genghini (SNG). from http://www.datenschutzzentrum.de/idmanage/study/ICPP_SNG_IMS-Study.pdf.

Juels, A. (2006). Technological Approaches to the RFID Privacy Problem. In S. Garfinkel & B. Rosenberg (Eds.), *RFID : Applications, Security, and Privacy* (pp. 329-339). Upper Saddle River, NJ: Addison-Wesley.

Karjoth, G., & Schunter, M. (2002). A Privacy Policy Model for Enterprises: Presentation at the 15th Computer Security Foundations Workshop (CSFW'02), Cape Breton, Nova Scotia, Canada, IBM Research Zurich Research Laboratory.

Kobsa, A., Chellappa, R. K., & Spiekermann, S. (Eds.). (2006). *Proceedings of CHI-2006 Workshop on Privacy-Enhanced Personalization.* Montréal, Canada. from http://www.isr.uci.edu/pep06/ papers/Proceedings_PEP06.pdf

Kobsa, A., & Cranor, L. (Eds.). (2005). *Proceedings of the UM05 Workshop on Privacy-Enhanced Personalization.* Edinburgh, Scotland. http://www.isr.uci.edu/pep05/papers/w9-proceedings.pdf

Mulligan, D., & Schwartz, A. (1999). *Your Place or Mine? Privacy Concerns and Solutions for Server and Client-Side Storage of Personal Information.* In proceedings of the Computers, Freedom & Privacy Conference (pp. 81-84).

Ramakrishnan, N., J.Keller, B., Mirza, B. J., Grama, A. Y., & Karypis, G. (2001). Privacy Risks in Recommender Systems. *IEEE Internet Computing* (Nov-Dec.), 54-62.

Reagle, J., & Cranor, L. (1999). The Platform for Privacy Preferences. *Communications of the ACM, 42*(2), 48-55.

Schreck, J. (2003). *Security and Privacy in User Modeling.* Dordrecht, Netherlands: Kluwer Academic Publishers.

Senicar, V., Jerman-Blazic, B., & Klobucar, T. (2003). Privacy-Enhancing Technologies: Approaches and Development. *Computer Standards & Interfaces, 25*(2), 147-158.

Tavani, H., & Moor, J. (2001). Privacy Protection, Control of Information, and Privacy-Enhancing Technologies. *ACM SIGCAS Computers and Society, 31*(1), 6-11.

Volokh, E. (2000). Personalization, Privacy, and the First Amendment. In CEI Staff (Ed.), *The Future of Financial Privacy: Private Choices versus Political Rules*: CEI.

Warren, S., & Brandeis, L. D. (1890). The Right to Privacy. *Harvard Law Review, 4*(5), 193-220. from http://www.lawrence.edu/fast/boardmaw/Privacy_brand_warr2. html.

Westin, A. F. (1967). *Privacy and Freedom.* New York, NY: Atheneum.

Compilation of References

Abidi, S. S. R. (2002). Designing adaptive hypermedia for internet portals: A personalization strategy featuring case base reasoning with compositional adaptation. In F.J. Garijo, J.C. Riquelme & M Toro (Ed.) *Lecture Notes in Artificial Intelligence 2527: Advances in Artificial Intelligence* (60-69). Berlin: Springer Verlag Press.

Abidi, S. S. R., & Chong, Y. H. (2003). E-healthcare via personalized information services: Addressing the need for factually consistent information. In M.E. Orlowska, S. Weerawarana, M. Papazoglou, J. Yang (Ed.), *Lecture Notes in Computer Science 2910: 1st International Conference on Service Oriented Computing* (pp. 132-148). Berlin: Springer Verlag Press.

Abidi, S. S. R., & Chong, Y. H. (2004). An adaptive hypermedia system for information customization via content adaptation. *IADIS International Journal of WWW/Internet*, 2(1), 79-94.

Abidi, S. S. R., & Zeng Y. (2006). Intelligent information personalization leveraging constraint satisfaction and association rule methods. *19th Canadian Conference on Artificial Intelligence* (pp. 134-145), Berlin: Springer Verlag Press.

Abidi, S. S. R., Chong, Y. H., & Zeng, Y. (2006). Generating customized yet factually consistent information: A constraint satisfaction approach. *Journal of Digital Libraries*, 6(3), 247-259.

Abidi, S. S. R., Han, C. Y., & Abidi, S. R. (2001). Patient empowerment via 'pushed' delivery of personalized healthcare educational content over the internet. *10th World Congress on Medical Informatics*. IOS Press.

Aciar, S., Zhang, D., Simoff, S., and Debenham, J. (2006). *Recommender system based on consumer product reviews*. In Proceedings of the IEEE/WIC/ACM International Conference on Web Intelligence.

Ackerman, M. S. (2000). The Intellectual Challenge of CSCW: The Gap between Social Requirements and Technical Feasibility. Human-Computer Interaction, 15 (2), 179-203.

ADL. (2001). *Sharable Content Object Reference Model Version 1.2: The SCORM Overview*. Retrieved Nov 25, 2007, from http://adlnet.gov/downloads/AuthNoReqd.aspx?FileName= SCORM_1_2_pdf.zip&ID=240.

ADL. (2004). *Sharable Content Object Reference Model (SCORM) Overview*. Retrieved Nov 25, 2007, from http://www.adlnet.gov/donloads/AuthNotReqd.aspx?FileName=SCORM.2004 .3ED.DocSuite.zip&ID=237

ADL. (2004). *Sharable Content Object Reference Model (SCORM) Run Time Environment*. Retrieved Nov 25, 2007, from http://www.adlnet.gov /dowloads/AuthNotReqd.aspx?FileName= SCORM.2004.3ED.DocSuite.zip&ID=237

ADL. (2004). *Sharable Content Object Reference Model (SCORM)*. Retrieved Nov 25, 2007, from http://www.adlnet.gov/dowloads/AuthNotReqd.aspx?FileName=SCORM.2004.3ED.DocSuit.zip&ID=237

Adomavicious, G., and Tuzhilin, A. (1999). User Profiling in Personalization Applications through Rule Discovery and Validation. *In Proceedings of the ACM Fifth International Conference on Data Mining and Knowledge Discovery (KDD'99)*, 377-381.

Agirre, E., Alfonseca, E., and de Lacalle, O. L. (2004). *Approximating hierarchy-based similarity for wordnet nominal synsets using topic signatures.*

Agrawal R. & Wimmers, E. L. (2000). A Framework for Expressing and Combining Preferences.. *Proceedings of ACM SIGMOD*, 297-306

Agrawal, R., Mannila, H., Srikant, R., Toivonen, H., & Verkamo., A. I. (1996). Fast Discovery of Association Rules in Large Databases. *Advances in knowledge discovery and data mining*, (pp. 307-328) MIT Press.

Alani, H., Kim, S., Weal, D. M. M., Hall, P. L. W., and Shadbolt, N. (2003). *Automatic extraction of knowledge from web documents.* In Proceedings of 2nd International Semantic Web Conference - Workshop on Human Language Technology for the Semantic Web abd Web Service.

Alani, H., O'Hara, K., and Shadbolt, N. (2002). *Ontocopi: Methods and tools for identifying communities of practice.*

Al-Khalifa, S., Jagadish H. V., Patel, J. M., Wu, Y., Koudas, N. & Srivastava, D. (2002). Structural Joins: A Primitive for Efficient XML Query Pattern Matching. In *Proceedings of the 18th International Conference on Data Engineering (ICDE)* (pp. 141–154). Los Alamitos, CA: IEEE Computer Society Press.

Alrifai, M., Dolog, P., & Nejdl, W. (2006). Learner profile management for collaborative adaptive eLearning application. *Joint International Workshop on Adaptivity, Personalization and the Semantic Web at 17th ACM Hypertext'06 conference.* ACM Press.

Anderson A. and Blockland A. (1997). Intelligibility of Speech Mediated by Low Frame-Rate Video, in C. Benoit (ed.) *Proceedings of the Audio-Visual Speech Processing Conference*, Rhodes, Greece.

Anderson, C., Domingos, P., & Weld, D. (2001). Adaptive Web Navigation for Wireless Devices. In *Proceedings of the 17th international joint conference on artificial intelligence (IJCAI'01)* (pp. 879-884).

Anderson, C., Domingos, P., & Weld, D. (2001). Personalizing web sites for mobile users. *10th International WWW Conference* (pp. 565-575). ACM Press.

Anderson, C., Domingos, P., & Weld, D. (2002). Relational markov models and their application to adaptive Web navigation. *Proceedings of the Eighth ACM SIGKDD International Conference on Knowledge Discovery and Data Mining* (KDD-2002), Edmonton, Alberta, Canada.

André, E., Rist, T., & Müller, J. (1998) WebPersona: A lifelike presentation agent for the world-wide web. *Knowledge-Based Systems, 11*(1), 25-36.

APEC-FIP. (2004). APEC Privacy Framework (No. 2004/AMM/014rev1): Asia-Pacific Economic Cooperation. from http://www.apecsec.org.sg/.

Apostolou, D., Feldkamp, D., Halaris, C., Hinkelmann, K., Magoutas, B., Papadomichelaki, X., Prackwieser, C., Probst, F., Schmidt, K.U., Stoiljkovic, B., Stoiljkovic, V., Stojanovic, L., Stojanovic, N., Thomas, S. M., Thönssen, B., Utz W., & Woitsch R. (2006). *Deliverable D2, framework for self-adaptive e-government of FIT IST Project.* Available at http://www.fit-project.org/Documents/D2.pdf

Apteker R.T., Fisher J.A., Kisimov V.S., and Neishlos H. Video Acceptability and Frame Rate, *IEEE Multimedia*, 2(3), pp. 32-40, 1995.

Arbanowski, S., Ballon, P., David., K., Droegehorn, O., Eetink, H., Kelleler, W., van Kranenburg, H., Raatikainen, K., & Popescu-Zeletin, R. (2004). I-centric Communications: Personalization, Ambient Awareness, and Adaptability for Future Mobile Services. *IEEE communications Magazine*, 42(9), 63-69

Ardissono, L., & Goy, A. (2000). Tailoring the interaction with users in web stores, *User Modelling and User Adapted Interaction, 10*(4), 251-303.

Arezki, R., Poncelet, P., Dray, G., & Pearson, D. W. (2004) Web information retrieval based on user profile. *Third International Conference on Adaptive Hypermedia and Adaptive Web-Based Systems,* pp. 275-278.

Arlein, R. M., Jai, B., Jakobsson, M., Monrose, F., & Reiter, M. K. (2000). Privacy-Preserving Global Customization. In proceedings of the 2nd ACM Conference on Electronic Commerce (pp. 176-184). Minneapolis, MN.

Armstrong, R., Freitag, D., Joachims, T., and Mitchel, T. (1995). Webwatcher: *A learning apprentice for the world wide web.* In AAAI Spring Synopsium on Information Gathering from Heterogenous, Distributed Environments.

Aroyo, L., Bellekens, P., Bjorkman, M., Broekstra, J., and Houben, G. (2006). *Ontology-based personalisation in user adaptive systems.* In 2nd International Workshop on Web Personalisation Recommender Systems and Intelligent User Interfaces in Conjunction with 7th International Conference in Adaptive Hypermedia.

Atzmueller, M. (2006). *Knowledge-Intensive Subgroup Mining - Techniques for Automatic and Interactive Discovery.* Dissertation, Department of Computer Science, University of Würzburg, Germany.

Ausubel, D. P. (1995). *Educational Psychology: A Cognitive View.* London: Routledge.

Ayersman, D., J. and Reed, W., M. (1998). Relationships among hypermedia-based mental models and hypermedia knowledge, *Journal of Research on Computing in Education*, 30 (3), pp.222-238.

Baader, F., Hoorocks, I. & Sattler, U. (2002). Description Logics for the Semantic Web. *Künstliche Intelligenz*, *16*(4), 57–59.

Baeza-Yates, R. and Ribeiro-Neto, B. (1999). *Modern Information Retrieval.* Addison Wesley.

Bailey C., Hall W., Millard D., & Weal M. (2002). Towards Open Adaptive Hypermedia. *In Proceedings of the Second International Conference on Adaptive Hypermedia and Adaptive Web Based Systems*, Malaga, Spain, LNCS 2347, Springer, pp. 36-46.

Balabanovic, M. (1997) An adaptive web page recommendation service. *First International Conference on Autonomous Agents.* ACM Press, pp. 378-385.

Balabanovic, M. (1998). *Learning to Surf: Multi-agent Systems for Adaptive Web Page Recommendation.* PhD thesis, Department of Computer Science, Stanford University.

Balabanovic, M. and Shoham, Y. (1997*). Fab: Content-based, collaborative recommendation.* Communications of the ACM, 40(3):6672.

Balabanovic, M.Bental, D., Cawsey, A., Pearson, J., & Jones, R. (2000) Adapting web-based information to the needs of patients with cancer. *Adaptive Hypermedia and Adaptive Web-based Systems*, Berlin: Springer-Verlag, pp. 27-37.

Bandura, A. (1986). Social foundations of thought and action: A social cognitive theory. Englewood Cliffs, NJ: Prentice-Hall.

Barlow, D. H. (2002). Anxiety and its disorders: The nature and treatment of anxiety and panic (2nd ed.). New York: The Guilford Press.

Barret, R., Maglio, P. and Kellem, D. (1997). How to Personalize the Web. *In Proceedings CHI 97.*

Barua, S. (2001). An interactive multimedia system on "Computer Architecture, Organization, and Design." *IEEE Transactions on Education, 44,* 41-46.

Basilico J., and Hofmann T. Unifying. (2004). Collaborative and content-based filtering. *In Proceedings of the 21st International Conference on Machine Learning*, Banff, Canada.

Bates, T. (2005). *Technology, e learning and distance education.* London: Routledge.

Bauer, M. and Deru, M. (2005) Motion-Based Adaptation of Information Services for Mobile Users. In L. Ardissono, P. Brna, and T. Mitrovic (Eds.), *LNAI 3538: Proceedings of the 10th International Conference on User Modeling (UM05)* (pp. 271–276). Berlin, Heidelberg: Springer.

Bauer, M., & Baldes, S. (2005). An Ontology-Based Interface for Machine Learning. In: J. Riedl, A. Jameson, D. Billsus, and T. Lau (Eds.), *Proceedings of the 2005 International Conference on Intelligent User Interfaces* (pp. 314–316). New York, NY: ACM Press.

Beaumont I. (1994). User modeling in the interactive anatomy tutoring system ANATOM-TUTOR. *User Models and User Adapted Interaction*, *4*(1), 21-45.

Belkin N.J., & Croft W.B. (1992). Information personalization and information retrieval: Two sides of the same coin? *Communications of the ACM*, *35*(12), 29-38.

Benjamins, V. R., Casanovas, P., Breuker, J. & Gangemi, A. (Eds.) (2005). *Law and the Semantic Web - Legal Ontologies, Methodologies, Legal Information Retrieval, and Applications*, Lecture Notes in Computer Science: Vol. 3369. Heidelberg, Germany: Springer-Verlag.

Berendt, B., & Spiliopoulou, M. (2000). Analysing navigation behaviour in Websites integrating multiple information systems. *VLDB Journal, Special Issue on Databases and the Web*, *9*(1), 56-75.

Berendt, B., Hotho, A., & Stumme, G. (2002). Towards semantic Web mining. *Proceedings of the First International Semantic Web Conference* (ISWC02), Sardinia, Italy.

Berens, L.V. (2002). Multiple models of personality types. *Australian Psychological Type Review*, *4*(1-2), 9-14.

Berkovsky, S., Eytani, Y., Kuflik, T., & Ricci, F. (2005). Privacy-Enhanced Collaborative Filtering. In proceedings of the PEP05, UM05 Workshop on Privacy-Enhanced Personalization (pp. 75-84). Edinburgh, UK.

Berkovsky, S., Eytani, Y., Kuflik, T., & Ricci, F. (2006). Hierarchical Neighborhood Topology for Privacy-Enhanced Collaborative Filtering In proceedings of the PEP06, CHI06 Workshop on Privacy-Enhanced Personalization (pp. 6-13). Montreal, Canada.

Berners-Lee, T., Hendler, J., & Lassila, O. (2001). The Semantic Web, *Scientific American*, *284*(5), 34–43.

Billsus, D. & Pazzani, M. J. (2000) User modeling for adaptive news access. *User Modeling and User Adapted Interaction*, *10*(2-3), 147-180.

Billsus, D., Pazzani, M., & Chen, J. (2000). A learning agent for wireless news access. In Proceedings of the ACM conference on intelligent user interfaces (pp. 33-36).

Blakowski, G. and Steinmetz R. A Media Synchronisation Survey: Reference Model, Specification, and Case Studies, *IEEE Journal on Selected Areas in Communications*, 14(1), pp. 5–35, 1996.

Blanco-Fernndez, Y., Gil-Solla, J. J. P.-A. A., Ramos-Cabrer, M., Barragns-Martnez, B., Garca-Duque, M. L.-N. J., FernndezVilas1, A., and Daz-Redondo, R. P. (2004). *Avatar: An advanced multi-agent recommender system of personalized TV contents by semantic reasoning.* In Web Information Systems WISE 2004, Springer-Verlag.

Blom, J. (2000) Personalization - a taxonomy. In *CHI 2000 Workshop on Designing Interactive Systems for 1-to-1 E-commerce* (pp. 313-314). ACM Press

Bogdanovych, A. & Bauer, M. (2007). *Using Trajectories of Avatars to Predict the Shopping Mood.* (paper submitted).

Bogonicolos N. et al. (1999). ARCHIMIDES : an intelligent agent for adaptive-personilized navigation within a WEB server, *In Proceedings of the 32nd Annual Hawaii Intl. Conf. On System Science, HICSS-32*, Vol 5.

Bollacker, K., Lawrence, S., & Giles, C.L. (1998). Citeseer: An autonomous Web agent for automatic retrieval and identification of interesting publications. *Proceedings of the Second International Conference on Autonomous Agents*, Minneapolis, Minnesota.

Bontcheva, K., Tablan, V., Maynard, D., and Cunningham, H. (2004). *Evolving gate to meet new challenges in language engineering.* Natural Language Engineering, 10.

Bork, A. (2001). Tutorial learning for the new century. *Journal of Science Education and Technology*, *10*(1), 57-71.

Boyle, C., & Encarnacion A. O. (1994). MetaDoc: An adaptive hypertext reading system. *User Models and User Adapted Interaction*, *4*(1), 1-19.

Boyle, E. A., Duffy, T., Dunleavy, K. (2003). Learning styles and academic outcome: The validity and utility of Vermunt's Inventory of Learning Styles in a British higher education setting, *British Journal of Educational Psychology*, 73, 267–290.

Bra, P. D., Aerts A., Berden, B., Lange, B., Rousseau, B., Santic, T., Smits, D., & Stash, N. (2003). *AHA! The Adaptive Hypermedia Architecture.* In Proceedings of the ACM Hypertext Conference, Nottingham, UK, pp 81-84

Bradberry, T., & Greaves, J. (2003). *Can you develop emotional intelligence online?* TalentSmart Inc. Retrieved October 15, 2006, from http://www.talentsmart.com/media/uploads/pdfs/Can%20You%20Develop%20Emotional%20Intelligence%20Online.pdf

Brafman, R, Domshlak, C., & Shimony, S. (2004). Qualitative decision making in adaptive presentation of structured information. *ACM Transactions on Information Systems*, *22*(4), 503-539.

Brannen K. (2001). *Intelligent use of metadata in the questionnaire design process.* In Proceedings of the 2001 New Techniques and Technologies for Statistics Conference.

Bransford, J. D., Brown, A. L., & Cocking, R. R. (Eds.). (2003). *How people learn: Brain, mind, experience, and school.* National Academy Press.

Bratman, M.E. (1987). *Intentions, plans, and practical reason.* Cambridge, MA: Harvard University Press.

Braubach, L., Pokahr, A., & Lamersdorf, W. (2004). Jadex: A short overview. In *Proceedings of the Net.ObjectDays 2004 Conference, AgentExpo* (pp. 195-207).

Braubach, L., Pokahr, A., Moldt, D., & Lamersdorf, W. (2004). Goal representation for BDI agent systems. In *Proceeding of the Second International Workshop on Programming Multiagent Systems (PROMAS-2004)* (pp. 9-20).

Breese, J., Heckerman, D., and Kadie, C. (1998). *Empherical analysis of predictive algorithms for collaborative filtering.* In Proceedings of the Fourteenth Conference on Uncertainty in Artificial Intelligence. Morgan Kaufmann Publisher.

Breuker, J., Tiscornia, D., Winkels, R. & Gangemi, A. (Eds.) (2004). *Journal of Artificial Intelligence and Law*, *12*(4): Special issue on Ontologies for Law.

Brooks, C., Greer, J., Melis, E., & Ullrich, C. (2006). Combining ITS and e-learning technologies: opportunities and challenges. In M. Ikeda, K. Ashley & T-W. Chan (Eds.), *Intelligent Tutoring Systems, 8th International Conference, ITS 2006* (pp. 278-287). Berlin: Springer.

Brooks, C., Winter, C. M., Greer, J., & McCalla, G. (2004). The massive user modelling system (MUMS). In J. C. Lester, R. M. Vicari & F. Paraguaçu (Eds.), *Intelligent Tutoring Systems, 7th International Conference, ITS 2004* (pp. 635-645). Berlin: Springer.

Brusilovsky, P. (1995) Intelligent tutoring systems for World-Wide Web. *Third International WWW Conference*, pp. 42-45

Brusilovsky, P. (1996). Methods and techniques of adaptive hypermedia. *User Modelling and User-Adapted Interaction, 6*(2-3), 87-129.

Brusilovsky, P. (2001). Adaptive hypermedia. *User Modelling and User-Adapted Interaction, 11*(1-2), 87-110.

Brusilovsky, P. (2003). From adaptive hypermedia to the adaptive Web. In J. Ziegler & G. Szwillus (Eds.), *Proceedings of Mensch & Computer 2003: Interaktion in Bewegung* (pp. 30-33). Stuttgart, Germany.

Brusilovsky, P. (2004). Adaptive educational hypermedia: From generation to generation. In M. Grigoriadou et al. (Eds.), *Proceedings of the 4th Hellenic Conference with International Participation in Information and Communication Technologies in Education* (pp. 19-33). New Technologies Publications.

Brusilovsky, P. (2004). *KnowledgeTree: A distributed architecture for adaptive e-learning.* Paper presented at the 13th International World Wide Web Conference, Alternate Track Papers & Posters.

Brusilovsky, P. and Pesin, L. (1998). Adaptive navigation support in educational hypermedia: An evaluation of the ISIS-Tutor, *Journal of Computing and Information Technology* 6 (1), 27-38.

Brusilovsky, P., A. Kobsa & Nejdl, W. (Ed).(2006). The adaptive web: Methods and strategies of web personalization. Berlin: Springer Verlag Press.

Brusilovsky, P., Eklund, J. and Schwarz, E. (1998). Web-based education for all: A tool for developing adaptive courseware. Computer Networks and ISDN Systems. Proceedings of the 7th International WWW Conference, 14-18 April, 30(1-7), 291-300.

Brusilovsky, P., Kobsa, A., & Vassileva, J. (Ed.) (1998). Adaptive hypermedia and hypertext. Dordrecht:Kluwer Academic Publishers.

Brusilovsky, P., Schwarz, E., & Weber, G. (1996). *ELM-ART: An Intelligent Tutoring System on World Wide Web.* In Third International Conference on Intelligent Tutoring Systems, ITS-96, Montreal, 1996

Brusilovsky, P.,and Peylo C. (2003). Adaptive and Intelligent Web-based Educational Systems, *International Journal of Artificial Intelligence in Education* 13, 156-169.

Buffett, S., Jia, K., Liu, S., Spencer, B., & Wang, F. (2004). Negotiating Exchanges of P3P-Labeled Information for Compensation. Computational Intelligence, 20 (4), 663-677.

Bull, S., & Kay, J. (2007). Student Models that Invite the Learner In: The SMILI Open Learner Modelling Framework. *International Journal of Artificial Intelligence in Education, 17*(3), 89-120.

Bull, S., Brna, P., & Pain, H. (1995). Extending the Scope of the Student Model. *User Modeling and User-Adapted Interaction, 5*(1), 45-65.

Bull, S., Quigley, S., & Mabbott, A. (2006). Computer-Based Formative Assessment to Promote Reflection and Learner Autonomy. *Engineering Education: Journal of the Higher Education Academy Engineering Subject Centre, 1*(1), 1-18.

Bulterman D.C.A., Rutledge L., Hardman L., & Ossenbruggen J. (1999). Supporting adaptive and adaptable hypermedia presentantion semantics, *Database Semantics* 8 Submission.

Buriano, L., Marchetti, M., Carmagnola, F., Cena, F., Gena, C., and Torre, I. (2006). *The role of ontologies in context-aware recommender systems.* In 7th International Conference on Mobile Data Management.

Burke, R. (2000). Knowledge-based recommender systems. In A. Kent (Ed.), *Encyclopedia of Library and Information Systems,* 69(32), New York: Marcel Dekker.

Burke, R. (2002) Hybrid recommender systems: Survey and experiments. *User Modeling and User-Adapted Interaction, 12*(4), 331-370.

Burke, R., Hammond, K., & Young, B. (1997). The FindMe Approach to Assisted Browsing. *Journal of IEEE Expert,* 12(4), 32-40.

Burton, L., & Goldsmith, D. (2002). *Students' experience in online course: A study using asychronous online focus groups.* Newington: Connecticut Distance Learning Consortium.

Buswell, S., Caprotti, O., Carlisle, D.P., Dewar, M. G., & Kohlhase, M. (2004). *The OpenMath Standard* (Standard): The OpenMath Society.

Callan, J., Smeaton, A., Beaulieu, M., Borlund, P., Brusilovsky, P., Chalmers, M., Lynch, C., Riedl, J., Smyth, B., Straccia, U. & Toms, E. (2003). *Personalization and recommender systems in digital libraries. Joint NSF-EU DELOS Working Group Report.* Sophia Antipolis, France: ERCIM. Retrieved January 15, 2008, from http://www.ercim.org/publication/ws-proceedings/Delos-NSF/Personalisation.pdf

Calvi, L. & Bra, P. D. (1997). Proficiency-adapted information browsing and filtering in hypermedia educational systems. *User Modeling and User Adapted Interaction, 7*(4), 257-277.

Camp, J., & Osorio, C. (2003). Privacy-Enhancing Technologies for Internet Commerce. In O. Petrovic, M. Ksela, M. Fallenböck & C. Kittl (Eds.), Trust in the Network Economy (pp. 317-331). Wien: Springer.

Canny, J. (2002). Collaborative Filtering with Privacy via Factor Analysis. In proceedings of the 25th Annual International ACM SIGIR Conference on Research and Development in Information Retrieval (SIGIR 2002) (pp. 238 - 245). Tampere, Finland.

Canny, J. (2002). Collaborative Filtering with Privacy. In proceedings of the IEEE Conference on Security and Privacy (pp. 45- 57). Oakland, CA.

Cantador, I. and Castells, P. (2006). *A multilayered ontology-based user profiles and semantic social networks for recommender systems.* In 2nd International Workshop on Web Personalisation Recommender Systems and Intelligent User Interfaces in Conjunction with 7th International Conference in Adaptive Hypermedia.

Cap Gemini (2006). *Online Availability of Public Services: How is Europe Progressing?* Web- based Survey on Electronic Public Services, Report of the 6th Measurement

CAP Gemini Ernst and Young. (2004). Online Availability of Public Services: How is Europe Progressing? European Commission DG Information Society.

Cappiello, C., Missier, P., Pernici, B., Plebani, P., & Batini, C. (2004). *Qos in multichannel IS: the mais approach.* In Proceedings of the International Workshop on Web Quality (WQ'04), Munich, Germany, 2004

Carbonell, J. R. (1970). AI in CAI: An artificial intelligence approach to computer assisted instruction. *IEEE Transactions on Man Machine Systems, MMS-11*(4), 190-202.

Card, S. K., Mackinlay J. D., & Shneiderman B. (1999). *Information Visualization: Using Vision to Think.* Morgan-Kaufmann, San Francisco, California.

Cardoso, J., Sheth, A., Miller, J., Arnold, J., & Kochut, K. (2002). *Modeling quality of service for workflows and web service processes.* Journal of Web Semantics

Carmagnola, F., Cena, F., Gena, C., and Torre, I. (2005). *A multidimensional approach for the semantic representation of taxonomies and rules in adaptive hypermedia systems.* In PerSWeb05 Workshop on Personalization on the Semantic Web in conjunction with UM05.

Carmichael, D. J., Kay, J. & Kummerfeld, B. (2005). Consistent modeling of users, devices and sensors in ubiquitious computing environment. *User Modeliing and User-Adapted Interaction, 15*, 197-234

Carter, E. W. (2002). Doing the best you can with what you have: Lessons learned from outcomes assessment. *Journal of Academic Librarianship 28*, 36-41.

Casanovas, P., Biasiotti, M. A., Francesconi, E. & Sagri, M.T. (2007). In *Proceedings of the Second ICAIL Legal Ontologies and Artificial Intelligence Techniques Workshop (LOAIT).* IAAIL Workshop Series. Oisterwijk, The Netherlands: Wolf Legal Publishers.

Cassady, C.C. (2004). The influence of cognitive test anxiety across the learning–testing cycle, *Learning and Instruction 14,* 569–592.

Chaffee J., & Gauch S. (2000). Personal Ontologies for Web Navigation, *ACM 2000*, 1-58113-320-0/00/11.

Chakrabarti, S., Dom, B., Gibson, D., Kleinberg, J., Raghavan, P., & Rajagopalan, S. (1998). Automatic resource list compilation by analyzing hyperlink structure and associated text. *Proceedings of the 7th International World Wide Web Conference*, Brisbane, Australia.

Chakrabarti, S., van den Berg, M., & Dom, B. (1999). Focused crawling: A new approach to topic-specific Web resource discovery. *Proceedings of the 3rd World Wide Web Conference*, Toronto.

Chan Núñez, M. E. (2004). *Modelo mediacional para el diseño educativo en línea.* Guadalajara, Jalisco: INNOVA, Universidad de Guadalajara.

Chandra, S.; Ellis, C., S.; & Vahdat, A., (2000). Application-level differentiated multimedia Web services using quality aware transcoding. *IEEE Journal on Selected Areas in Communications,* 18(12), pp. 2544-2565.

Chang, H.H., Henriquez, A., Honey, M., Light, D., Moeller, B., & Ross, N. (1998). *The Union City story:*

Education reform and technology students' performance on standardized tests. New York: Center for Children and Technology.

Chang, S. E. (2005). Computer anxiety and perception of task complexity in learning programming-related skills, *Computers in Human Behavior 21,* 713–728.

Chedrawy, Z. & Abidi, S. S. R. (2006). An adaptive personalization recommendation strategy featuring context-sensitive content adaptation. *International Conference on Adaptive Hypermedia and Adaptive Web-based Systems*, Springer Verlag Press.

Chedrawy, Z. & Abidi, S. S. R. (2006). Case based reasoning for information personalization: Using a context-sensitive case Adaptation Approach. *IEEE International Conference on Engineering of Intelligent Systems*, IEEE Press.

Chen, L. and Sycara, K. (1998). *Webmate: A personal agent for browsing and searching.* In 2nd International Conference on Autonomous Agents, Minneapolis MN USA.

Chen, S.Y. (2002). A cognitive model for non-linear learning in hypermedia programmes. *British Journal of Educational Technology, 33*, 449-460.

Chen, S.Y. and Macredie, R.D. (2002). Cognitive Styles and Hypermedia Navigation: Development of A Learning Model. *Journal of the American Society for Information Science and Technology* 53 (1) 3-15.

Chen, S.Y., & Ford, N.J. (1998). Modelling user navigation behaviours in a hypermedia-based learning system: An individual differences approach. *International Journal of Knowledge Organization, 25*(3), 67-78.

Cheverst, K., Mitchell, K., & Davies, N. (2002). The role of adaptive hypermedia in a context-aware tourist guide. *Communications of the ACM, 45*(5), 47-51.

Chi, E. H. (2000). A Taxonomy of Visualization Techniques using the Data State Reference Model. *Proceedings of the IEEE Symposium on Information Visualization 2000 (InfoVis'00)*, 69-75

Chittaro, L. & Ranon R. (2002). Dynamic Generation of Dynamic VRML Content: a General Approach and its Application to 3D E-Commerce. Proceedings of Web3D Conference, pp. 145-154.

Chittaro, L. & Ranon, R. (2000) Adding adaptive features to virtual reality interfaces for e-commerce. *Adaptive Hypermedia and Adaptive Web-based Systems*, Berlin: Springer-Verlag, pp. 86-91.

Chittaro, L., & Cin, P. D. (2002). Evaluating interface design choices on wap phones: Navigation and selection. *Personal and ubiquitous computing*, 6 (4), 237–244.

Chopra, V., Bakore, A., Eaves, J., Galbraith, B., Li, S., & Wiggers, C. (2004). *Professional Apache Tomcat 5.* Published by Wrox, ISBN 0764559028, May 17, 2004

Chuang, Y-R. Teaching in a Multimedia Computer Environment: A study of effects of learning style, gender, and math achievement, 1999. Available: http://imej.wfu.edu./articles/1999/1/10/index/asp [21/12/2001]

Church, K., Smyth, B., Cotter, P., & Bradley, K. (2007). Mobile Information Access: A Study of Emerging Search behaviour on the Mobile Internet. ACM Transactions on the Web, 1 (1).

Cingil I., Dogac A., and Azgin A. (2000). A broader approach to personalization, *Communications of the ACM*, Vol. 43, No. 8.

Clark, R., & Lyons, C. (1999). Using Web-based training wisely. *Training, 36*(7), 51-61.

Clarkson, B. (2002). *Life Patterns: structure from wearable sensors.* PhD thesis, School of Architecture and Planning, Massachusetts Institute of Technology, Cambridge, MA, USA.

Claypool, M., Gokhale, A., Miranda, T., Murnikov, P., Netes, D., & Sartin, M. (1999). Combining content-based and collaborative filters in an online newspaper. *Proceedings of the ACM SIGIR '99 Workshop on Recommender Systems: Algorithms and Evaluation*, Berkeley, California.

Clerkin, P., Cunningham, P., & Hayes, C. (2001). Ontology discovery for the semantic Web using hierarchical clustering. *Semantic Web Mining Workshop at ECML/PKDD-2001*, Freiburg, Germany.

Composite Capability/Preference Profiles (CC/PP): Structure and Vocabularies 2.0. The World Wide Web Consortium (W3C) (2007). Retrieved from http://www.w3.org/TR/2007/WD-CCPP-struct-vocab2-20070430/

Cook, R., & Kay, J. (1994). The Justified User Model: A Viewable, explained user model. In *Proceedings of the Fourth International Conference on User Modeling* (pp. 145 - 150). Hyannis MA, The MITRE Corporation.

Cooley, R., Mobasher, B., & Srivastava, J. (1997). Web mining: Information and pattern discovery on the World Wide Web. *Proceedings of the International Conference on Tools with Artificial Intelligence*, 558-567, Newport Beach. IEEE Press.

Cooley, R., Mobasher, B., & Srivastava, J. (1999). Data preparation for mining World Wide Web browsing patterns. *Journal of Knowledge and Information Systems, 1*(1), 5-32.

Cornelis, B. (2003). *Personalizing search indigital libraries.* Unpublished master's thesis, University of Maastricht, Maastricht, The Netherlands.

Corradini, F., Angelis, F. D., Polzonetti, A., Re, B., & Brugnoni, E. (2006). *e-GovQoS: an Ontology for Quality of e-Government Services.* In 5th International EGOV Conference 2006, DEXA, Krakow (Poland), pp. 171-178, September 2006.

Couper, M. (2001). *Web Surveys: The Questionnaire Design Challenge.* In Proceedings of the 53rd session of the ISI, http://134.75.100.178/isi2001/

Coyle, M., & Smyth, B. (2005). Explaining Search Results. In *Proceedings of the 19th international joint conference on artificial intelligence (IJCAI '05)* (pp. 1553-1555). Edinburgh, Scotland.

Coyle, M., & Smyth, B. (2007). On the community-based explanation of search results. In D. N. Chin, M. X. Zhou, T. A. Lau, & A. R. Puerta (Eds.), *Proceedings of the ACM conference on Intelligent user interfaces* (pp. 282-285). ACM.

Coyle, M., & Smyth, B. (2007). Supporting intelligent navigation in web search. ACM Transactions on Internet Technology (TOIT). Dourisboure, Y., Geraci, F., & Pellegrini, M. (2007). Extraction and classification of dense communities in the web. In *WWW '07: Proceedings of the 16th international conference on world wide web* (pp. 461–470). New York, NY, USA: ACM.

Cranley, N., Murphy, L., & Perry, P. (2003). User-perceived quality-aware adaptive delivery of MPEG-4 content, *Proceedings of the 13th international workshop on Network and operating systems support for digital audio and video*, 42-49, Monterey, CA.

Cranor, L. F. (2003). 'I Didn't Buy it for Myself': Privacy and Ecommerce Personalization. In proceedings of the 2003 ACM Workshop on Privacy in the Electronic Society. Washington, DC.

Craven, M., DiPasquo, D., Freitag, D., McCallum, A., Mitchell, T., Nigam, K., & Slattery, S. (2000). Learning to construct knowledge bases from the World Wide Web. *Artificial Intelligence, 118*(1-2), 69-113.

Dai, H., & Mobasher, B. (2002). Using ontologies to discover domain-level Web usage profiles. *Proceedings of the 2nd Semantic Web Mining Workshop at ECML/PKDD 2002*, Helsinki, Finland.

Damasio, A. (1999). *The feeling of what happens: Body and emotion in the making of consciousness.* Hartcourt.

Damasio, A. R. (1994). Descartes' error: Emotion, reason, and the human brain. New York: Putnam Publishing Group.

Damjanovic, V., Kravcik, M., & Devedzic, V. (2005). An approach to the realization of personalized adaptation by using eQ agent system. In *Proceedings of UM'2005 Workshop on Personalized Adaptation on the Semantic Web (PerSWeb'05)* (pp. 116-125).

Damjanovic, V., Kravcik, M., & Gasevic, D. (2005). eQ through the FOSP method. In *Proceedings of the ED-MEDIA 2005 World Conference on Educational Multimedia, Hypermedia and Telecommunications* (pp. 3080-3088). Montreal, Canada.

Daugherty, M., & Funke, B.L. (1998). University faculty and student perceptions of Web-based instruction. *Journal of Distance Education, 13*(1), 21-39.

Davidson, J., & Coward, D. (1999). *Java servlet specification v2.2*. Sun Press, 1999.

Davis, B., Sumara, D., & Luce-Kapler, R. (2000). *Engaging minds: Learning and teaching in a complex world.* Lawrence Erlbaum Associates.

Davis, S., & Abidi, S. S. R. (2006). Adaptive patient education framework featuring personalized cardiovascular risk management interventions. *International Conference on Adaptive Hypermedia and Adaptive Web-based Systems,* Berlin: Springer Verlag Press.

Davis, S., & Abidi, SSR (2006). Tailoring cardiovascular risk management educational interventions: A synergy of SCORE risk assessment and behavior change model. *11th International Symposium for Health Information Management Research*, pp. 66-78.

Dawes, S. (2002). *The Future of E-Governmen.t* Center for Technology in Government, Albany, NY: Center for Technology in Government.

De Bra P., Brusilovsky P., and Houben G. (1999). Adaptive Hypermedia: From systems to framework, *ACM Computing Surveys* 31(4).

De Bra, P. and Calvi, L. (1998). AHA ! An open Adaptive Hypermedia Architecture. *The New Review of Hypermedia and Multimedia*, 4, Taylor Graham Publishers, pp. 115-139.

De Carolis, B., Cozzolongo, G., & Pizzutilo, S. (2005). Generating personalized tourist map descriptions. In M. Ali and F. Esposito (Ed.): *Lecture Notes in Artificial Intelligence 3533*, Berlin: Springer Verlag, pp. 259–268.

de Paula, R. r., Ding, X., Dourish, P., Nies, K., Pillet, B., Redmiles, D. F., et al. (2005). In the Eye of the Beholder: A Visualization-based Approach to Information System Security. International Journal of Human-Computer Studies, 63 (1-2), 5-24.

De Roure, D., & Hendler, J.A. (2004). E-science: The grid and the Semantic Web. *IEEE Intelligent Systems, 19*(1), 65-71.

De Roure, D., Jennings, N.R., & Shadbolt, N.R. (2005). The semantic grid: Past, present and future. *Proceedings of the IEEE, 93*(3), 669-681.

Delicato F., Pirmez L., and Carmo L. (2001). Fenix–personalized information filtering system for WWW pages, Internet Research: Electronic Networking Applications and Policy, Vol. 11, No. 1, pp. 42-48.

Demetriadis, S., Triantafilou, E., and Pombortis, A. A Phenomenographic Study of Students' Attitudes Toward the Use of Multiple Media for Learning, *ACM SIGCSE Bulletin, Proceedings of the 8th annual conference on Innovation and technology in computer science education*, June 30 – July 2 2003, Thessaloniki, Greece, pp 183 – 187, 2003.

Demetriou, A. and Kazi, S. (2001). Unity and modularity in the mind and the self: Studies on the relationships between self-awareness, personality, and intellectual development from childhood to adolescence. London: Routdledge.

Demetriou, A., Efklides, A. and Platsidou, M. (1993). The architecture and dynamics of developing mind: Experiential structuralism as a frame for unifying cognitive development theories. *Monographs of the Society for Research in Child Development*, 58 (Serial No. 234), 5-6.

Denaux, R., Dimitrova, V., & Aroyo, L. (2004). *Interactive Ontology-based User Modeling for Personalized Learning Content Management.* In Workshop on Applications of Semantic Web technologies for E-Learning (SWEL) held in conjunction with Adaptive Hypermedia 2004

Derry, S. J. (1990). Learning strategies for acquiring useful knowledge. In B.F. Jones & L. Idol (Eds.), *Dimensions of thinking and cognitive instruction* (pp. 347-379). Hillsdale: Lawrence Erlbaum Associates.

DE-TML. (2007). German Telemedia Law. from http://www.gesetze-im-internet.de/tmg/.

Devedzic, V. B. (2003). Key issues in next-generation Web-based education. *IEEE Transactions on Systems, Man, and Cybernetics - Part C: Applications and Reviews, 33*(3), 339-349.

Device Management Working Group. Open Mobile Alliance (2007). Retrieved from http://www.openmobilealliance.org/tech/wg_committees/dm.html

Devitt, A., Danev, B., & Matusikova, K. (2006, December). *Constructing Bayesian Networks Automatically using Ontologies.* Paper presented at the Second Workshop Formal Ontologies Meet Industry (FOMI), Trento, Italy

Dichev, C., & Dicheva, D. (2005). Contexts in Educational Topic Maps. In C.K. Looi, G. McCalla, B. Bredeweg & J. Breuker (Eds.), *12th International Conference on Artificial Intelligence in Education* (pp. 789–791). Amsterdam: IOS Press.

DiGioia, P., & Dourish, P. (2005). Social Navigation as a Model for Usable Security. In proceedings of the Symposium on Usable Privacy and Security SOUPS 2005 (pp. 101-108). Pittsburgh, PA.

Dilley, R. (1999). The Problem of Context. New York: Berghahn Books.

Dobson, G., Lock, R., & Sommerville, I. (2005). *QoSOnt: a QoS ontology for service-centric systems.* In: EUROMICRO-SEAA'05.

Dobson, S., Massacci, F., Denazis, S., Nixon, P., Fernandez, A., Saffre, F., Gaiti, D., Schmidt, N., Gelenbe, E., & Zambonelli, F., (2006). A Survey of Autonomic Communications. *ACM Transactions on Autonomous and Adaptive Systems*, 1(2), 223–259.

Dolog, P, Henze, N, Nejdl, W., & Sintek, M. (2004). The personal reader: Personalizing and enriching learning resources using semantic web technologies. *International Conference on Adaptive Hypermedia and Adaptive Web-Based Systems*, Berlin: Springer Verlag.

Dolog, P. and Schafer, M. (2005). *Learner modelling on the semantic web.* In PerSWeb05 Workshop on Personalization on the Semantic Web in conjunction with UM05.

Dolog, P., Henze, N., Nejdl, W., & Sintek, M. (2003). Towards the adaptive semantic Web. In *Proceedings of Principles and Practice of Semantic Web Reasoning, International Workshop, PPSWR 2003,* Mumbai, India.

Dolog, P., Henze, N., Nejdl, W., & Sintek, M., (2004). *Personalization in distributed e-learning environments.* In WWW Alt. '04: Proceedings of the 13th International World Wide Web Conference on Alternate Track Papers & Posters, New York, NY (pp. 170–179). New York, NY: ACMvPress.

Domik G. O., & Gutkauf B (1994). User modeling for adaptive visualization systems. In R. Daniel Bergeron and Arie E. Kaufman, editors, *Proceedings of the IEEE Conference on Visualization.*

Dourish, P., & Anderson, K. (2006). Collective Information Practice: Exploring Privacy and Security as Social and Cultural Phenomena. Human-Computer Interaction, 21 (3), 319-342.

Dourish, P., Grinter, R. E., Dalal, B., Flor, J. D. d. l., & Joseph, M. (2004). Security Day-to-Day: User Strategies for Managing Security as an Everyday, Practical Problem. Personal Ubiquitous Computing, 8 (6), 391-401.

Doyle, D., Cunningham, P., Bridge, D., & Rahman, Y. (2004). Explanation Oriented Retrieval. In P. A. G. Calero & P. Funk (Eds.), *Proceedings of the European conference on case-based reasoning (ECCBR-04).* Springer. (Madrid, Spain)

Drucker, P. (1989). *New realities.* New York: Harper & Row.

Dumais, S., Cutrell, E., Cadiz, J.J., Jancke, G., Sarin, R., & Robbins, D.C. (2003). Stuff I've seen: a system for personal information retrieval and re-use. In *SIGIR '03: Proceedings of the 26th annual international ACM SIGIR conference on Research and development in information retrieval* (pp. 72–79). New York, NY: ACM Press.

ECeG Project (2003). The "Semantic web techniques for the management of digital identity and the access to norms" PRIN Project Home Page. Retrieved January 15, 2008, from http://www.cirsfid.unibo.it/eGov03/

ECeGov (n.d.). The European Commission e-Government Home Page. Retrieved January 15, 2008, from http://europa.eu.int/information_society/eeurope/2005/all_about/egovernment/index_en.htm

eGovernment Unit, DG Information Society, European Commission, (2004). *Top of the web: user satisfaction and usage survey of egovernment services.* Available online from Europe's Information Society Thematic Portal Web site: http://europa.eu.int/information_society/activities/egovernment_research/doc/top_of_the_web_report_2004.pdf

Eirinaki M., & Vazirgiannis M. (2003). Web Mining for Web Personalization, *ACM Transactions on Internet Technology*, Vol. 3, No. 1, Pages 1-27.

Eklund J. and Sinclair K. (2000). An empirical appraisal of the effectiveness of adaptive interfaces of instructional systems. *Educational Technology and Society* 3 (4), ISSN 1436-4522.

Ellis, R. D., & Kurniawan, S.H. (2000). Increasing the usability of online information for older users. A case study in participatory design. *International Journal of Human-Computer Interaction, 12*(2), 263-276.

Erickson, T. (2002). Some problems with the notion of context-aware computing. *Communications of the ACM*, 45(2), pp. 102-104.

ETSI OSA Phase 4 (Draft Parlay 6.0 Specifications) (2007). ETSI Retrieved from http://portal.etsi.org/docbox/TISPAN/Open/OSA/Parlay60.html

EU. (1995). Directive 95/46/EC of the European Parliament and of the Council of 24 October 1995 on the Protection of Individuals with Regard to the Processing of Personal Data and on the Free Movement of such Data. Official Journal of the European Communities (23 November 1995 No L. 281), 31ff. from http://158.169.50.95:10080/legal/en/dataprot/directiv/directiv.html.

EU. (2002). Directive 2002/58/EC of the European Parliament and of the Council Concerning the Processing of Personal Data and the Protection of Privacy in the Electronic Communications Sector. from http://register.consilium.eu.int/pdf/en/02/st03/03636en2.pdf.

Evans, C., Gibbons, N.J., Shah, K., & Griffin, D.K. (2004). Virtual learning in the biological sciences: Pitfalls of simply putting notes on the Web. *Computers and Education, 43*, 49-61.

Evans, D., W.Hersh, Monarch, I., Lefferts, R., and Henderson, S. (1991). *Automatic indexing of abstracts via natural-language processing using a simple thesaurus.* Medical Decision Making, 11(3):108-115.

Farzan, R., Coyle, M., Freyne, J., Brusilovsky, P., & Smyth, B. (2007). Assist: adaptive social support for information space traversal. In S. Harper et al. (Eds.), *Proceedings of International conference on hypertext* (pp. 199-208). ACM.

Felder, R.M., and Silverman, L.K. (1988). Learning and Teaching Styles in Engineering Education, *Engineering Education* 78: 674-681.

Feldman, S., & Sherman, C. (2000). The High Cost of Not Finding Information. In (IDC White Paper). IDC Group. Fu, X., Budzik, J., & Hammond, K. (2000). Mining Navigation History for Recommendation. In *Proceedings of conference on intelligent user interfaces* (pp. 106-112).

Fensel, D. (2001): Ontologies: a silver bullet for knowledge management and electronic commerce. Springer, Berlin.

Finch, S. and Chater, N. (1994). *Learning syntactic categories: A statistical approach.* In Oaksford, M. and Brown, G., editors, Neurodynamics and Psychology. Academic Press.

Fink, J. & Kobsa, A. (2002). User modeling in personalized city tours. *Artificial Intelligence Review, 18*, 33-74,

Fink, J., & Kobsa A. (2002). Putting personalization into practice, *Communications of the ACM, 45*(5), 41-42.

Fischer G., Lemke A., Mastaglio T., & Morch A. (1991). The role of Critiquing in Coorporative Problem Solving. *ACM Transactions on Information Systems* (9), 123 – 151

Flavell, J. H. (1979). Metacognition and Cognitive Monitoring: A New Area of Cognitive-Development. *American Psychologist, 34*(10), 906-911.

Flechsig, K.-H. (1996). *Kleines Handbuch didaktischer Modelle (Small manual of didactical models)*. Eichenzell: Neuland.

Foner, L. N. (1997). Yenta: A Multi-Agent Referral-Based Matchmaking System. In proceedings of the International Conference on Autonomous Agents (pp. 301-307). Marina del Rey, CA.

Ford, N., & Miller, D. (1996). Gender differences in Internet perceptions and use. *Aslib Proceedings, 48*, 183-192.

Ford, N.,Wood, F.,Walsh, C. (1994). Cognitive styles and searching. Online CD-ROM Rev. 18(2), 79–86.

Fox, M.S., Gruninger, M. (1998). Enterprise Modelling. *AI Magazine, American Association for AI*, pp. 109-121

Frankowski, D., Cosley, D., Sen, S., Terveen, L., & Riedl, J. (2006). You Are What You Say: Privacy Risks of Public Mentions. In proceedings of the 29th Annual International ACM SIGIR Conference on Research and Development in Information Retrieval (pp. 565-572). Seattle, WA.

Freire, P. (1999). *Psicología del Oprimido*. México City: Editorial Siglo XXI.

Frias-Martinez, E., Magoulas, G., Chen, S. & Macredie, R. (2006). Automated user modeling for personalized digital libraries. *International Journal of Information Management*, *26*(3), 234–248.

FTC. (2000). Online Profiling: A Report to Congress. from http://www.ftc.gov/os/2000/07/ onlineprofiling.pdf.

FTC. (2000, May 2000). Privacy Online: Fair Information Practices in the Electronic Marketplace. A Report to Congress. from http://www.ftc.gov/reports/privacy2000/privacy2000.pdf.

FTC. (2000). The Seven Safe Harbor Principles. from http://europa.eu.int/comm/internal_ market/en/media/dataprot/news/shprinciples.pdf.

Fukuda, K., Wakamiya, N., Murata, M., and Miyahara, H., QoS Mapping between User's Preference and Bandwidth Control for Video Transport, in *Proceedings of the 5th International Workshop on QoS*, Paris, France, pp. 291-301, 1997.

Furnas, G. W., Landauer, T. K., Gomez, L. M., & Dumais, S. T. (1987). The vocabulary problem in human-system communication. *Communications of the ACM*, 30(11), 964-971.

Gabber, E., Gibbons, P. B., Matias, Y., & Mayer, A. (1997). How to Make Personalized Web Browsing Simple, Secure, and Anonymous. In Financial Cryptography'97 (Vol. 1318). Berlin - Heidelberg - New York: Springer Verlag.

Ganesan, P., Garcia-Molina, H., & Widom, J. (2003). Exploiting hierarchical domain structure to compute similarity. *ACM Transactions on Information Systems, 21*(1), 63-94.

Garofalakis, M. N., Ozden B. Ä, and Silberschatz A. (1998). On Periodic Resource Scheduling for Continuous Media Databases, *In Proceedings of the 8th International Workshop on Research Issues in Data Engineering*, February.

Gauch, S., Chaffee, J. & Pretschner, A. (2003). Ontology-Based User Profiles for Search and Browsing. *Web Intelligence and Agent Systems, 1*(3-4), 219–234.

Gay, G. (1986). Interaction of learner control and prior understanding in computer-assisted video instruction. *Journal of Educational Psychology, 78*(3), 225-227.

Gemmell D.J., Vin H.M., Kandlur D.D., Rangan P.V., and Rowe L.A. (1995). Multimedia Storage Servers: *A Tutorial. IEEE Computer*, 28(5):40{49, May.

Gemmell, J., Bell, G., Lueder, R., Drucker, S., & Wong, C. (2002). MyLifeBits: Fulfilling the Memex Vision. In *Proceedings of ACM Multimedia '02* (pp. 235–238), Juan-les-Pins, France.

Germanakos, P, Tsianos, N, Lekkas, Z, Mourlas, C, and Samaras, G. (2007). Capturing Essential Intrinsic User Behaviour Values for the Design of Comprehensive Web-based Personalized Environments, *Computers in Human Behavior Journal*, Special Issue on Integration of Human Factors in Networked Computing, doi:10.1016/j.chb.2007.07.010.

Germanakos, P, Tsianos, N, Lekkas, Z, Mourlas, C, Belk, M, & Samaras, G. (2007). An AdaptiveWeb System for Integrating Human Factors in Personalization of Web Content. *Demonstration in the Proceedings of the 11th International Conference on User Modeling (UM2007)*, Corfu, Greece, June 25-29.

Germanakos, P., Tsianos, N., Mourlas, C., and Samaras, G. (2005). New Fundamental Profiling Characteristics for Designing Adaptive Web-based Educational Systems, *In Proceeding of the IADIS International Conference on Cognition and Exploratory Learning in Digital Age (CELDA2005)*, Porto, December 14-16, pp. 10-17.

Getoor, L., Friedman, N., Koller, D., & Taskar, B. (2001). Learning probabilistic models of relational structure. *Proceedings of the 18th International Conference on Machine Learning.*

Ghani, R., & Fano, A. (2002). Building recommender systems using a knowledge base of product semantics. *Proceedings of the Workshop on Recommendation and Personalization in E-Commerce*, 2nd International Conference on Adaptive Hypermedia and Adaptive Web Based Systems, Malaga, Spain.

Ghinea, G and Thomas, J P., QoS Impact on User Perception and Understanding of Multimedia Video Clips, in *Proceedings of ACM Multimedia '98*, Bristol, United Kingdom, pp. 49-54, 1998.

Gibbons, A. S., & Fairweather, P. G. (2000). Computer-based instruction. In S. Tobias & J. D. Fletcher (Eds.), *Training & Retraining: A Handbook for Business, Industry, Government, and the Military*: MacMillan Reference Books.

Gilburd, B., Schuster, A., & Wolff, R. (2004). k-TPP: A New Privacy Model for Large-Scale Distributed Environments. In proceedings of the 10th ACM SIGKDD International Conference on Knowledge Discovery and Date Mining (KDD'04) (pp. 563-568). Seattle, WA.

Giugno, R., & Lukasiewicz, T. (2002). P-SHOQ(D): A probabilistic extension of SHOQ(D) for probabilistic ontologies in the semantic Web. *Proceedings of the 8th European Conference on Logics in Artificial Intelligence*, Cosenza, Italy.

Godoy, D. & Amandi, A. (2005). User Profiling for Web Page Filtering. *IEEE Internet Computing, 9*(4), 56–64.

Godoy, D. and Amandi, A. (2006). *Modeling user interests by conceptual clustering.* Information Systems. Elsevier Science, 31(4):247265.

Goggins, S. P., Laffey, J., & Tsai, I.-C. (2007). Cooperation and groupness: community formation in small online collaborative groups. In *Group '07: Proceedings of the 2007 International ACM conference on conference on supporting group work* (pp. 207–216). New York, NY, USA: ACM.

Goleman, D. (1995). Emotional Intelligence: why it can matter more than IQ, New York: Bantam Books.

Golemati, M., Katifori, A., Vassilakis, C., Lepouras, G. & Halatsis, C. (2007). Creating an Ontology for the User Profile: Method and Applications. In *Proceedings of the First IEEE International Conference on Research Challenges in Information Science (RCIS)* (pp. 407–412). Los Alamitos, CA: IEEE Computer Society Press.

Gomes, P., B. Antunes, L. R., Santos, A., Barbeira, J., and Carvalho, R. (2006). *Using ontologies for elearning personalization.* In eLearning Conference.

Gonczi, A., & Athanasou, J. (1996). Instrumentación de la educación basada en competencias. Perspectivas de la teoría y la práctica en Australia. In A. Argüelles (Ed.), *Competencia laboral y educación basada en normas de competencia* (pp. 265-288). México: Limusa y Noriega Editores.

Gong, Z., Cheang, C. W., and U, L. H. (2005). *Web query expansion by wordnet.* In Database and Expert Systems Applications, Springer Verlag, pages 166-175.

Grandi, F., Mandreoli, F., & Tiberio, P. (2005). Temporal Modelling and Management of Normative Documents in XML Format. *Data & Knowledge Engineering, 54*(3), 327–354.

Grandi, F., Mandreoli, F., Bergonzini, M. & Tiberio, P. (2003). A Temporal Data Model and Management System for Normative Texts in XML Format. In R. H. L. Chiang, A. H. F. Laender & E.-P. Lim (Eds.), *Proceedings of the Fifth ACM Intlernational Workshop on Web Information and Data Management (WIDM)* (pp. 29–36). New York, NY: ACM Press.

Grandi, F., Mandreoli, F., Martoglia, R., Ronchetti, E., Scalas, M. R. & Tiberio, P. (2006). An eGovernment System for Temporal- and Semantic-aware Access to Norms. In A. Abecker, A. Sheth, G. Mentzas & L. Stojanovic (Eds.), *Semantic Web meets eGovernment: Papers from the AAAI Spring Symposium (SWEG)* (pp. 80–86). Menlo Park, CA: AAAI Press.

Grandi, F., Mandreoli, F., Scalas, M. R. & Tiberio, P. (2004). *Management of the Citizen's Digital Identity and Access to Multi-version Norm Texts on the Semantic Web*. Paper presented at the International Symposium on Challenges in the Internet and Interdisciplinary (IPSI), Pescara, Italy.

Grandi, F., Scalas, M. R., Mandreoli, F. & Martoglia, R. (2005). Personalized Access to Multi-version Documents for E-Government Applications. In P. Isaías, P. Kommers & M. McPherson, *Proceedings of IADIS International Conference e-Society 2005* (pp. 553–558). Lisbon, Portugal: IADIS Press.

Gruber T. (1993). *A Translation Approach to Portable Ontology Specifications*. Knowledge Acquisition, 5(2), 199-220.

Grust, T. (2002). Accelerating XPath Location Steps. In M. J. Franklin, B. Moon & A. Ailamaki, *Proceedings of the 2002 ACM SIGMOD International Conference on Management of Data* (pp. 109–120). New York, NY: ACM Press.

Guarino, N. (1998). *Formal Ontology in Information Systems*. Amsterdam, The Netherlands: IOS Press.

Guinness, D. L. & Harmelen E. F. (2003). *OWL Web Ontology Language Overview*. W3C Proposed Recommendation, http://www.w3.org/TR/2003/PR-owl-ref-20031215/, December 15, 2003.

Gulliver, S., R., and Ghinea, G. (2004). Stars in their Eyes: What Eye-Tracking Reveals about Multimedia Perceptual Quality, *IEEE Transactions on Systems*, Man and Cybernetics, Part A, 34(4), 472-482.

Haarslev, V., & Möller, R. (2001). *RACER System Description*. In: Goré R., Leitsch A., Nipkow T. (Eds.) International Joint Conference on Automated Reasoning (IJCAR 2001), Siena. Springer-Verlag, 2001, pp. 701–705.

Han, J., & Fu, Y. (1995). Discovery of multiple-level association rules from large databases. *Proceedings of the 1995 International Conference on Very Large Data Bases* (VLDB95), Zurich, Switzerland.

Hanani, U., Shapira, B., & Shoval, P. (2001). Information filtering: Overview of issues, research and systems. *User Modeling and User-Adapted Interaction, 11*, 203-259.

Hedberg, J.G., & Corrent-Agostinho, S. (2000). Creating a postgraduate virtual community: Assessment drives learning. *Educational Media International, 37*(2), 83-90.

Henderson, L. (1972). Spatial and verbal codes and the capacity of STM. *Quarterly Journal of Experimental Psychology*, 24, (pp. 485-495).

Henke, H. (2001). Applying Kolb's Learning Style Inventory with Computer Based Training.

Henze, N., & Nejdl, W. (2003). *Logically characterizing adaptive educational hypermedia systems*. In *Proceeding of the International Workshop of Adaptive Hypermedia and Adaptive Web-based Systems (AH 2003),* Budapest, Hungary.

Herder, E. (2003). Modelling User Navigation. In *Proceedings of the 9th International Conference on User Modelling* (pp. 417-419). Springer-Verlag.

Herlocker, J. L., Konstan, J. A., & Riedl, J. (2000). Explaining collaborative filtering recommendations. In *Proceedings of the International conference on computer supported cooperative work*. 241–250.

Herlocker, J., & Konstan, J. (2001). Content-Independent Task-Focused Recommendation. IEEE Internet Computing, 5(6), 40 - 47.

Herlocker, J., Konstan, J., Borchers, A., & Riedl, J. (1999). An algorithmic framework for performing collaborative filtering. *Proceedings of the 22nd ACM Conference on Research and Development in Information Retrieval* (SIGIR'99), Berkeley, CA.

Herlocker, J., Konstan, J., Borchers, A., and Reidl, J. (1999). *An algorithmic framework for performing collaborative filtering.* In Proceedings of the Conference on Research and Development in Information Retrieval.

Hicks M., Nagarjan A., and Renesse R.. User-specified Adaptive Scheduling in a Streaming Media Network. OpenARCH'03. San Francisco, CA. April 2003.

Hitchens, M., Kay, J., Kummerfeld, B., & Brar, A. (2005). Secure Identity Management for Pseudo-Anonymous Service Access. In proceedings of the Security in Pervasive Computing: Second International Conference (pp. 48-55). Boppard, Germany.

Hjelsvold R., Vdaygiri S., and Leaute Y. (2001). Web –based personalization and management of interactive video, ACM 1-58113-348-0/01/0005.

Hodgins, W. (2005). *Grand challenges for learning objects.* Presentation at Learntec, Karlsruhe, Germany.

Hohl, H., Bocker, H., Gunzenhauser, R. (1996). HYPADAPTER: An adaptive hypertext system for exploratory learning and programming, *User Modelling & User Adapted Interaction*, *6*(2), 131-156.

Holz, H., Maus, H., Bernardi, A., & Rostanin, O. (2005). A lightweight approach for proactive, task-specific information delivery. In *Proceedings of I-KNOW 2005 –Special Track on Business Process Oriented Knowledge Infrastructures BPOKI.*

Hong H. and Kinshuk. (2004). Adaptation to Student Learning Styles in Web Based Educational Systems, *In L. Cantoni & C. McLoughlin, (Eds.) Proceedings of ED-MEDIA 2004–World Conference on Educational Multimedia, Hypermedia & Telecommunications* (June 21-26, 2004, Lugano, Switzerland).

Horrocks, I. & Patel-Schneider, P. F. (2003). Reducing OWL Entailment to Description Logic Satisfiability. In D. Fensel, K. P. Sycara & J. Mylopoulos (Eds.), *The Semantic Web - ISWC 2003, Second International Semantic Web Conference* (pp. 17–29). Lecture Notes in Computer Science: Vol. 2870. Heidelberg, Germany: Springer-Verlag.

Horrocks, I. (2002). DAML+OIL: A description logic for the semantic Web. *IEEE Data Engineering Bulletin, 25*(1), 4-9.

Horrocks, I., & Sattler, U. (2001). Ontology reasoning in the SHOQ(D) description logic. *Proceedings of the 17th International Joint Conference on Artificial Intelligence*, Seattle, WA.

Horvitz, E., Dumais, S., & Koch, P. (2004). Learning predictive models of memory landmarks. In *Proceedings of the CogSci 2004: 26th Annual Meeting of the Cognitive Science Society.* Chicago, USA.

Hotho, A., Maedche, A., & Staab, S. (2001). Ontology-based text clustering. *Proceedings of the IJCAI-2001 Workshop Text Learning: Beyond Supervision*, Seattle, WA.

Houssos, N., Alonistioti, N., & Merakos, L. (2005). Specification and dynamic introduction of 3rd party, service-specific adaptation policies for mobile applications. *Mobile Networks and Applications*, 10(4), pp. 405-421.

Houssos, N., Gazis, E., Panagiotakis, S., Gessler, S., Schuelke, A., & Quesnel, S., (2002). *Value Added Service Management in 3G networks.* Paper presented at Network Operations and Management Symposium, Florence, Italy.

Hu, Z., Chin, W., & Takeichi, M. (2000). Calculating a New Data Mining Algorithm for Market Basket Analysis. *Lecture Notes in Computer Science*, (Vol. 1753, pp.169–175) Springer-Verlag.

Huber, M. J. (1999). JAM: A BDI-theoretic mobile agent architecture. In *Proceedings of the 3rd Conference on Autonomous Agents* (pp. 236–243). New York, NY: ACM Press.

Hudson, L. Contrary Imaginations, Penguin, Harmondsworth, 1966.

Huedo E. , Montero R. , Llorente I., A framework for adaptive execution in grids, In Software: Practice and Experience, Vol. 34, No 7, pp. 631 - 651, 2004, John Wiley & Sons.

Hui, S., & Cheung, K.P. (1999). Developing a Web-based learning environment for building energy efficiency and solar design in Hong Kong. *Solar Energy, 67*(1-3), 151-159.

Hull, C. L. (1943). *Principles of behavior.* New York: Appleton-Century-Crofts.

IBM. (2003). IBM Tivoli Privacy Manager for E-Business. from http://www-306.ibm.com/software/ tivoli/products/ privacy-mgr-e-bus/.

IEEE PAPI. (2001). IEEE 1484.2.1, Standard for Learning Technology - Public and Private Information (PAPI) for Learners (PAPI Learner) - Core Features.

IEEE. (2002). *1484.12.1 Draft Standard for Learning Object Metadata.*

Igel, C., & Daugs, R. (2002). Mehrwertpotenziale Internetbasierter Lehre (Added value capabilities of Internet-based teaching). In K. P. Jantke, W. S. Wittig, & J. Herrmann (Eds.), *Vom e-Learning bis e-Payment: Das Internet als sicherer Marktplatz (From e-learning to e-payment: The Internet as a safe marketplace)* (pp. 8–19). Berlin: infix.

Igel, C., & Daugs, R. (2003). eLearning in der Bewegungs- und Trainingswissenschaft: Das Engineering des BMBF-Projektes "eBuT" (eLearning in movement and training science: The engineering of the project eBut backed by the Federal Ministry of Education and Resarch). *dvs Informationen, 18*(3), 5–8.

Igel, C., & Daugs, R. (2003). Zur Individualisierung Internetbasierter Lehr-Lern-Prozesse: Didaktische Überlegungen und technologische Entwicklungen im BMBF-Projekt "eBuT" (Individualization of Internet-based teaching-learning processes: Didactical considerations and technological developments in the eBUT). In U. Beck & V. Sommer (Eds.), *Learntec 2003: 11. Europäischer Kongress und Fachmesse für Bildungs- und Informationstechnologie* (pp. 253–258). Karlsruhe: Holler Verlag.

Igel, C., & Daugs, R. (Eds.). (2005). *eLearning in der Sportwissenschaft: Strategien, Konzeptionen, Perspektiven (eLearning in sports science: Strategies, conceptual design, prospects).* Schorndorf: Hofmann.

Igel, C., & Sturm, R. (2003). Server-Architektur, Autorensystem, Datenbanken, Assets: Die Informations infrastruktur des Projektes "eBuT" (Server architecture, authoring tool, databases, assets: The information infrastructure of the eBut). *dvs Informationen, 18*(3), 9–13.

Ishitani, L., Almeida, V., & Wagner, M., Jr. (2003). Masks: Bringing Anonymity and Personalization Together. IEEE Security & Privacy Magazine, 1 (3), 18-23. from DOI 10.1109/MSECP.2003. 1203218.

Jadav D., Srinilta C., and Choudhary A. (1997). Batching and dynamic allocation techniques for increasing the stream capacity of an on-demand media server. *Parallel Computing - Special Issue on parallel processing and multimedia*, 23(12):1727{1742, December.

Jadav D., Srinilta C., Choudhary A., and Berra Bruce P.(1997). An evaluation of design tradeo®s in a high performance media-on-demand server. *Multimedia Systems*, 5(1):53{68, 1997b 17.

Jameson, A., & Smyth, B. (2007). Recommendation to groups. In P. Brusilovsky, A. Kobsa, & W. Nejdl (Eds.), *The adaptive web* (Vol. 4321, pp. 596-627). Springer-Verlag.

Jank, W., & Meyer, H. (2002). *Didaktische Modelle (Didactical models).* Frankfurt a.M.: Cornelsen.

Jankun, T. J., & Kwan, L. M. (2003). MoireGraphs: Radial Focus+Context Visualization and Interaction for Graphs with Visual Nodes, *IEEE Symposium on Information Visualization, Seattle, Washington*

Jantke, K. P. (2003, June 13). Knowledge discovery & data mining: Lehren und Lernen im Internet (Knowledge discovery & dat mining: Teaching and learning in the Internet). In *Köthener Informatik-Tag*. Köthen: FH Anhalt.

Jantke, K. P. (2004, June 3-4). Neue Technologien: Potentiale und Probleme illustriert an Anwendungen des e-Learning (eingeladener Hauptvortrag) (New technologies: Potentials and problems illustrated on eLearning applications – invited speech). In *Wismarer Wirtschaftsinformatik-Tage, WIWITA 2004*.

Jantke, K. P. (2004, June 3-4). ROI: Das unlösbare Problem des e-Learning (ROI: The unsolvable problem of eLearning). In *Wismarer Wirtschaftsinformatik-Tage, WIWITA 2004*.

Jantke, K. P. (2005). Informatik und Künstliche Intelligenz: Beiträge zur Adaptivität einer kommenden Generation intelligenter eLearning-Systeme (Information technology and artificial intelligence: Contributions on adptivity of a coming generation of intelligent eLearning systems). In C. Igel & R. Daugs (Eds.), *eLearning in der Sportwissenschaft: Strategien, Konzeptionen, Perspektiven (eLearning in sports science: Strategies, conceptual design, prospects)* (pp. 49–70). Schorndorf: Hofmann.

Jantke, K. P., & Knauf, R. (2005, January 3-6). Didactic design through storyboarding: Standard concepts for standard tools. In *Proceedings of the First International Workshop on Dissemination of E-Learning Technologies and Applications,* Cape Town, South Africa.

Jantke, K. P., & Lunzer, A. (2005). Search, comparison and evaluation in exploratory e-learning with subjunctive interfaces. In *Proceedings of the 3rd Conference on Professional Knowledge Management, 1st Workshop on Learner-Oriented Knowledge Management and KM-Oriented E-Learning,* Kaiserslautern, Germany.

Jantke, K. P., Degel, G., Grieser, G., Memmel, M., Rostanin, O., & Tschiedel, B. (2004, September 29 - October 1). Technology enhanced dimensions in e-learning. In M.E. Auer & U. Auer (Eds.), *International Conference on Interactive Computer Aided Learning, ICL 2004* (CD). Villach, Austria.

Jantke, K. P., Grieser, G., & Lange, S. (2004, September 29 - October 1). Adaptation to the learners' needs and desires by induction and negotiation of hypotheses. In M.E. Auer & U. Auer (Eds.), *International Conference on Interactive Computer Aided Learning, ICL 2004* (CD), Villach, Austria.

Jantke, K. P., Grieser, G., & Memmel, M. (2004, October 4-6). DaMiT: Data Mining lernen und lehren (Learning and teaching data mining). In *Lernen, Wissensentdeckung und Adaptivität (Learning, Knowledge detection and adaptivity)* (LWA-2004), Fachgruppentreffen Maschinelles Lernen (FGML). Berlin.

Jantke, K. P., Lange, S., Grieser, G., Grigoriev, P., Thalheim, B., & Tschiedel, B. (2004, April 14-17). Learning by doing and learning when doing. In I. Seruca, J. Filipe, S. Hammoudi, & J. Cordeiro (Eds.), *Proceedings of the International Conference on Enterprise Information Systems* (Vol. 5, pp. 238–241), Porto, Portugal. INSTICC.

Jantke, K. P., Lange, S., Grieser, G., Grigoriev, P., Thalheim, B., & Tschiedel, B. (2004, September 27-30). Work-integrated e-learning: The DaMiT approach. In O. Sawodny & P. Scharff (Eds.), *Proceedings of the 49 Internationales Wissenschaftliches Kolloquium, TU* (Vol. 2, pp. 333–339). Shaker Verlag.

Jantke, K. P., Memmel, M., Rostanin, O., & Rudolf, B. (2004, November 1-5). Media and service integration for professional e-learning. In *Proceedings of the E-Learn 2004, World Conference on E-Learning in Corporate, Government, Healthcare & Higher Education,* Washington, DC.

Jantke, K. P., Memmel, M., Rostanin, O., Thalheim, B., & Tschiedel, B. (2003). Decision support by learning-on-demand. In *CAiSE Workshop 2003*, Klagenfurt, Österreich.

Jin, X., & Mobasher, B. (2003). Using semantic similarity to enhance item-based collaborative filtering. *Proceedings of The 2nd IASTED International Conference on Information and Knowledge Sharing,* Scottsdale, Arizona.

Joachims, T., Freitag, D., & Mitchell, T. (1997). Webwatcher: A tour guide for the World Wide Web. *Proceedings of the 15th International Conference on Artificial Intelligence*, Nagoya, Japan.

Jonassen, D.H., & Grabowski, B.L. (1993). *Handbook of individual differences, learning, and instruction.* Hillsdale: Lawrence Erlbaum Associates.

Jørstad, I., Van Thanh, D., & Dustdar, D. (2006). *Personalisation of Next Generation Mobile Services.* Paper presented at Ubiquitous Mobile Information and Collaboration Systems (UMICS2006), Luxembourg, June 5-6.

Jørstad, I., Van Thanh, D., (2006). Service Personalisation in Mobile Heterogeneous Environmnents. In *Advanced International Conference on Telecommunications AICT-ICIW '06. International Conference on Internet and Web Applications and Services* (pp. 70-70). IEEE Computer Society

Kaplan, B., Farzanfar, R. and Friedman R.H. (1999). Research and Ethical Issues Arising from Ethnographic Interviews of Patients' Reactions to an Intelligent Interactive Telephone Health Behavior Advisor System, *In: Ngwenyama, O., Introna, L.D., Myers, M.D. and DeGross, J.I. (Eds) New Information Technologies in Organizational Processes: Field Studies and Theoretical Reflections on the Future of Work*, Boston: Kluwer Academic Publishers, 67-77.

Karat M.C., Brodie C., Karat J., Vergo J., and Alpert S.R. (2003). Personalizing the user experience on ibm.com. *IBM Systems Journal*, Vol. 42, No. 4, 2003

Karat, J., Karat, C.-M., Brodie, C., & Feng, J. (2005). Privacy in Information Technology: Designing to Enable Privacy Policy Management in Organizations. International journal of Human-Computer Studies, 63, 153-174. from DOI 10.1016/j.ijhcs.2005.04.011.

Katifori, A., Halatsis, C., Lepouras, G., Vassilakis, C. & Giannopoulou, E. (2007). Ontology Visualization Methods-A Survey. *ACM Computing Surveys* (39) 4, 2007.

Kautz, H., Selman, B., and Shah, M. (1997). *Referral web: Combining social networks and collaborative filtering.* Communications of the ACM, 40(3):6365.

Kay, J. (2006). Scrutable Adaptation: Because We Can and Must. In Adaptive Hypermedia and Adaptive Web-Based Systems (pp. 11-19): Springer Berlin / Heidelberg.

Kay, J., & Lum, A. (2004). Ontologies for scrutable student modelling in adaptive e-learning. In L. Aroyo & D. Dicheva (Eds.), *Proceedings of the AH (Adaptive Hypermedia and Adaptive Web-Based Systems) 2004 Workshop on Applications of Semantic Web Technologies* (pp. 292-301). Department of Mathematics and Computer Science, TU/e Technische Universiteit Eindhoven, 2004.

Kay, J., Kummerfeld, B., & Lauder, P. (2003). Managing private user models and shared personas. In proceedings of the Workshop on User Modelling for Ubiquitous Computing, 9th International Conference on User Modeling (pp. 1-11).

Ke, H., Kwakkelaarb, R., Taic, Y., & Chenc, L. (2002) Exploring behavior of e-journal users in science and technology: Transaction log analysis of Elsevier's ScienceDirect OnSite in Taiwan. *Library & Information Science Research*, *24*(3), 265-291.

Keeffe, I., Conlan, O., Dagger, D., & Wade V. (2005). *Dynamically Adapting Multimedia Content using Strategically-driven Generic Adaptive Services.* ACM Multimedia 2005, Singapore, November (Submitted)

Kellerer, W., Hirschfeld, R., Tarlano, A. & Wagner, M. (2003, June). *Towards a Personalized Service Provisioning Environment.* Paper presented at the IST Mobile Communications Summit Aveiro, Portugal.

Kellerer, W., Wagner, M., Balke, W., Schulzrinne H. (2003). Preference-based Session Management for Personalized Services. *European Transactions on Telecommunications*, 15(4), pp. 415-427.

Khaleel A. and Reddy A. (1999). Evaluation of data and request distribution policies in clustered servers, *In Proceedings of the High Performance Computing*, 1999.

Khalifa, M., & Lam R. (2002). Web-based learning: Effects on learning process and outcome. *IEEE Transactions on Education, 45*, 350-356.

Kim W. (2002). Personalization: Definition, Status, and Challenges Ahead, Published by ETH Zurich, Chair of Software Engineering JOT, ©2002, Vol. 1, No. 1.

Klavans, J., Chodrow, M., and Wacholder, N. (1992). *Building a knowledge base from parsed definitions.* In Jansen, K., Heidorn, G., and Richardson, S., editors, Natural Language Processing: The PLNLP Approach. Kluwer Academic Publishers.

Klein, B., & Weber, G. (2002, March 3-5). Die Realisierung von Adaptivität mit dem Internet-Autorensystem NetCoach (The realization of adaptivity with the Internet authoring tool NetCoach). In U. Rinn & J. Wedekind (Eds.), *Referenzmodelle netzbasierten Lehrens und Lernens (Models of reference on net-based teaching and learning)* (pp. 101–118). Münster: Waxmann.

Klein, M. C. A. & Fensel, D. (2001). *Ontology versioning on the Semantic Web.* In I. F. Cruz, S. Decker, J. Euzenat & D. L. McGuinness (Eds.), *Proceedings of SWWS 2001, The first Semantic Web Working Symposium* (pp. 75–91). Amsterdam, The Netherlands: IOS Press.

Knight, K. and Luk, S. (1994*). Building a large scale knowledge base for machine translation.* In Proceedings of the Thirteenth National Conference on Artificial Intelligence, pages 773-778. AAAI Press.

Knostan, J., Miller, B., D.Maltz, Herlocker, J., Gordon, L., and Riedl, J. (1997). *Grouplens: Applying collaborative filtering to Usenet news.* Communications of the ACM, 40(3):7787.

Knublauch, H. & Horridge, M. (2005). *The Protégé-OWL API.* Available at http://protege.stanford.edu/plugins/owl/api/index.html

Knublauch, H., Fergerson, R.W., Noy, N.F., & Musen, M.A. (2004). *The Protege OWL Plugin: An open development environment for Semantic Web applications.* Semantic Web - Iswc 2004, Proceedings 2004;3298:229-243.

Kobsa, A. (2001) Tailoring privacy to user's needs. In: M. Bauer, P. J. Gmytrasiewicz, J. Vassileva (Ed.), *Lecture Notes on Artificial Intelligence 2109*, Berlin: Springer-Verlag, pp. 303-313.

Kobsa, A. (2001). Generic User Modeling Systems. *User Modeling and User-Adapted Interaction, 11*(1-2), 49–63.

Kobsa, A. (2002). Personalization and International Privacy. Communications of the ACM, 45 (5), 64-67. from DOI 10.1145/767193.767196.

Kobsa, A. (2003). A Component Architecture for Dynamically Managing Privacy in Personalized Web-based Systems. In proceedings of the Privacy Enhancing Technologies: Third International Workshop (Vol. LNCS 2760, pp. 177-188). Dresden, Germany. from DOI: 10.1007/b94512.

Kobsa, A. (2007). *Privacy-enhanced web personalisation.* In Brusilovsky P., Kobsa A., Nejdl W. (Eds.): The Adaptive Web: Methods and Strategies of Web Personalisation, Springer-Verlag, Heidelberg, Germany, pp. 628-670

Kobsa, A. (2007). Privacy-Enhanced Personalization. *Communications of the ACM, 50*(8), 24-33.

Kobsa, A., & Pohl, W. (1995). The BGP-MS User Modeling System. *User Modeling and User-Adapted Interaction, 4*(2), 59-106.

Kobsa, A., & Schreck, J. (2003). Privacy through Pseudonymity in User-Adaptive Systems. ACM Transactions on Internet Technology, 3(2), 149-183.

Kobsa, A., Koenemann, J., & Pohl, W. (2001). Personalized Hypermedia Presentation Techniques for Improving Online Customer Relationships. *The Knowledge Engineering Review, 16*(2), 111-155.

Kobsa, A., Muller, D., & Nill, A. (1994). KN-AHS: An adaptive hypermedia client of the user modeling system BGP-MS. *Fourth International Conference on User Modeling*, pp. 99-105.

Koch, M. (1994). No girls allowed! *Technos, 3,* 14-19.

Kohlhase, M. (2006). *OMDoc—An Open Markup Format for Mathematical Documents (version 1.2)*: Springer Verlag.

Kolb, A.Y., and Kolb, D.A. (2005). The Kolb Learning Style Inventory–Version 3.1 2005 Technical Specifications, Experience Based Learning Systems, Inc.

Konstan, J., Miller, B., Maltz, D., Herlocker, J., Gorgan, L., & Riedl, J. (1997). GroupLens: Applying collaborative filtering to usenet news. *Communications of the ACM*, 40(3), 77-87.

Kort, B., and Reilly, R. (2002). Analytical Models of Emotions, Learning and Relationships: Towards an Affect-Sensitive Cognitive Machine. *Conference on Virtual Worlds and Simulation (VWSim 2002),* [on-line]: http://affect.media.mit.edu/projectpages/lc/vworlds.pdf.

Kouvelas, I., Hardman, V., and Watson, A., Lip Synchronisation for use over the Internet: Analysis and Implementation, in *Proceedings of IEEE Globecom '96*, London, United Kingdom, retrieved from the World Wide Web: http://www-mice.cs.ucl.ac.uk/multimedia/publications.

Kraigher-Hozo, M. (1991). *Painting / Painting methods / Materials*. Sarajevo: Svjetlost Publications.

Krause, M., Hochstatter, I. (2005). Challenges in Modelling and Using Quality of Context (QoC). In *Mobility Aware Technologies and Applications, Second International Workshop, MATA* 17-19 October 2005, Montreal, Canada

Kravcik, M. (2004). The specification of adaptation strategy by FOSP method. In *Proceedings of AH2004 Conference,* Eidhoven, The Netherlands.

Kravcik, M., Specht, M., & Oppermann, R. (2004). Evaluation of WINDS authoring environment. In *Proceedings of the Adaptive Hypermedia 2004 Conference* (pp. 166-175). Eidhoven, The Netherlands.

Kröner, A., & Basselin, N. (2006). Situated Views on Augmented Memories. In P. Isaias, M.B. Nunes, I.J. Martinez (Eds.), *Proceedings of the IADIS International Conference WWW/Internet 2006* (vol. 2, pp. 272–277), Murcia, Spain.

Krüger, A., Baus, J., Heckmann, D., Kruppa, M., & Wasinger, R. (2007). *Adaptive Mobile Guides*. In Brusilovsky P., Kobsa A., Nejdl W. (eds.): The Adaptive Web: Methods and Strategies of Web Personalization. Berlin, Heidelberg, New York: Springer (ISBN: 978-3540720782), 2007, pp. 521-549.

Kuo, F. F., & Shan, M. K. (2002). A personalized music filtering system based on melody style classification. *IEEE international Conference on Data Mining*, pp. 649–652.

Kuwahara, N., Noma, H., Kogure, K., Hagita, N., Tetsutani, N., & Iseki, H. (2003). Wearable autoevent-recording of medical nursing. In *Proceedings of the Ninth IFIP TC13 International Conference on Human-Computer Interaction (INTERACT 2003).*

Laing, M. Teaching Learning and Learning Teaching: An Introduction to Learning Styles. *New Frontiers in Education* 31(4), 463-475, 2001.

Lamming, M., & Flynn, M. (1994). Forget-Me-Not: Intimate computing in support of human memory. In *Proceedings of FRIEND21, the 1994 International Symposium on Next Generation Human Interface*, Meguro Gajoen, Japan.

Lang, K. (1995). *Newsweeder: Learning to filter Netnews.* In 12th International Conference on Machine Learning.

Lankhorst M.M., Kranenburg, Salden A., and Peddemors A.J.H. (2002). Enabling Technology for Personalizing Mobile Services, *In Proceedings of the 35th Annual Hawaii International Conference on System Sciences* (HICSS-35'02).

Larson, K., & Czerwinski, M. (1998). Web Page Design: Implications of memory, structure and scent for information retrieval. In *Proceedings of the CHI'98 human factors in computer systems* (pp. 25-32). ACM Press.

Last, D.A., O'Donnell, A.M., & Kelly, A.E. (2001). The effects of prior knowledge and goal strength on the use of hypermedia. *Journal of Educational Multimedia and Hypermedia, 10*(1), 3-25.

Laukkanen, M. (2004). *Semantic Web Technologies in Context-Aware Systems* (Seminar Paper). Department of Computer Science, University of Helsinki.

Lawrence, S., & Giles, C. L. (1998). Context and page analysis for improved web search. *IEEE Internet Computing*, July-August, 38-46.

Lawrie, D. and Croft, W. (2000). *Discovering and comparing topic hierarchies.* In Proceedings of RIAO.

LeActiveMath Consortium. (2007). Language-Enhanced, User-Adaptive, Interactive eLearning for Mathematics. Retrieved June 22, 2007, from http://www.leactivemath.org

Lecolinet, E., Likforman-Sulem, L., Roberrt, L., Role, F., & Lebrave, J-L, (1998). An Integrated Reading and Editing Environment for Scholarly Research on Literary Works and their Handwritten Sources. *Proceedings of ACM Digital Libraries Conference.*

Lee B.Y.J. (1998). Parallel video servers: A tutorial. IEEE Multimedia, 5(2):20{28, 1998.

Lee, B., Klemmer, S. R., & Brafman, R. (2006). *Adaptive interfaces for declarative presentation of heterogeneous content.* Technical Report CSTR 2006-10 09/29/06, Stanford University, HCI Group, Stanford, CA, USA.

Lehmann, J., Biasiotti, M. A., Francesconi, E. & Sagri, M. T. (Eds.) (2005). *Proceedings of the First ICAIL Legal Ontologies and Artificial Intelligence Techniques Workshop (LOAIT)*, IAAIL Workshop Series. Oisterwijk, The Netherlands: Wolf Legal Publishers.

Lerner, J. S., & Keltner, D. (2000). Beyond valence: Toward a model of emotion specific influences on judgment and choice. *Cognition and Emotion*, 14, 473–493.

Lewis, C., & Polson, P.G. (1990). Theory-based design for easily learned interfaces. *HCI, 5*, 191-220.

Lewis, D., Feeney, K., Tiropanis, T., & Courtenage, S. (2004). Semantic-based Policy Engineering for Autonomic Systems. In: Smirnov, Michael, (Ed.), *Autonomic Communication: First International IFIP Workshop, WAC 2004: revised selected papers* (pp. 152-164). Lecture Notes in Computer Science (3457). Springer, Berlin, Germany.

Liaw, S.-S. (2002). An Internet survey for perceptions of computers and the World Wide Web: Relationship, prediction, and difference. *Computers in Human Behavior, 18,* 17-35.

Lieberman, H. (1995). Letizia: An Agent That Assists Web Browsing. *In 1995 International Joint Conference on Aritifical Intelligence*, Montreal, CA.

Likert, R. (1932). *A Technique for the Measurement of Attitudes.* Archives of Psychology 140, 55.

Lin C-S, Shu W., and Wu Y. M. (1999). Performance study of synchronization schemes on parallel cbr video servers, *In Proceedings of the Seventh ACM International Multimedia Conference*, November.

Lin, D. and Pantel, P. (2001*). Induction of semantic classes from natural language text.* In Knowledge Discovery and Data Mining, pages 317-322.

Linard, M., & Zeillger, G. (1995). Designing navigational support for educational software. *Proceedings of Human Computer Interactions* (pp. 63-78).

Liu Y. and Ginther, D. (1999). Cognitive Styles and Distant Education. *Online Journal of Distance Learning Administration*, Vo. 2(3)..

Loh, S., Wives, L.K., & de Oliveira, J.P. (2000). Concept-based knowledge discovery in texts extracted from the Web. *SIGKDD Explorations, 2*(1), 29-39.

Lyman, P., & Varian, H. R. (2003). How much information. Retrieved from http://www.sims.berkeley.edu/how-much-info-2003 on January 14th, 2005.

Maamar, Z.,Al Khatib, G., Mostefaoui, S., K. (2004), *Context-based Personalization of Web Services Composition and Provisioning,* Paper presented at the Euromicro Conference, Rennes, France.

Maedche, A. and Staab, S. (2001). *Ontology learning for the semantic web.* IEEE Intelligent Systems, 18(2):72-79.

Maedche, A., & Staab, S. (2000). Discovering conceptual relations from text. *Proceedings of the European Conference on Artificial Intelligence* (ECAI00), Berlin.

Maedche, A., Ehrig, M., Handschuh, S., Volz, R., & Stojanovic, L. (2002). Ontology-focused crawling of documents and relational metadata. *Proceedings of the 11th International World Wide Web Conference* (WWW02), Honolulu, Hawaii.

Maglio P., and Barret, R. (2000). Intermediaries Personalize Information Streams, Communications of the ACM, Vol. 43(8), pp. 96-101.

Magoutas, B., Halaris, C., & Mentzas, G. (2007). *An Ontology for the Multi-Perspective Evaluation of Quality in E-government Services.* In Sixth International EGOV Conference 2007, Regensburg (Germany), September 3-7, 2007.

Malin, B., Sweeney, L., & Newton, E. (2003). Trail Re-Identification: Learning Who You Are From Where You Have Been (Technical Report No. LIDAP-WP12). Pittsburgh, PA: Carnegie Mellon University, Laboratory for International Data Privacy. from http://privacy.cs.cmu.edu/ people/sweeney/trails1.pdf.

Mamoulis, N., Yiu, M., L., Cheng K. H. & Cheung D. W. (2007). Efficient top-k aggregation of ranked inputs. *ACM Transactions on Database Systems* (32) 3.

Mandreoli, F., Martoglia, R., & Ronchetti, E. (2006). Supporting Temporal Slicing in XML Databases. In Y. E. Ioannidis, M. H. Scholl, J. W. Schmidt, F. Matthes, M. Hatzopoulos, K. Böhm, A. Kemper, T. Grust & C. Böhm (Eds.), *Advances in Database Technology - EDBT 2006. 10th International Conference on Extending Database Technology* (pp. 295–312). Lecture Notes in Computer Science: Vol. 3896. Heidelberg, Germany: Springer-Verlag.

Mandreoli, F., Martoglia, R., Grandi, F., & Scalas, M. R. (2007). Efficient Management of Multi-version XML Documents for e-Government Applications. In J. Filipe, J. Cordeiro & V. Pedrosa (Eds.), *Web Information Systems and Technologies – International Conferences WEBIST 2005/2006. Revised Selected Papers* (pp. 283–294). Lecture Notes in Business Information Processing: Vol. 1. Heidelberg, Germany: Springer-Verlag.

Maneewatthana, T., Wills, G., & Hall W. (2006). *Adaptation in Adaptable Personal Information Environment.* In Adaptive Hypermedia and Adaptive Web-Based Systems, June 20th - June 23rd, 2006, Dublin, Ireland.

Marian, A., Amer-Yahia, S., Koudas, N., Srivastava, D. (2005). Adaptive Processing of Top-k Queries in XML. Proceedings of the 21st International Conference on Data Engineering, 162-173.

Marrison, D. L. and Frick, M. J. The Effect of Agricultural Students' Learning Styles on Academic Achievement and Their Perceptions of Two Methods of Instruction. *Journal of Agricultural Education*, 35 (1) 26-30, 1994.

Marsden, G., & Jones, M. (2001). Ubiquitous computing and cellular handset interfaces are menus the best way forward? In *Proceedings of the south african institute of computer scientists and information technologists annual conference (SAICSIT)* (pp. 111–119).

McCallum, A., Rosenfeld, R., Mitchell, T., & Ng, A. (1998). Improving text classification by shrinkage in a hierarchy of classes. *Proceedings of the 15th International Conference on Machine Learning*, Madison, Wisconsin.

McCarthy, K., Reilly, J., McGinty, L., & Smyth, B. (2004). On the Dynamic Generation of Compound Critiques in Conversational Recommender Systems. In *P. D. Bra (Ed.), Proceedings of the 3rd International conference on adaptive hypermedia and adaptive web-based systems (AH-04).* (Eindhoven, The Netherlands)

McCarthy, K., Reilly, J., McGinty, L., & Smyth, B. (2004). Thinking Positively–Explanatory Feedback for Conversational Recommender Systems. In P. Cunningham & D. McSherry (Eds.), *Proceedings of the European conference on case-based reasoning*

(ECCBR-04): Explanation workshop (pp. 115-124). (Madrid, Spain)

McCarthy, K., Salamo, M., Coyle, L., McGinty, L., & Nion, B. S. . P. (2006). Group Recommender o Systems: A Critiquing Based Approach. In *Proceedings of the FLAIRS 2006 Conference* (pp. 1-16). Springer Verlag. (Florida, USA.)

McDonald, C. J., Stodel, E. J., Farres, L. G., Breithaupt, K., & Gabriel, M. A. (2001). The demand-driven learning model: A framework for Web-based learning, the Internet and higher education, *4*(1), 9-30.

McGilly, K. (1994). *Classroom lesson: Integrating cognitive theory and classroom practice.* Cambridge: MIT.

McGinty, L., & Smyth, B. (2002). Comparison-Based Recommendation. In S. Craw (Ed.), *Proceedings of the th European conference on case-based reasoning (ECCBR-02)* (pp. 575-589). Springer. (Aberdeen, Scotland.)

McGinty, L., & Smyth, B. (2003). The Role of Diversity in Conversational Systems. In D. Bridge & K. Ashley (Eds.), *Proceedings of the 5th International conference on case-based reasoning (ICCBR-03).* Springer-Verlag. (Trondheim, Norway.)

McGinty, L., & Smyth, B. (2003). Tweaking critiquing. In *Proceedings of the workshop on personalization and web techniques at the International joint conference on artificial intelligence (IJCAI-03).* Morgan-Kaufmann. (Acapulco, Mexico)

McLoughlin C. (1999). The implications of the research literature on learning styles for the design of instructional material. *Australian Journal of Educational Technology,* 15(3), p. 222-241.

McMahon, J. and Smith, F. (1996). *Improving statistical language model with performance with automatically generated word hierarchies.* Computational Linguistics, 2(22):217-247.

McSherry, D. (2003). Explanation in case-based reasoning: An evidential approach. . In B. Lees (Ed.), *Proceedings of the 8th UK workshop on case-based reasoning.* (Cambridge, UK)

McSherry, D. (2003). Similarity and compromise. In K. D. Ashley & D. G. Bridge (Eds.), *Proceedings of the 5th International conference on case-based reasoning* (pp. 291-305). SpringerVerlag.

McSherry, D. (2004). Explaining the pros and cons of conclusions in CBR. . In P. A. G. Calero & P. Funk (Eds.), *Proceedings of the European Conference on Case-Based Reasoning (ECCBR04).* Springer. (Madrid, Spain)

Melis, E., Andrès, E., Büdenbender, J., Frischauf, A., Gogaudze, G., Libbrecht, P., et al. (2001). ActiveMath: A Generic and Adaptive Web-Based Learning Environment. *International Journal of Artificial Intelligence in Education, 12,* 385-407.

Melville, P., Mooney, R.J., & Nagarajan, R. (2002). Content-boosted collaborative filtering for improved recommendations. *Proceedings of the 18th National Conference on Artificial Intelligence* (AAAI02), Edmonton, Alberta, Canada.

Messick, S. (1984) The nature of cognitive style: problems and promise in educational practice, *Educational Psychologist* 19, 59–74.

Micarelli, A., Gasparetti, F., Sciarrone, F. & Gauch, S. (2007). Personalized Search on the World Wide Web. In P. Brusilovsky, A. Kobsa & W. Nejdl (Eds.), *The Adaptive Web - Methods and Strategies of Web Personalization* (pp. 195–230). Lecture Notes in Computer Science: Vol. 4321. Heidelberg, Germany: Springer-Verlag.

Middleton, S. E., Shadbolt, N. & De Roure, D. C. (2004). Ontological user profiling in recommender systems. *ACM Transactions on Information Systems, 22*(1), 54–88.

Middleton, S., Alani, H., Shadbolt, N., and Roure, D. D. (2002). *Exploiting synergy between ontologies and recommender systems.* In Semantic Web Workshop.

Miller, B., Konstan, J., & Riedl, J. (2004). PockLens: Toward a Personal Recommender System. ACM Transactions on Information Systems, 22 (3), 437-476.

Miller, D. (1981). The depth/breadth tradeoff in hierarchical computer menus. In *Proceedings of the 25th annual meeting of the human factors and ergonomics society* (pp. 296-300).

Miller, G. A. (1956). The magical number seven, plus or minus two: Some limits on our capacity for processing information. *Psychological Review, 63* (pp. 81–97).

Miller, G. A., Beckwith, R., Fellbaum, C., Gross, D., and Miller, K. J. (1990). *Introduction to wordnet: An on-line lexical database*. International Journal of Lexicography, 3(4):235-244.

Miller, G., Beckwith, R., Fellbaum, C., Gross, D., and Miller, K. (1990). *Introduction to wordnet: An online lexical database*. Journal of Lexicography, 3(4):235-244.

Milosavljevic, M., & Oberlander, J. (1998). Dynamic hypertext catalogues: Helping users to help themselves. *9th ACM International Hypertext Conference*, ACM Press, pp. 123-131.

Mitchell, T. J. F., Chen, S. Y., & Macredie, R. D. (2005). Hypermedia learning and prior knowledge: Domain expertise vs. system expertise. *Journal of Computer Assisted Learning, 21*, 53-64.

Mitrovic, A., & Martin, B. (2007). Evaluating the Effect of Open Student Models on Self-Assessment. *International Journal of Artificial Intelligence in Education, 17*(3), 121-144.

Mladenic, D. (1996). *Personal WebWatcher: design and implementation*. Technical report, Department for Intelligent Systems, J. Stefan Institute, Jamova 39, 11000 Ljubljana, Slovenia.

Mobasher B, Anand S.S., and Kobsa A. (2007). Intelligent Techniques for Web Personalization. *Proceedings of the 5th workshop ITWP 2007*, held in conjunction with the 22nd National Conference in Artificial Intelligence (AAAI2007).

Mobasher B., Dai H., Luo T., Nakagawa M., and Wiltshire J. (2002). Discovery of aggregate usage profiles for Web personalization. *Data Mining and Knowledge Discovery*, Vol. 6 (1), pp. 61–82.

Mobasher, B. (2005). Web usage mining and Personalization. In Munindar P. Singh (ed.) *The Practical Handbook of Internet Computing*. CRC Press.

Mobasher, B., Cooley, R., & Srivastava, J. (2000). Automatic personalization based on Web usage mining. *Communications of the ACM, 43*(8), 142-151.

Mobasher, B., Dai, H., Luo, T., & Nakagawa, M. (2001). Effective personalization based on association rule discovery from Web usage data. *Proceedings of the 3rd ACM Workshop on Web Information and Data Management* (WIDM01), Atlanta, Georgia.

Mobasher, B., Dai, H., Luo, T., & Nakagawa, M. (2002). Discovery and evaluation of aggregate usage profiles for Web personalization. *Data Mining and Knowledge Discovery, 6,* 61-82.

Mobasher, B., Dai, H., Luo, T., Sun, Y., & Zhu, J. (2000). Integrating Web usage and content mining for more effective personalization. *E-Commerce and Web Technologies: Proceedings of the EC-WEB 2000 Conference*, Lecture Notes in Computer Science (LNCS) 1875, 165-176. Springer.

Mobasher, B., Jin, X., and Zhou, Y. (2004). *Semantically enhanced collaborative filtering on the web*. In Web Mining: FromWeb to SemanticWeb: First EuropeanWeb Mining Forum, pages 57-76.

Modjeska, D. (2000). View vs. Overview: Hierarchical Data Visualization in Desktop Virtual Reality. *Proceedings of NordiCHI 2000*.

Moe, M., & Blodgett, H. (2000). *The knowledge Web*. Merrill Lynch.

Morales, R., Pain, H., Bull, S., & Kay, J. (1999). Open, interactive, and other overt approaches to learner modelling. *AIED Resources, 10*, 1070-1079.

Morales, R., Van Labeke, N., & Brna, P. (2006). Approximate Modelling of the Multi-dimensional Learner. In M. Ikeda, K. Ashley, & T-W. Chan (Eds.), *Intelligent Tutoring Systems, 8th International Conference, ITS 2006* (pp. 555-564). LNCS 4053. Berlin: Springer-Verlag.

Mori, J., Matsuo, Y., and Ishizuka, M. (2005). *Finding user semantics on the web using word co-occurrence information*. In PerSWeb05 Workshop on Personalization on the Semantic Web in conjunction with UM05.

Mostefaoui, S., K., Hirsbrunner, B., (2004). *Context Aware Service Provisioning.* Paper presented at the International Conference on Pervasive Services ICPS, Beirut, Lebanon.

Moukas, A. (1996). *Amalthaea: Information discovery and filtering using a multi-agent evolving ecosystem.* In Proc. 1st Intl. Conf. on the Practical Application of Intelligent Agents and Multi Agent Technology, London.

Mulvenna, M. D., Anand S. S., and Buchner, A. G. (2002). Personalization on the net 23using Web mining. *Communications of the ACM*, 43, 8 (August), 123–125.

Mustière, S., Zucker, J.-D., & Saitta, L. (2000). *An Abstraction-based Machine Learning approach to Cartographic Generalization.* Paper presented at the 9th International Symposium on Spatial Data Handling (SDH 2000), Beijing, China.

Mylonas, P., Vallet, D., Fernndez, M., Castells, P., and Avrithis, Y. (2006). *Ontology-based personalization for multimedia content.* In 3rd European Semantic Web Conference - Semantic Web Personalization Workshop.

Nakashima, E. (2006). AOL Search Queries Open Window Onto Users' Worlds. from http://www.washingtonpost.com/wp-dyn/content/article/2006/08/16/AR2006081601751_pf.html.

Nanas, N., Uren, V., and Roeck, A. D. (2003). *Building and applying a concept hierarchy representation of a user profile.* In Proceedings of the 26th annual international ACM SIGIR conference on Research and development in information retrieval, pages 198-204. ACM Press New York, NY, USA.

Nébel, I.-T. (2005). Patient and learner adaptation in e-learning by induction based on medical context. In R. Kaschek (Ed.), *Perspectives of Intelligent Systems' Assistance, International Workshop,* Palmerston North, New Zealand.

Neo, T. and Neo, M. Classroom innovation: engaging students in interactive multimedia learning, *Campus-Wide Information Systems*, 21(3), pp 118 – 124, 2004.

Ng, W., & Gunstone, R. (2002). Students' perceptions of the effectiveness of the World Wide Web as a research and teaching tool in science learning. *Research in Science Education, 32*(4), 489-510.

Oard, D. (1997). *The state of the art in text filtering.* User Modeling and User-Adapted Interaction, 7.

OASIS. (2005). eXtensible Access Control Markup Language (XACML), Version 2.0; OASIS Standard, February 1, 2005. .

OECD. (1980). Recommendation of the Council Concerning Guidelines Governing the Protection of Privacy and Transborder Flows of Personal Data. from http://www.oecd.org/dsti/sti/it/secur/ prod/PRIV-EN.HTM.

OECD. (2003). *The PISA 2003 Assessment Framework*: Organisation for Economic Co-Operation and Development. Paris, France: OECD Press.

Olsson, T. (1998). Decentralised Social Filtering based on Trust. In proceedings of the The AAAI-98 Recommender Systems Workshop (Working Notes) (pp. 84-88). Madison, Wisconsin.

OMA Service Environment (Approved version 1.0.4) (2007). Open Mobile Alliance Retrieved from http://www.openmobilealliance.org/release_program/ose_v1_0.html

Oppermann, R., & Specht, M. (2000). A context sensitive nomadic information system as an exhibition guide, *2nd International Symposium on Handheld and Ubiquitious Computing,* pp. 127-142.

OSA Application Programming Interface (API) version 7 (2007). 3GPP TS 29.198-X. Retrieved from http://www.3gpp.org/ftp/Specs/html-info/29198.htm

Owen, M. B., & Liles, R. (1998). *Factors contributing to the use of Internet by educators.* Retrieved from http://outreach.missouri.edu/netc98/manuscripts/owen-liles.html

OWL (2004). The Web Ontology Language Home Page. W3C Consortium. Retrieved January 15, 2008, from http://www.w3.org/2004/OWL/

P.Cimiano, Hotho, A., and Staab, S. (2005). *Learning concept hierarchies from text corpa using formal concept hierarchies.* Journal of Artificial Intelligence Research, (24):305-339.

Paiva, A., & Self, J. A. (1995). TAGUS - A User and Learner Modeling Workbench. *User Modeling and User-Adapted Interaction, 4*(3), 197-226.

Palme, J. (1998). Information filtering. *4th International Conference on Intelligent Tutoring Systems.* ACM Press.

Palmirani, M., & Brighi, R. (2002). Norma-system: A legal document system for managing consolidated acts. In A. Hameurlain, R. Cicchetti & R. Traunmüller (Eds.), *Database and Expert Systems Applications: 13th International Conference, DEXA 2002* (pp. 310-320). Lecture Notes in Computer Science: Vol. 2453. Heidelberg, Germany: Springer-Verlag.

Palopoli, L., Sacca, D., Terracina, G., & Ursino, D. (2003). Uniform techniques for deriving similarities of objects and subschemes in heterogeneous databases. *IEEE Transactions on Knowledge and Data Engineering, 15*(1), 271-294.

Palpanas, T., & Mendelzon, A. (1999). Web prefetching using partial match prediction. *Proceedings of the 4th International Web Caching Workshop* (WCW99), San Diego, CA.

Panayiotou C., and Samaras G. (2004). mPersona: Personalized Portals for the Wireless User: An Agent Approach. *Journal of ACM/ Baltzer Mobile Networking and Applications* (MONET), special issue on "Mobile and Pervasive Commerce", (6), 663-677.

Panayiotou C., and Samaras G. (2006). Mobile User Personalization with Dynamic Profiles: Time and Activity. *On the Move to Meaningful Internet Systems 2006: OTM 2006 Workshops*, PerSys 2006, Montpellier, France, October 29 - November 3, 2006. Proceedings, Part II, pp. 1295-1304.

Papadomichelaki, X., Magoutas, B., Halaris, C., Apostolou, D., & Mentzas, G. (2006). *A Review of Quality Dimensions in E-government Services.* In M.A. Wimmer et al. (Eds.): EGOV 2006, LNCS 4084, pp. 128–138, 2006.

Papagelis M., Plexousakis D., Rousidis D., and Theoharopoulos E. (2004). Qualitative Analysis of User-based and Item-based Prediction Algorithms for Recommendation Systems, CIA 2004: 152-166.

Papanikolaou K.A., Grigoriadou M., Kornilakis H., and Magoulas G.D. (2003). Personalizing the Interaction in a Web-based Educational Hypermedia System: the case of INSPIRE. User-Modeling and User-Adapted Interaction, 13(3), 213-267.

Parent, S., Mobasher, B., & Lytinen, S. (2001). An adaptive agent for Web exploration based on concept hierarchies. *Proceedings of the International Conference on Human Computer Interaction*, New Orleans, LA.

Parlay X Web Services (2002). The Parlay Group white paper. Retrieved from http://www.parlay.org/imwp/idms/popups/pop_download.asp?contentID=7103

Parlay/ OSA specifications release 6 (2007). The Parlay Group Retrieved from http://www.parlay.org/en/specifications/apis.asp

Parry, D. (2004). *A fuzzy ontology for medical document retrieval.* In ACSW Frontiers '04: Proceedings of the second workshop on Australasian information security, Data Mining and Web Intelligence, and Software Internationalisation, pages 121-126, Darlinghurst, Australia, Australia. Australian Computer Society, Inc.

Patouni E. et al. (2006). *E²R Scenario on Autonomic Communication Systems for Seamless Experience.* E²R II White Paper. Retrieved from http://e2r2.motlabs.com/whitepapers/E2RII_ScenarioAutonomic_White_Paper.pdf

Patterson, D. J., Liao, L., Gajos, K., Collier, M., Livic, N., Olson, K., Wang, S., Fox, D. & Kautz, H. A. (2004). Opportunity Knocks: A System to Provide Cognitive Assistance with Transportation Services. In N. Davies, E. D. Mynatt, I. Siio (Eds.), *LNCS 3205: UbiComp 2004: Ubiquitous Computing: 6th International Conference* (pp. 433–450). Berlin, Heidelberg: Springer.

Pazzani, M. (1999). A framework for collaborative, content-based and demographic filtering. *Artificial Intelligence Review, 13*(5-6), 393-408.

Pazzani, M. and Billsus, D. (1997). *Learning and revising user profiles: The identification of interesting web sites.* Machine Learning, 27:313-331.

Perkowitz M, and Etzioni O. (2003). Adaptive Websites, Towards Adaptive Web sites: Conceptual Framework and case study, [on-line]: http://www.cse.buffalo.edu/~sbraynov/ seninar2003/presenttations/adaptive.pdf.

Perkowitz, M. (2001). Adaptive web sites: Cluster mining and conceptual clustering for index page synthesis. PhD Thesis, Department of Computer Science and Engineering. University of Washington.

Perkowitz, M., & Etzioni, O. (1998). Adaptive Websites: Automatically synthesizing Web pages. *Proceedings of the 15th National Conference on Artificial Intelligence*, Madison, WI.

Perkowitz, M., & Etzioni, O. (2000). Towards adaptive web sites: Conceptual framework and case study. *Journal of Artificial Intelligence*, 18(1-2), 245-275.

Perugini, S., Gonçalves, M. A., & Fox, E.A. (2004). Recommender Systems Research: A Connection-Centric Survey. *Journal of Intelligent Information Systems, 23*(2), 107-143.

Picard, R. W., Kort, B., & Reilly, R. (2007). Exploring the Role of Emotion in Propelling the SMET Learning Process. *NSF Project Summary and Description* Retrieved Nov 23, 2007, from http://affect.media.mit.edu/projectpages/lc/nsf1.html

Pierrakos D., Paliouras G., Papatheodorou C., and Spyropoulos C.D. (2001). KOINOTITES: A Web Usage Mining Tool for Personalization, *Proceedings of the Panhellenic Conference on Human Computer Interaction*, Patra.

Pithers R. T. (2002). Cognitive Learning Style: A review of the field dependent- field independent approach. *Journal of Vocational Education and Training*, Vol. 54 (11), pp. 117-8.

Pitkow, J., & Pirolli, P. (1999). Mining longest repeating subsequences to predict WWW surfing. *Proceedings of the 2nd USENIX Symposium on Internet Technologies and Systems*, Boulder, Colorado.

Plate, C., Basselin, N., Kröner, A., Schneider, M., Baldes, S., Dimitrova, V., & Jameson, A. (2006). Recomindation: New functions for augmented memories. In V. Wade, H. Ashman (Eds.), *LNCS 4018: Adaptive hypermedia and adaptive web-based systems – Proceedings of AH 2006* (pp. 141–150). Berlin, Heidelberg: Springer.

Polat, H., & Du, W. (2003). Privacy-Preserving Collaborative Filtering Using Randomized Perturbation Techniques. In proceedings of the Third IEEE International Conference on Data Mining (ICDM'03) (pp. 625-628). Melbourne, FL.

Polat, H., & Du, W. (2005). Privacy-Preserving Collaborative Filtering. The International Journal of Electronic Commerce (IJEC), 9 (4), 9-35.

Polat, H., & Du, W. (2005). SVD-based Collaborative Filtering with Privacy. In proceedings of the 20th ACM Symposium on Applied Computing (pp. 791-795). Santa Fe, NM.

Pollack, M. E., Brown, L., Colbry, D., McCarthy, C. E., Orosz, C., Peintner, B.,Ramakrishnan, S., & Tsamardinos, I.. (2003). Autominder: An intelligent cognitive orthotic system for people with memory impairment. *Robotics and Autonomous Systems*, 44 (pp. 273–282).

Polson, M. C., & Richardson, J. J. (Eds.). (1988). *Foundations of Intelligent Tutoring Systems.* New Jersey: Lawrence Erlbaum Associates.

Powell, T., & Schneider, F. (2004). *JavaScript: The Complete Reference*. McGraw Hill, 2004, iSBN: 0072253576

Power, D. J., & Roth, R. M. (1999). Issues in designing and using Web-based teaching cases. *Proceedings of the Fifth Americas Conference on Information System (AMCIS 1999)* (pp. 936-938).

Powers, A. (2006). *Web Survey Toolbox Home Page.* Available online at: https://hciresearch.hcii.cs.cmu.edu/

docs/display/wst/Home (accessed 01 June 2007).

Preibusch, S. (2006). Personalized Services with Negotiable Privacy Policies. In proceedings of the PEP06, CHI 2006 Workshop on Privacy-Enhanced Personalization (pp. 29-38). Montreal, Canada.

Pretschner, A. (1998). *Ontology based personalized search.* Unpublished master's thesis, University of Kansas, Lawrence, Kan.

Pretschner, A. and Gauch, S. (2004). *Ontology based personalized search and browsing.* Web Intelligence and Agent Systems, 1(4):219-234.

Pu P., and Faltings B. (2002). Personalized Navigation of Heterogeneous Products Spaces using SmartClient, © 2002 ACM 1-58113-459-2/02/0001.

Quan, D., Huynh, D., & Karger, D.R. (2003). Haystack: A platform for authoring end user semantic web applications. In *Proceedings of the 2nd International Semantic Web Conference (ISWC 2003)* (pp. 738–753). Florida, USA.

Quan, T. T., Hui, S. C., and Cao, T. H. (2004). Foga: A fuzzy ontology generation framework for scholarly semantic web. In Workshop on Knowledge Discovery and Ontologies In conjunction with ECML/PKDD.

Quintana, Y. (1996). *Evaluating the value and effectiveness of Internet-based learning.* Retrieved from www.crim.ca/inet96/pa pers/cl/cl_4.htm

Rafter, R., Bradley, K., & Smyth, B. (2000). Automatic collaborative filtering applications for online recruitment services. *In O. S. P. Brusilovsky & C. Strapparava (Eds.), Proceedings of the International conference on adaptive hypermedia and adaptive web-based systems* (pp. 363-368). Springer-Verlag.

Ralph, P., & Parsons, J., (2006). *A Framework for Automatic Online Personalization.* Paper presented at the 39th Hawaii International Conference on System Sciences—2006, Kauai, HI.

Ramsey, M., & Nielsen, J. (2000). The wap usability report. Neilsen Norman Group. Reiken, D. (2000). Special issue on personalization. Communications of the ACM, 43(8).

Rao, J. R., & Rohatgi, P. (2000). Can Pseudonymity Really Guarantee Privacy? In proceedings of the 9th USENIX Security Symposium (pp. 85–96).

Razmerita, L., & Gouarderes, G. (2004). *Ontology-based user modeling for personalization of grid learning services.* In Proceedings of ITS'04 GRID Learning Services Workshop, Maceio, Brazil.

Razmerita, L., Angehrn, A. & Maedche, A. (2003). Ontology-based User Modeling for Knowledge management Systems. In P. Brusilovsky, A. T. Corbett & F. de Rosis (Eds.), *User Modeling 2003, 9th International Conference, UM 2003* (pp. 213–217). Lecture Notes in Computer Science: Vol. 2702. Heidelberg, Germany: Springer-Verlag.

Reddy N.L.A. (1995). Scheduling and data distribution in a multiprocessor video server, *In Proceedings of the 2nd IEEE Int'l Conference on Multimedia Computing and Systems*, pp. 256{263, 1995.

Reed W. M., Ayersman D. J. and Liu M. (1996). The effects of students' computer-based prior experiences and instructional exposures on the application of hypermedia-related mental models. *Journal of Educational Computing Research*, 14 (2), pp. 175-187.

Reed, W. M., & Oughton, J. M. (1997). Computer experience and interval-based hypermedia navigation. *Journal of Research on Computing in Education, 30*, 38-52.

Reigeluth, C. M. (1999). *Instructional-Design Theories and Models: A New Paradigm of Instructional Theory*: Lawrence Erlbaum Associates.

Reilly, J., McCarthy, K., McGinty, L., & Smyth, B. (2004). Dynamic Critiquing. In P. G. Calero & P. Funk (Eds.), *Proceedings of the European conference on case-based reasoning (ECCBR04).* Springer-Verlag. (Madrid, Spain)

Reilly, J., McCarthy, K., McGinty, L., & Smyth, B. (2005). Explaining compound critiques. *Artificial Intelligence Review*, 24 (2), 199-220. Roush, W. (2004). Search Beyond Google. MIT Technology Review, 34–45.

Resnick, P. and Varian, H. (1997). Recommender systems. *Communications of the ACM.*, *40*(3):56-58.

Resource Description Framework (RDF). The World Wide Web Consortium (W3C) (2007). Retrieved from http://www.w3.org/RDF/

Rich, E. (1999). Users are individuals: individualizing user models. *International Journal on Human-Computer Studies*, *51*(2), 323–338.

Riding R. (2001). Cognitive Style Analysis–Research Administration, Published by Learning and Training Technology.

Riding R.J. and Douglas, G.. The effect of cognitive style and mode of presentation on learning performance, *British Journal of Educational Psychology*, 63, 297-307, 1993.

Riding, R. J. *Cognitive Styles Analysis*, Birmingham: Learning and Training Technology, 1991.

Riding, R.J, and Cheema, I.. Cognitive styles: An overview and integration. *Educational Psychology*, 11(3 & 4), 193-215, 1991.

Riding, R.J. and Grimley, M. Cognitive style and learning from multimedia materials in 11 year old children. *British Journal of Educational Technology* 30 (2) 43-56, 1999..

Riding, R.J. and Rayner, S.G. Cognitive Styles and Learning Strategies, London: David Fulton Publisher, 1998.

Riecken, D. (2000). Personalized views of personalization. *Communications of the ACM*, *43*(8), 27–28.

Robertson G., Czerwinski M., Larson K., Robbins D., Thiel D. & van Dantzich M. (1998). Data Mountain: Using Spatial Memory for Document Management, *Proceedings of ACM UIST '98 Symposium on User Interface Software& Technology*

Robertson, G. G., Van Dantzich, M., Robbins, D., Czerwinski, M., Hinckley, K., Risden, K., Thiel, D. & Gorokhovsky, V. (2000). The Task Gallery: A 3D Window Manager. *CHI Letters, 2(1),* 494-501.

Robertson, G., Mackinlay, J., & Card, S. (1991). Cone Trees: Animated 3D Visualizations of Hierarchical Information. *Proceedings of CHI '91*, 189-194.

Robinson, R. (2000). *Context management in mobile environments.* PhD thesis, University of Queensland, Australia.

Rodotà, S. (2001). Introduction to the "One world, one privacy" session. *Proceedings of 23rd Data Protection Commissioners Conf.*, Paris, France. Retrieved January 15, 2008, from http://www.paris-conference-2001.org/eng/contribution/rodota_contrib.pdf

Rodriguez, M.A., & Egenhofer, M.J. (2003). Determining semantic similarity among entity classes from different ontologies. *IEEE Transactions on Knowledge and Data Engineering, 15*(2), 442-456.

Rosenblatt, W., Trippe, W., & Mooney, S. (2001). Digital Rights Management: Business and Technology. Indianapolis, IN: Hungry Minds, Inc.

Rossi G., Schwade D., & Guimaraes M.R. (2001). Designing Personalized Web Applications, ACM 1-58113-348-0/01/0005.

Rothwell, W. J., & Kazanas, H. C. (2004). *Mastering the instructional design process: A systematic approach* (3rd ed.). Pfeiffer.

Rottmann V., Berenbrink P., and Lauling I.R. (1997). A simple distributed scheduling policy for parallel interactive continuous media servers. *Parallel Computing - Special Issue on parallel processing and multimedia,* 23(12):1757{1776, December.

Rottmann V., Berenbrink P., and Luling R. (1996). A comparison of data layout schemes for multi- media servers, *In European Conference on Multimedia Applications, Services, and Techniques* (ECMAST'96), pages 345{364, 1996.

Roy, M., & Chi, M. T. C. (2003). Gender differences in patterns of searching the Web. *Journal of Educational Computing Research*, *29*, 335-348.

Sadler-Smith E. & Riding R., (1999). Cognitive style and instructional preferences. Instructional Science Volume 27, Number 5, September 1999, 355-371.

Salovey, P., & Mayer, J.D. (2000). Emotional intelligence. *Imagination, Cognition and Personality, 9*(3), 185-911.

Sanchez, D. and Moreno, A. (2005). A multi-agent system for distributed ontology learning. In EUMAS, pages 504-505.

Sanderson, M. and Croft, W. B. (1999). *Deriving concept hierarchies from text.* In Research and Development in Information Retrieval, pages 206-213.

Sapp M. (1993). Test anxiety: Applied research, assessment, and treatment intervention. Lanham, MD: University Press of America.

Sarkin, J. A., Johnson, S. S., Prochaska, J. O. & Prochaska, J. M. (2001). Applying the transtheoretical model to regular moderate exercise in an overweight population: validation of a stages of change measure. *Preventive Medicine, 33*, 462-469.

Sarwar, B., Karypis, G., Konstan, J., & Riedl, J. (2001). Item-based collaborative filtering recommendation algorithms. *10th International World Wide Web Conference*, ACM Press, pp. 285-295.

Sarwar, B.M., Karypis, G., Konstan, J., & Riedl, J. (2000). Analysis of recommender algorithms for e-commerce. *Proceedings of the 2nd ACM E-Commerce Conference* (EC'00), Minneapolis, MN.

Schacter, D. L. (2001). *The seven sins of memory: how the mind forgets and remembers.* Boston, Houghton Mifflin.

Schank, R.C. (2002). Are we going to get smarter? In J. Brockman (Ed.), *The next fifty years: Science in the first half of the twenty-first century* (pp. 206-215). New York: Vintage.

Schneider, M. (2006). RDF:Stores – A Lightweight Approach on Managing Shared Knowledge. In *Proceedings of the 3rd International Conference on Ubiquitous Intelligence and Computing (UIC)*, Wuhan, China.

Schwarz, J. (2001). *Lost in virtual space: Gender differences are magnified.* Retrieved October 15, 2002, from www.washington.edu/newsroom/news/2001archive/06-01archive/k061301.html

Schwarzer R. (1984). Worry and emotionality as separate components in test anxiety. *International Review of Applied Psychology*, 33, 205-220.

Searle, J. R. (1980). *Mind, brains, and programs: Vol. 3 of The Behavioral and Brain Sciences*. Cambridge University Press.

Self, J. (1988). Bypassing the intractable problem of student modelling. In C. Frasson (Ed.), *Proceedings of the 1st International Conference on Intelligent Tutoring Systems ITS'88* (pp. 18-24). Montreal, Canada.

Self, J. (1999). The Defining Characteristics of Intelligent Tutoring Systems Research: ITSs Care, Precisely. *International Journal of Artificial Intelligence in Education, 10*, 350-364.

Seunghwa, L. & Eunseok, L. (2007). A Collective User Preference Management System for U-Commerce. In *Managing Next Generation Networks and Services*, Springer Berlin / Heidelberg, 21-30.

Shafer, G. (1976). *A Mathematical Theory of Evidence*: Princeton University Press.

Shahabi C. and Chen Y. (2003). Web Information Personalization: Challenges and Approaches, *In the 3nd International Workshop on Databases in Networked Information Systems* (DNIS 2003), Aizu-Wakamatsu, Japan.

Shardanand U. and Maes. (1995). Social information filtering: Algorithms for automating "Word of Mouth", *Proceedings of CHI'95 -- Human Factors in Computing Systems*, 210-217.

Sharp, J. E. (1998). Learning Styles and Technical Communication: Improving Communication and Teamwork Skills.

Sharples, M., Hogg, D., Hutchison, C., & Torrance, S. (1989). *Computers and Thought: A Practical Introduction to Artificial Intelligence*. Bradford Book.

Shashaani, L. (1994). Gender differences in computer experience and its influence on computer attitudes. *Journal of Educational Computing Research, 11*(4), 347-367.

Shen, X., Tan, B. & Zhai, CX. (2007). Privacy protection in personalized search, *ACM SIGIR Forum*, *41*(1), 4–17.

Shih, C., & Gamon, J. (1999). *Student learning styles, motivation, learning strategies, and achievement in Web-based courses.* Retrieved from http://iccel.wfu.edu/publications/journals/jcel/jcel990305/ccshih.htm

Shneiderman, B. (1996). The eyes have it: a task by data type taxonomy for information visualization. *Proceedings of the IEEE Visual Languages.*

Shneiderman, B., Feldman, D., Rose, A., & Ferre G., X. (2000). Visualizing Digital Library Search Results with Categorical and Hierarchical Axes. *Proceedings of the 5th ACM International Conference on Digital Libraries*, 57-66.

Sieg, A., Mobasher, B., Burke, R., Prabu, G., and Lytinen, S. (2005). *Representing user information context with ontologies.* In Proceedings of the 3rd International Conference on Universal Access in Human-Computer Interaction.

Sigg, S., Haseloff, S., & David, K. (2006). The Impact of the Context Interpretation Error on the Context Prediction Accuracy. In *Third Annual International Conference on Mobile and Ubiquitous Systems: Networking & Services*, 17-21 July, San Jose, California

Smaldino, S. (1999). Instructional design for distance education. *Techtrends, 43*(5), 9-13.

Smith B., Caputi P. (2005). Cognitive interference model of computer anxiety: Implications for computer-based assessment, *Computers in Human Behavior 21*, 713-728.

Smyth, B. (2007). Case-based recommendation. In P. Brusilovsky, A. Kobsa, & W. Nejdl (Eds.), *The adaptive web* (Vol. 4321, pp. 342-376). Springer.

Smyth, B. and Cotter, P. (2000). A personalised television listings service. *Communications of the ACM*, *43*(8).

Smyth, B., & Cotter, C. (2000). Wapping the Web: A Case-Study in Content Personalization for WAP-enabled Devices. *In Proceedings of the International conference on adaptive hypermedia and adaptive web-based systems (AH'00)* (pp. 98-108). Springer-Verlag

Smyth, B., & Cotter, P. (2002). Personalized adaptive navigation for mobile portals. *15th European Conference on Artificial Intelligence*, IOS Press, pp. 608-612.

Smyth, B., & Cotter, P. (2002). Personalized adaptive navigation for mobile portals. In *Proceedings of the 15th European conference on artificial intelligence - prestigious applications of artificial intelligence.* IOS Press.

Smyth, B., & Cotter, P. (2002). The Plight of the Navigator: Solving the Navigation Problem for Wireless Portals. In *Proceedings of the 2nd International Conference on Adaptive Hypermedia and Adaptive Web-Based Systems (AH'02)* (pp. 328-337). Springer-Verlag.

Smyth, B., Balfe, E., Boydell, O., Bradley, K., Briggs, P., Coyle, M., et al. (2005). A live-user evaluation of collaborative web search. In *Proceedings of the 19th International joint conference on artificial intelligence (IJCAI '05)* (pp. 1419–1424). Morgan Kaufmann. (Edinburgh, Scotland)

Smyth, B., Balfe, E., Freyne, J., Briggs, P., Coyle, M., & Boydell, O. (2004). Exploiting query repetition and regularity in an adaptive community-based web search engine. *User Modeling and User-Adapted Interaction: The Journal of Personalization Research,* 14 (5), 383-423.

Smyth, B., Cotter, P., & Oman, S. (2007). Enabling intelligent content discovery on the mobile internet. In *Proceedings of the conference on innovative applications of artificial intelligence (IAAI/AAAI)* (pp. 1744-1751).

SOAP/XMLP (2000). The XML Protocol Working Group Home Page. W3C Consortium. Retrieved January 15, 2008, from http://www.w3.org/2000/xp/Group/

Solove, D. (2006). A Taxonomy of Privacy. University of Pennsylvania Law Review, 154 (3), 477-564.

Specht, M. (1998). *Adaptive Methoden in computerbasierten Lehr/Lernsystemen (Adaptive methods in computer-based teaching-learning systems).* Doctoral thesis, Universität Trier, FB Psychologie.

Spencer, L., Pagell, F., Hallion, M. E. & Adams, T. B. (2002). Applying the transtheoretical model to tobacco cessation and prevention: a review of literature. *American Journal of Health Promotion, 17*, 7-71.

Sperling, G. (1960). The information available in brief visual presentations. *Psychology Monographs, 74*(11) (pp. 1–29).

Spielberger C. D. (1972). Conceptual and methodological issues in anxiety research. *In C. D. Spielberger (Ed.), Anxiety. Current trends in theory and research (Vol. 2).* New York: Academic Press.

Spielberger C. D. (1983). Manual for the State-Trait Anxiety Inventory (STAI). PaloAlto, CA: Consulting Psychologists Press.Spielberger, C. D. (1972). Conceptual and methodological issues in anxiety research. *In C. D. Spielberger (Ed.), Anxiety. Current trends in theory and research (Vol. 2).* New York: Academic Press.

Spielberger C. D., andVagg P. R. (1995). Test anxiety: A transactional process model. *In C. D. Spielberger and P. R. Vagg (Eds.), Test anxiety: Theory, assessment, and treatment (pp. 3-14).* Washington, DC: Taylor & Francis.

Spiliopoulou, M. (2000). Web usage mining for Web site evaluation. *Communications of ACM, 43*(8), 127-134.

Sridharan, K. (2004). A course on Web languages and Web-based applications. *IEEE Transactions on Education, 47*(2), 254-260.

Srivastava, J., Cooley, R., Deshpande, M., & Tan, P. (2000). Web usage mining: Discovery and applications of usage patterns from Web data. *SIGKDD Explorations, 1*(2), 12-23.

Steinmetz, R. Human Perception of Jitter and Media Synchronisation, *IEEE Journal on Selected Areas in Communications*, 14(1), pp. 61 –72, 1996.

Stone, P. (1997). *Multiagent systems.* Retrieved October 15, 2006, from http://www-2.cs.cmu.edu/afs/cs/usr/pstone/public/papers/97MAS-survey/node2.html

Stumme, G., Taouil, R., Bastide, Y., Pasquier, N., & Lakhal, L. (2000). Fast computation of concept lattices using data mining techniques. *Proceedings of the Knowledge Representation Meets Databases Conference* (KRDB00), Berlin.

Sumi, Y., & Mase, K. (2002). Supporting awareness of shared interests and experiences in community. *International Journal of Human-Computer Studies*, 14(6) (pp. 127–146).

Sweeney, L. (2002). k-Anonymity: A Model for Protecting Privacy. International Journal on Uncertainty, Fuzziness, and Knowledge-based Systems, 10 (5), 557-570. from DOI 10.1142/ S0218488502001648.

Tallon, S. (2005). *Adaptive Ontology-Driven Personalised News Services.* A dissertation submitted to the University of Dublin, available at https://www.cs.tcd.ie/publications/tech-reports/reports.05/TCD-CS-2005-87.pdf

Tchetagni, J., Nkambou, R., & Bourdeau, J. (2007). Explicit Reflection in Prolog-Tutor. *International Journal of Artificial Intelligence in Education, 17*(3), 169-215.

Tchienehom, P. L. (2005). Profiles semantics for personalized information access. In PerSWeb05 Workshop on Personalization on the Semantic Web in conjunction with UM05.

Teltzrow, M., & Kobsa, A. (2004). Impacts of User Privacy Preferences on Personalized Systems: a Comparative Study. In C.-M. Karat, J. Blom & J. Karat (Eds.), Designing Personalized User Experiences for eCommerce (pp. 315-332). Dordrecht, Netherlands: Kluwer Academic Publishers. from DOI 10.1007/1-4020-2148-8_17.

Tergan, S.-O., & Schenkel, P. (Eds.). (2004). *Was macht E-Learning erfolgreich? Grundlagen und Instrumente der Qualitätsbeurteilung (How does eLearning become successful? Basics and tools of quality-assessment).* Springer.

Terveen, L., Hill, W., Amento, B., McDonald, D., and Creter, J. (1997). Phoaks: A system for sharing recommendations. Communications of the ACM, 40(3):5962.

The Operators Vision on Systems Beyond 3G, (2003), EURESCOM Project P1203. http://www.eurescom.de

The Virtual Home Environment. 3GPP TR 22.121 V5.3.1 (2002-06). Retrieved from http://www.3gpp.org/

Tho, Q. T., Hui, S. C., Fong, A., and Cao, T. H. (2006). Automatic fuzzy ontology generation for semantic web. IEEE Transactions on Knowledge and Data Engineering, 18(6):842856.

Thomas C. and Fischer G. (1997). Using agents to personalize the Web, *In proceedings ACM IUI'97*, pp. 53-60, Florida Usa.

Thorndike, E. L. (1913). *Educational psychology* (Vol. 1 & 2). New York: Columbia University Press.

TopicMaps.org. (2001). *XML Topic Maps (XTM) 1.0* (Specification): TopicMaps.org.

Torkzadeh, G., & Van Dyke, T.P. (2002). Effects of training on Internet self-efficacy and computer user attitudes. *Computers in Human Behavior, 18,* 479-494.

Toulmin, S. (1959). *The Uses of Arguments*: Cambridge University Press.

t-Protégé (n.d.). The t-Protégé Project Home Page. University of Peloponnese. Retrieved January 15, 2008, from http://t-protege.uop.gr/

Trajkova, J. & Gauch, S. (2004). Improving ontology-based user profiles. In *RIAO 2004 Conference Proceedings* (pp 380–389). Paris, France: C.I.D. Retrieved January 15, 2008, from http://www3.riao.org/Proceedings-2004/papers/0290.pdf

Ubiquitous Web Applications Working Group (UWAWG). The World Wide Web Consortium (W3C) (2007). Retrieved from http://www.w3.org/2007/uwa/

UDDI (n.d.). The Universal Description Discovery and Integration Specification, OASIS Organization. Retrieved January 15, 2008, from http://www.oasis-open.org/committees/tc_home.php?wg_abbrev=uddi-spec

UDG Virtual. (2004). *El modelo educativo de UDGVirtual*. Guadalajara, Jalisco: Universidad de Guadalajara.

Universal Description, Discovery and Integration (UDDI) (2005) OASIS, v3.0.2, retrieved from http://www.oasis-open.org/specs/index.php#uddiv3.0.2

Uren, V., Cimiano, P., Iria, J., Handschuh, S., Vargas-Vera, M., Motta, E., & Ciravegna, F. (2006). *Semantic Annotation for Knowledge Management: Requirements and a Survey of the State of the Art.* Web Semantics, 4(1), pp. 14-28.

USACM. (2006). USACM Policy Recommendations on Privacy. New York, NY: U.S. Public Policy Committee of the Association for Computing Machinery. from http://www.acm.org/usacm/ Issues/Privacy.htm.

USeGov (2006). The U.S. President's e-Government Initiatives Home Page. Retrieved January 15, 2008, from http://www.whitehouse.gov/omb/egov/

Van den Hoven, E. (2004). *Exploring graspable cues for everyday recollecting.* Paper presented at the PERVASIVE 2004 Workshop on "Memory and Sharing of Experience", Vienna, Austria.

van Kranenburg, H., Bargh, M.S., Iacob, S., Peddemors, A. (2006). A Context Management Framework for Supporting Context-Aware Distributed Applications. *IEEE Comunications. Magazine*, August 2006, vol. 44, no. 8, 67-74.

Van Labeke, N., Brna, P., & Morales, R. (2007). Opening up the Interpretation Process in an Open Learner Model. *International Journal of Artificial Intelligence in Education, 17*(3), 305-338.

Visser, P. R. S & Bench-Capon, T. J. M. (1998). A Comparison of Four Ontologies for the Design of Legal Knowledge Systems. *Artificial Intelligence and Law, 6*(1), 27–57.

Vozalis E., Nicolaou A., and Margaritis K. G. (2001). Intelligent Techniques for Web Applications: Review and Educational Application, *presented at the Fifth Hellenic-European Conference on Computer Mathematics and its Applications* (HERCMA), Athens, Greece.

Vygotsky, L. (1996). *Thought and Language*: Cambridge, MA: MIT Press.

Wagner, M., Kellerer, W., Tarlano, A., & Hirschfeld R.(2003, October). *From Personal Mobility to Mobile Personality.* Paper presented at the Eurescom Summit, Heidelberg, Germany

Wahlster, W. (2007). Digital Product Memory: Embedded Systems Keep a Diary. In D. Harting, *tec.News 15* (pp. 6–9). Retrieved June 4, 2007, from http://www.harting.com/.

Wahlster, W., Kröner, A., & Heckmann, D. (2006). SharedLife: Towards Selective Sharing of Augmented Personal Memories. In O. Stock, M. Schaerf (Eds.), *Reasoning, Action and Interaction in AI Theories and Systems. Essays Dedicated to Luigia Carlucci Aiello*, LNAI 4155 (pp. 327–342). Berlin, Heidelberg: Springer.

Wang J., and Lin J. (2002). Are personalization systems really personal?–Effects of conformity in reducing information overload, *Proceedings of the 36th Hawaii International Conference on Systems Sciences* (HICSS'03), 0-7695-1874-5/03, © 2002 IEEE.

Wang K. H., Wang T. H., Wang W. L., Huang S. C. (2006). Learning styles and formative assessment strategy: enhancing student achievement in Web-based learning. *Journal of Computer Assisted Learning*, 22, 207-217. (SSCI).

Wang, H., Lee, M. K. O., & Wang, C. (1998). Consumer Privacy Concerns about Internet Marketing. Communications of the ACM, 41 (3), 63-70.

Wang, S. R., & Jonassen, D. H. (1993, April). *Investigating the effects of individual differences on performance in cognitive flexibility hypertexts.* Annual Meeting of the American Educational Research Association. Atlanta, GA.

Wang, Y., & Kobsa, A. (2006). Impacts of Privacy Laws and Regulations on Personalized Systems. In proceedings of the PEP06, CHI06 Workshop on Privacy-Enhanced Personalization (pp. 44-46). Montréal, Canada. http://www.ics.uci.edu/~kobsa/papers/2006-PEP-wang-kobsa.pdf

Wang, Y., & Kobsa, A. (2007). Respecting Users' Individual Privacy Constraints in Web Personalization In proceedings of the UM07, 11th International Conference on User Modeling (pp. 157–166). Corfu, Greece. from DOI 10.1007/978-3-540-73078-1.

Wang, Y., Kobsa, A., van der Hoek, A., & White, J. (2006). PLA-based Runtime Dynamism in Support of Privacy-Enhanced Web Personalization. In proceedings of the 10th International Software Product Line Conference (pp. 151-162). Baltimore, MD. from DOI 0.1109/ SPLINE.2006.1691587.

Wang, Y., Zhaoqi, C., & Kobsa, A. (2006). A Collection and Systematization of International Privacy Laws, with Special Consideration of Internationally Operating Personalized Websites. from http://www.ics.uci.edu/~kobsa/privacy/intlprivlawsurvey.html.

Watson A and Sasse, M.A. Measuring Perceived Quality of Speech and Video in Multimedia Conferencing Applications, in *Proceedings of ACM Multimedia '98*, Bristol, United Kingdom, pp. 55-60, 1998.

Weber G. & Specht M. (1997). User Modeling and Adaptive Navigation Support in WWW-Based Tutoring Systems. *In Proceedings of User Modeling '97*, pp. 289-300.

Weber, G. (1996). Episodic learner modelling. *Cognitive Science, 20*, 195–236.

Weber, G. (1999). Adaptive learning systems in the World Wide Web. In *User Modeling; Proceedings of the Seventh International Conference UM'99* (pp. 371–378). Springer.

Weber, G. (2005). Mediendidaktik: Varianten virtueller Lehr-/Lernformen (Versions of virtual teaching-learning forms). In C. Igel & R. Daugs (Eds.), *eLearning in der Sportwissenschaft: Strategien, Konzeptionen, Perspektiven (eLearning in sports science: Strategies, conceptual design, prospects)* (pp. 71-98). Schorndorf: Hofmann.

Weber, G., Kuhl, H.-C., & Weibelzahl, S. (2001). Developing adaptive Internet based courses with the authoring system NetCoach. In S. Reich, M.M. Tzagarakis, & P.M.E. De Bra (Eds.), *Hypermedia: Openness, structural awareness and adaptivity* (pp. 226–238). Springer.

Wenger, E. (1987). *Artificial intelligence and tutoring systems.* California: Morgan Kaufmann.

White, S., Fisher, M., Kattell, R., Hamilton, & G., Hapner, M. (2001). *JDBC API Tutorial and Reference, Second edition.* Addison Wesley, 2001

Widyantoro, D. H. and Yen, J. (2002). Using fuzzy ontology for query refinement in a personalized abstract search engine. In 10th IEEE International Conference on Fuzzy Systems, pages 705-708.

Wijayaratne R., and Reddy N.L.A. (2000). Providing QOS guarantees for disk I/O. *Multimedia Systems*, 8(1):57{68.

Wijesekera, D. and Srivastava, J. Quality of Service (QoS) Metrics for Continuous Media, *Multimedia Tools and Applications*, 3(1), pp. 127-166, 1996.

Williams, H., M., Roussaki, I., Strimpakou, M., Yang, Y., MacKinnon, L., Dewar, R., Milyaev, N., Pils, C., & Anagnostou, M., (2005). *Context-Awareness and Personalisation in the Daidalos Pervasive Environment.* Paper presented at International Conference on the International Conference on Pervasive Services, ICPS, Santorini, Greece.

Witkin H., Moore C., Gooddenough D., Cox P. (1977). Field- dependent and field- independent cognitive styles and their educational implications. *Review of Educational Research* 47, pp 1-64.

Wiza W., K. Walczak & W. Cellary (2004). Periscope - A System for Adaptive 3D Visualization of Search Results, *Web3D 2004 Symposium - the 9th International Conference on 3D Web Technology, Monterey, California (USA), ACM SIGGRAPH*, 29-39.

WS-BPEL (n.d.). The Web Services Business Process Execution Language, OASIS Organization. Retrieved January 15, 2008, from http://www.oasis-open.org/committees/tc_home.php?wg_abbrev=wsbpel

Wu Y.M. and Shu W. (1996). Scheduling for large-scale parallel video servers, *In Proceedings of the Sixth Symposium on the Frontiers of Massively Parallel Computation*, pp. 126{133, October.

XML (n.d.). The eXtensible Markup Language Home Page. W3C Consortium. Retrieved January 15, 2008, from http://www.w3.org/XML/

XPDL (n.d.). The XML Process Definition Language. WfMC Coalition. Retrieved January 15, 2008, from http://www.wfmc.org/standards/docs.htm

XQuery (n.d.). The XML Query Home Page.W3C Consortium. Retrieved January 15, 2008, from http://www.w3c.org/XML/Query

XSL/XSLT (n.d.). The eXtensible Stylesheet Language Family Home Page. W3C Consortium. Retrieved January 15, 2008, from http://www.w3.org/Style/XSL/

Yuliang, L. and Dean, G. (1999). Cognitive Styles and Distance Education. *Online Journal of Distance Learning Administration*, Vol. 2 (3).

Zapata-Rivera, D., Hansen, E., Shute, V. J., Underwood, J. S., & Bauer, M. (2007). Evidence-based Approach to Interacting with Open Student Models. *International Journal of Artificial Intelligence in Education, 17*(3), 273-303.

Zapata-Rivera, J.-D., & Greer, J. (2004). Inspectable Bayesian Student Modelling Servers in Multi-agent Tutoring Systems. *International Journal of Human-Computer Studies, 61*(535-563).

Zaphirs, P. (2000). Depth vs. breadth in the arrangement of web links. In *Proceedings of 44th annual meeting of the human factors and ergonomics society* (pp. 139-144).

Zeimpekis, V., Giaglis, G.M., & Lekakos, G. (2003). A Taxonomy of Indoor and Outdoor PositioningTechniques for Mobile Location Services. In *ACM SIGecom Exchanges*, 3(4) (pp. 19–27).

Zhang, J., Ackerman, M. S., & Adamic, L. (2007). Expertise networks in online communities: structure and algorithms. In *WWW '07: Proceedings of the 16th international conference on world wide web* (pp. 221–230). New York, NY, USA: ACM.

Zhou, D., Manavoglu, E., Li, J., Giles, C. L., & Zha, H. (2006). Probabilistic models for discovering e-communities. In *WWW '06: Proceedings of the 15th international conference on world wide web* (pp. 173–182). New York, NY, USA: ACM.

Zimmermann A., Specht M. & Lorenz A. (2005). Personalization and Context Management. *User Modleing and User-Adapted Interaction.* 15, 275-302.

Zwyno, M. S. Student Learning Styles, Web Use Patterns and Attitudes Towards Hypermedia-Enhanced Instruction, *Proceedings of the 33rd ASEE/IEEE Frontiers in Education Conference*, Colorado, USA, pp 1-6, 2003.

About the Contributors

Costas Mourlas is assistant professor in the National and Kapodistrian University of Athens (Greece), Department of Communication and Media Studies since 2002. He obtained his PhD from the Department of Informatics, University of Athens in 1995 and graduated from the University of Crete in 1988 with a diploma in computer science. In 1998 was an ERCIM fellow for post-doctoral studies through research in STFC, UK. He was employed as lecturer at the Univeristy of Cyprus, Department of Computer Science from 1999 till 2002. His previous research work focused on distributed multimedia systems with adaptive behaviour, quality of service issues, streaming media and the Internet. His current main research interest is in the design and the development of intelligent environments that provide adaptive and personalized context to the users according to their preferences, cognitive characteristics and emotional state. He has several publications including edited books, chapters, articles in journals and conference contributions. Dr. Mourlas has taught various undergraduate as well as postgraduate courses in the Dept. of Computer Science of the University of Cyprus and the Dept. of Communication and Media Studies of the University of Athens. Furthermore, he has coordinated and activelly participated in numerous national and EU funded projects.

Panagiotis Germanakos, PhD, is a research scientist, in the Laboratory of New Technologies, Faculty of Communication & Media Studies, National & Kapodistrian University of Athens and of the Department of Computer Science, University of Cyprus. He obtained his PhD from the University of Athens in 2008 and his MSc in international marketing management from the Leeds University Business School in 1999. His BSc was in Computer Science and also holds a HND diploma of technician engineer in the field of computer studies. His research interest is in Web adaptation and personalization environments and systems based on user profiling/filters encompassing amongst others visual, mental and affective processes, implemented on desktop and mobile / wireless platforms. He has several publications, including co-edited books, chapters, articles in journals, and conference contributions. Furthermore, he actively participates in numerous national and EU funded projects that mainly focus on the analysis, design and development of open interoperable integrated wireless/mobile and personalized technological infrastructures and systems in the ICT research areas of e-Government, e-Health and e-Learning and has an extensive experience in the provision of consultancy of large-scaled IT solutions and implementations in the business sector.

* * *

Nancy Alonistioti has a BSc degree and a PhD degree in informatics and telecommunications (University of Athens). She had been working for 7 years at the Institute of Informatics and Telecommunications of NCSR "Demokritos" in the areas of protocol and service design and test, mobile systems (UMTS), open architectures, and software defined radio systems and networks. She specializes in reconfigurable mobile systems and networks for beyond 3G and adaptable services, pervasive computing and context awareness. Moreover, she has wide experience in formal specification and testing of communication protocols and services, design of object oriented, mobile applications. She has participated in several national and European projects, (CTS, SS#7, ACTS RAINBOW, EURESCOM, IST E^2R etc) and was Technical manager of the IST-MOBIVAS and IST-ANWIRE projects, which had a focus on reconfigurable mobile systems, networks and respective service provision. She is co-editor and author in "Software defined radio, Architectures, Systems and Functions", published by John Wiley in May 2003. She is TPC member in many conferences in the area of mobile communications and mobile applications for systems and networks beyond 3G. She has over 55 publications in the area of mobile communications and reconfigurable systems and networks.

Nathalie Basselin is junior researcher at DFKI. She studied computer science in France and then at a French-German institute (ISFATES) in collaboration with the HTW des Saarlandes, Germany, and the IUP HCI in Metz, France. Her master's thesis "*Usability Study for an Adaptive Collaborative Context- and Affect-Aware Shopping Assistant*" conducted in the context of the Specter project has been awarded a German national prize as the best diploma thesis of 2004 in business computer science from an applied sciences university. She then integrated a master in HCI in Toulouse, France and joined DFKI and the SharedLife project. Her work focuses on the design and evaluation of intelligent user interfaces for mobile computing in instrumented environments. She researches on situated user-support, memories exploitation, and learning communities.

Mathias Bauer holds a diploma and a PhD in computer science from Saarland University. After several years of research in the areas of user modeling and machine learning at DFKI, he became one of the co-founders and CEO of mineway, a startup company developing adaptive and self-learning systems mainly for industrial applications. He will be one of the two Conference Co-Chairs of IUI2009, the International Conference on Intelligent User Interfaces.

Paul Brna, Professor, obtained his PhD in artificial intelligence, University of Edinburgh (1987). He was director of the Computer Based Learning Unit at Leeds University before taking up a professorial chair at the University of Northumbria. Most recently, he was the director of the Scottish Council for Research in Education (SCRE) Centre at Glasgow University. He has a strong interest in the use of open learner modelling to promote learning and is a founder member of the Learner Modelling for Reflection (LeMoRe) research network. He is now an educational consultant in technology enhanced learning.

Christos Chalaris is adjunct lecturer at the University of Thessaly, teaching e-commerce and senior researcher at the Information Management Unit/National Technical University of Athens (NTUA). He holds a PhD in e-business and virtual organizations (2000) and a diploma degree in electrical & computer engineering (1995), both from NTUA. He also holds an MBA degree (1999) from NTUA and AUEB (Athens University of Economics and Business). He has worked for more than 10 years as business consultant and thus acquired solid experience in the areas of project and program management,

E-Government service development and business planning (development and evaluation).He has also worked on various ESPRIT and IST research projects. During his military service he worked at the Hellenic Navy for the development and establishment of an ISO 9001:2000 quality management system in Salamis Technical Base.

María Elena Chan obtained her PhD in education from the University of Guadalajara in 2004, following previous studies in pedagogy and communication. She is a member of the Mexican National Research System and currently director of the Institute for Management of Knowledge and Learning in Virtual Environments at the University of Guadalajara. She has been involved in training academics on curriculum design and non conventional educational modalities since 1988, and in multidisciplinary research and development projects in Mexico and Latin America, including projects partially funded by the European Union.

Sherry Y. Chen received the PhD degree from the University of Sheffield, U.K., in 2000. Currently, she is a reader in the Department of Information Systems and Computing, Brunel University, U.K. She is the co-editor of the books, *Adaptive and Adaptable Hypermedia Systems* and *Advances in Web-Based Education: Personalized Learning Environments.* Her current research interests include human–computer interaction, data mining, and multimedia learning. She is a member of the editorial board of six computing journals. Dr. Chen has given numerous invited talks, such as the Engineering and Physical Sciences Research Council Network of Women in Computer Science Colloquium.

Rafael Morales Gamboa, PhD, has a first degree in mathematics from Universidad Nacional Autónoma de México (UNAM) and a Masters in Computer Science from Instituto Tecnológico y de Estudios Superiores de Monterrey (ITESM), both Mexican Universities. His PhD in Artificial Intelligence is from the University of Edinburgh (2000). He worked for more than two years as a Research Fellow at the Universities of Northumbria and Glasgow (2004-2006) in the UK, before joining the University of Guadalajara as a lecturer in 2006. His main area of interest is student modelling for intelligent learning environments, and he is broadly interested in web technologies, technology enhanced learning and cognitive science.

Gheorghita Ghinea received the BSc and BSc (Hons) degrees in computer science and mathematics, in 1993 and 1994, respectively, and the MSc degree in computer science, in 1996, from the University of the Witwatersrand, Johannesburg, South Africa; he then received the PhD degree in computer science from the University of Reading, United Kingdom, in 2000. He is a reader in the Department of Information Systems and Computing at Brunel University, United Kingdom. His research interests span perpetual aspects of multimedia, quality of service and multimedia resource allocation, as well as computer networking and security issues.

Maria Golemati was born in Athens, Greece in 1971. She received a BSc degree in informatics (1996) from the Athens University of Economics and Business and an MSc in cognitive science from the University of Athens-Faculty of Philosophy and History of Science. Ms. Golemati is currently a PhD candidate in the Department of Informatics and Telecommunications of the National and Kapodistrian University of Athens. Her research interests include information visualization, cognitive issues in human-computer interaction, ontologies, and context-awareness in graphical interfaces.

Fabio Grandi is currently an associate professor in the Faculty of Engineering of the University of Bologna, Italy. Since 1989 he has worked at the CSITE center of the Italian National Research Council (CNR) in Bologna, initially supported by a CNR fellowship. In 1993 and 1994 he was an adjunct professor at the Universities of Ferrara, Italy, and Bologna. He joined his current department (Dept. of Electronics, Computer Science and Systems) as a research associate in 1994. His scientific interests include temporal databases, version management, Web information systems, knowledge representation. He is a member of the TSQL2 language design committee. He received a Laurea degree cum laude in electronics engineering and a PhD in electronics engineering and computer science from the University of Bologna.

Christos Halaris, PhD, is adjunct lecturer at the University of Thessaly, teaching e-commerce and senior researcher at the Information Management Unit/National Technical University of Athens (NTUA). He holds a PhD in e-business and virtual organizations (2000) and a diploma degree in electrical & computer engineering (1995), both from NTUA. He also holds an MBA degree (1999) from NTUA and AUEB (Athens University of Economics and Business). He has worked for more than 10 years as business consultant and thus acquired solid experience in the areas of project and program management, e-government service development and business planning (development and evaluation).He has also worked on various ESPRIT and IST research projects. During his military service he worked at the Hellenic Navy for the development and establishment of an ISO 9001:2000 quality management system in Salamis Technical Base.

Constantinos Halatsis, professor, was born in Athens, Greece in 1941. He received the BSc degree in physics in 1964, and the MSc in electronics in 1966, both from the University of Athens. In 1971 he received the PhD degree in computer science from the University of Manchester, England. From 1971 to 1981 he was with the Computer Center of NCR Democritos in Athens. In 1981 he became full professor in computer science at the Aristotle University of Thessaloniki, Greece, and in 1988 he moved to the Department of Informatics, University of Athens, where he continues to be. His research interests include computer architecture, logic design, logic programming and Prolog machines, data and knowledge bases, optimization of scheduling and planning, computer networks, multimedia and hypermedia systems, virtual reality, parallel computing, software engineering, systems analysis and design.

Akrivi Katifori was born in Athens, Greece in 1977. She holds a BSc in informatics and telecommunications (2000) and an MSc in signal processing for telecommunications and multimedia (2003) from the University of Athens and is currently a PhD student of the same department. She has participated in European and national RTD projects and has authored several papers in different research areas of computer science. Her scientific interests include ontologies and semantic web technologies, virtual museums, information visualization and personal information management.

Alexander Kröner has studied computer science at Saarland University, where he has been awarded a diploma in computer science in 1996 and a PhD in 2000. His field of experience comprises the application of constraints, web technology, and ontologies for adaptive user support, with a particular focus on personalized and situated information presentation. Currently, he is employed as senior researcher at the DFKI; his current research is focusing on the exploitation of digital memories for user support. In this context, he led the project SPECTER and is now guiding SharedLife.

Alfred Kobsa is a professor in the Donald Bren School of information and computer sciences of the University of California, Irvine. His research lies in the areas of user modeling and personalized systems, privacy, and information visualization. He is the editor of *User Modeling and User-Adapted Interaction*, editorial board member of the *Springer Lecture Notes in Computer Science (LNCS), World-Wide Web, and Universal Access in the Information Society.* Dr. Kobsa edited several books and authored numerous publications in the areas of user-adaptive systems, human-computer interaction and knowledge representation. He received research awards from the Humboldt Foundation, Google, and several other organizations.

Zacharias Lekkas is currently a PhD candidate and research associate in the Laboratory of New Technologies at the Department of Communication and Media Studies of the National & Kapodistrian University of Athens. He holds a BA in philosophy and psychology from the University of Athens and a PGDip in psychology and MSc in occupational psychology from the University of Nottingham. His main research interests lie in the area of individual differences and personalization techniques in knowledge management. Moreover, he focuses on emotions, personality theories and decision making approaches using advanced statistical analysis and quantitative methods.

George Lepouras, PhD, was born in Athens, Greece in 1967. He received a degree in mathematics from the University of Athens in 1991, an MSc in information technology systems in 1992 from the University of Strathclyde, and a PhD in human-computer interaction from the University of Athens in 2000. Dr. Lepouras has participated in numerous European and national RTD projects, including the SmartGov and CB-Business projects of the IST framework. Dr. Lepouras has authored more than 40 papers for international conferences and journals in various subject areas, including e-government, user interfaces and web technologies. Currently Dr. Lepouras is an assistant professor in the University of Peloponnese and a research fellow for the University of Athens. His scientific interests include human-computer interaction, e-Government, and virtual reality systems.

Babis Magoutas is a PhD candidate and researcher at the Information Management Unit/National Technical University of Athens (NTUA). He holds a diploma degree in electrical & computer engineering (2003) and a master in business administration degree (2006), both from NTUA. During 2004-2005 he worked as telecom engineer in the company INTRACOM S.A He is currently working in IST Research Projects and his research interests include the emerging semantic web, quality management, e-Government and semantically adaptive interfaces.

Federica Mandreoli is a research associate at the Department of Information Engineering of the University of Modena and Reggio Emilia, Italy. She holds a Laurea degree in computer science and a PhD in electronics engineering and computer science from the University of Bologna. Her scientific interests are in the field of information and knowledge management and, currently, mainly concerns data sharing in P2P networks and personalized access to great quantity of graph-based information. As to those research themes, she is author of publications and book chapters dealing with query processing in P2P networks, structural disambiguation for semantic-aware applications and personalized accesses to XML data and ontologies.

Gregoris Mentzas is professor of information technology management at the School of Electrical and Computer Engineering of the National Technical University of Athens (NTUA) and director of the Information Management Unit (IMU) a multidisciplinary research unit at the University. His area of expertise is information technology management and his research concerns the integration of knowledge management, semantic web and e-service technologies. He was/is principal investigator in more than 30 international research projects in his areas of expertise and has published 50 research papers in international scientific journals, 60 papers in international conferences and is the lead author of the book "*Knowledge Asset Management*" published by Springer in the series "*Advanced Information and Knowledge Processing.*" He serves on the editorial board of four journals and has been on the program committees of more than 20 international conferences.

Riccardo Martoglia is a research associate at the Faculty of Mathematical, Physical and Natural Sciences of the University of Modena e Reggio Emilia. He received his Laurea degree (*cum Laude*) and his PhD in computer engineering from the same university. He teaches a number of subjects in the area of databases, information systems, information retrieval and Semantic Web. His current research is about studying new methodologies for efficiently and effectively querying and managing large amounts of semi-structured and multi-version data. He is author of many publications and book chapters about the above mentioned topics. He is a member of ACM and IEEE Computer Society.

Costas Polychronopoulos holds an MSc (with honours) in information systems from the Athens University of Economics & Business (AUEB). Prior to that, he graduated from the Department of Informatics & Telecommunications at the National & Kapodistrian University of Athens (NKUA) having also studied in the Department of Business Informatics at the University of Vienna on a Socrates-Erasmus grant. Mr. Polychronopoulos has also received a scholarship from AUEB on his postgraduate exceptional performance. For the past 3 years, he serves as a research fellow in the Communication Networks Laboratory at the NKUA for the European IST-FP6 integrated projects "E^2R", "E^2R II" (End-to-End Reconfigurability phase I and II) and "LIAISON" (LocatIon bAsed serviceS for the enhancement of wOrking enviroNment). His research interests lie in the intersection of beyond 3G wireless communications systems and service-oriented architectures, with a special focus on situation awareness and location-based services.

Syed Sibte Raza Abidi is a professor at the Faculty of Computer Science and director of Health Informatics at Dalhousie University. He leads the NICHE research group that conducts research in the areas of knowledge management, health informatics and information and web-service personalization. He holds a BEngg degree in electronic engineering from NED University of Engineering & Technology, Karachi, Pakistan (1986), MSc degree in computer engineering from University of Miami, Florida, USA (1989), and a PhD degree in computing sciences from University of Surrey, UK (1994). He is involved in both government and industry-funded research projects, whereby his research has been funded by the National Science and Engineering Research Council, Canadian Foundation for Innovation, Nova Scotia Health Research Foundation, Agfa Inc. Canada, European Strategic Program for Research in Information Technology (ESPRIT), WHO, UN, the Malaysian Government's program on intensified research in priority areas, and various industry-funded projects. He has served as an invited reviewer for a number of computer science and health informatics journals, conferences, and research grants proposals. He is the recipient of the VHK International Award for Innovation in Medical Informatics (Hannover, 2000) for his work on the intelligent personalization of healthcare information. He has twice received the Best Paper Award in the "IT for Healthcare" track at the IEEE Hawaii International Conference on System Sciences (HICSS-38 and HICSS-39) in 2005 and 2006.

Enrico Ronchetti is a PhD student in computer science at the Research Doctorate in Information Engineering of the University of Modena and Reggio Emilia. His scientific interests are in the field of efficient and effective access to XML data. In particular, his research activity focuses on personalized access to multi-version XML documents using temporal database and semantic Web techniques for e-government applications. Moreover, He is author of publications on international and national conferences about the above mentioned topics, with particular reference to temporal slicing in XML databases.

George Samaras is a professor of computer science, University of Cyprus. He received a PhD in computer science from Rensselaer Polytechnic Institute, USA, in 1989. He was previously at IBM Research Triangle Park, USA and taught at the University of North Carolina at Chapel Hill (adjunct assistant professor, 1990-93). He served as the lead architect of IBM's distributed commit architecture (1990-94) and co-authored the final publication of the architecture (IBM Book, SC31-8134-00, September 1994). He was member of IBM's wireless division and participated in the design/architecture of IBM's WebExpress, a wireless Web browsing system. He co-authored a book on data management for mobile computing (Kluwer A.P). He has a number of patents relating to transaction processing technology and numerous (over 100) technical conference and journal publications. His work on utilizing mobile agents for Web database access has received the best paper award of the 1999 IEEE International Conference on Data Engineering (ICDE′99). He also participates in EC and locally funded projects (e.g. HealtheService24, DBGlobe, SeLeNe, MEMO, SEACORN, MB-NET, INTELCITIES, PRISMA, BEEP, e-MINDER, eNLARGE, DITIS, MATHWN). He is a voting member of the ACM and IEEE Computer Society.

Makis Stamatelatos has received a BSc and a MSc degree from the Department of Informatics and Telecommunications at the University of Athens. He has participated IST-E2R-I and E2R-II working in the area of end-to-end reconfigurability and beyond 3G mobile communication networks. He is currently participating in the ICT E3 project in cognitive systems and efficiency and the ICT Self-Net working in the area cognitive self-managed elements of the future Internet. Since 2006 he has been serving as designated representative (DR) of NKUA at IEEE P1900.4 working group. His research interests include beyond 3G mobile communication systems, context and knowledge management, information modeling and business (meta-)modeling. He is currently pursuing a PhD in context and knowledge management in OO environments.

Maria Rita Scalas is currently a full professor in the Faculty of Engineering of the University of Bologna, Italy. From 1975 to 1979 she worked at the Universities of Pisa and Bologna supported by a fellowship from the Italian Ministry of Education. In 1980 she became a research assistant in Computer Science at the University of Bologna and a consultant at the CIOC center of the National Research Council in Bologna. In 1986 she was a visiting scientist at the IBM Scientific Center in Heidelberg, Germany, where she took part in the AIM-P project. In 1987 she became an associate professor at the University of Trieste, Italy. She holds a Laurea degree in Physics from the University of Bologna. Her research interests are in the area of temporal data management and schema versioning.

Michael Schneider, as a high school student, has won the German Federal Competition in Informatics (BWINF) in 1997. After high school, he studied computer science at Saarland University, where he has been awarded a Diploma (MSc) in 2003. Currently he is a PhD student at the intelligent user interface group at DFKI and is working as a researcher in the project SharedLife. His research interests include ubiquitous computing and plan recognition

Barry Smyth received a BSc in computer science from University College Dublin in 1991 and a PhD from Trinity College Dublin in 1996. His research interests includes artificial intelligence, case-based reasoning, information retrieval, and user profiling & personalization. He has published over 250 scientific articles in journals and conferences and has received a number of international awards for his research. He also co-founded ChangingWorlds Ltd. to commercialise personalization technologies in the mobile Internet sector. ChangingWorlds now employs more than 120 people, and has deployed personalization technologies across 50 of the world's leading mobile operators, and has offices in Europe, Asia and the US.

Nikos Tsianos is a PhD candidate at the Faculty of Communication and Mass Media of the University of Athens, and research assistant of the New Technologies Laboratory, located at the aforementioned department. He has a bachelor degree in communication and mass media and Msc in political communication and new technologies. His main research area is the personalization of educational adaptive web hypermedia on the basis of psychological individual differences, such as cognitive and emotional parameters. He has participated in the design and development of Web-applications and corresponding psychometric tools, as well as in assessment procedures. His research interests also include the social impact of locative media and mobile appliances, both in terms of psychological research and HCI design.

Paolo Tiberio received the Laurea in electronic engineering cum laude from the University of Pisa, Italy in 1967. At present he is full professor of computer science at the Engineering Faculty of the University of Modena and Reggio Emilia where from 2004 to 2007 he was faculty dean. He was also research associate from 1970 and professor from 1976 to 1998 at the University of Bologna. In 1971 he was visiting scientist at the University of Michigan, Ann Arbor, and in 1978, 1979, 1981 and 1984 with "System R" and related projects of the IBM Research Center, San Jose, California. His past research activity was in the fields of computer aided design, operating systems , relational database design while at present his research interests are multimedia databases, digital libraries and P2P systems.

Gulden Uchyigit has a PhD in artificial intelligence from Department of Computing, Imperial College. She also has BSc and MSc in computer science from King's College, University of London. Her research interests are in the area of machine learning, personalization, intelligent user interfaces and recommender systems. She has authored over 30 papers in refereed, books, journals, conferences and workshops. She serves on the programme committee's of several international conferences and has organised and chaired several workshops all related to the area of personalization and recommender systems.

Nicolas Van Labeke, PhD, is a postdoctoral research assistant at the School of Computer Science and Information Systems, Birkbeck College. He has a PhD in computer science from the University of Nancy, France (1999), and was a research associate at the University of Nottingham (2000-2003) and a research fellow at Northumbria University, then at Glasgow University (2004-2006). His research interests are in artificial intelligence in education (learner modelling, personalisation and adaptation, multiple external representations). He is currently working on the MyPlan project, developing, deploying and evaluating techniques and tools that allow personalised planning of lifelong learning.

Costas Vassilakis, PhD, was born in Arta, Greece in 1968. He holds a BSc in informatics (1990) and a PhD in design and implementation of an historical DBMS (1995). Dr. Vassilakis has authored more than 70 papers for international conferences and journals in subject areas including e-government, Web technologies and databases; he has also participated in numerous European and national RTD projects. Currently Dr. Vassilakis is an assistant professor in the University of Peloponnese and a research fellow for the University of Athens. His scientific interests include semantic web technologies, e-government, databases, user interaction and distributed systems.

Yang Wang is a PhD candidate in the Donald Bren School of Information and Computer Sciences of the University of California, Irvine. His broad research interests span across the fields of human-computer interaction (HCI), software engineering (SE), e-commerce and applied statistics. His PhD research focuses on mechanisms of reconciling web personalization with privacy constraints imposed by legal restrictions and by users' privacy preferences. He was a visiting researcher at Institute of Information Systems at Humboldt University in Berlin. He has performed research with several organizations, including CommerceNet, Fuji Xerox Palo Alto Lab (FXPAL), and Intel Research.

Index

D

E

F

G

H

I

K

L

Q

R

S

T

U

V

W